ATLAS OF THORACIC SURGERY

VOLUME TWO

ATLAS OF

Thoracic Surgery

VOLUME TWO

EDITED BY

Academician Boris V. Petrovsky

Translated from the Russian by

Ludmila Aksenova

With a foreword to the English language edition by

Michael E. DeBakey, M.D.

810 figures, including 284 in color

The C. V. Mosby Company

ST. LOUIS • TORONTO • LONDON 1979

TWO VOLUMES

Originally published as *Atlas Grudnoĭ Khirurgii,* © 1974 by Meditsina Publishing House, USSR

Printed in the United States of America

The C. V. Mosby Company
11830 Westline Industrial Drive, St. Louis, Missouri 63141

Library of Congress Cataloging in Publication Data

Main entry under title:

Atlas of thoracic surgery.

Translation of Atlas grudnoĭ khirurgii.
1. Chest—Surgery—Atlases. I. Petrovskiĭ, Boris Vasil'evich, 1908- [DNLM: 1. Thorax—Surgery—Atlases. WF17 A881]
RD536.A7813 617'.54 78-23699
ISBN 0-8016-3832-1

GW/U/B 9 8 7 6 5 4 3 2 1 03/C/300

Foreword

This *Atlas of Thoracic Surgery,* originally published in Russian in 1974, is based on the extensive experience of Professor Boris V. Petrovsky, who has long been the Director of the Research Institute of Clinical and Experimental Surgery and is now Minister of Public Health of the USSR. A pioneer in this field of endeavor, Professor Petrovsky has developed this Institute into one of the great centers of thoracic and cardiovascular surgery. The experience gained in this Institute provides the basis of this *Atlas*.

The first portion of the *Atlas* is devoted to a detailed anatomic description of the thoracic wall and the organs of the thoracic cavity. This section is well illustrated with many color plates that are clear, precise, and well presented in terms of anatomic relationships. Although the actual anatomic presentations are fairly standard, emphasis is placed on the surgical approach to anatomy.

The subsequent chapters deal with technical principles of surgical procedures, first on the chest wall, including those related to trauma, thoracoplasty, and operation on the breast. Other chapters are devoted to technical consideration of various operations on the lungs, esophagus, and heart and great vessels. These are described in considerable detail, with extensive illustrations of each step of the operation. Several technical methods are presented for certain conditions, as exemplified in the approach to coarctation, consisting in resection and end-to-end anastomosis, resection and graft replacement, patch-graft angioplasty, and subclavian-artery bypass.

Although most of the operations described are based on the methods used by Professor Petrovsky and his associates, in general they represent surgical principles that are now fairly standard and universally employed. Accordingly, the *Atlas* serves a useful purpose as a general reference source for surgical anatomy of the thorax and for technical principles of surgical procedures that are applicable to this region of the body.

Michael E. DeBakey, M.D.
President and Chancellor,
Chairman of the Department of Surgery
Baylor College of Medicine
Houston, Texas

Preface to Volume One

The creation of illustrated works on surgery in the Russian literature dates back to the publication of the original atlases compiled by I. Buyalsky and N. Pirogov, eminent surgeons of the nineteenth century. They endeavored to provide physicians with visual aids demonstrating the anatomical and technical aspects of the performance of surgical operations.

The successes achieved in the development of Soviet surgery and the growth of specialized medical service called for the compilation of an authoritative practical atlas reflecting modern surgical techniques in such an expanding field as thoracic surgery. In creating such an atlas, the authors spared no effort to make not only a handy guide for experienced surgeons but, in equal measure, an indispensable manual for young surgeons just beginning to practice the specialty of thoracic surgery.

The *Atlas of thoracic surgery* we are offering to the reader comprises two volumes. The first deals with the surgical anatomy of the thorax and operations on the thoracic wall, the lungs, and the heart, and the second is devoted to operations on the major vessels of the thorax, on the esophagus, and on the diaphragm.

The material in the *Atlas* is based on the experience in the surgical treatment of diseases of the thoracic organs accumulated at the Institute of Clinical and Experimental Surgery, under the USSR Ministry of Public Health, headed by Academician Boris V. Petrovsky. This is why, from among the great variety of operations, preference has been given in the *Atlas* to modifications used by the authors. The modifications that are original are indicated in the text by an asterisk. Most of the drawings were made in the operating room. Drawings copied from other atlases or manuals are acknowledged in the legends.

The text accompanying the drawings explains the main principles of the methods and describes the techniques of the surgical operations as a whole.

The first volume of the *Atlas* was prepared for publication by specialists of the respective departments of the Institute (the section dealing with operations on the lungs by M. I. Perelman and V. A. Klimansky and the section concerned with operations on the heart by G. M. Solovyev) as well as by G. E. Ostroverkhov, Yu. M. Lopukhin, and N. S. Zheltikov, specialists in topographic anatomy and operative surgery, who have been closely collaborating with our Institute for many years.

The authors hope that the *Atlas* will prove valuable to all surgeons operating on the thoracic organs and will be grateful for any critical remarks in regard to this work.

Preface to Volume Two

The second volume of the *Atlas of thoracic surgery* is a continuation of Volume I which was published in 1971. This volume provides descriptions of surgical interventions undertaken in treating diseases of the major vessels of the thorax, the esophagus, and the diaphragm. Among the great variety of existing surgical techniques, the *Atlas* gives preference to those modifications that were elaborated at the Institute of Clinical and Experimental Surgery, under the USSR Ministry of Public Health, headed by Academician Boris V. Petrovsky. Most of the drawings were made in the operating room. This made it possible to reproduce the techniques of different stages of each operation as they were accomplished under the real conditions.

Contributions to the second volume of the *Atlas* were made by specialists of the respective departments of the Institute: the section dealing with operations on the major vessels of the thorax was contributed by N. N. Malinovsky and M. D. Knyazev, the section describing operations on the esophagus by E. N. Vantsyan and R. A. Toshchakov, and the section on operations on the diaphragm by N. O. Nikolaev and N. N. Kanshin.

Upon completing many years of work devoted to the *Atlas of thoracic surgery,* its authors hope that it will become a useful aid to surgeons operating on the thoracic organs. It is only natural that the first illustrated practical guide of this kind published in our country (USSR) will have its shortcomings, so the authors will be grateful for any critical remarks made by the readers of this work.

Contents

VOLUME ONE

VOLUME TWO

ATLAS OF THORACIC SURGERY

VOLUME TWO

The drawings in this volume were made by A. Gurevich (Operations on the Major Vessels of the Thorax), B. Shkuratov (Operations on the Esophagus), and R. Dostyan (Operations on the Diaphragm).

OPERATIONS ON THE MAJOR VESSELS OF THE THORAX

General principles of operations on the aorta and coronary arteries

Operations on the thoracic aorta and its branches are carried out through various approaches: total or partial median sternotomy, transbipleural approach with transection of the sternum, and thoracotomy with transection of the rib cartilages. Various combinations of these approaches are sometimes used.

Median sternotomy is the universal approach to the coronary vessels, ascending aorta, and the brachiocephalic trunk. The transbipleural approach is used for creating a shunt of the whole arch of the aorta in cases with aneurysms; prosthetics of the descending aorta may be conduced through left thoracotomy.

Various types of manual sutures applied with atraumatic needles and synthetic threads are used in surgical interventions on the thoracic aorta and its branches. A blanket suture is the commonly applied suture to the aorta and its branches. This type of suture is represented schematically in Fig. 474. Special care should be exercised in making a vascular suture, and maximum airtightness of the anastomosis should be ensured. In some cases arteries may be anastomosed by means of a mechanical suture applied with a vessel-stitching instrument (Fig. 475). In creating an anastomosis between an altered aorta and a prosthesis, it is sometimes necessary to perform endarterectomy to remove calcified masses. This manipulation is carried out with a special spade, with which the involved intima is carefully detached and then removed under visual control. In atherosclerotic occlusion of the aorta and arteries, endarterectomy from the distal part of an artery also has to be carried out. Endarterectomy by the eversion method is most convenient in such cases; its techniques are illustrated in Fig. 476.

Operations on the coronary arteries, particularly when performed with extracorporeal circulation, are carried out with strict adherence to the main principles of heart surgery (Volume I, pp. 000-000).

Reconstructive operations on coronary arteries marked by atherosclerotic occlusion or stenosis have the purpose of restoring adequate coronary blood flow. An aortico-coronary shunt is created with the use of venous or arterial autografts. When the atherosclerotic process spreads to smaller branches of the coronary artery, endarterectomy by eversion or gas endarterectomy is performed first. The proximal anastomosis between the aorta and the shunt is formed by the end-to-side method. The type of distal anastomosis is determined by the character of the atherosclerotic process in the coronary artery. In total occlusion the coronary artery is transected distal to the blockage, and end-to-end anastomosis is formed between it and the autograft. When the coronary artery is stenosed, an end-to-side distal anastomosis is formed. After the coronary artery has been opened, retrograde blood flow must be checked without fail. If necessary, endarterectomy or bougienage of the coronary artery is performed (Fig. 477).

The proximal and distal anastomoses are formed both with interrupted and continuous vascular sutures.

Before performing a reconstructive operation it is necessary to inspect the coronary arteries visually and by palpation. If there is no doubt as to the location of the pathological process and its boundaries are clearly defined, longitudinal incision of the coronary artery may be carried out without its preliminary separation from the epicardial bed. If doubt exists, however, the artery is freed from the epicardial bed for a certain distance, so that its location may be defined exactly. In this case the small branches should be preserved as much as possible to avoid microfocal changes in the myocardium and to preserve the collateral communications in the arterial system. After the blood flow in the coronary artery has been restored, fluometry should be conducted without fail to check the restoration and adequacy of the coronary circulation.

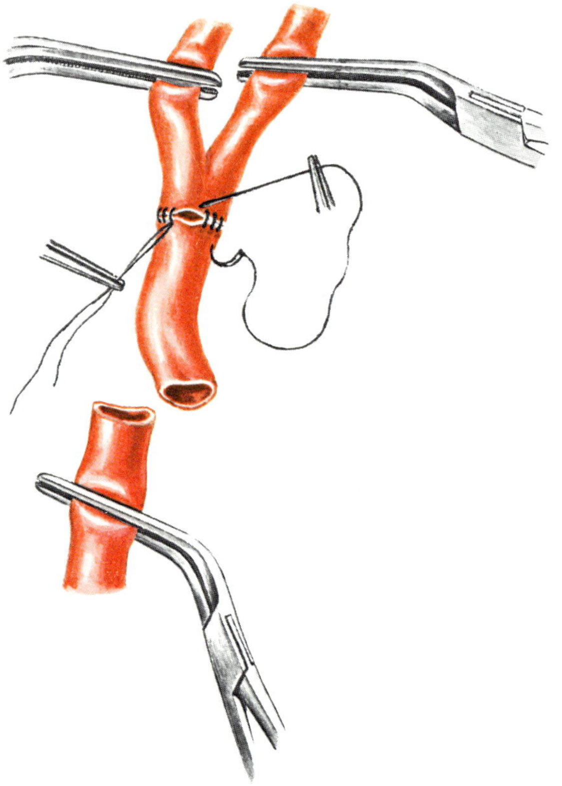

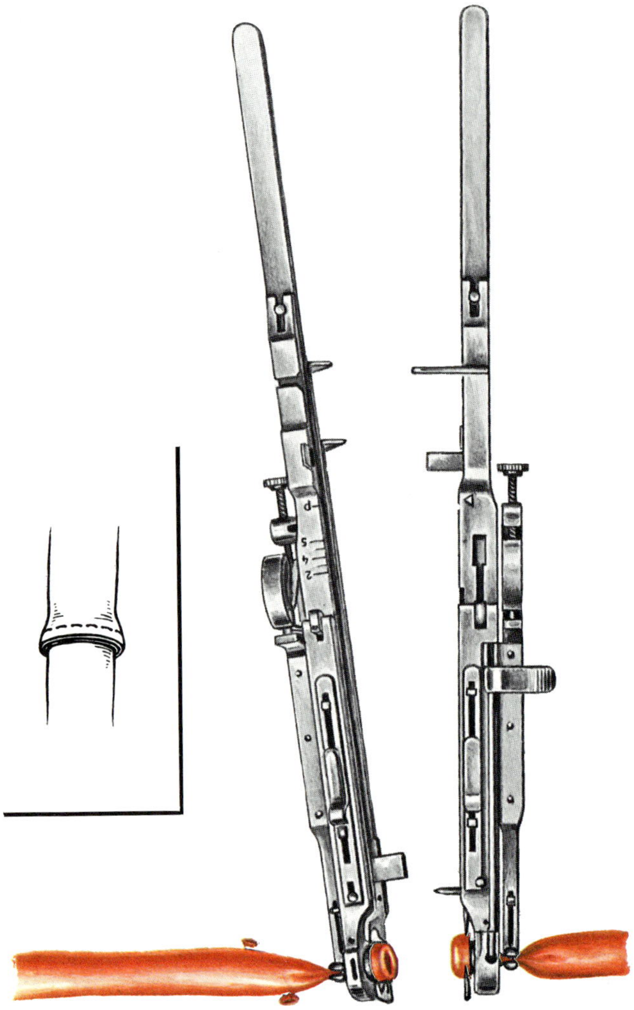

Fig. 474. Suture for carotid artery. Application of vascular blanket suture in prosthesis with arterial autograft.

Fig. 475. Application of vascular suture by means of vessel-stitching instrument.

Reconstructive operations on the coronary arteries may be performed with or without applying extracorporeal circulation. The former variant is preferable in stenosis of the main trunks of the coronary arteries. Irrespective of the character of the pathological process, however, it is necessary to cannulate the superior and inferior venae cavae through the right atrium as well as the femoral artery so that should complications occur (cardiac fibrillation or arrest), the heart-lung machine can be immediately connected.

Surgical interventions in aneurysms of the thoracic aorta and its branches are marked by certain peculiarities. The aneurysmal sac is fused with the surrounding organs and tissues, as a rule. The aneurysm pushes them aside and disturbs the normal anatomical relationships. That is why separation of the aneurysmal sac calls for extreme caution. It is a matter of principle to begin the operation with the mobilization of the aorta proximal and distal to the aneurysm. Strong tapes are looped around the aorta so that it may be compressed with vessel clamps above and below the aneurysm in the event of injury to the aneurysmal sac. Since the blood flow in the thoracic aorta is arrested while it is clamped, it is essential to apply extracorporeal circulation or a temporary shunt for this period. Hypothermia may also be used. After the aneurysm has been disconnected from the circulation, it is widely cut and the orifices of the intercostal arteries are stitched from within and ligated. The next step is prosthetic replacement of the aorta. Because of the possibility of considerable blood loss through the wall of the prosthesis after the blood begins to flow along it, particularly in heparinization, it is preferable to use impermeable or semibiological prostheses with zero surgical porosity.

When the vascular suture has been completed, the atraumatic vessel clamps are removed from the distal

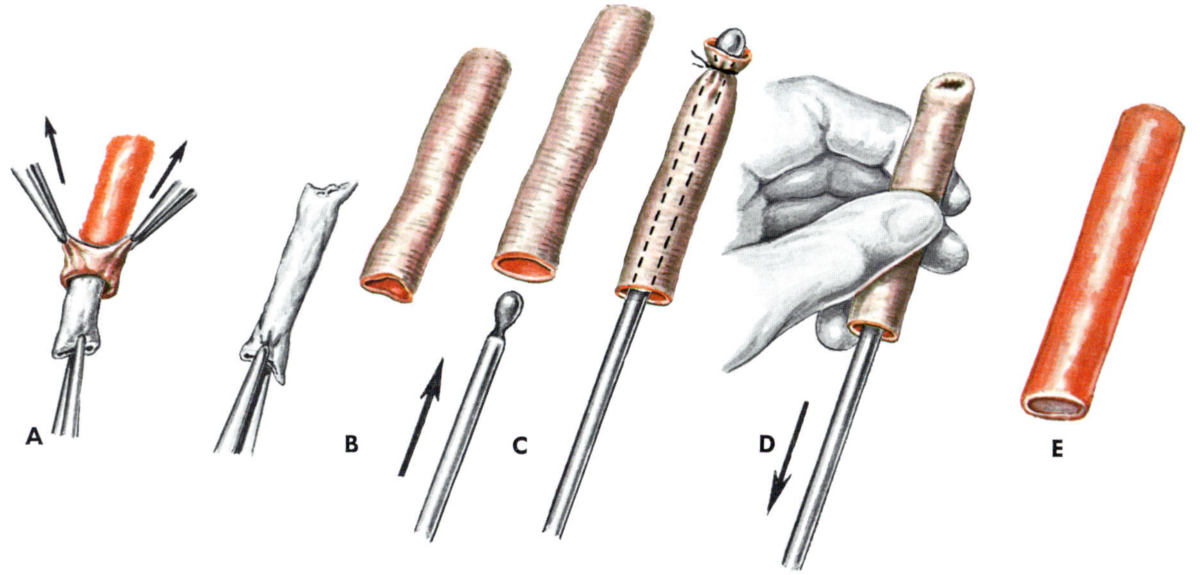

Fig. 476. Endarterectomy by eversion method. **A** Diseased intima is grasped with forceps; muscular coat and adventitia are everted. **B** Vascular segment is turned inside out; pathological masses are removed. **C** Bougie is introduced into vessel, and one end of vascular segment is fastened to it. **D** By pulling bougie, vessel is returned to its initial state by inversion. **E** Lumen of vessel is restored after endarterectomy and inversion.

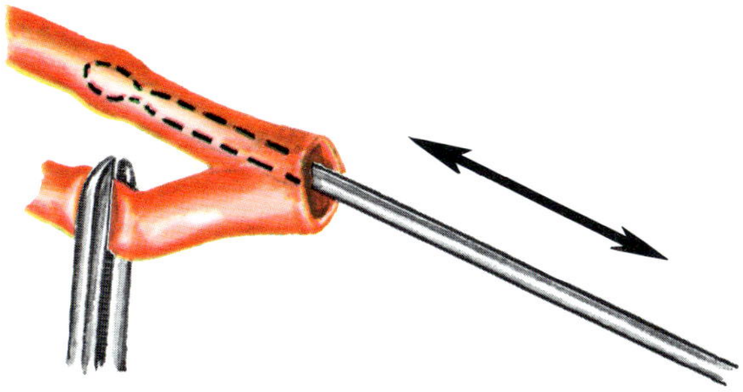

Fig. 477. Dilation of vascular lumen with bougie.

parts of the vessels. The prosthesis is filled with blood, which pushes the air out of it. After that the clamp is slowly taken off the proximal part of the aorta. The pulsatile blood flow is restored. Careful hemostasis and inspection of the distal parts of the vascular channel are necessary to be convinced that the flow of blood is sufficient.

For objective quantitative appraisal of the blood flow, intraoperative electromagnetic flurometry is widely used.

Revascularization of the myocardium in ischemic heart disease

SURGICAL ANATOMY OF CORONARY ARTERIES

With the development of reconstructive surgery of the coronary arteries, the knowledge of their anatomy has acquired great practical significance. The possibilities of intravital coronarography have provided for the precise identification of their anatomy both in health and in involvement in various pathological processes (atherosclerosis, developmental anomalies, aneurysms, fibrous muscular dysplasia, etc.). A new field, roentgen anatomy of the coronary arteries, has been created. This has naturally brought with it a new terminology, because of which the International (Paris) Anatomical Nomenclature of 1955 cannot fully satisfy surgeons engaged in coronary surgery.

Unfortunately, there is still no standard anatomical nomenclature of the coronary arteries. This is why we are obliged to resort to the motley terms commonly used in the special literature.

The sources of blood supply to the myocardium are two coronary arteries of the heart arising at the very origin of the ascending aorta from its right and left sinuses (Valsalva's sinuses).

On branching off from the aorta, the right coronary artery extends at the base of the right auricle. To separate its initial portion from the epicardial bed, it is necessary to pull the auricle of the right atrium upward and draw it to the right (Fig. 478). At this level the artery is 3 to 4 mm in diameter. In this part it gives off branches to the right ventricle and anterior branches to the right atrial auricle. On reaching beyond the right auricle, the right coronary artery divides into two large branches, one of which stretches along the right anterior contour of the heart and is called the marginal branch; its diameter in the proximal part is 1 or 1.5 to 2 mm. The other branch, which is like a continuation of the main vessel, makes a right turn along the coronary sulcus and then back, reaching the posterior longitudinal sinus and descending along it to the apex of the heart. It is called the posterior interventricular branch (Fig. 479). It gives off the right posterior ventricular branches and a posterior branch to the cardiac septum.

Thus, the branches of the right coronary artery mainly supply blood to the right half of the heart: the posterior wall of the right ventricle and its papillary muscles, the right atrium, the posterior third of the interventricular septum, and also a small area of the posterior wall of the left ventricle and its posterior papillary muscle.

The terminal branches of the right coronary arteries anastomose widely with the branches of the left coronary artery, particularly in atherosclerotic stenosis or occlusion. It should be noted that the coronary arteries also form anastomoses between each other in normal conditions not being terminal and, together with the venous vessels, form "a third circulation system" in a human being.

The left coronary artery stretches between the origin of the pulmonary trunk at the left atrium and soon, on emerging from under the pulmonary trunk, divides into two main branches: the anterior descending (or the anterior interventricular) branch and the circumflex branch. The main trunk of the left coronary artery is therefore covered by the pulmonary trunk. To gain access to it and perform any manipulations upon it, one has to transect the pulmonary trunk.

The anterior interventricular branch extends along the anterior longitudinal sulcus to the apex of the heart, giving off diagonal branches on the left, and branches to the interventricular septum to the right.

The circumflex branch stretches along the coronary sulcus under the left auricle to the left, to the posterior surface of the heart and gives off the first, second, and third posterior interventricular branches (see Fig. 479). The diameter of the main trunk of the left coronary artery is 3 to 4.5 mm, that of its anterior descending branch 2 to 1.5 mm, and that of the circumflex branch in the proximal segment also 2 to 1.5 mm, on the average.

The left coronary artery and its branches mainly supply blood to the left half of the heart: the anterior and most of the posterior walls of the left ventricle and its papillary muscles, the left atrium and auricle, and the anterior two thirds of the interventricular septum. The zones of the heart supplied with blood by the arteries should not be regarded absolute, since they depend on the degree to which the system of this or that coronary artery develops; this is precisely what determines the three types (or forms) of vascularization of the heart.

1. The left type with predominant development of the left coronary artery and its branches. In this form the circumflex branch of the left coronary artery extends to

the left ventricle and part of the right ventricle and stretches in the posterior interventricular sulcus. It supplies the entire cardiac septum and the papillary muscles of the left and part of the right sides.

2. The right type. The right coronary artery supplies with blood part of the posterior wall of the left ventricle.

3. The uniform type, which is characterized by the equal development of both coronary arteries that supply the corresponding halves of the heart with nutrients.

A knowledge of the types of blood supply to the heart in atherosclerosis of the coronary arteries is of utmost practical significance in the interpretation of coronarograms, which in the long run determines the proper surgical tactics.

The coronary arteries stretch in fatty epicardial sheaths and are accompanied by veins not enclosed in these sheaths. The great cardiac vein is found on the anterior surface of the heart (see Fig. 478). It originates at the apex and ascends in the anterior longitudinal sulcus in attendance to the anterior descending branch of the left

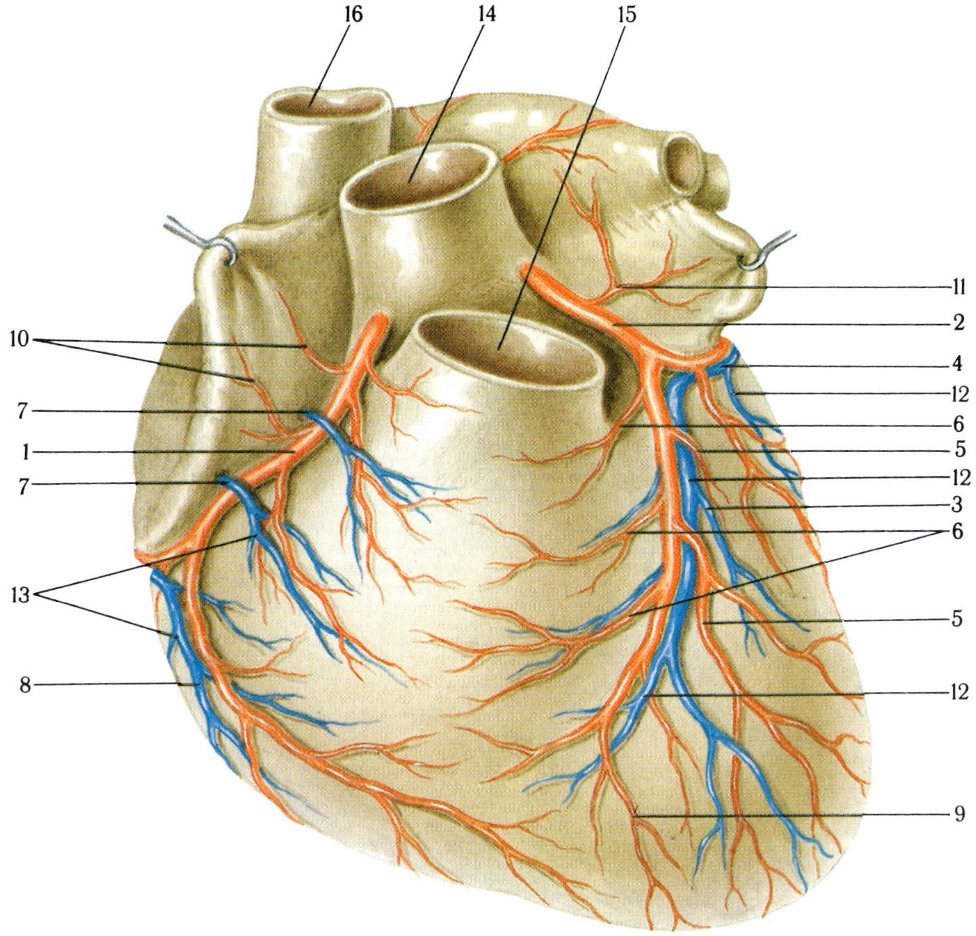

Fig. 478. Ventral surface of heart.

1 Right coronary artery
2 Left coronary artery
3 Anterior descending (anterior interventricular) branch of left coronary artery
4 Circumflex branch of left coronary artery
5 Diagonal branches of anterior descending artery
6 Branches of descending artery to interventricular septum
7 Right ventricular branches of right coronary artery
8 Marginal branch of right coronary artery
9 Apical branch of anterior descending artery
10 Anterior branches of right coronary artery to right atrial auricle
11 Anterior branch for left atrial auricle
12 Great cardiac vein
13 Anterior cardiac veins
14 Aorta
15 Pulmonary trunk
16 Superior vena cava

coronary artery. Having reached the coronary sulcus, it passes to the posterior surface of the heart and drains into the coronary sinus (see Fig. 479).

The anterior veins of the heart accompany the marginal branch and the right ventricular branches of the right coronary artery and drain into the right atrium.

The middle vein ascends from the apex of the heart along the posterior longitudinal sulcus and drains into the coronary sinus just like the left posterior ventricular vein of the heart attendant to the left posterior ventricular branches of the circumflex artery. The small cardiac vein passes on the posterior surface of the heart in the right part of the coronary sulcus and drains into the coronary sinus.

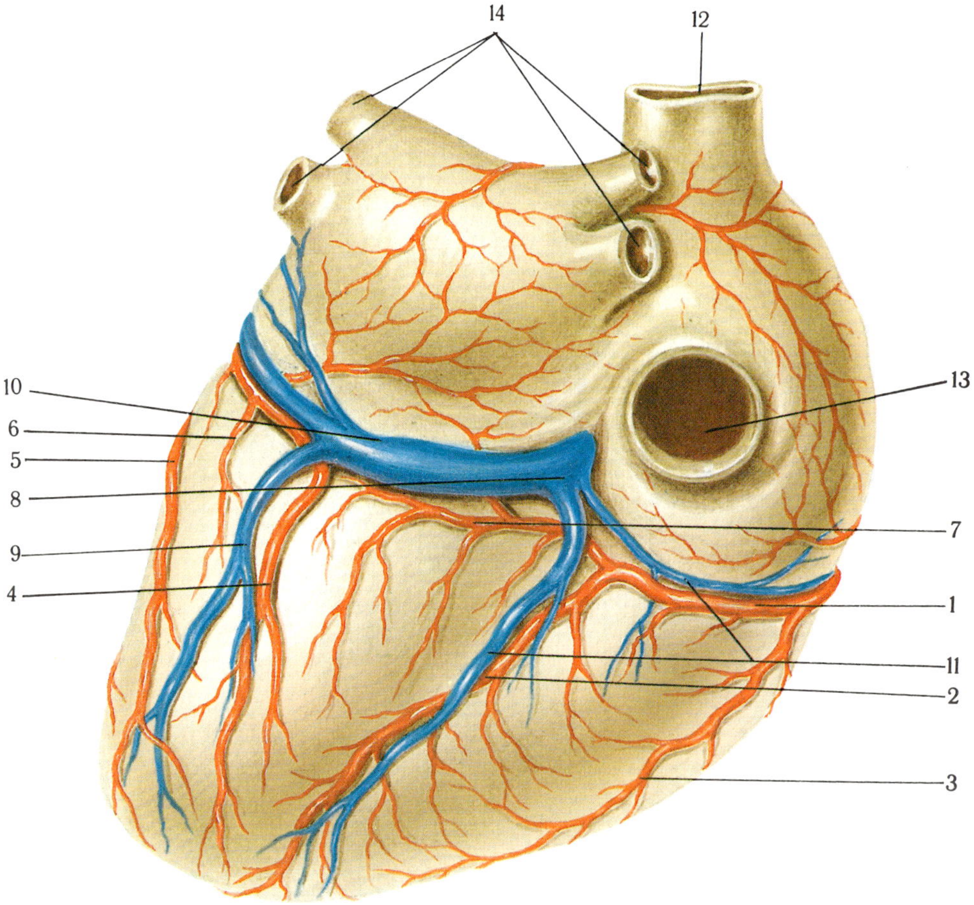

Fig. 479. Dorsal surface of heart.

1 Right coronary artery
2 Posterior interventricular branch of right coronary artery
3 Third posterior right ventricular branch
4 Third posterior left ventricular branch
5 Anterior posterior left ventricular branch
6 Second posterior left ventricular branch
7 Left ventricular branch (from right coronary artery)
8 Coronary sinus
9 Posterior left ventricular vein
10 Middle vein
11 Small cardiac vein
12 Aorta
13 Superior vena cava
14 Pulmonary veins

IMPLANTATION OF INTERNAL THORACIC ARTERY INTO MYOCARDIUM (VINEBERG'S OPERATION)

The essence of the surgical intervention consists in the implantation of the internal thoracic artery into the thickness of the myocardium of the left or right ventricle.

The left anterolateral approach in the fifth intercostal space is used in implantation of the left internal thoracic artery, and the transsternal approach when both arteries are to be implanted.

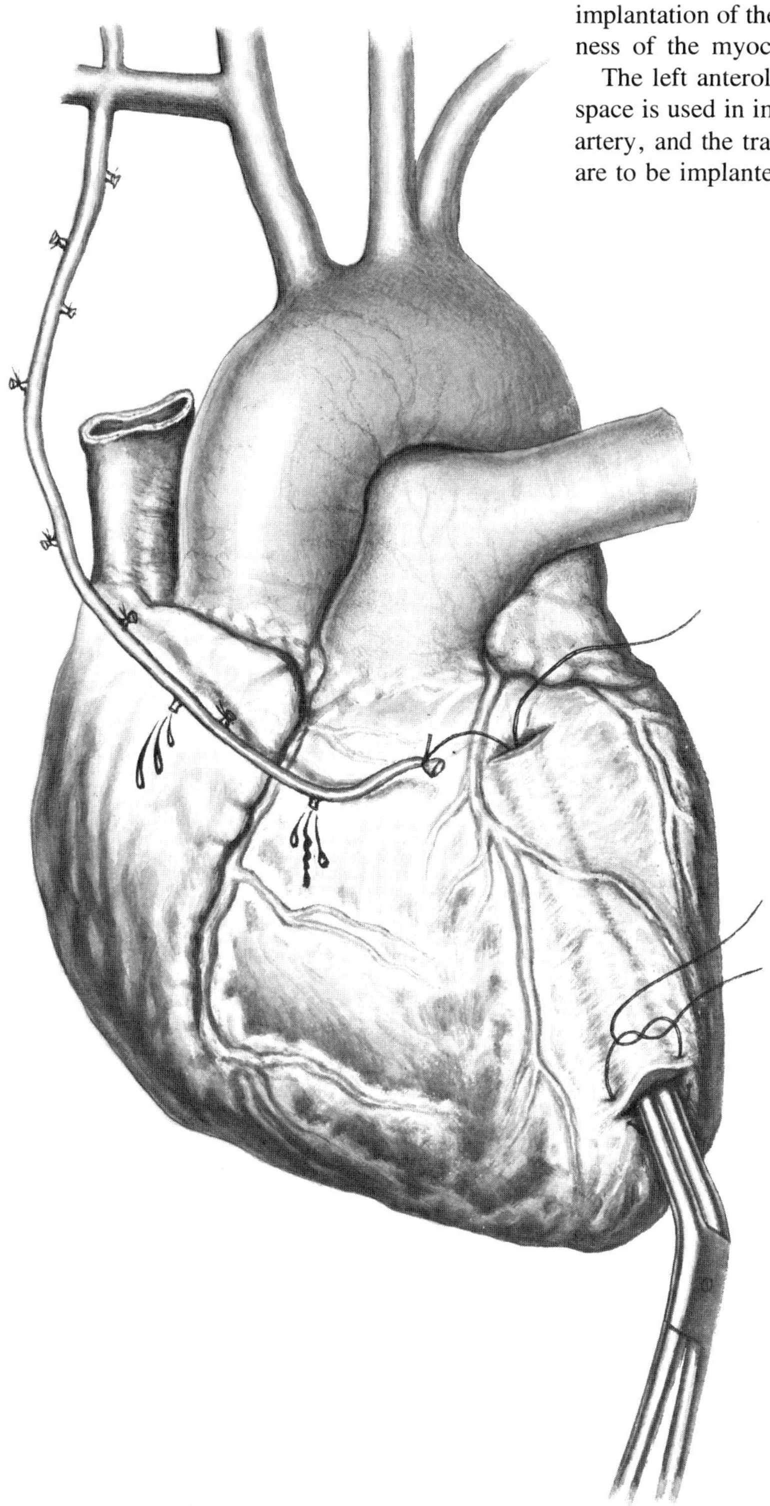

Fig. 480. By pulling ligature, bleeding part of internal thoracic artery is implanted into myocardium of left ventricle.

The artery is mobilized almost along its entire length so that it may be implanted into the thickness of the myocardium without stretching. The small bleeding branches are ligated one by one, and their stumps are left on that part of the artery that will be submerged into the myocardium. Some of these vessels at the peripheral end of the artery need not be ligated because they will be sunk in the thickness of the myocardium. The artery is transected between two ligatures as low as possible. The pericardium is opened; a cut is made in the epicardium at the base of the left ventricle; a purse-string suture is applied to the apex of the ventricle; and a tunnel is formed by means of a thin instrument. The ligature applied to the end of the artery is grasped with the same instrument and, by pulling on this ligature, the bleeding portion of the vessel is fitted into the myocardium

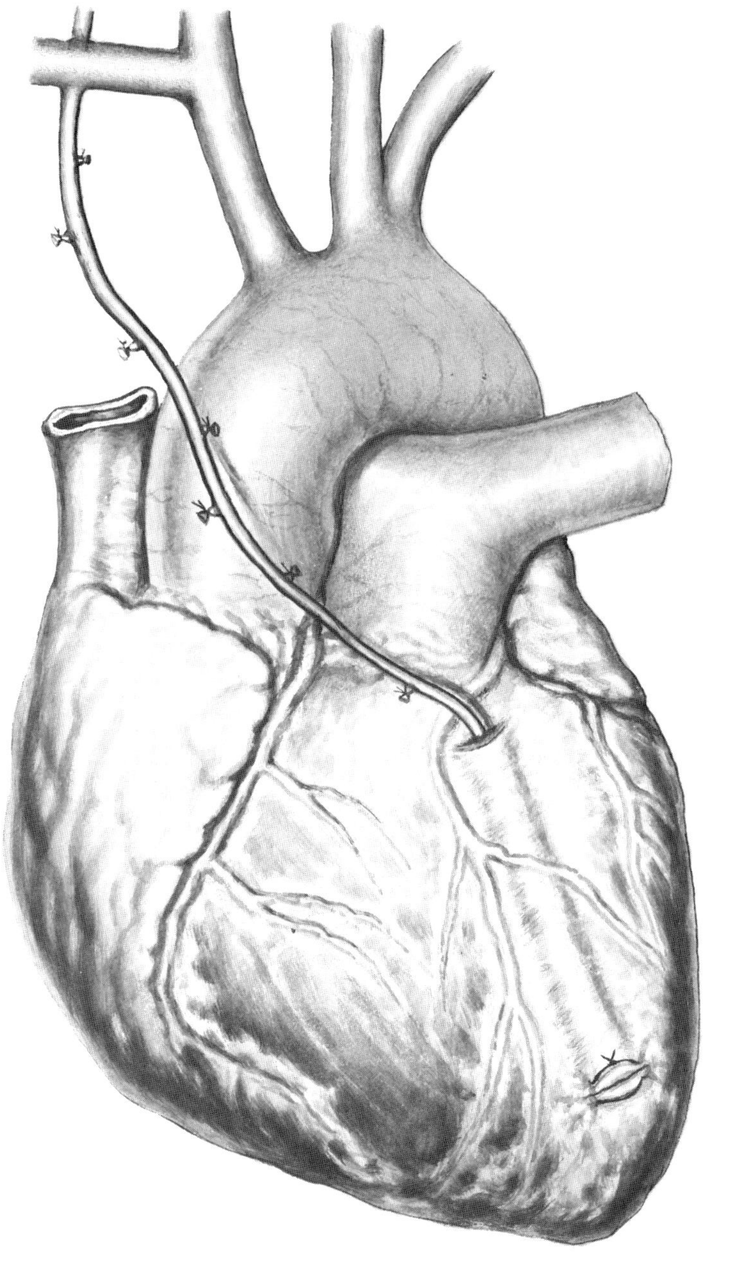

Fig. 481. Artery is fitted into myocardium; purse-string suture on apex of heart is tied.

(Fig. 480). The end of the artery is fastened by tightening the purse-string suture on the apex of the ventricle (Fig. 481).

A venous autograft may be implanted instead of the internal thoracic artery. The great saphenous vein of the thigh may be used for the purpose. One of its ends is stitched into the arch of the aorta as in the aorticocoronary shunt, while the other is implanted into the myocardium (Fig. 482). This modification of Vineberg's operation, however, is comparatively rarely applied.

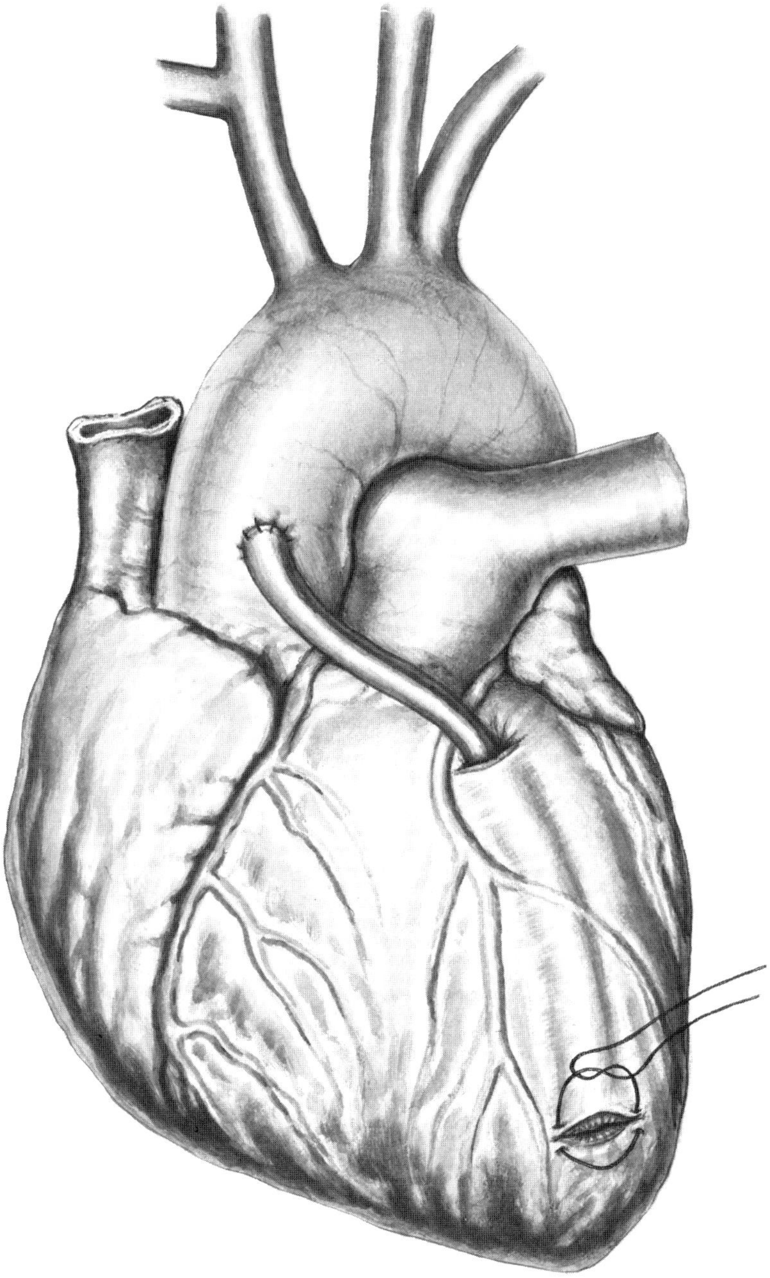

Fig. 482. Implantation of venous autograft into thickness of myocardium of left ventricle (modification of Vineberg's operation).

SHUNTING OF RIGHT CORONARY ARTERY

Median sternotomy is carried out. The pericardium is opened longitudinally and with additional transverse cuts. The right coronary artery is inspected by palpation. The auricle of the right atrium is pulled cranially and laterally with fenestrated forceps. The right coronary artery is separated from the epicardial bed, ligated distal to the site of the occlusion, and transected (Fig. 483). In total occlusion of the right coronary artery the operation may be performed without applying extracorporeal circulation. If the retrograde bleeding after transection of

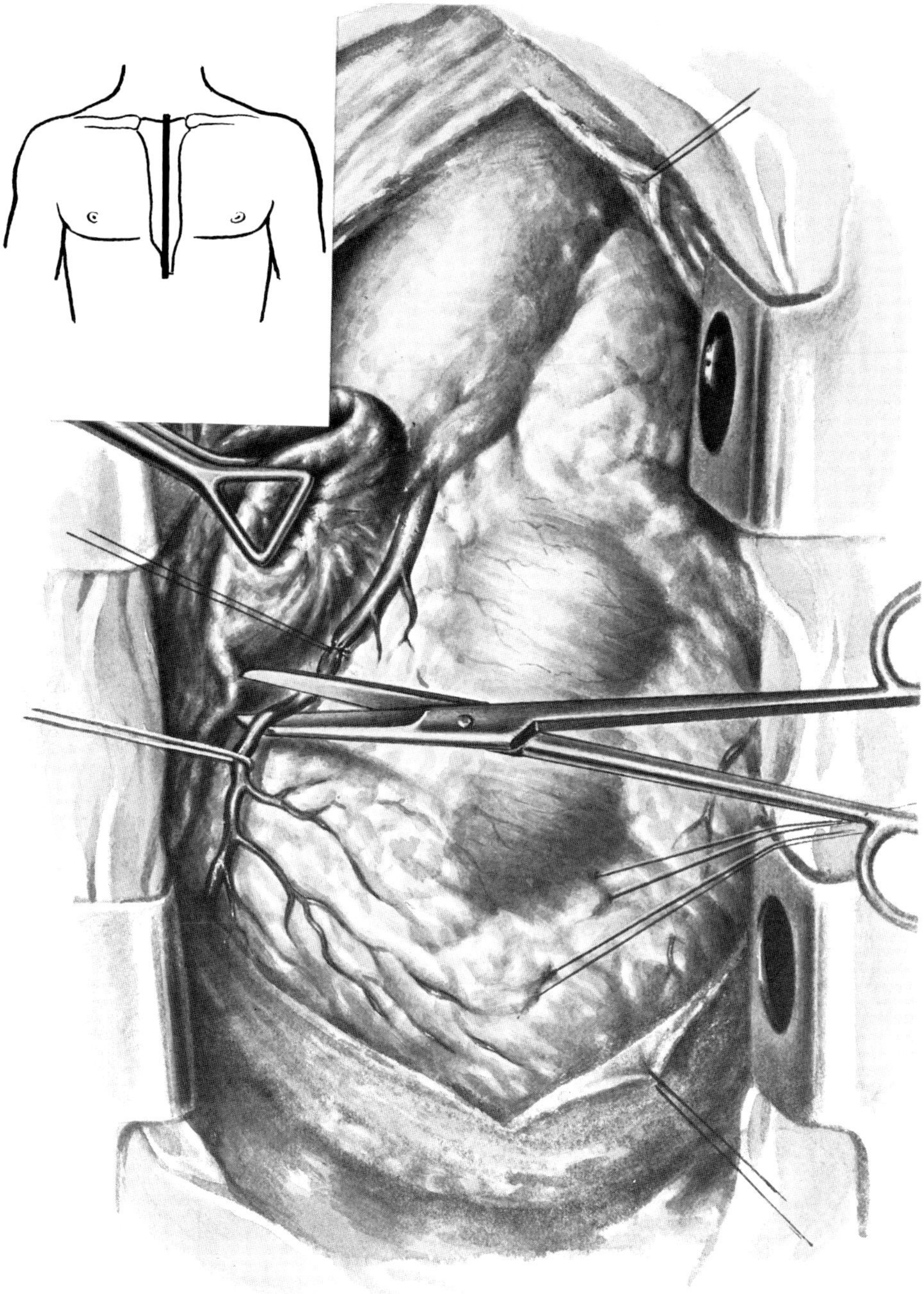

Fig. 483. Right auricle is drawn away laterally and cranially with fenestrated forceps. Mobilized right coronary artery is transected. Artery is ligated distal to occlusion and held with a loop below the site of its transection.

the artery is mild or absent, endarterectomy from the distal part of the coronary artery is conducted additionally by the eversion method (Fig. 484) till a good retrograde blood flow appears.

By the time these manipulations on the coronary arteries are completed, the second team of surgeons prepares the venous autograft from the great saphenous vein of the thigh. The anastomosis between the coronary artery and the venous graft may be created end to end with a circular vascular suture on a special bougie introduced into the lumen of the coronary artery (Fig. 485). With the distal anastomosis formed, the ascending aorta is

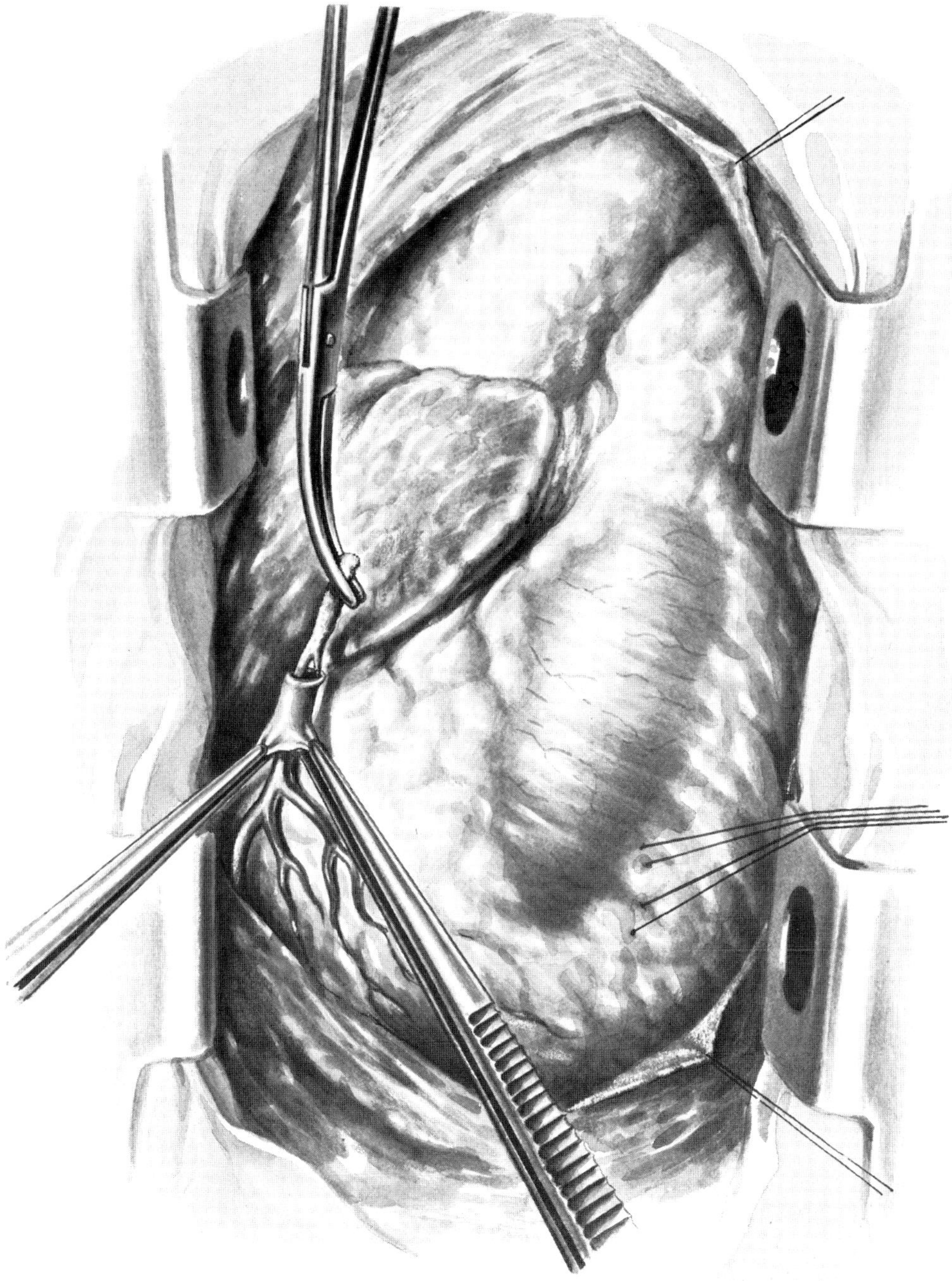

Fig. 484. Endarterectomy from stenosed distal part of right coronary artery by eversion method.

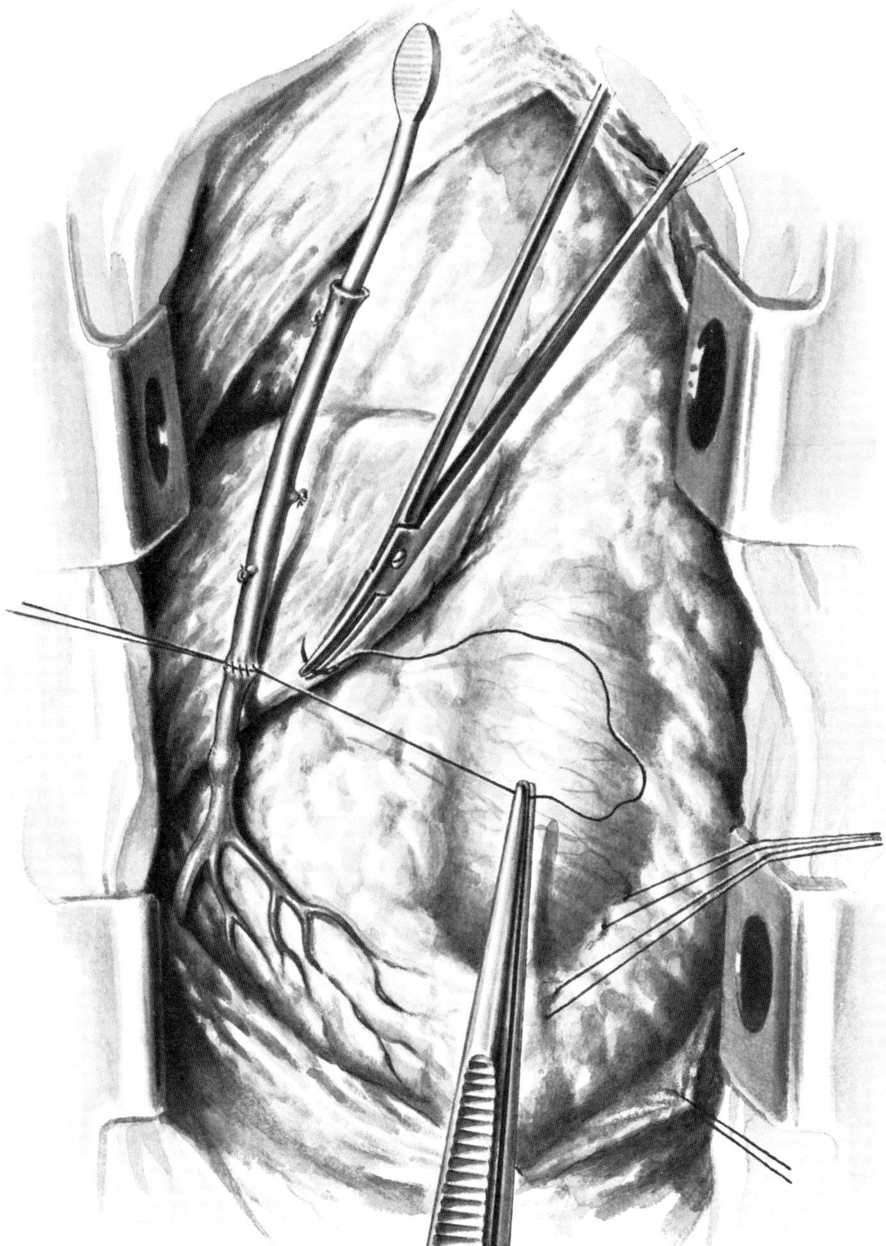

Fig. 485. Creation of end-to-end anastomosis between venous autograft and right coronary artery on bougie. Distal end of bougie is outlined in lumen of coronary artery. Circular vascular suture is applied.

clamped along its wall, in which an oval opening is then made (Fig. 486).

End-to-side anastomosis is created between the venous autograft and the aorta. The clamp is taken off the aorta, and the blood flow in the coronary artery restored. The volumetric blood flow in the coronary shunt is measured with a flow meter (Fig. 487).

The final stage of the operation is represented schematically in Fig. 488.

Two or three widely spaced sutures are placed on the pericardium. A drain is left in the anterior mediastinum. The wound is sutured layer by layer.

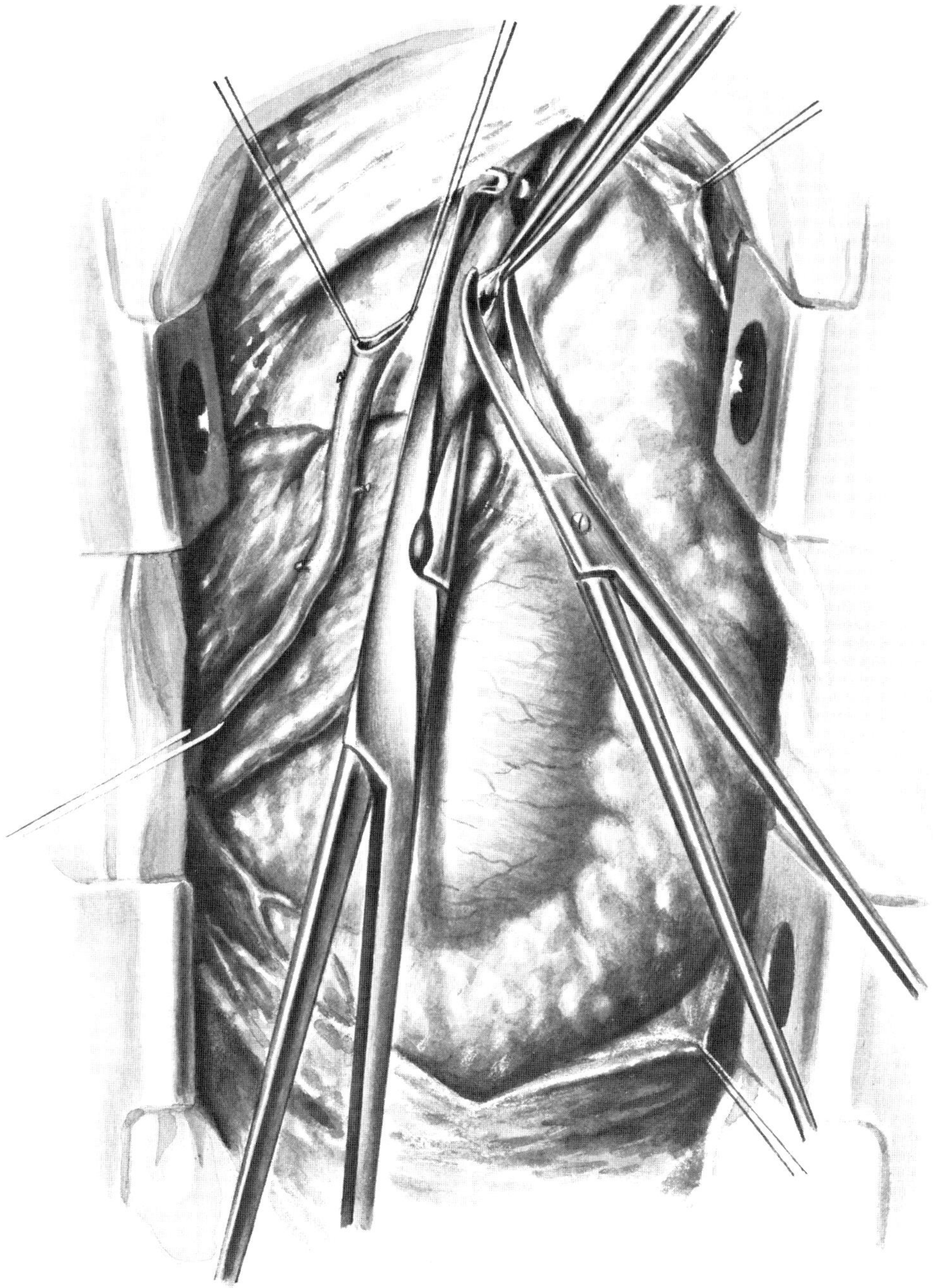

Fig. 486. Clamp is applied along wall of ascending aorta. Oval opening is cut in it. Two separate traction threads are stitched through central end of venous autograft.

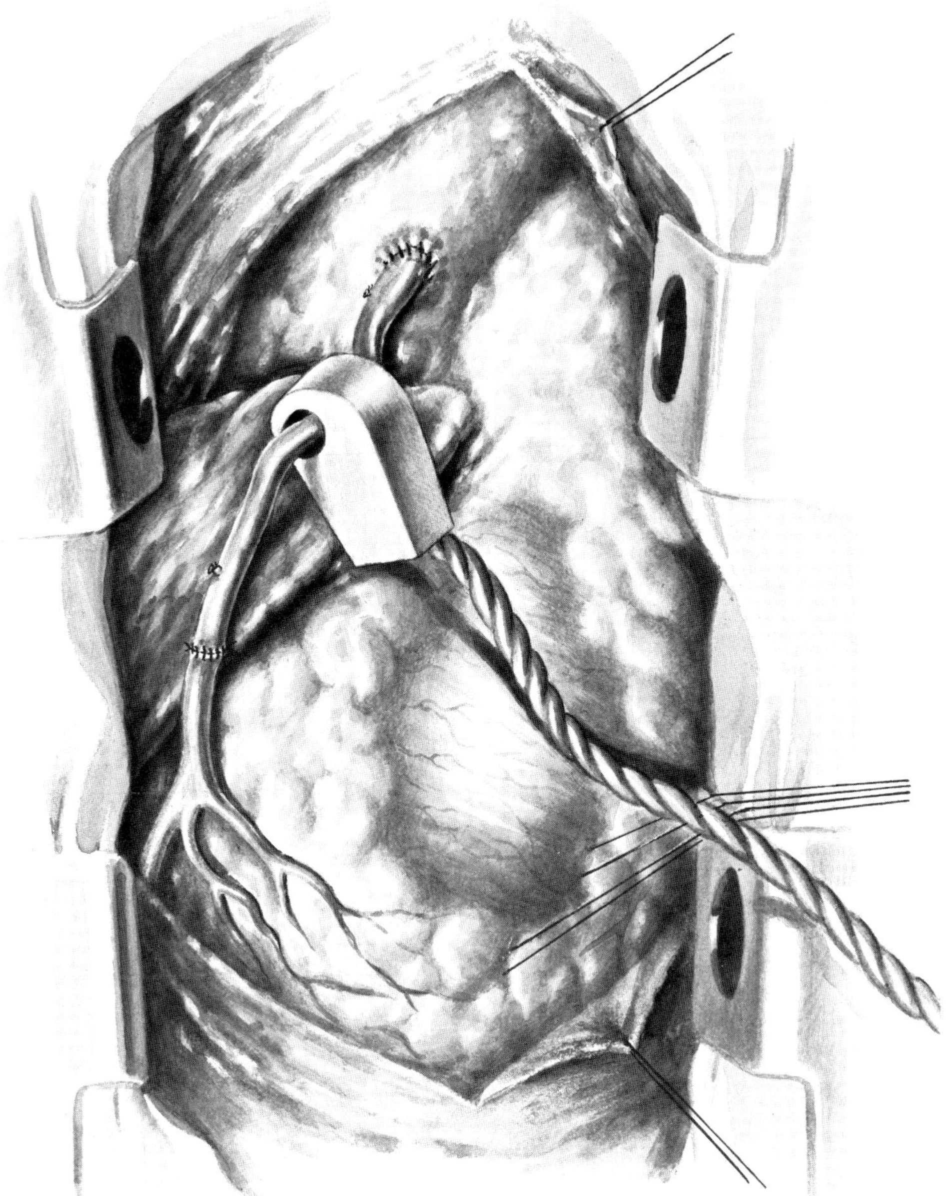

Fig. 487. Volumetric blood flow in aorticocoronary shunt by way of venous autograft is measured with flow meter.

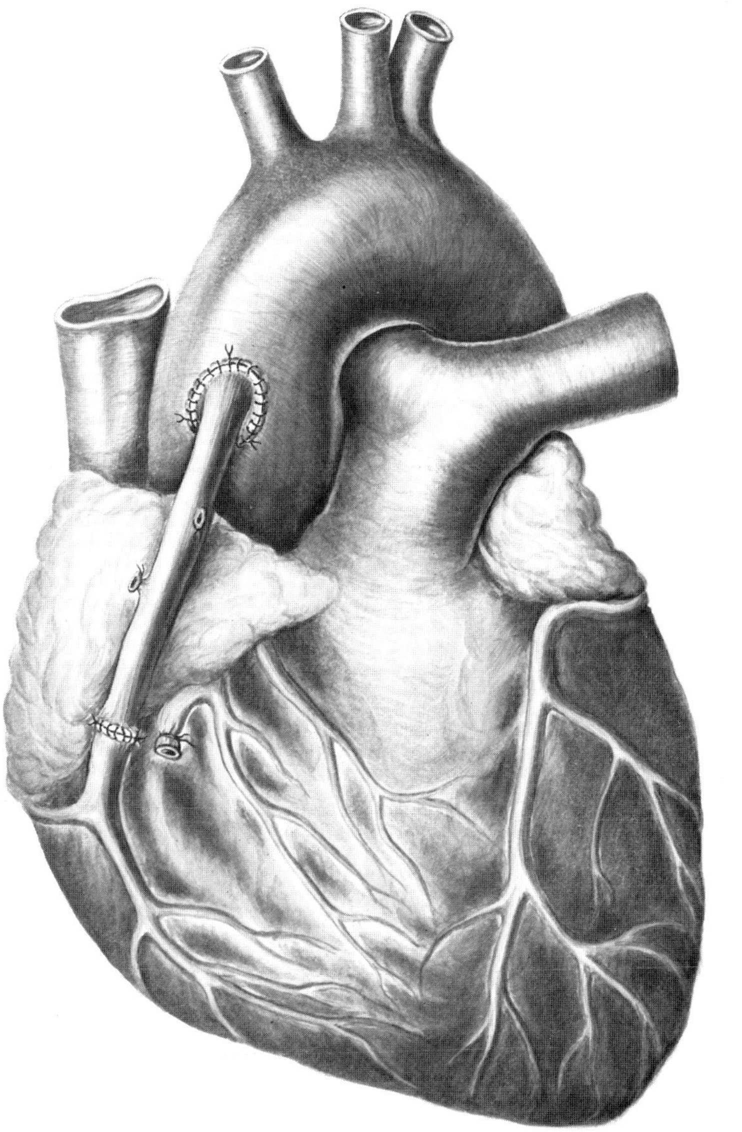

Fig. 488. Schema of reconstructed right coronary artery.

SHUNTING OF ANTERIOR INTERVENTRICULAR BRANCH OF LEFT CORONARY ARTERY

The operative approach is the same as in reconstruction of the right coronary artery. The anterior interventricular artery is inspected by palpation. It is then separated from the epicardial bed, ligated distally to the site of the occlusion, raised by loops (Fig. 489), and transected. In total occlusion of the vessel the operation may be conducted without the use of the heart-lung machine. A graft is formed from the great saphenous vein of the thigh or the deep femoral artery (Fig. 490).

To provide good access to the anterior intraventricular artery, the apex of the heart may be raised, the heart turned somewhat to the right, and a napkin placed under it. It should be borne in mind that as the heart is turned, disorders of rhythm to the point of ventricular fibrillation may develop. That is why in operations on the anterior interventricular artery, even when it is occluded, it is advisable to cannulate the venae cavae and the femoral artery beforehand so that the heart-lung machine may be immediately connected should the need arise.

The autologous venous or arterial graft is anastomosed

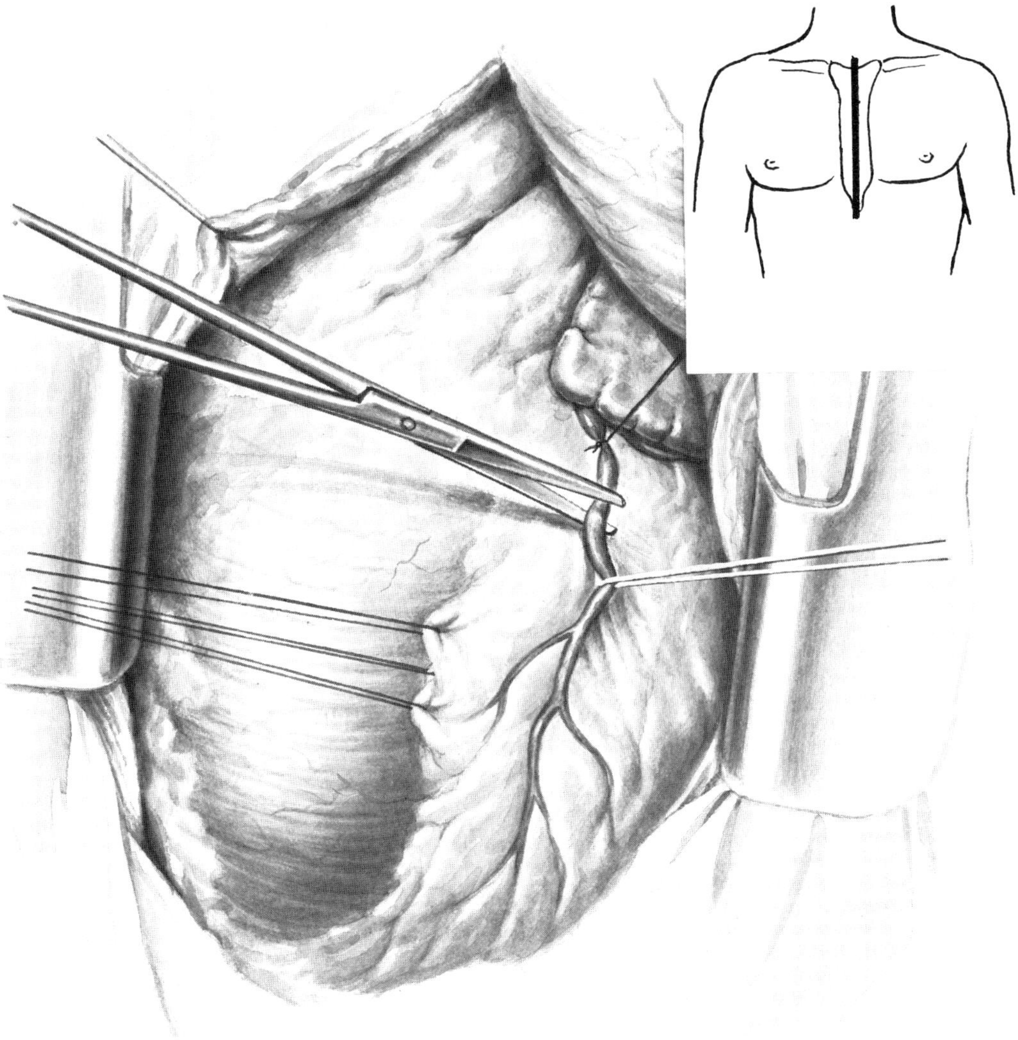

Fig. 489. Transection of anterior interventricular artery ligated distal to occlusion.

end to end with the distal stump of the coronary artery (Fig. 491). The aorta is clamped along the wall, and an oval opening is made in it (Fig. 492). The central anastomosis is formed end to side. The clamps are removed from the aorta, and the blood flow in the coronary artery is restored (Fig. 493). A drain is left in the anterior mediastinum. The wound is sutured layer by layer.

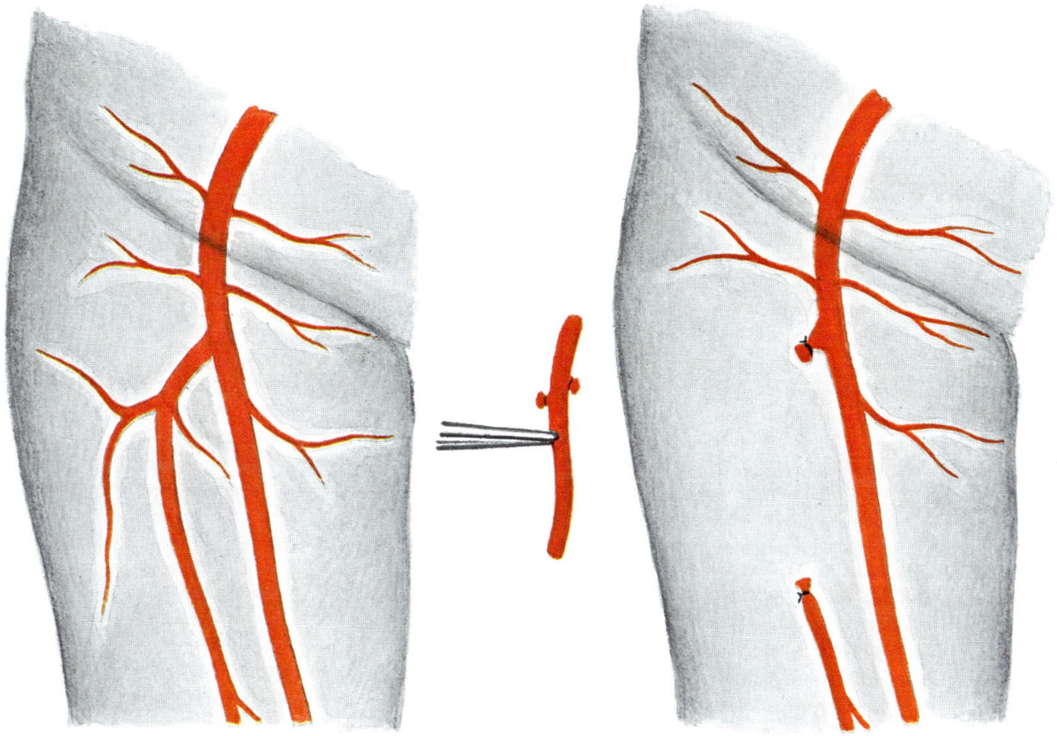

Fig. 490. Schema of resection of segment of deep femoral artery to be used as graft.

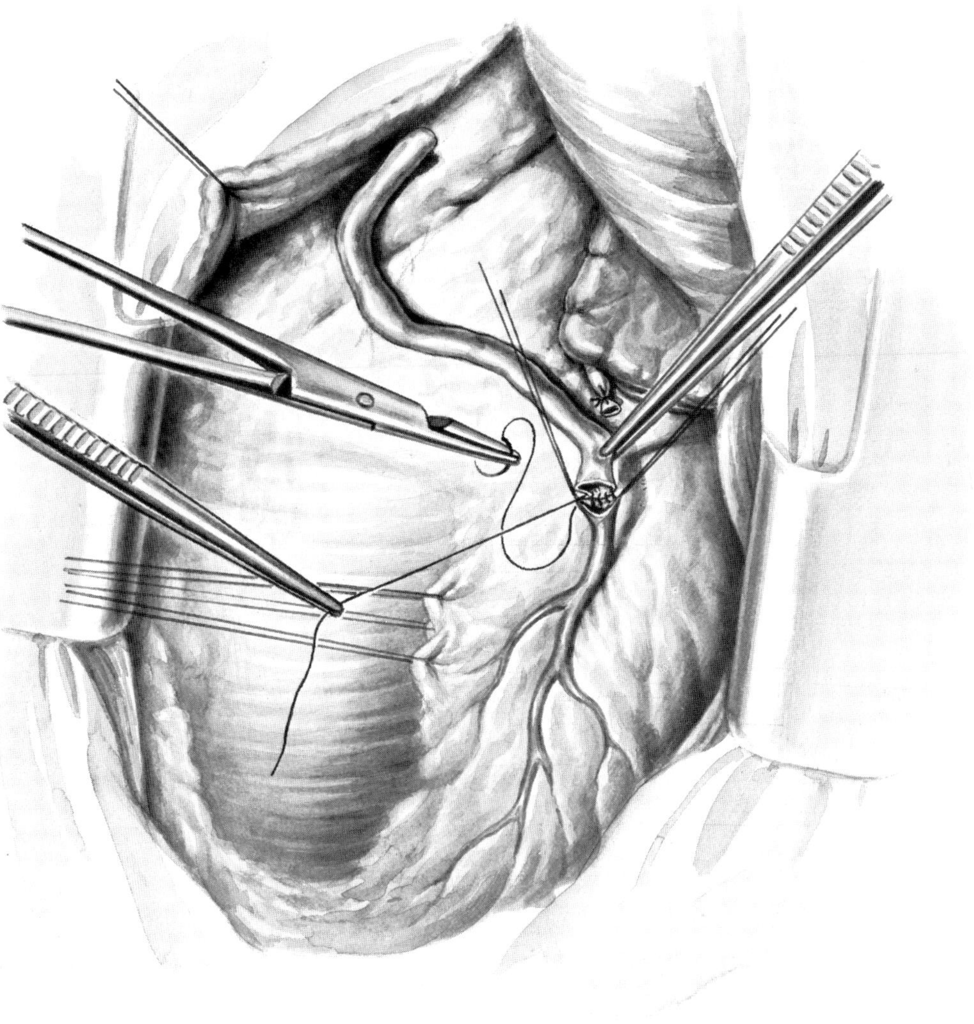

Fig. 491. Formation of end-to-end distal anastomosis between venous autograft and anterior interventricular artery with continous suture.

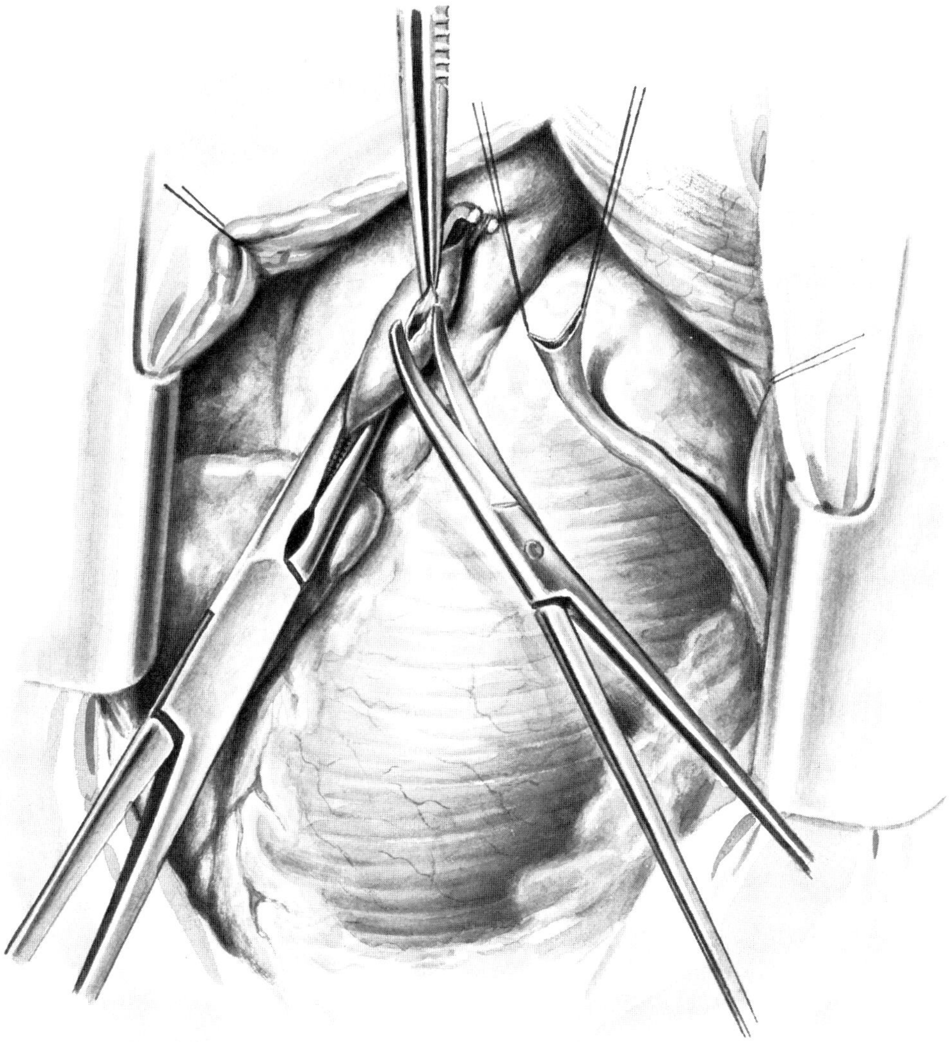

Fig. 492. Preparation of aorta for creation of central anastomosis.

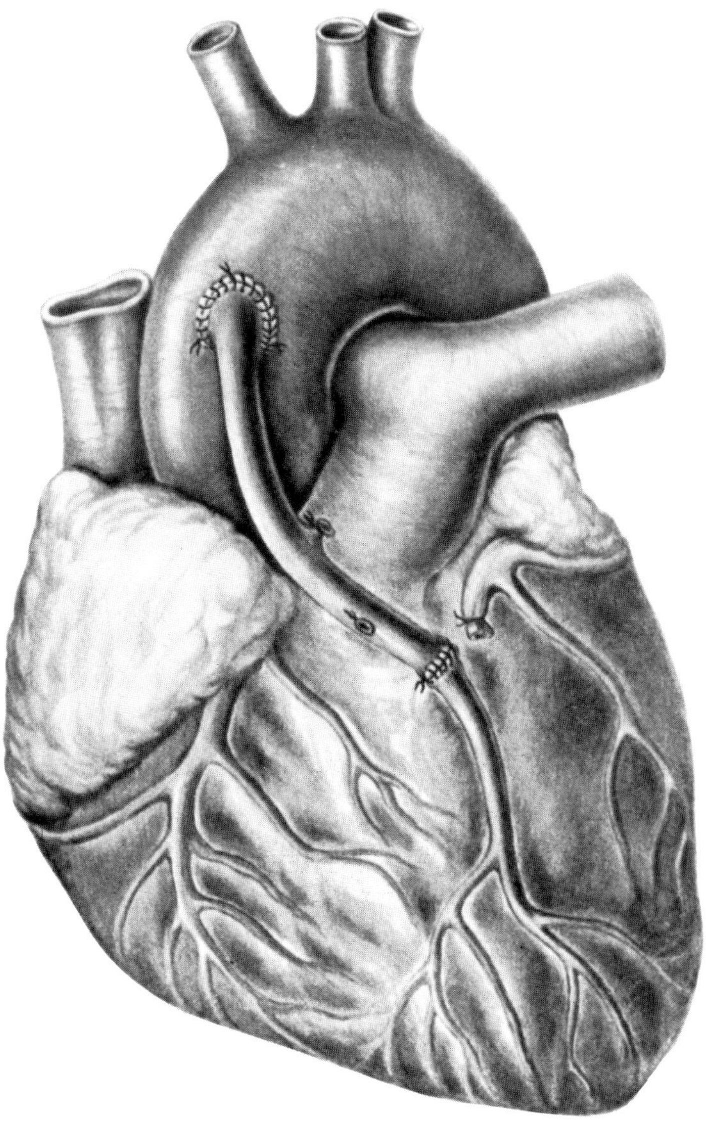

Fig. 493. Reconstructed anterior interventricular artery is represented schematically.

ONE-STAGE SHUNTING OF RIGHT CORONARY ARTERY AND ANTERIOR INTERVENTRICULAR BRANCH OF LEFT CORONARY ARTERY

Approach is gained by median sternotomy. The superior and inferior venae cavae and the femoral artery are cannulated. The heart-lung machine is connected. The aorta is clamped along the wall, and an oval opening is made in it (Fig. 494). An end-to-side anastomosis is created between the autologous venous graft and the aorta by means of a continuous vascular suture (Fig. 495). The clamp is taken off the aorta, and the venous

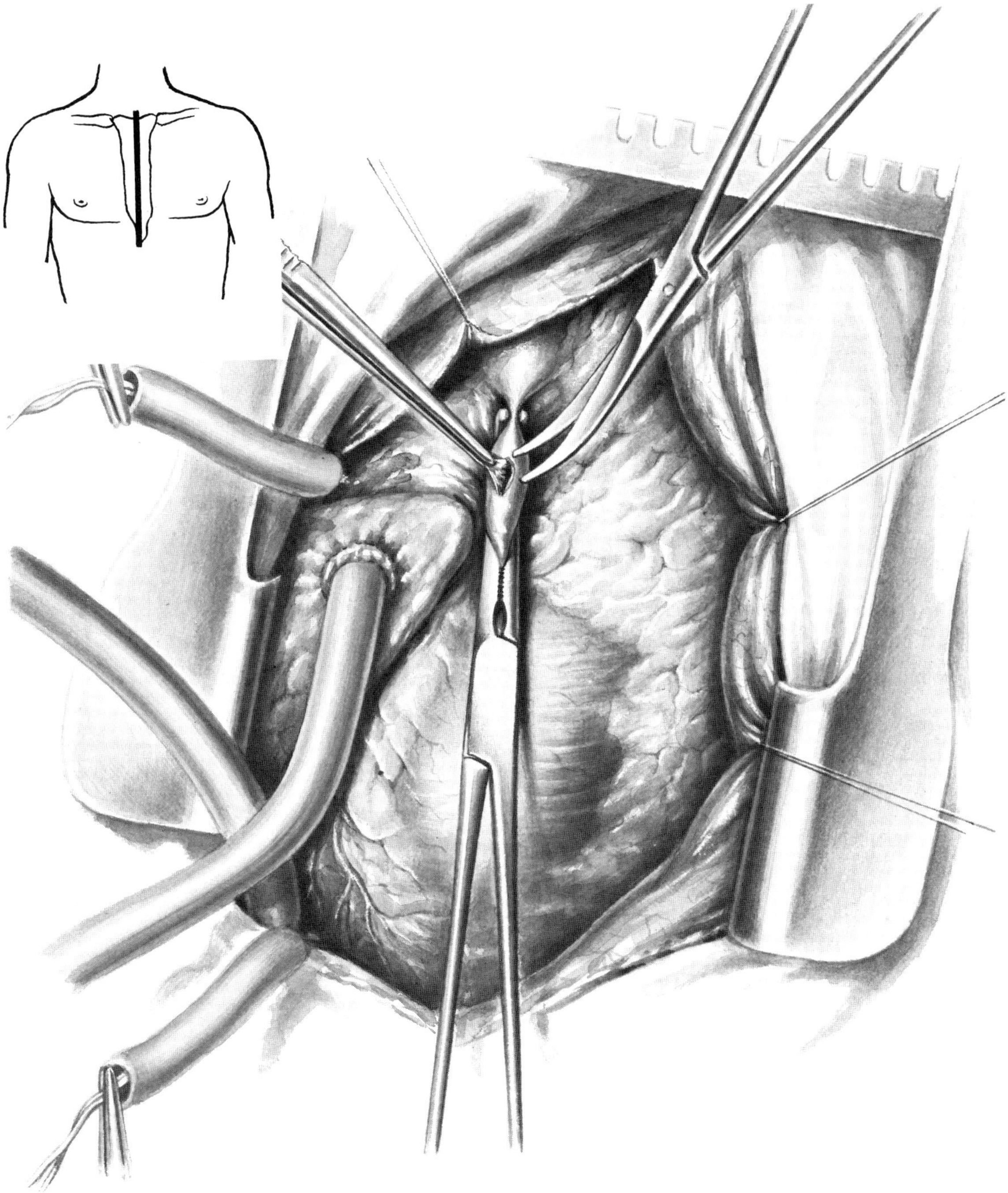

Fig. 494. Superior and inferior venae cavae are cannulated. Clamp has been applied along wall of aorta. Oval opening is made in it.

graft is clamped nearer the aorta (Fig. 496). The central end of the second venous autograft is anastomosed somewhat distally to the anastomosis formed (Fig. 497) and is also temporarily clamped (Fig. 498). The anterior interventricular artery is raised with two loops without separating it from the epicardial bed. The artery is cut lengthwise, distal to the site of the stenosis (Fig. 499), and an end-to-side anastomosis is formed between the first venous graft and the coronary artery with a continuous suture (Fig. 500). The clamp is removed from

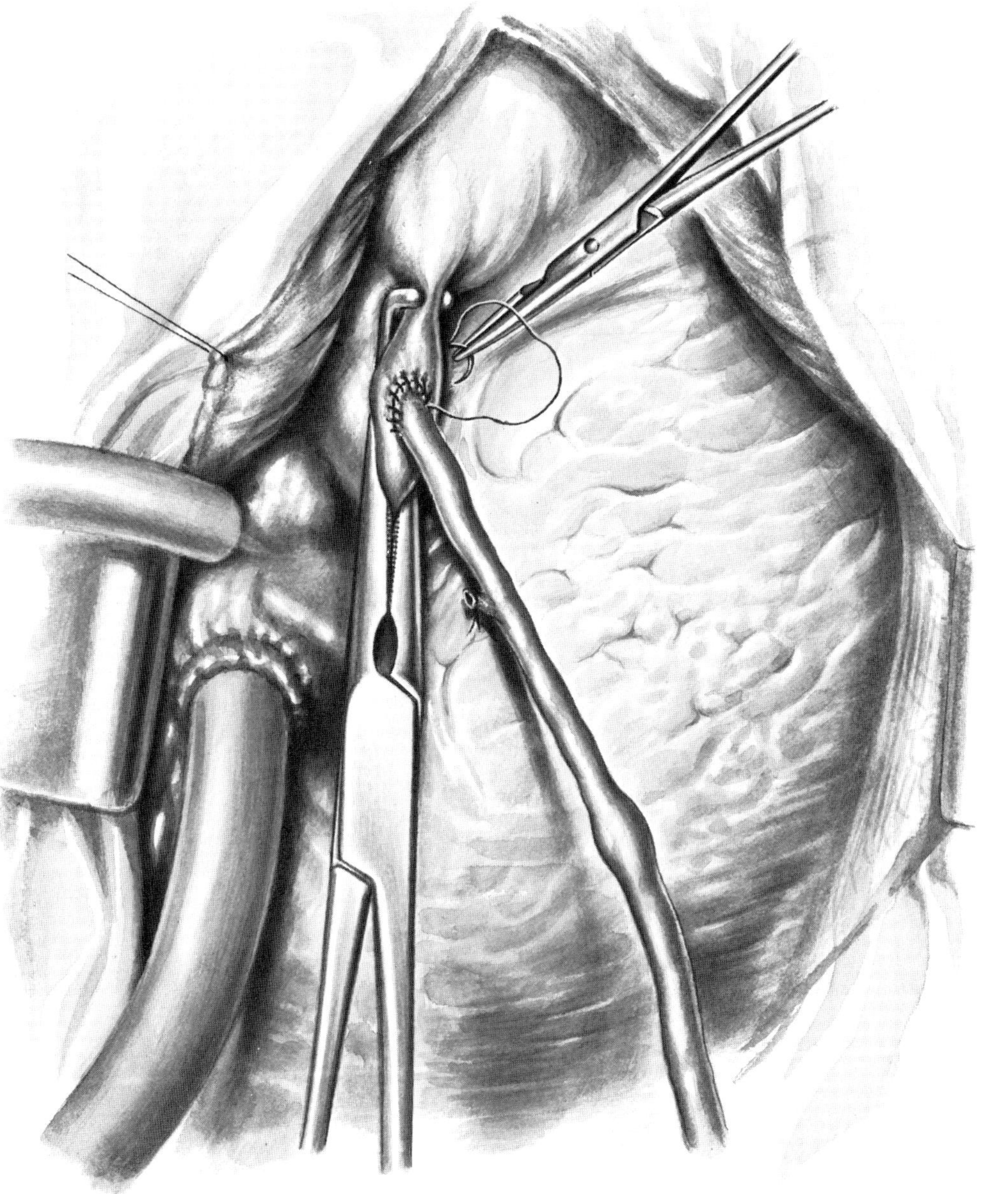

Fig. 495. Proximal anastomosis between aorta and venous autograft is formed with continuous suture.

the venous graft, and the blood flow is restored in the anterior interventricular artery.

The right coronary artery is mobilized distal to the site of the stenosis, cut lengthwise, and anastomosed end to side with the second venous graft (Fig. 501). The clamp is taken off the venous graft, and the blood flow in the right coronary artery is restored. The heart-lung machine is disconnected (Fig. 502). The anterior mediastinum is drained.

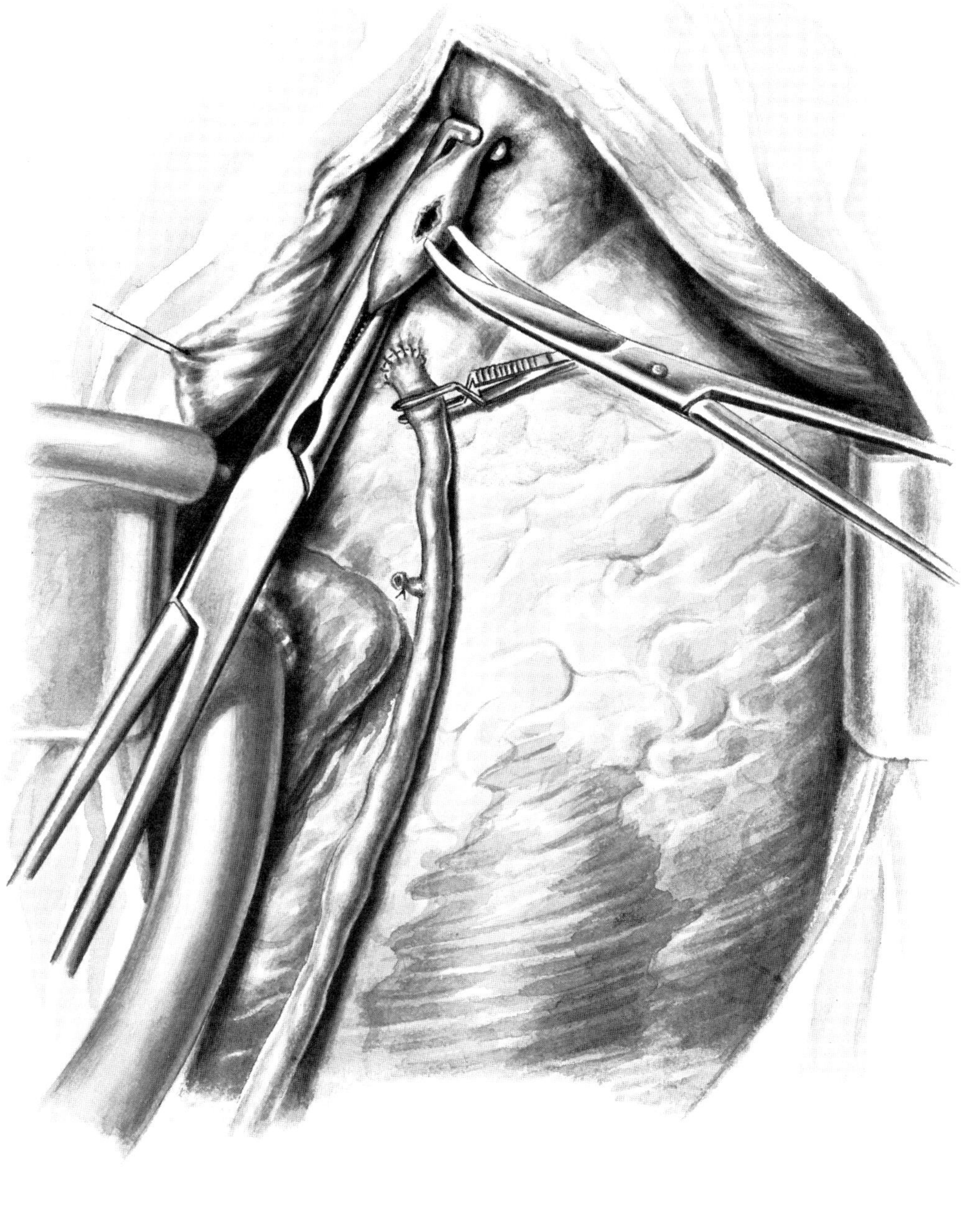

Fig. 496. Part of aorta distal to first anastomosis is prepared for creating second anastomosis with venous autograft.

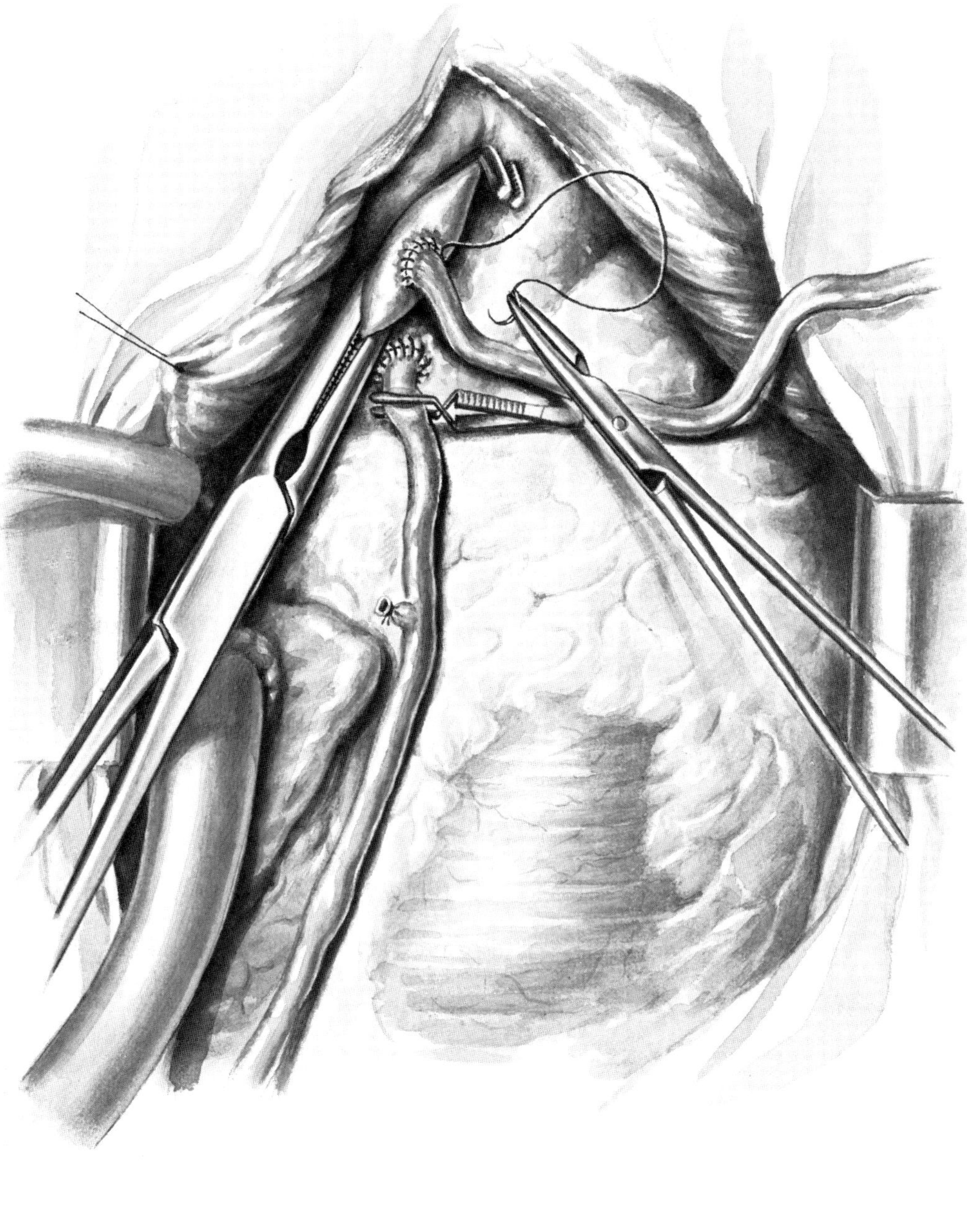

Fig. 497. Second anastomosis between aorta and venous autograft is formed with continuous suture.

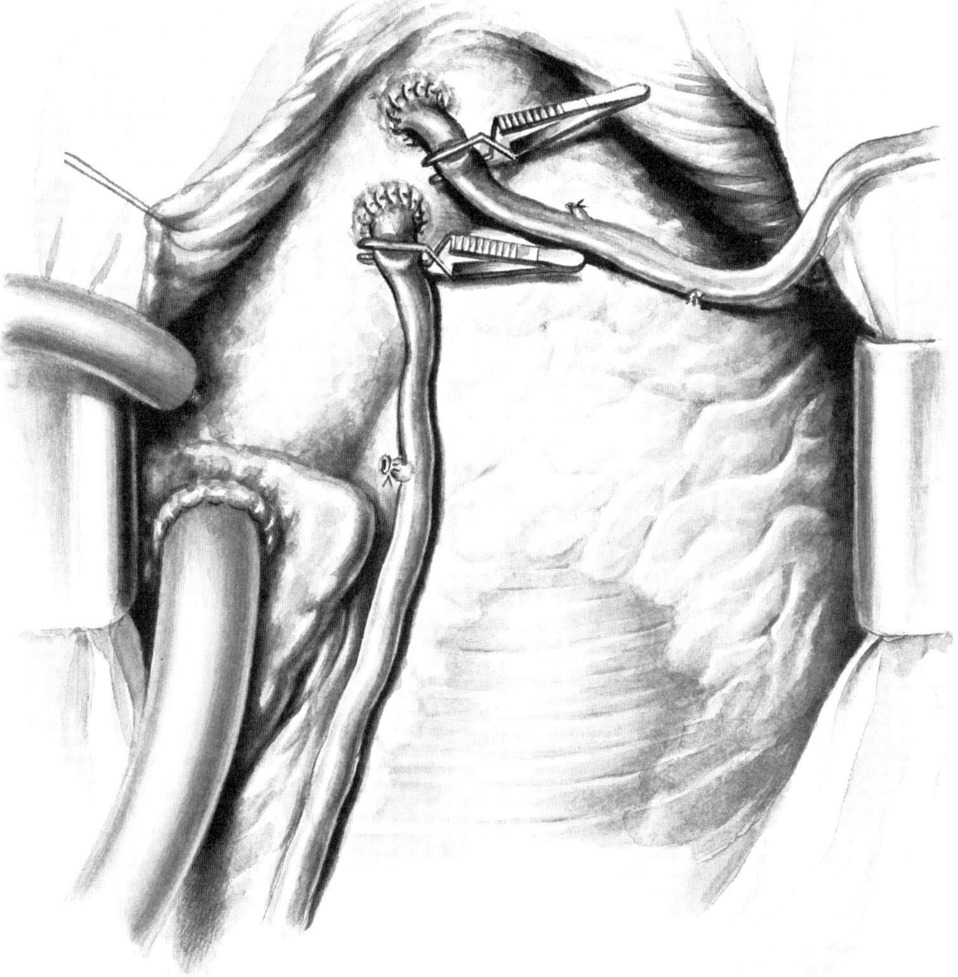

Fig. 498. Anastomoses between aorta and venous autografts are formed.

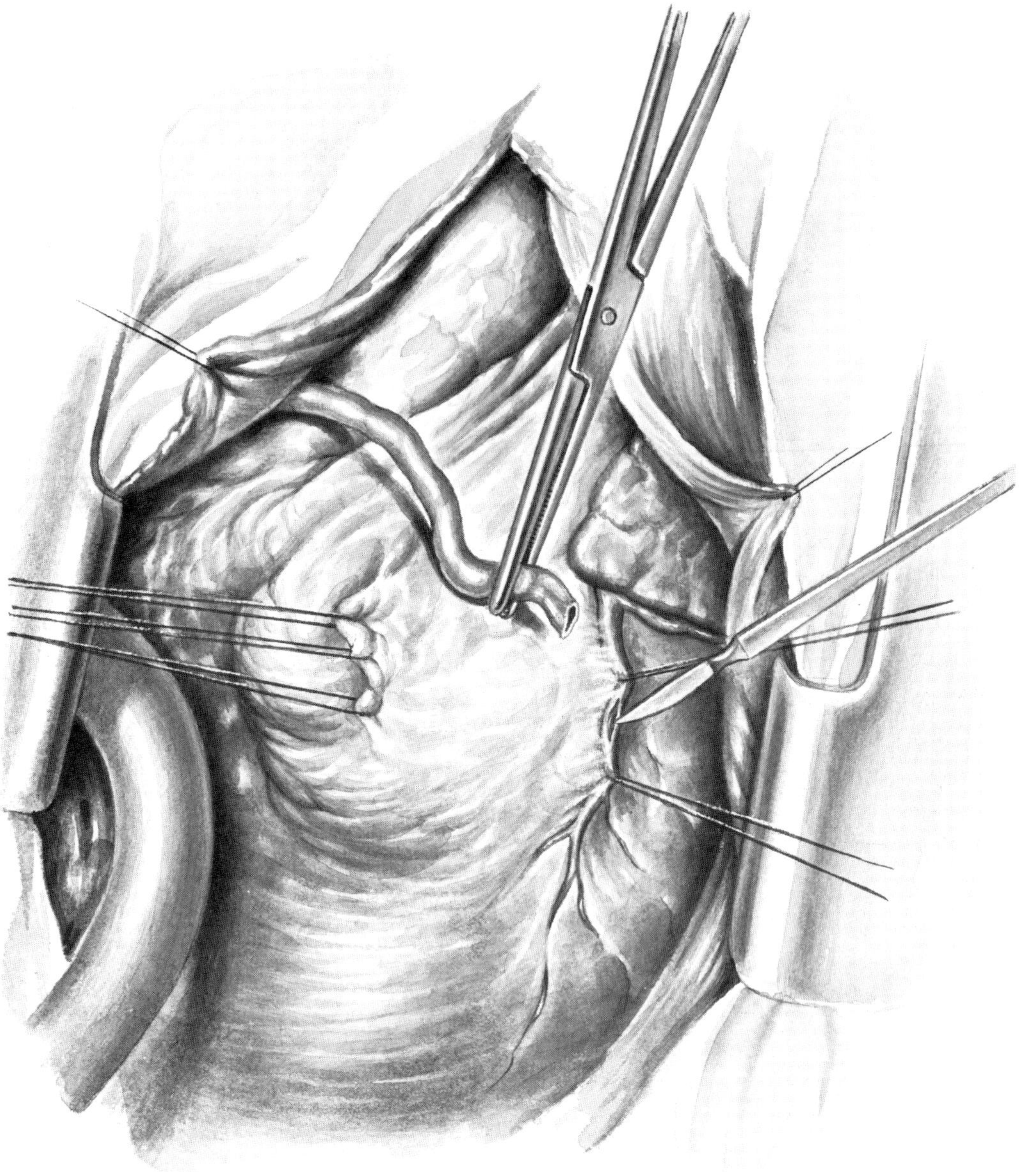

Fig. 499. Anterior interventricular artery is cut lengthwise. Distal end of one venous autograft is brought up to it.

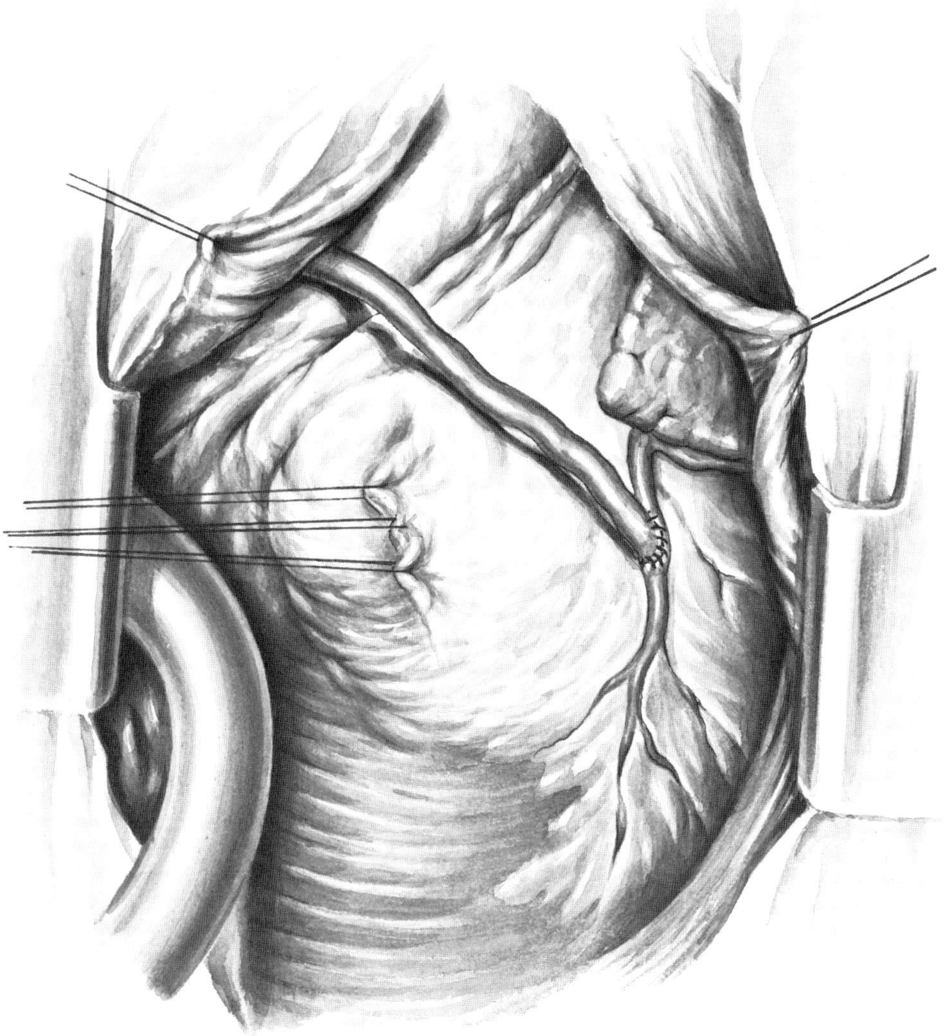

Fig. 500. End-to-side anastomosis between venous autograft and anterior interventricular artery has been formed and blood flow restored.

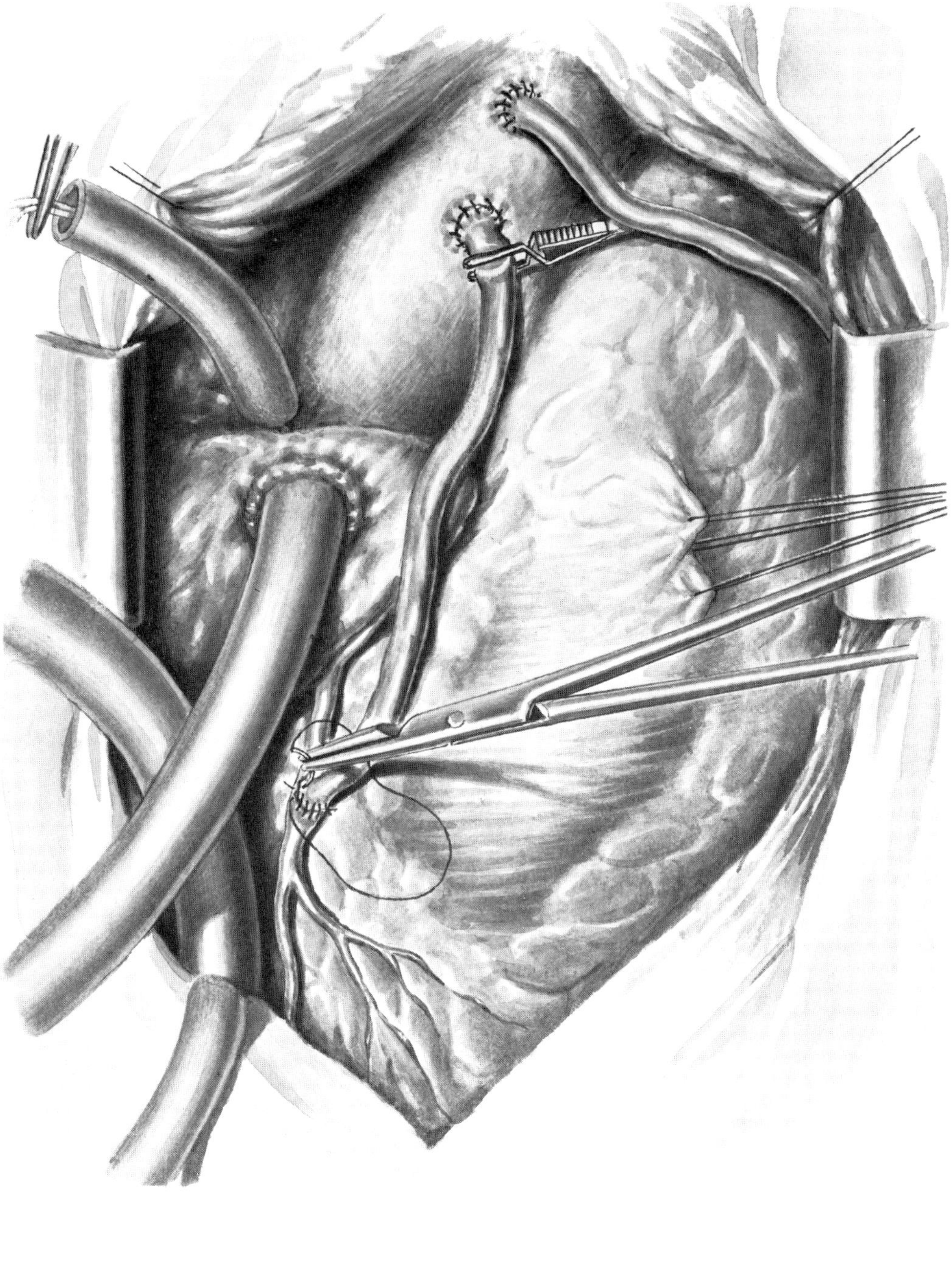

Fig. 501. End-to-side anastomosis between venous autograft and right coronary artery formed with continuous suture.

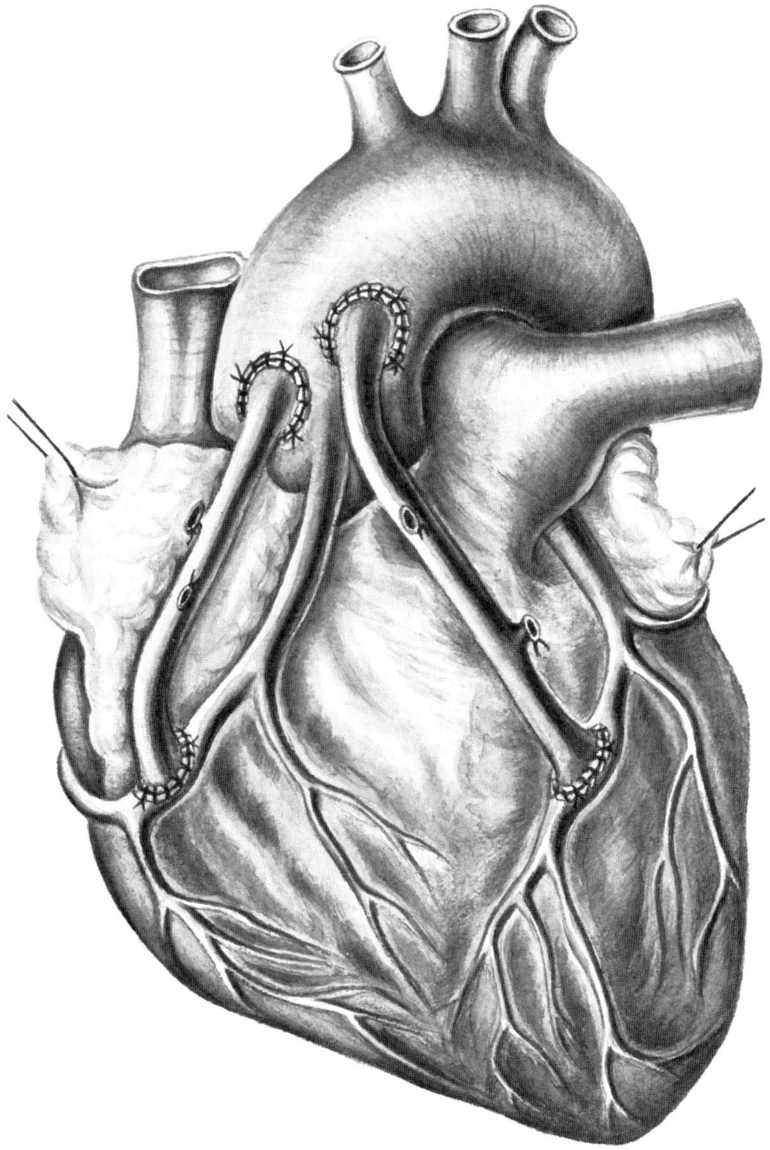

Fig. 502. Schema of double aorticocoronary shunt.

Operations in aneurysms of the thoracic aorta

RESECTION OF SACCULATED ANEURYSM OF ASCENDING AORTA

The anatomical features of a sacculated aneurysm make it possible to apply a clamp laterally along the wall of the aorta without disturbing circulation in its brachiocephalic branches and the segments stretching distally. That is why the operation may be conducted without using extracorporeal circulation.

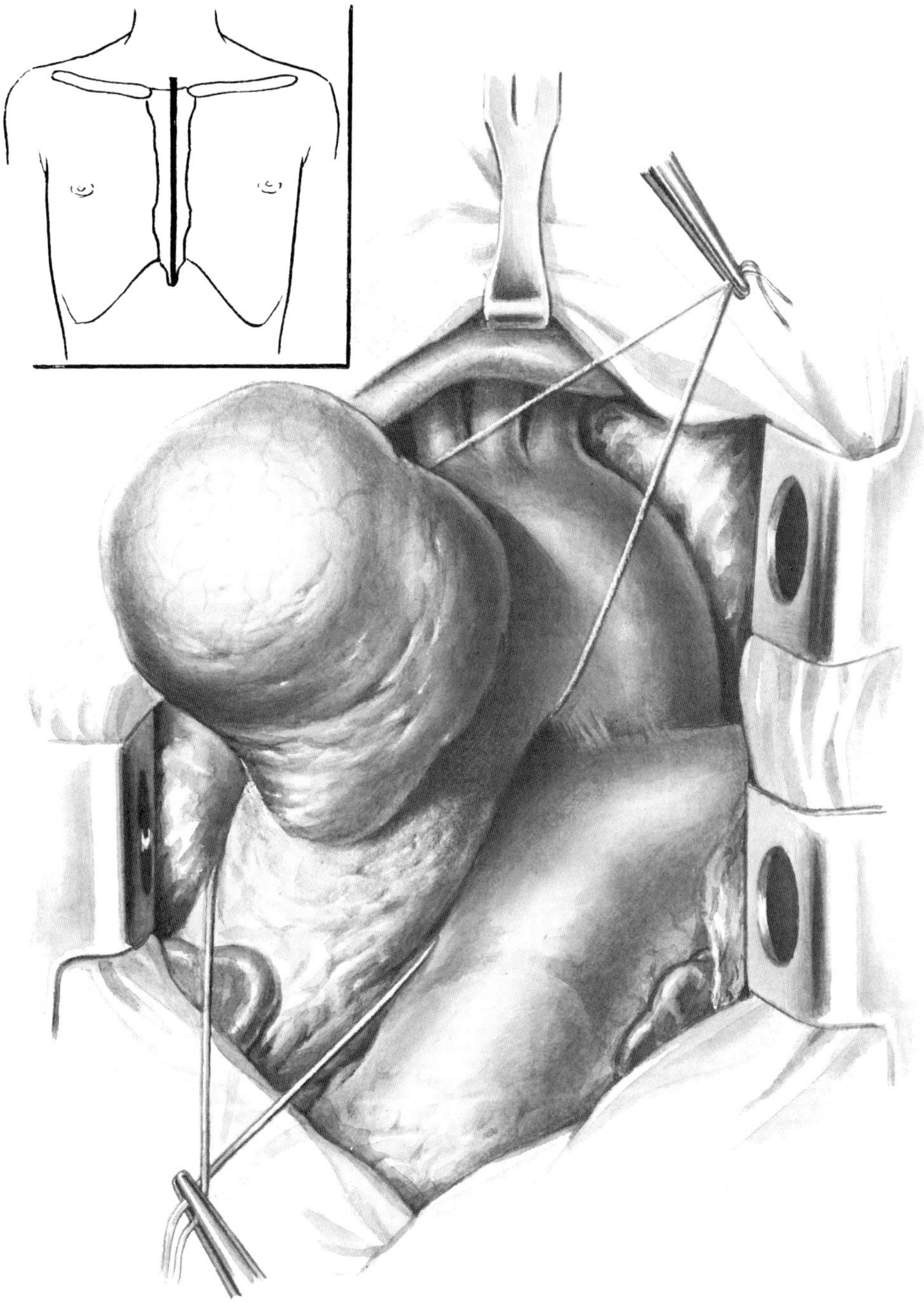

Fig. 503. Aorta is held with loops. General view of sacculated aneurysm in operative wound after edges of sternum had been drawn apart and pericardium opened. *Inset;* schema of operative approach.

Median sternotomy is performed, and the pericardium is opened wide. The ascending aorta and the aneurysmal sac are carefully freed from the adhesions (Fig. 503). There is no need to free the apex of the aneurysm when the adhesions are extensive.

The principal stage of the operation consists in freeing the base of the aneurysm so that the ascending aorta may be reliably clamped along its wall (Fig. 504). The aneurysmal sac is excised. Two rows of continuous sutures (mattress and blanket sutures) are applied to the aortic wall, making it sufficiently airtight and strong (Fig. 505). The clamp is taken off the aorta (Fig. 506). Widely spaced sutures are applied to the pericardium. The anterior mediastinum is drained.

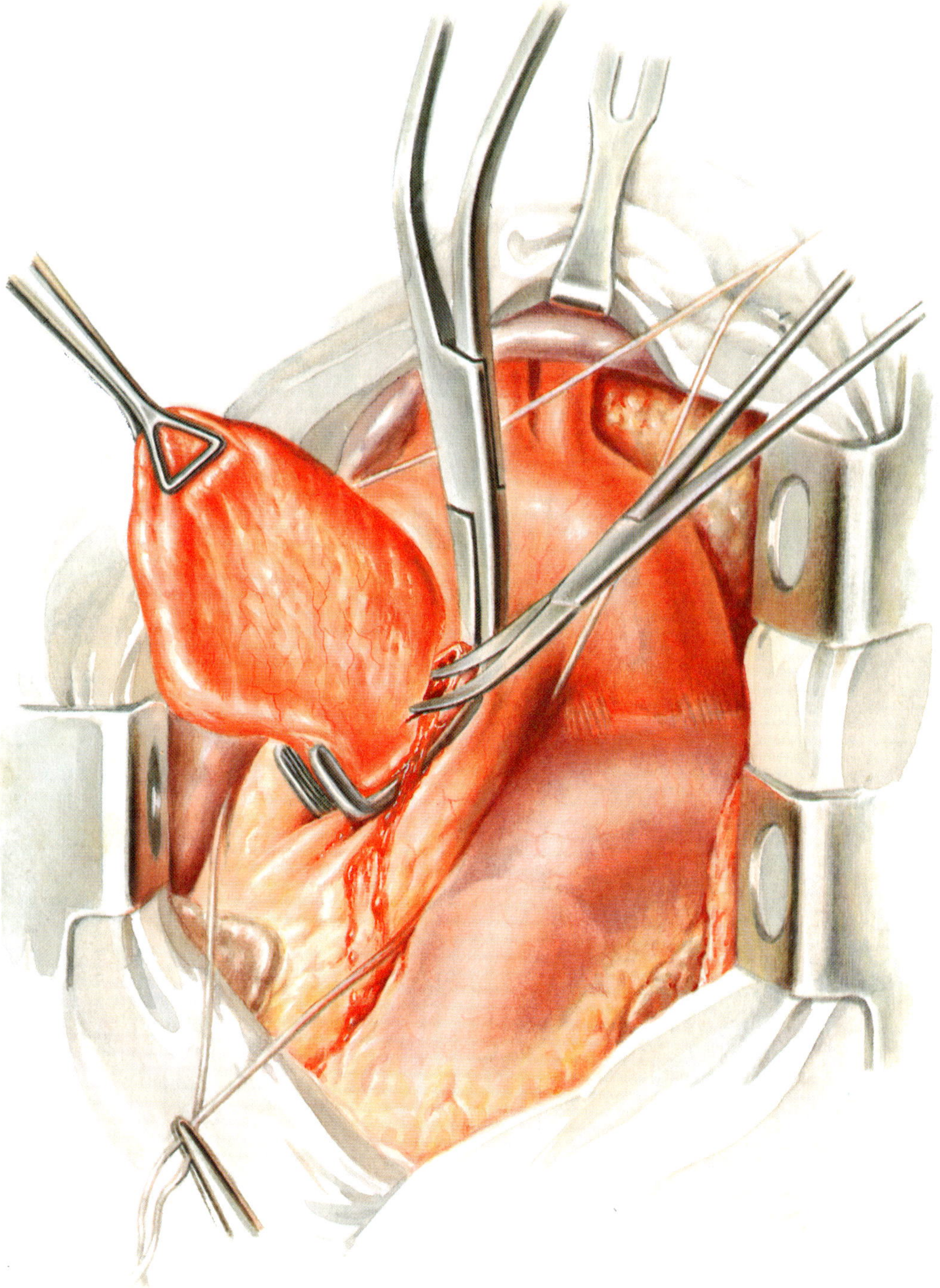

Fig. 504. Clamp is applied to aorta at base of aneurysm. Aneurysmal sac is excised.

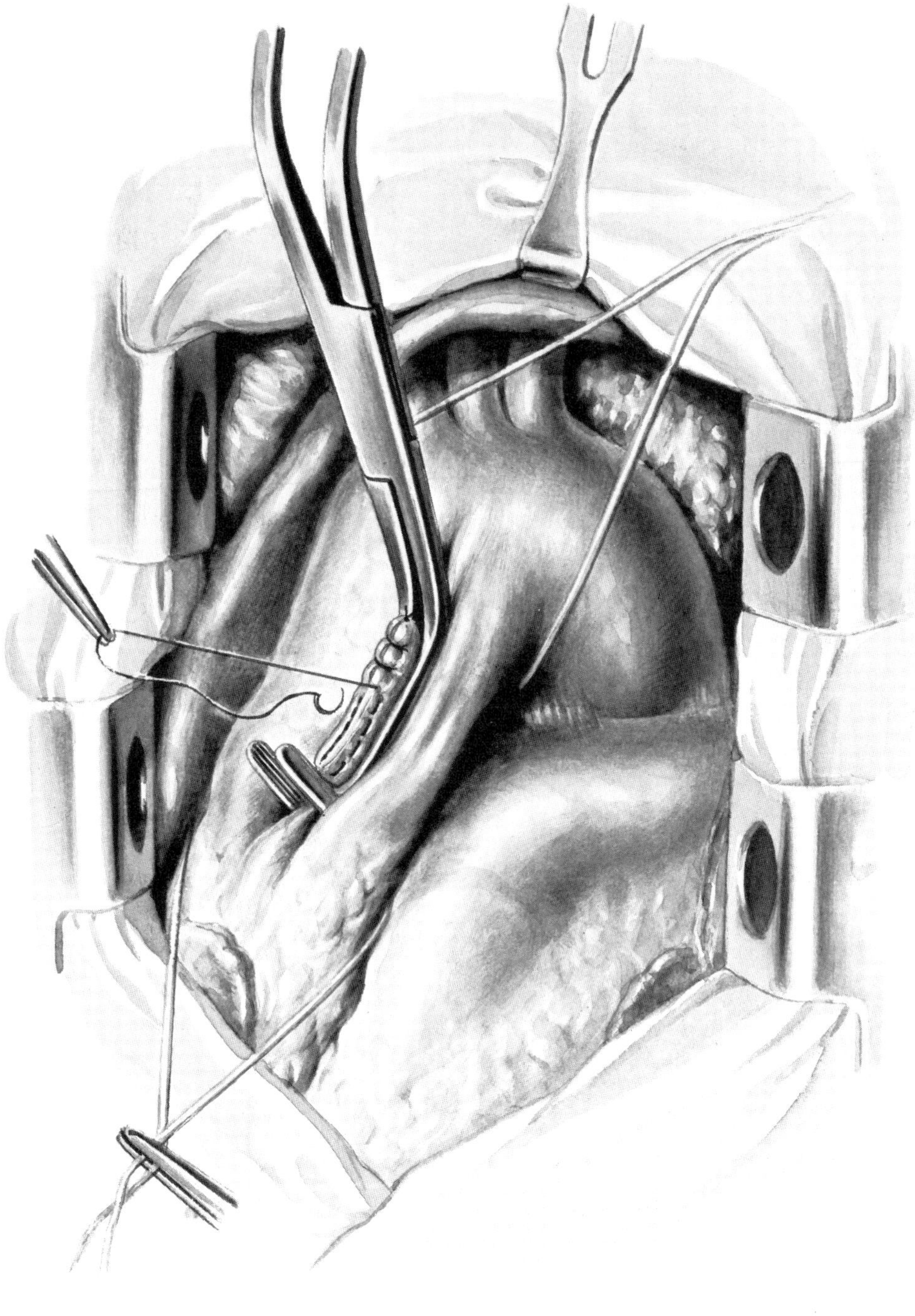

Fig. 505. Application of sutures to aortic wall after removal of aneurysm.

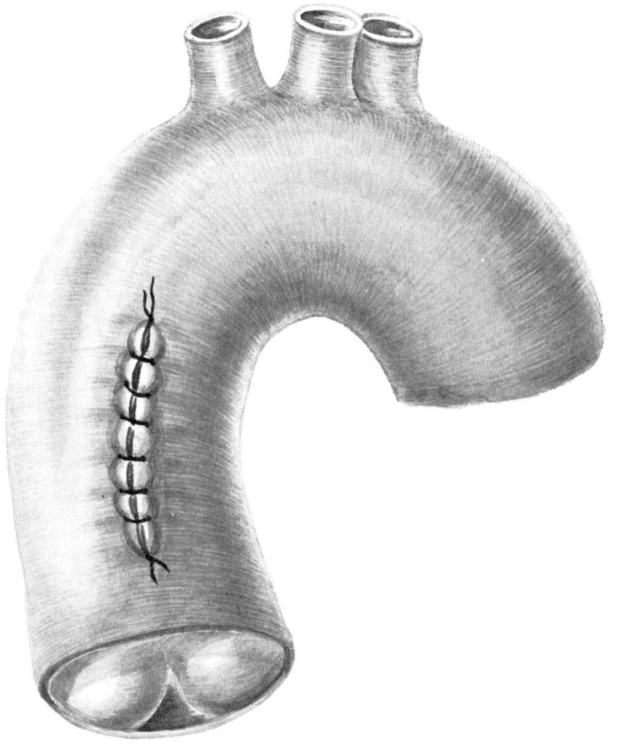

Fig. 506. Schema of aorta after removal of sacculated aneurysm.

PLASTIC SURGERY OF ASCENDING AORTA IN DISSECTING ANEURYSM

The operation is conducted under conditions of extracorporeal circulation. Median sternotomy is performed, and the pericardium is opened wide. The ascending aorta with the aneurysm is mobilized, and loops are drawn around it (Fig. 507). The superior and inferior venae cavae and the femoral artery are cannulated, and the heart-lung machine is connected.

Two clamps are applied to the aorta, which is tran-

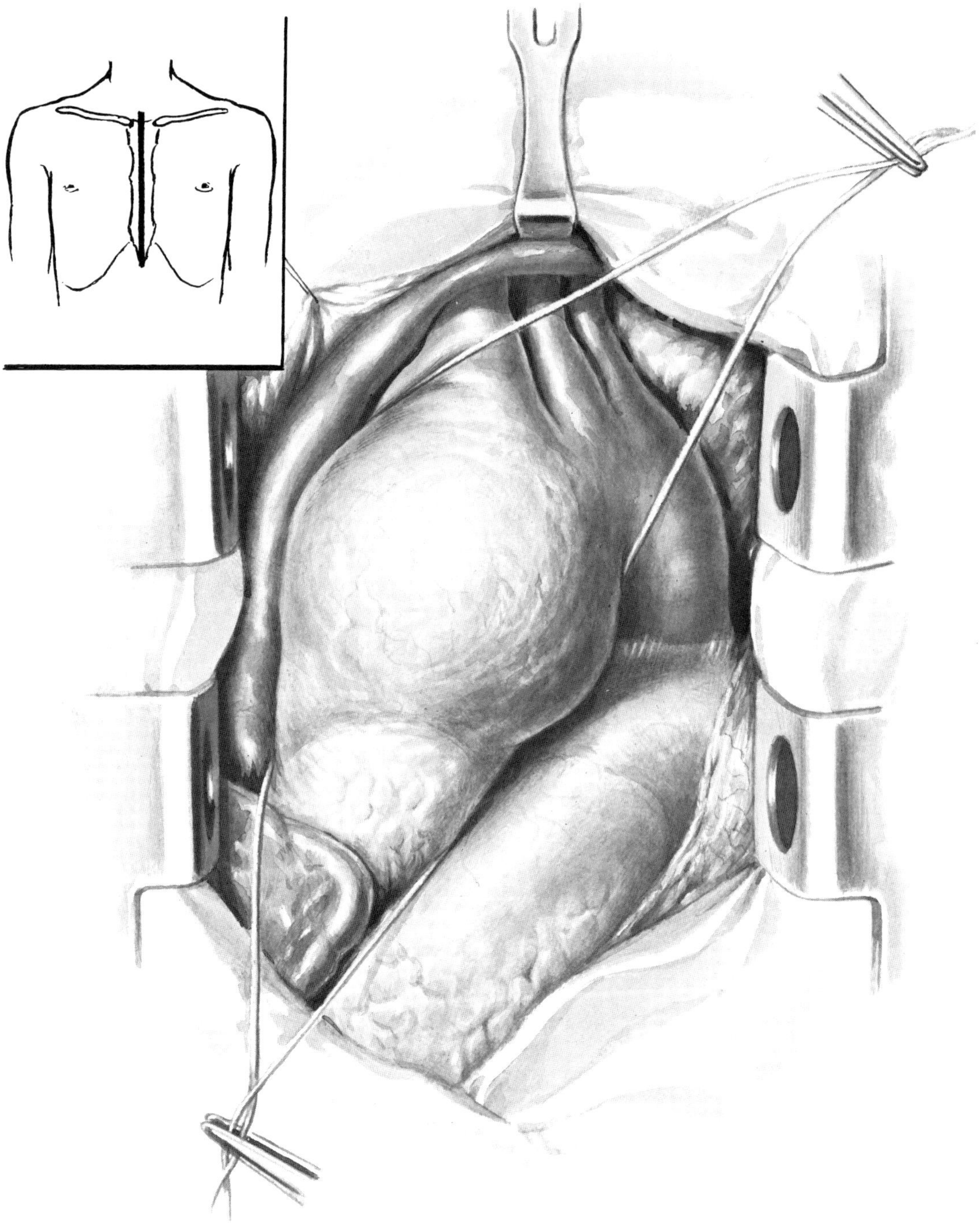

Fig. 507. Loops are drawn under aorta. *Inset;* operative approach.

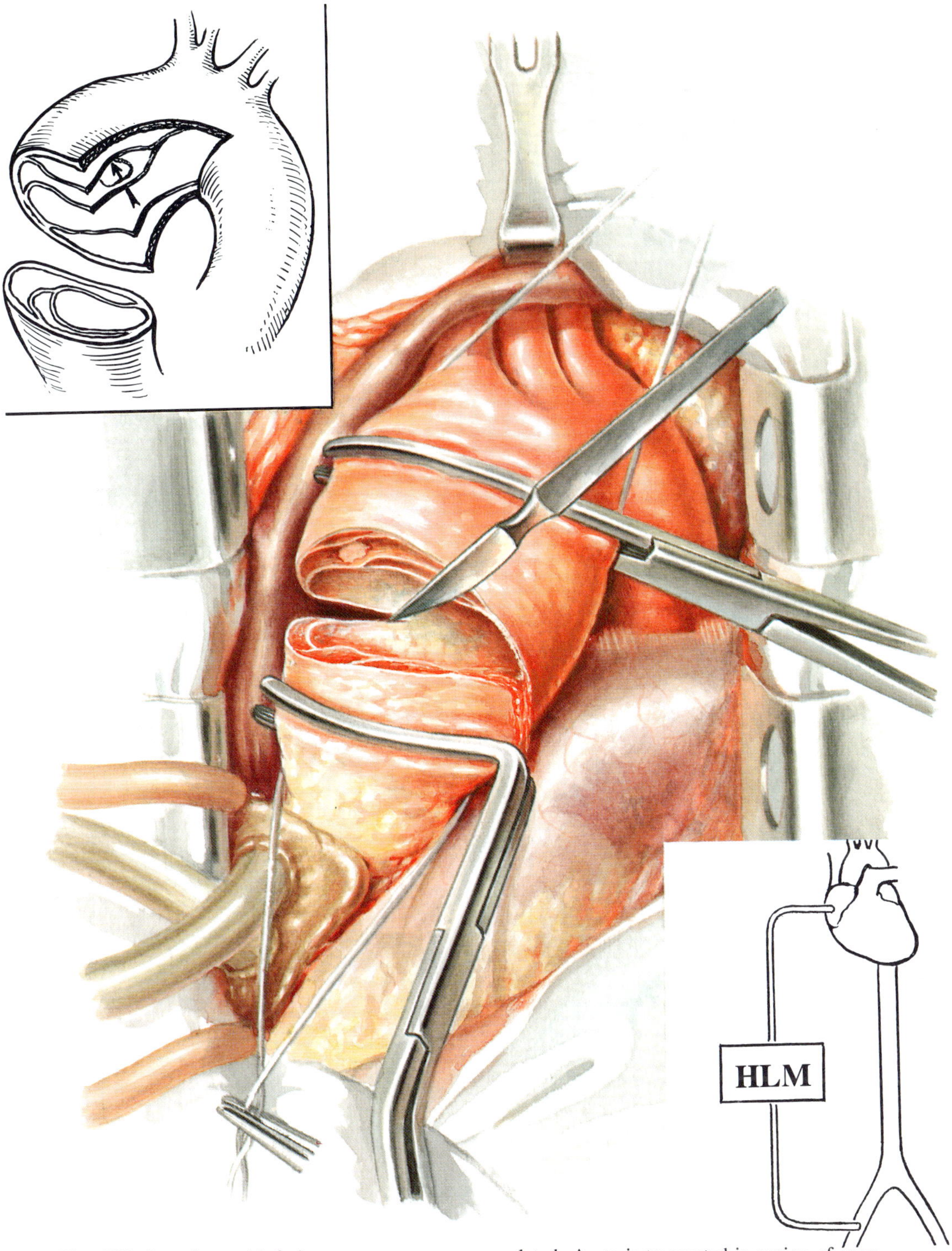

Fig. 508. Superior and inferior venae cavae are cannulated. Aorta is transected in region of aneurysm between two clamps. *Top inset,* defect in aortic intima through which blood escapes under coats of aorta and separates them. *Lower inset,* heart-lung machine (HLM).

sected between them (Fig. 508). The central clamp is removed and coronary perfusion is begun. After transection of the aneurysm the aneurysmal sac is emptied of blood; it collapses. It becomes easy to discern the dissected aortic wall and the defect in the intima through which the blood enters the aorta, separating its coats.

The defect in the intima is repaired with a continuous blanket suture stitched through the edge of the transected aorta, after which the proximal and distal ends of the aorta are anastomosed by means of a continuous circular suture (Fig. 509). The distal clamp is removed, and the blood flow in the aorta is restored (Fig. 510). The heart-lung machine is disconnected, and the cannulas are removed from the venae cavae and the femoral artery. Widely spaced sutures are placed on the pericardium, and a drain is left in the anterior mediastinum.

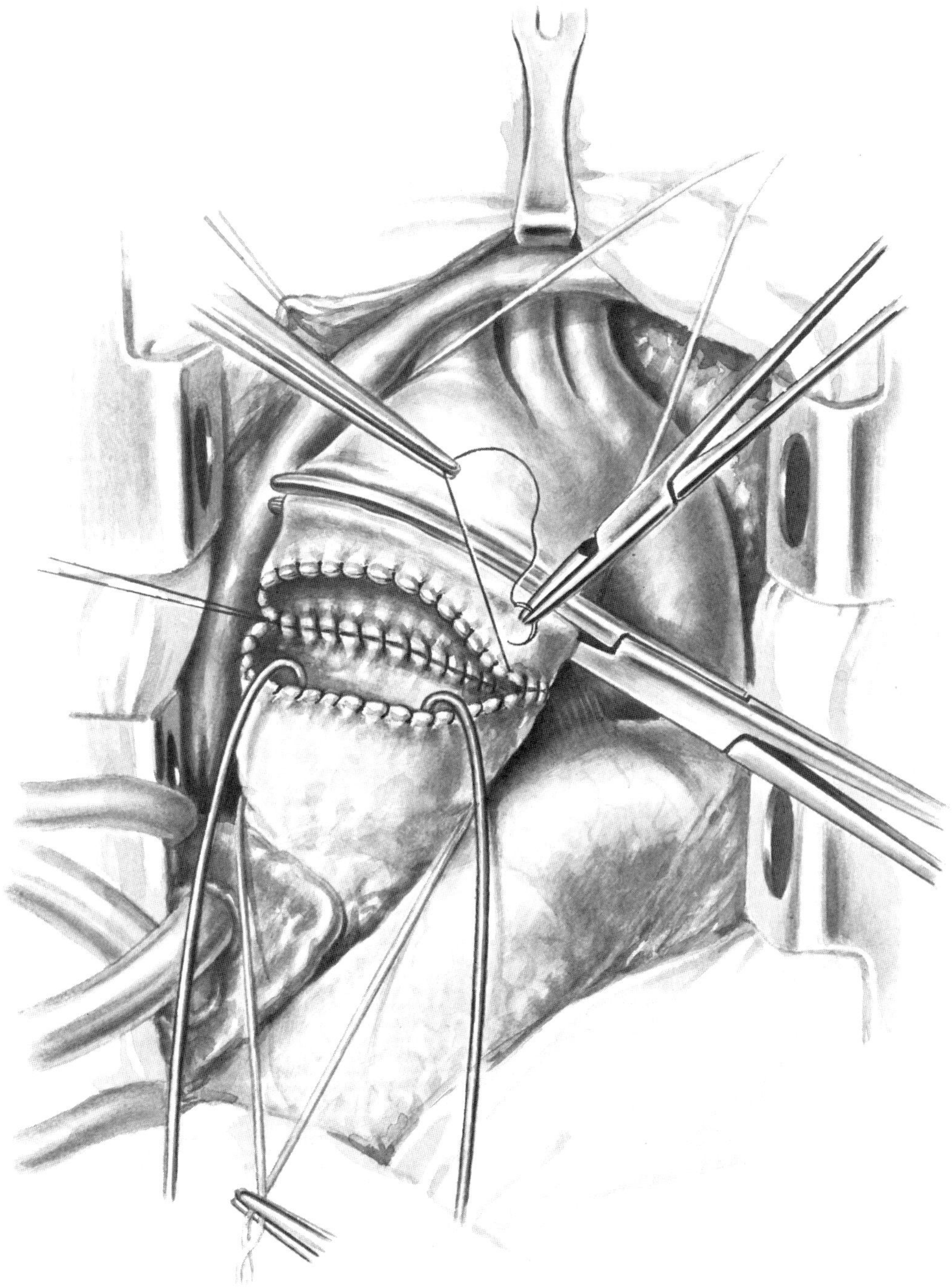

Fig. 509. Circular blanket suture has been applied to entire circumference of aorta. Proximal and distal ends of aorta are being stitched to each other.

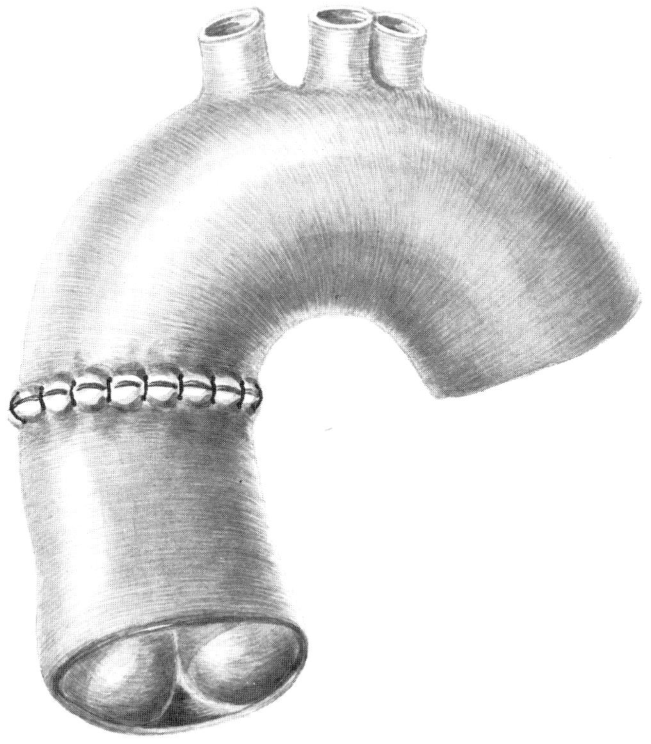

Fig. 510. View of reconstructed aorta after removal of dissecting aneurysm. (Schema.)

RESECTION OF DIFFUSE ANEURYSM AND PROSTHETIC REPLACEMENT OF ASCENDING AORTA

Partial longitudinal sternotomy is performed with the incision continued in the left fourth intercostal space, and the pleural cavity is opened. The pericardium is incised widely. The superior and inferior venae cavae and the femoral artery are cannulated, and the heart-lung machine is connected. The ascending aorta with the aneurysm is carefully mobilized, and loops are brought under the brachiocephalic branches (Fig. 511). Clamps

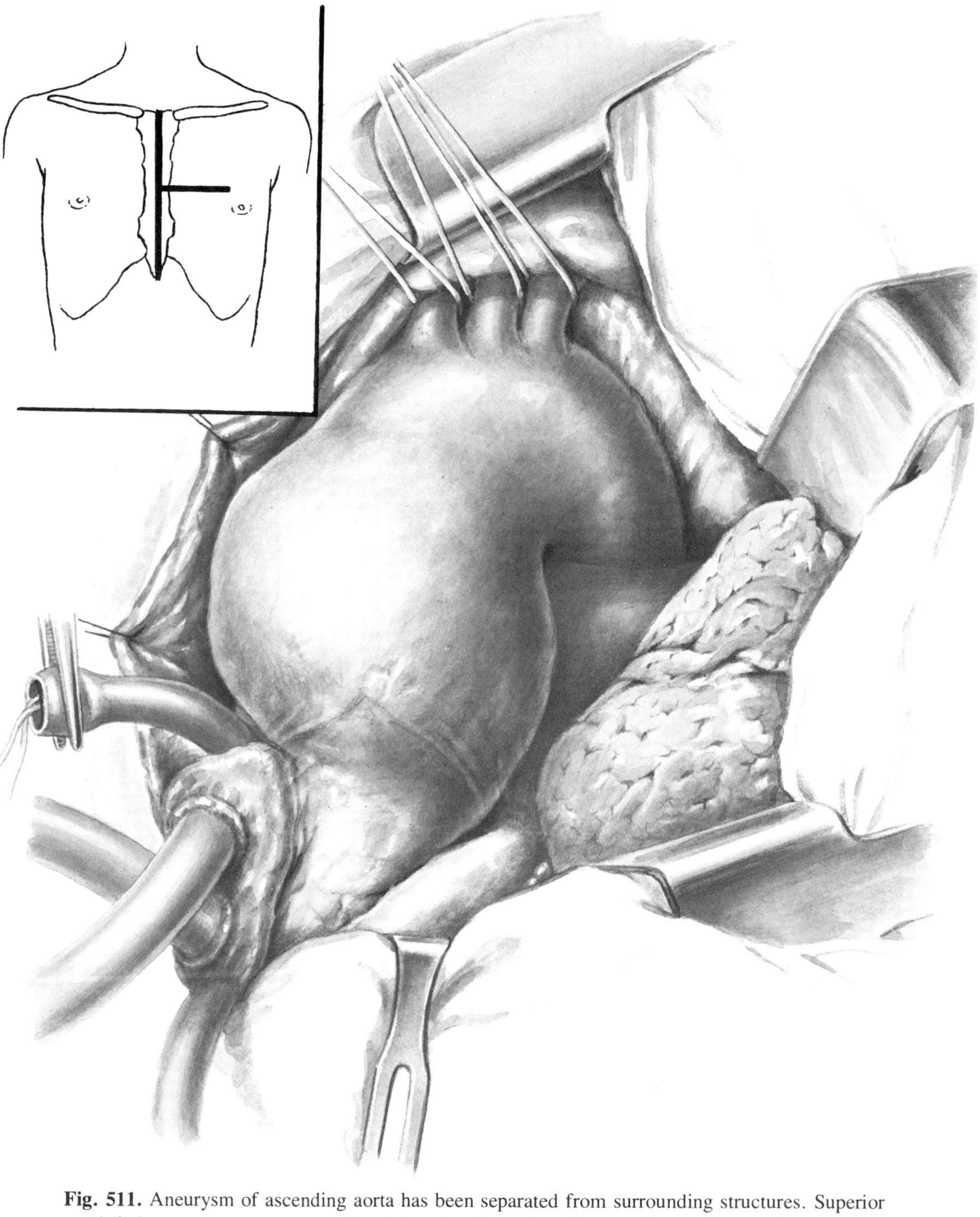

Fig. 511. Aneurysm of ascending aorta has been separated from surrounding structures. Superior and inferior venae cavae are cannulated through right atrium. *Inset;* schema of operative approach.

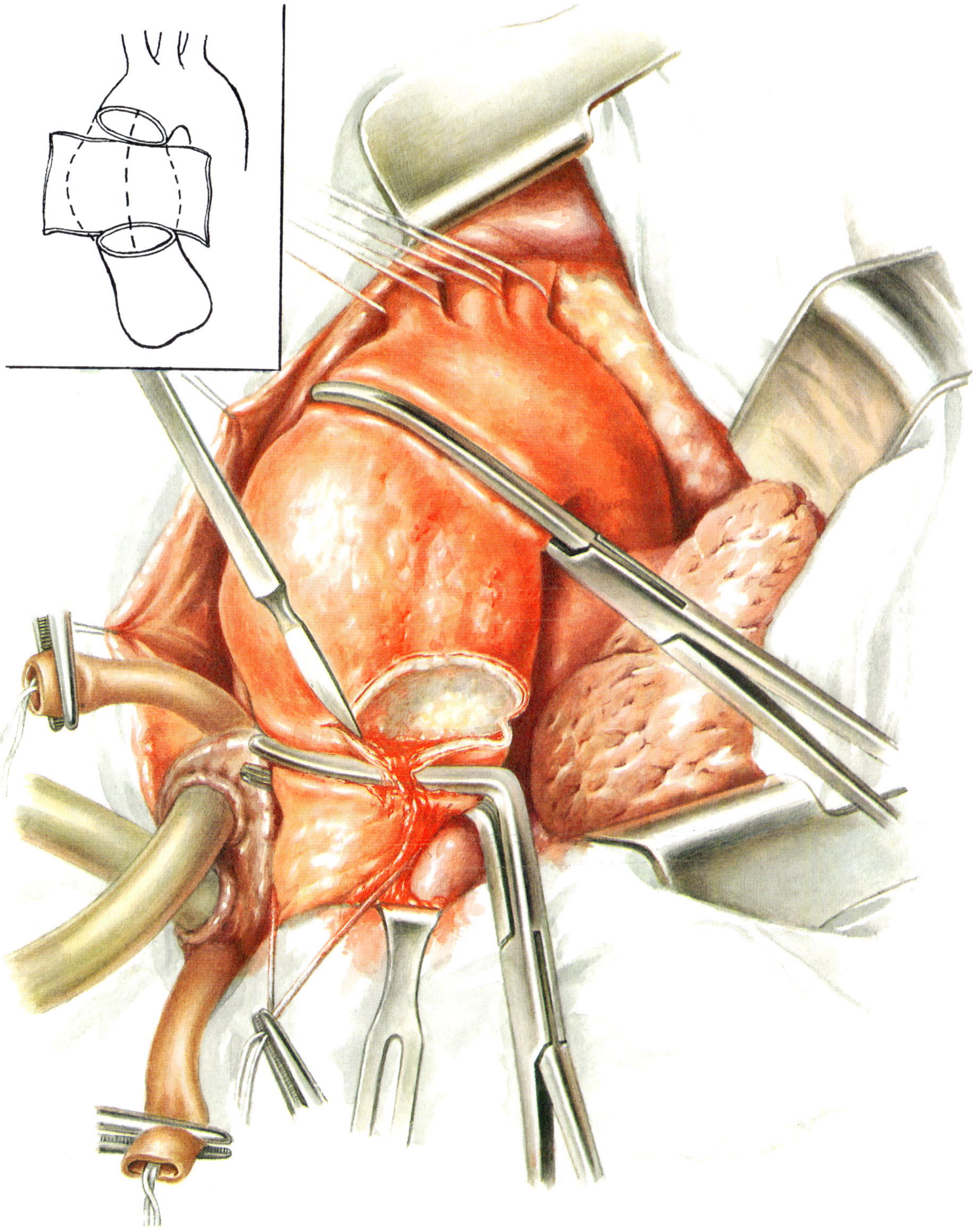

Fig. 512. Aorta is clamped proximal and distal to aneurysm. Aneurysm is cut away. *Inset;* part of posterior wall of aneurysmal sac is left in place and is used later to reinforce prosthesis.

are applied to the aorta below and above the aneurysm. The aneurysm is resected, leaving the posterior part of the wall of the aneurysmal sac (Fig. 512). Immediately after the aneurysm has been cut off from the central part of the aorta, perfusion of the coronary arteries is begun and anastomoses are formed between the aorta and the prosthesis (Figs. 513 and 514). Before the proximal anastomosis is completed, coronary perfusion is discontinued. The preserved wall of the aneurysmal sac is cleansed of thrombotic and calcified atheromatous

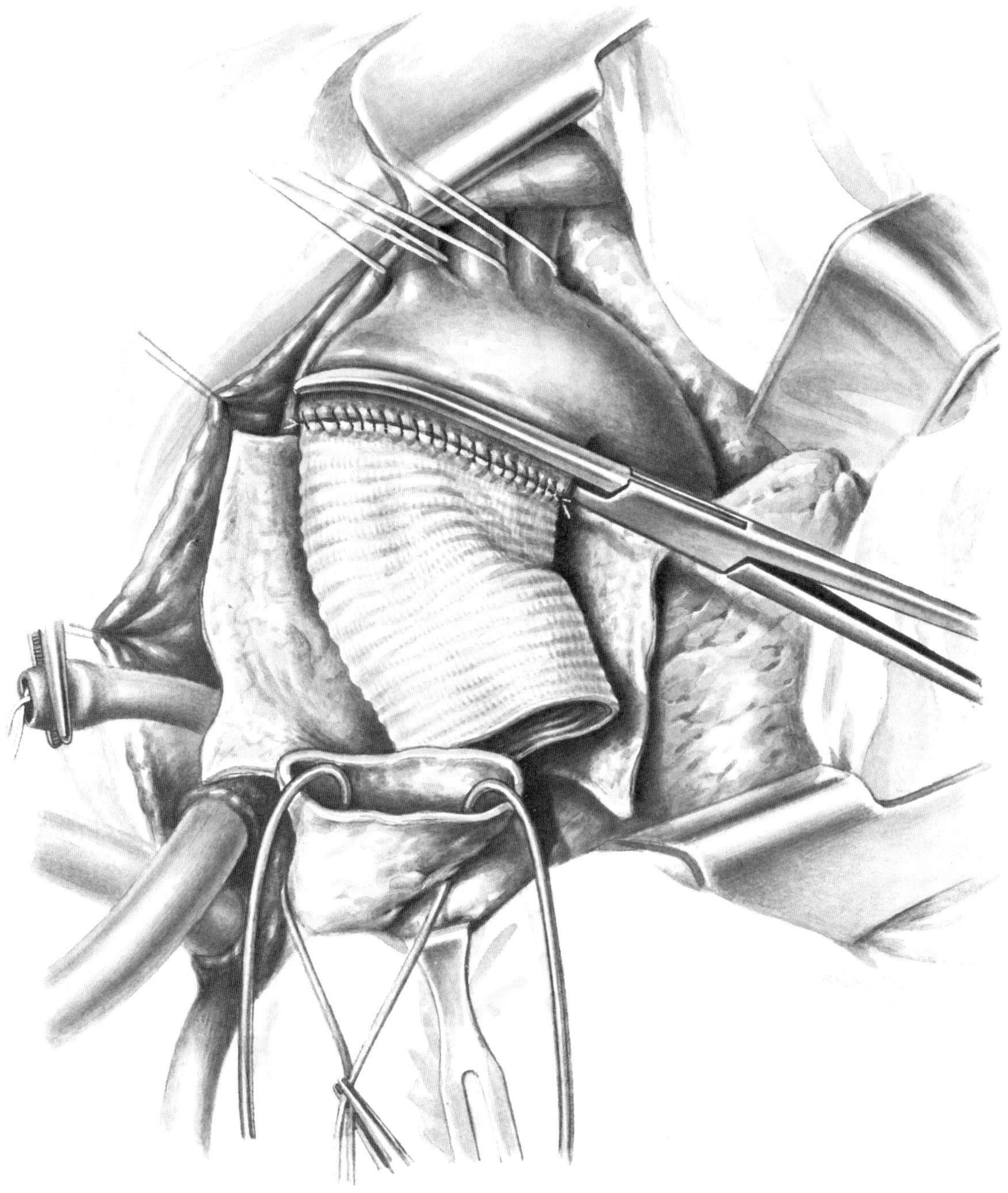

Fig. 513. Reconstruction of aorta with prosthesis. Peripheral anastomosis has been formed. Coronary perfusion is conducted.

masses with a Volkmann-type spoon. It is then used as a cuff to wrap the prosthesis, which is reinforced with additional sutures (Fig. 515).

The clamps are removed from the aorta, and the blood flow is restored. The heart-lung machine is disconnected.

Widely spaced sutures are placed on the pericardium, and drains are left in the pleural cavity and the anterior mediastinum.

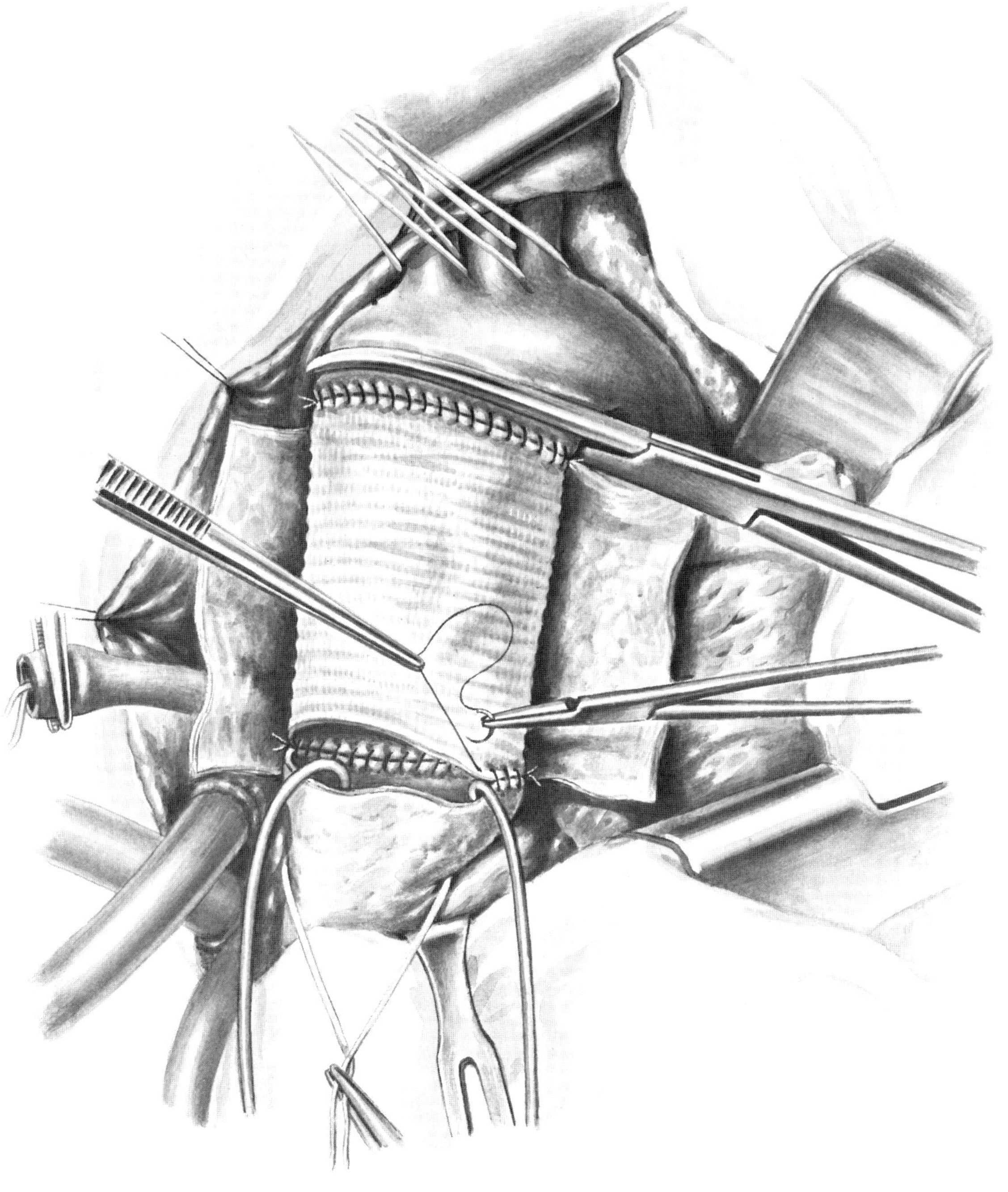

Fig. 514. Anterior wall of central anastomosis is sutured. Coronary perfusion is continued. Prosthesis is placed into remnants of aneurysmal sac.

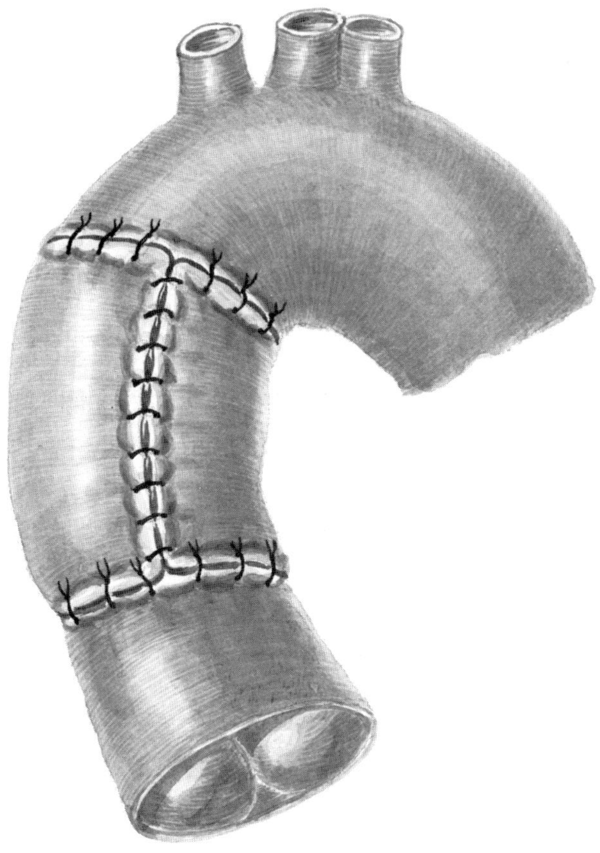

Fig. 515. View of aorta after reconstruction with prosthesis. Prosthesis is wrapped in remnants of aneurysmal sac. (Schema.)

PROSTHETIC REPLACEMENT OF DESCENDING PART OF AORTIC ARCH

An operation for aneurysm of the descending part of the aortic arch is conducted by left lateral approach in the fourth intercostal space under conditions of extracorporeal circulation.

The left lung is moved caudally and ventrally, exposing the posterior mediastinum and the arch of the aorta. The mediastinal pleura is opened wide (Fig. 516). The part of the aorta central to the aneurysm is first mobilized and held with a loop; then the part caudal to the aneurysm is mobilized, and a loop is also brought under it. The left subclavian artery is quite often involved in the aneurysm, so it is likewise held with a loop (Fig. 517).

The heart-lung machine is connected. The venous cannula is introduced into the auricle of the left atrium; the arterial cannula into the femoral artery.

The aorta is clamped proximal and distal to the aneu-

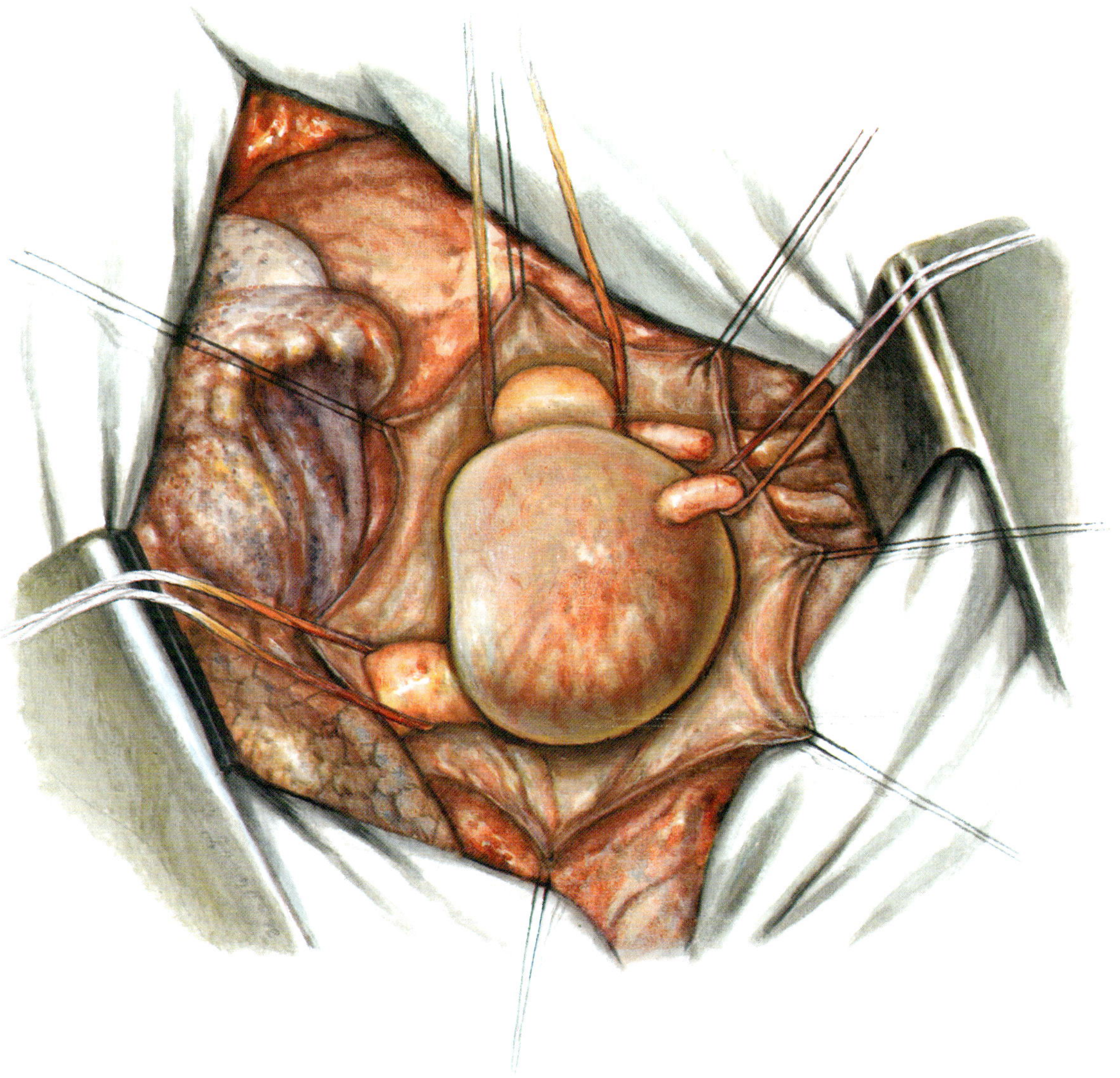

Fig. 516. View of aneurysm of descending part of aortic arch.

rysm, and a clamp is applied to the left subclavian artery. The wall of the aneurysm is cut lengthwise, and the thrombotic masses are removed.

The cavity of the aneurysm is inspected, and the aneurysm is then cut away from the aorta together with the healthy parts of the vessel (Fig. 518). Whenever necessary, the subclavian artery is also resected.

The resected part of the aorta is replaced with a plastic prosthesis. The central anastomosis is formed first by applying a continuous Halsted suture to the dorsal wall. When the entire dorsal semicircumference of the aorta and prosthesis has been stitched through, the suture is tightened and its ends are tied with applied lateral interrupted sutures. Then the ventral wall of the aorta and the prosthesis are stitched with a continuous Halsted or blanket suture, with each stitch tightened. The proximal end of the subclavian artery is stitched into the wall of the prosthesis (Fig. 519). First the caudal and then the cranial clamps are taken off the aorta. Extracorporeal circulation is discontinued.

The plastic prosthesis is wrapped with the coats of the resected aneurysm, which are stitched with a continuous suture (Figs. 520 and 521).

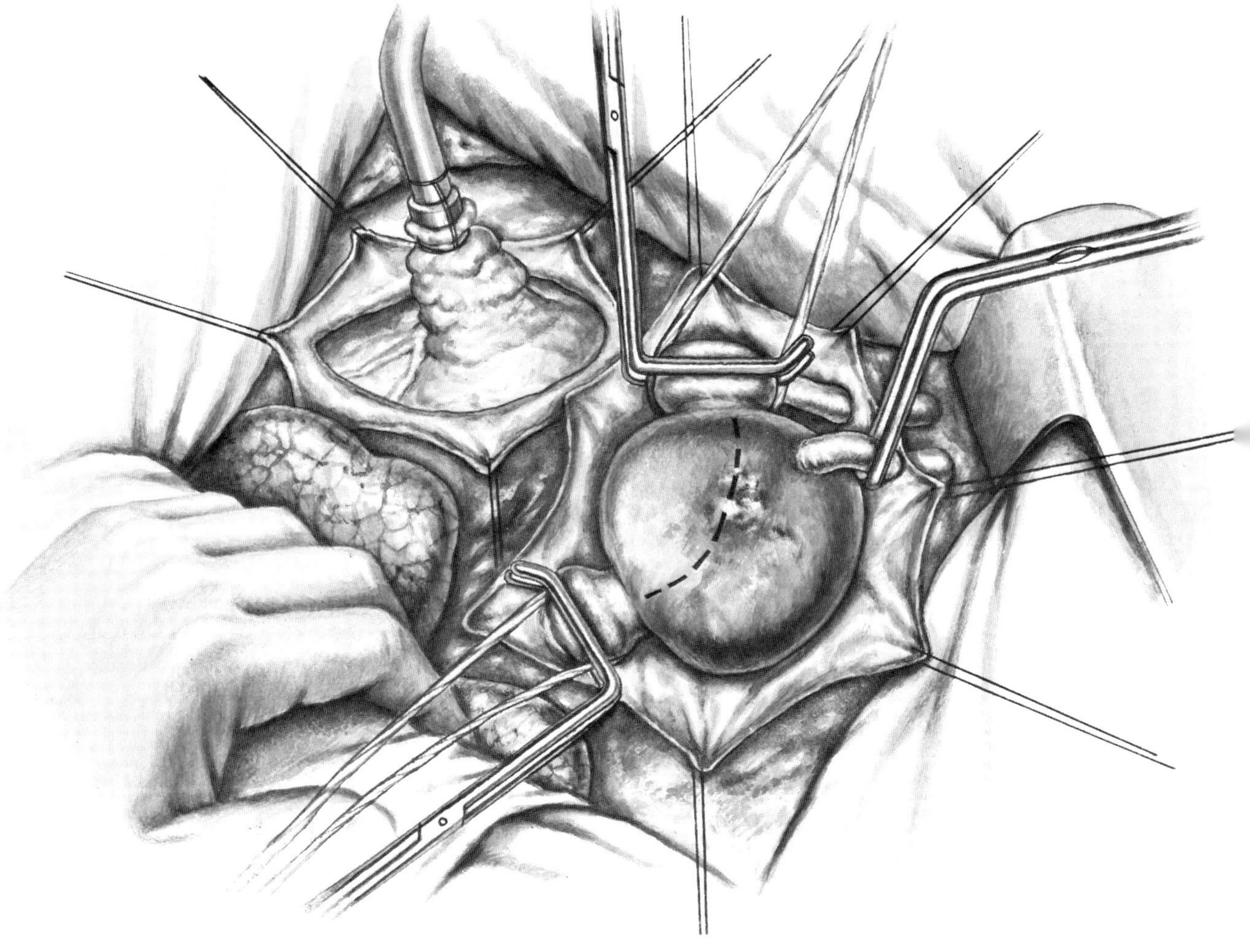

Fig. 517. Aneurysm is freed from surrounding structures, and aorta is clamped above and below it.

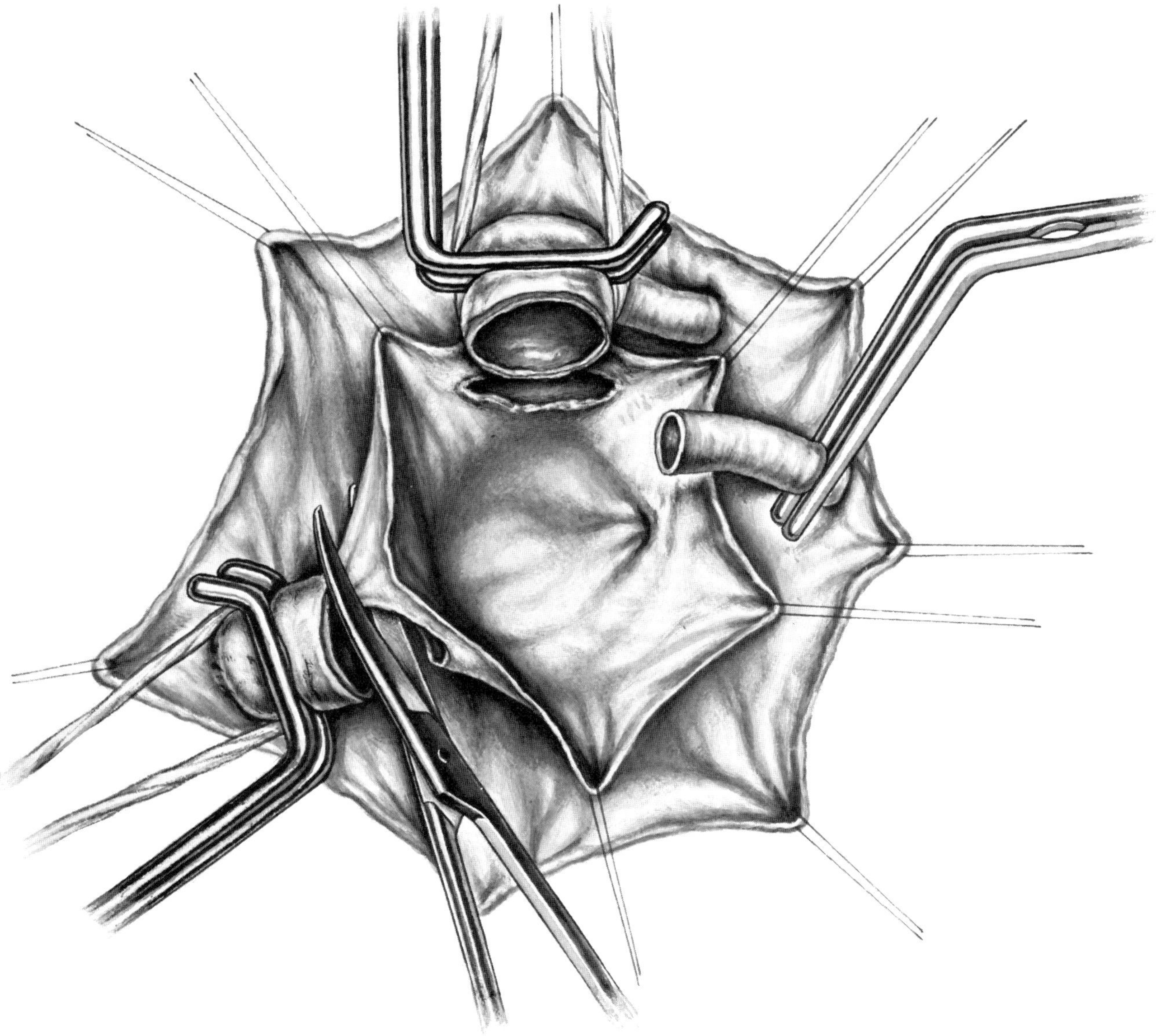

Fig. 518. Aneurysm is resected from aorta.

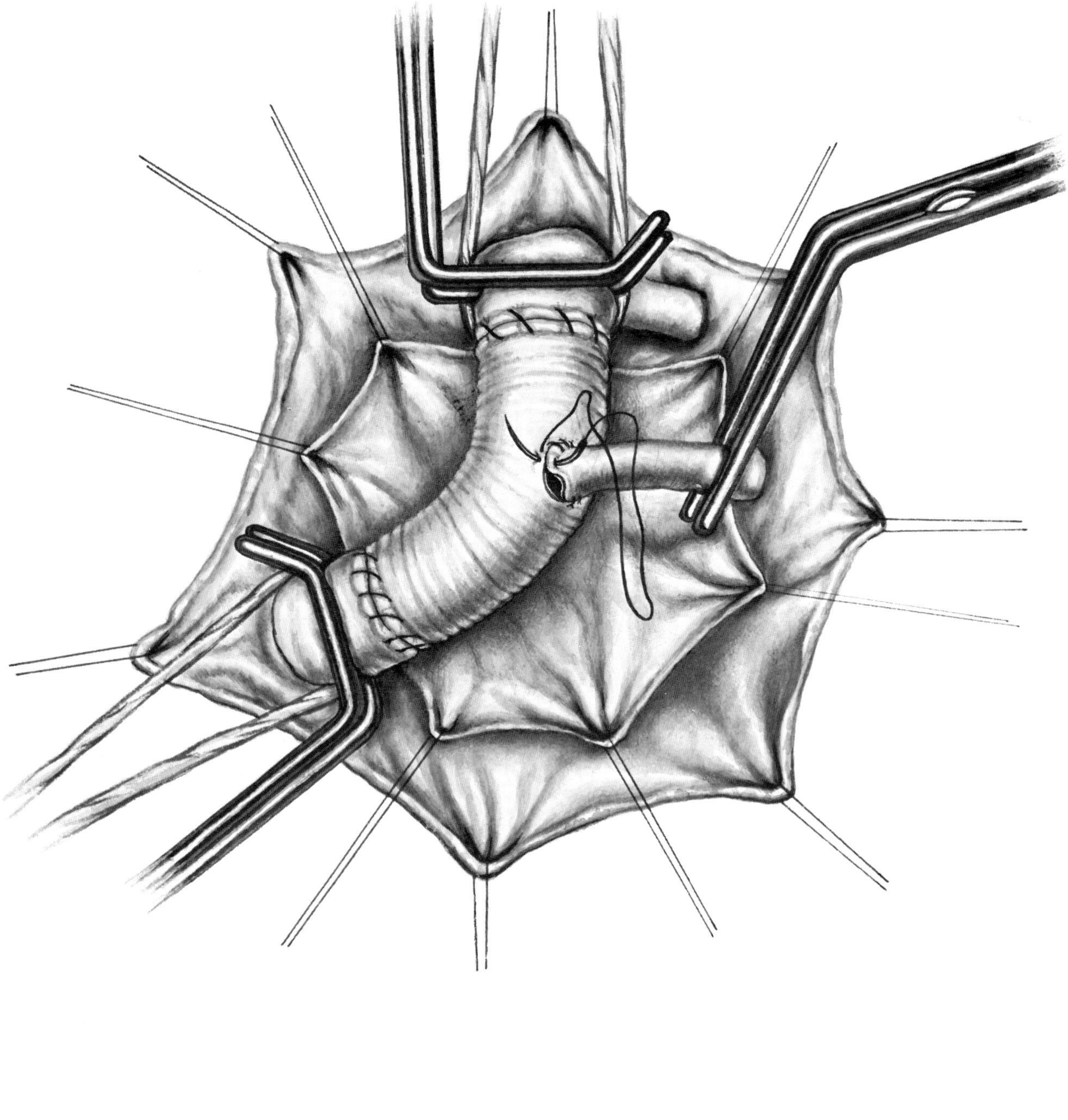

Fig. 519. Defect in descending aorta is repaired with prosthesis. Subclavian artery is anastomosed with prosthesis.

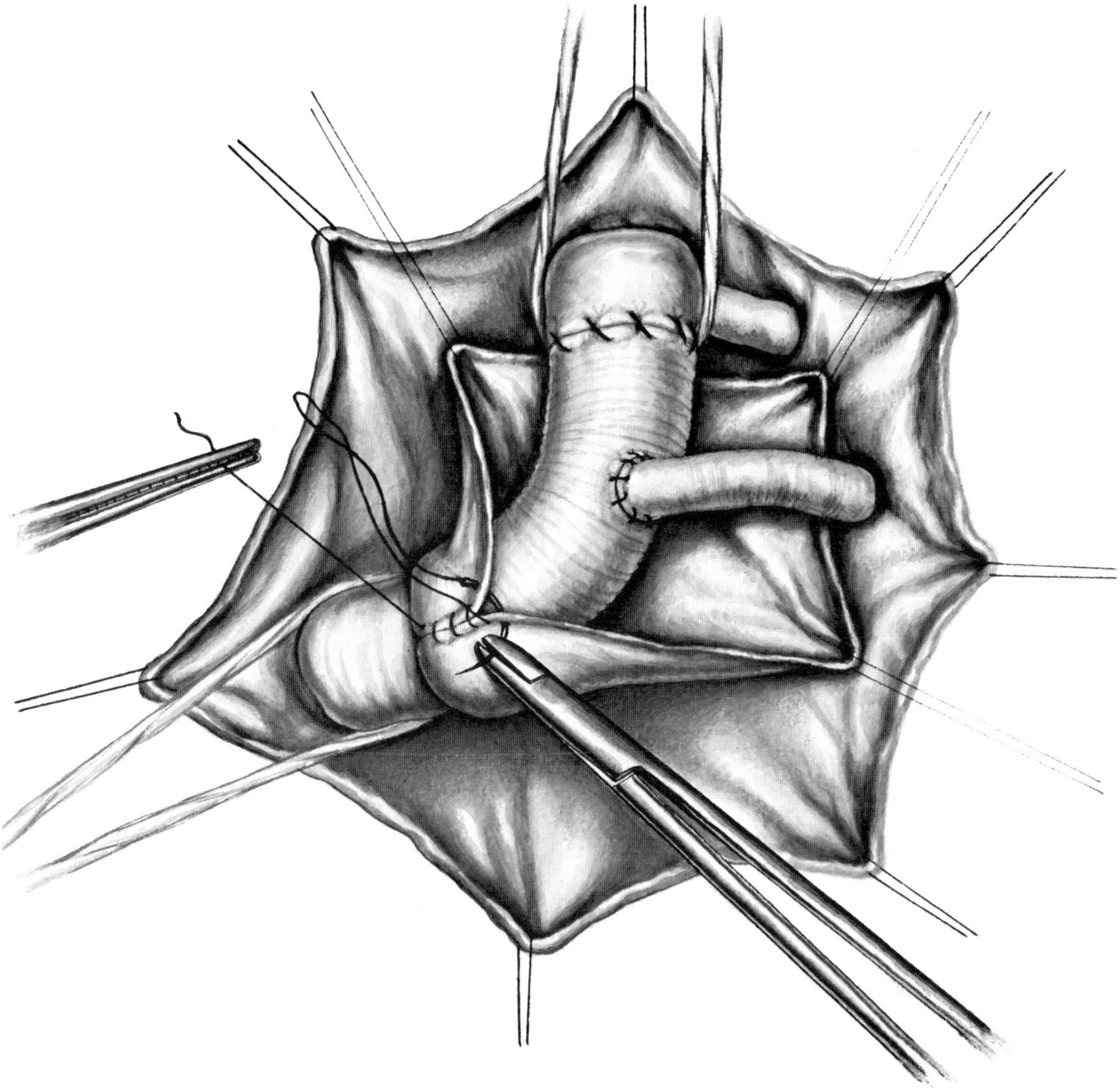

Fig. 520. Plastic prosthesis is wrapped in aneurysmal coats.

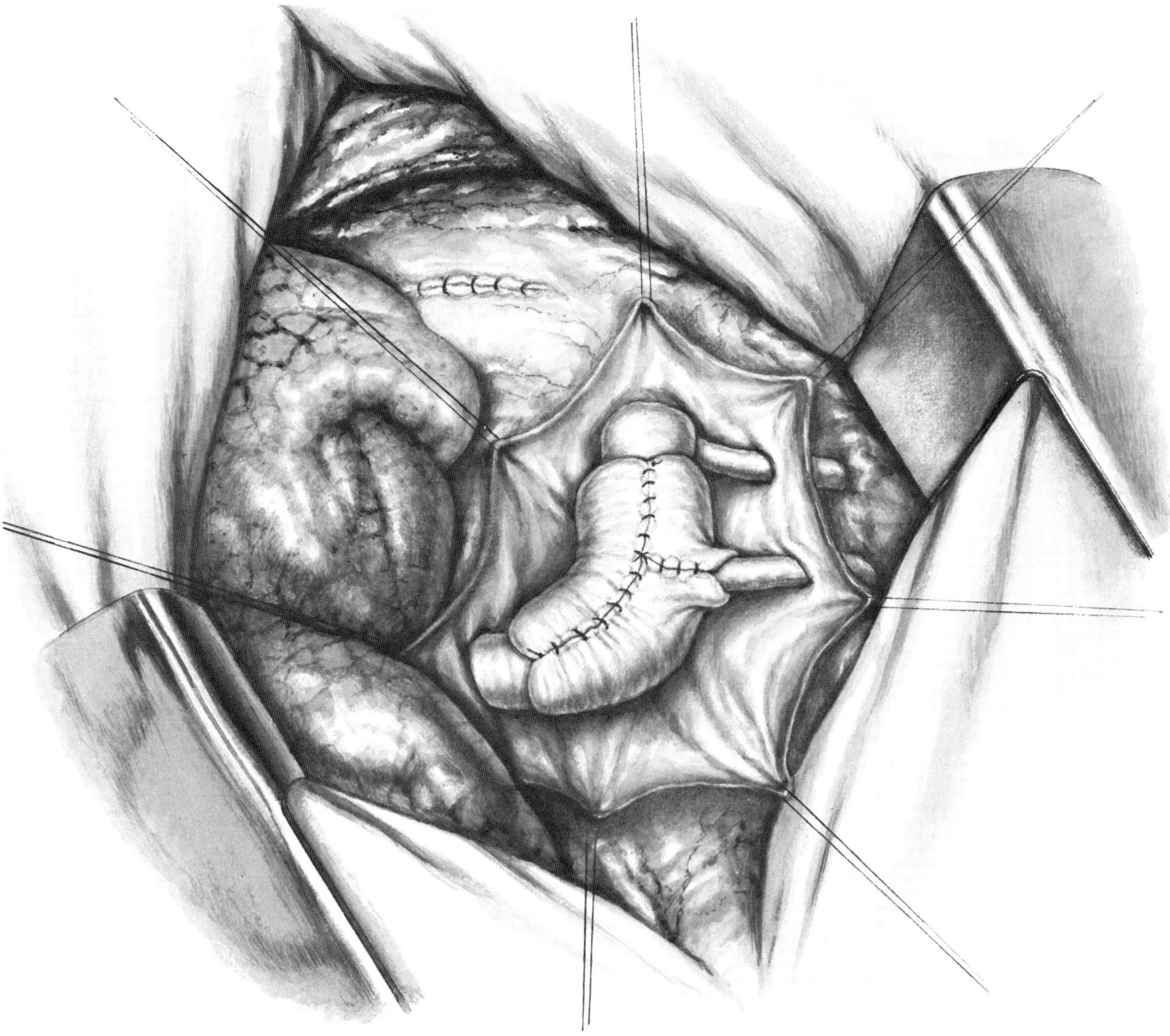

Fig. 521. View of aorta after prosthetic replacement.

RESECTION OF ANEURYSM OF DESCENDING AORTA AND ITS PROSTHETIC REPLACEMENT WITHOUT EXTRACORPOREAL CIRCULATION

Longitudinal median sternotomy and anterolateral thoracotomy in the left fifth intercostal space are carried out. The left lung is pulled medially and caudally. The descending aorta is separated, and the overlying pleura and adventitia are cut; care must be taken not to injure the vagus nerve (Fig. 522). A clamp is placed along the

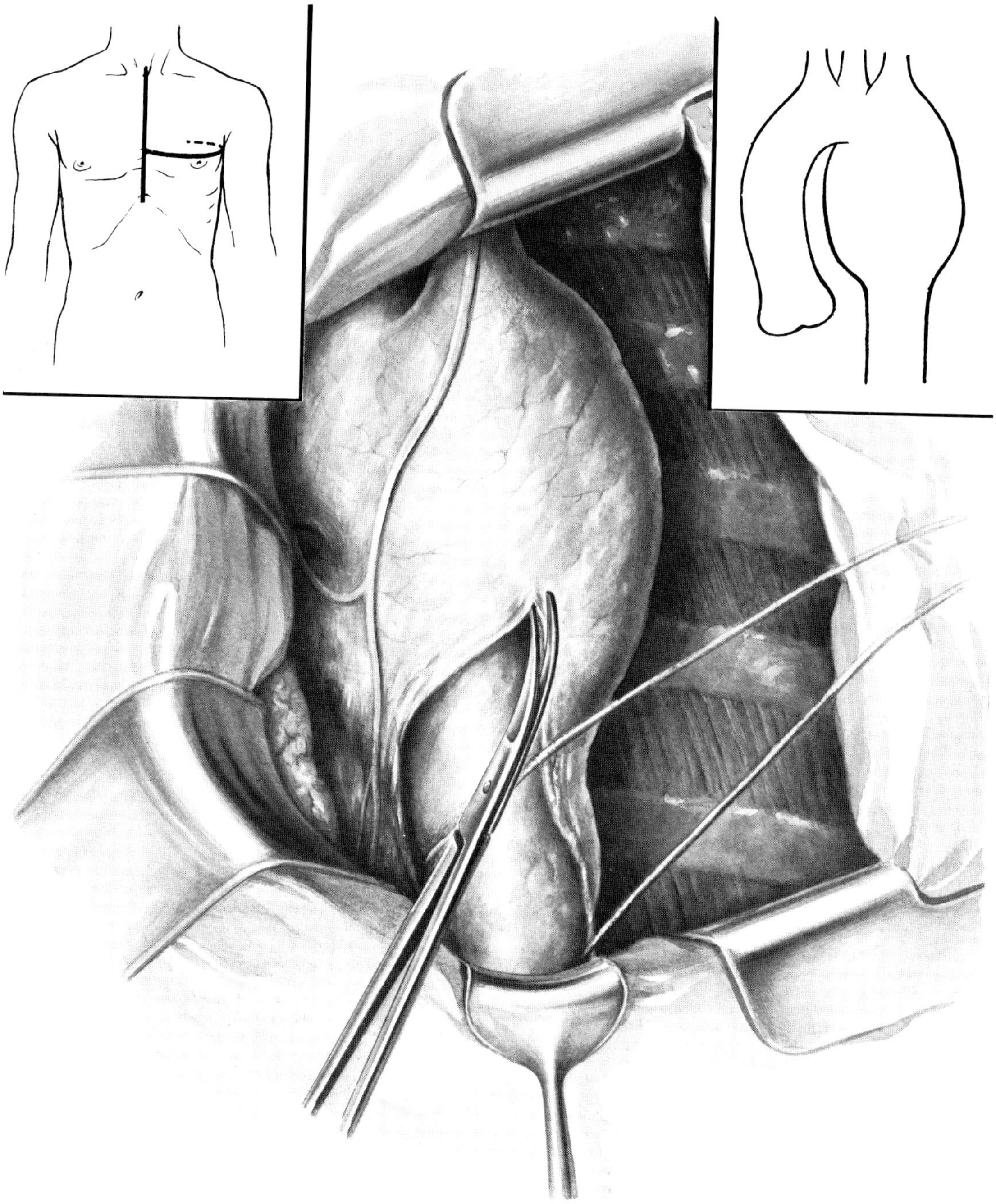

Fig. 522. Left lung is pulled medially and caudally. Parietal pleura is cut over descending aorta caudally to aneurysm. *Right inset,* schema of operative approach. *Left, inset,* schema of aneurysm of descending aorta.

anterior wall of the descending aorta; a longitudinal cut is made in the wall; and an end-to-side anastomosis is formed between the synthetic prosthesis and the aorta with a continuous vascular suture (Fig. 523). Another prosthesis of smaller diameter is stitched beforehand into the side of the prosthesis, which will be used as a temporary shunt between the ascending and descending aorta during resection of the aneurysm and will ensure the supply of blood to the abdominal organs and the kidneys.

When this stage of the operation has been concluded, the ascending aorta is mobilized, a clamp is applied

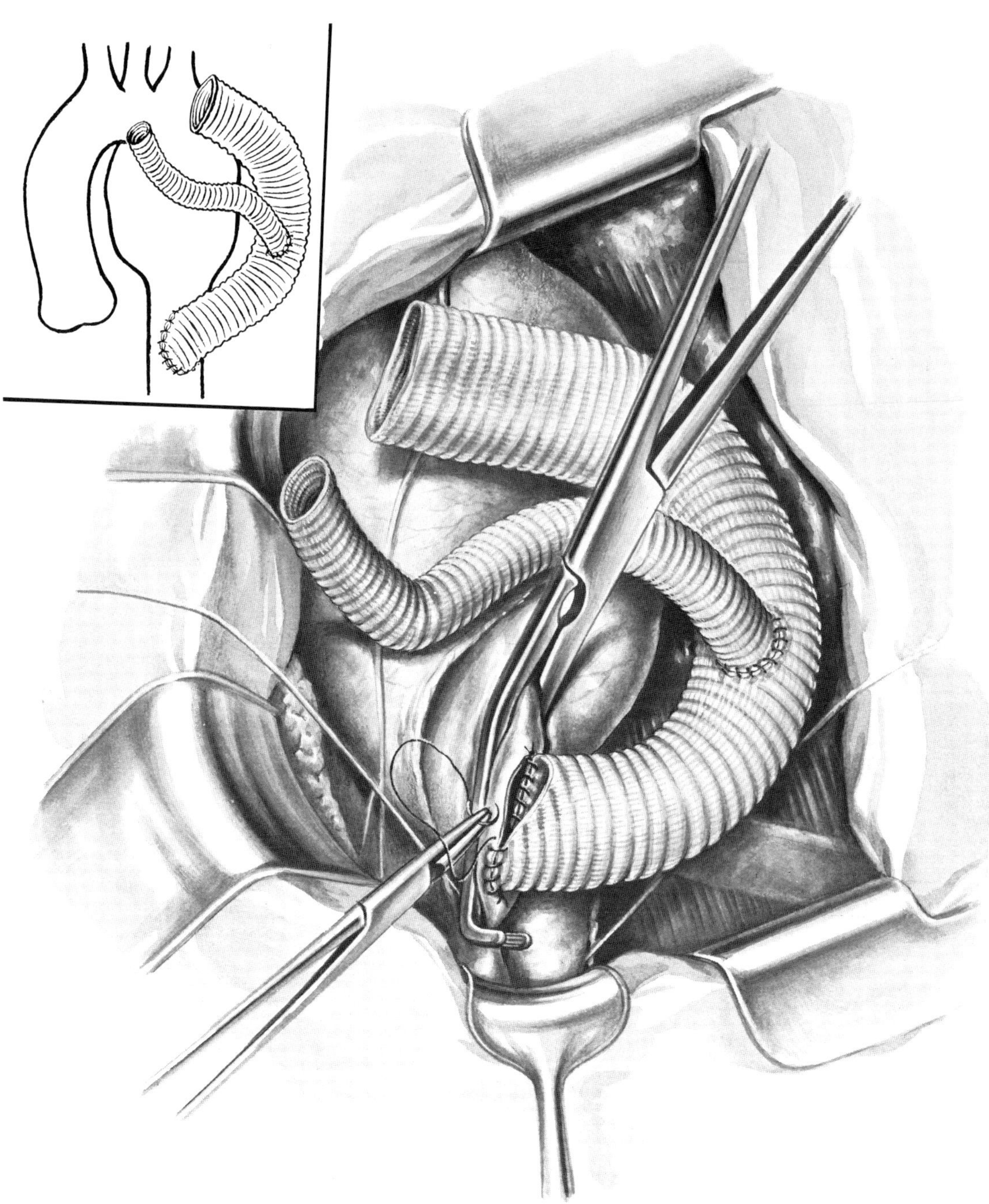

Fig. 523. Clamp is applied along wall of descending aorta caudally to aneurysm, and end-to-side anastomosis is formed between synthetic prosthesis and aorta. For shunting aorta, antoher prosthesis of smaller diameter is stitched into side of first prosthesis beforehand. *Inset,* schema of this stage of operation.

along its anterior wall, and a cut is made in it. A temporary end-to-side anastomosis is formed between the shunt-prosthesis and the ascending aorta (Fig. 524). Clamps are applied to the aorta below and above the aneurysm. The left subclavian artery and the prosthesis above the shunt stitched into it are also clamped (Fig. 525). The blood flow in the descending and abdominal aorta is restored by way of the shunt, and the aneurysmal sac is resected. Its dorsal wall is left in place for the subsequent reinforcement of the prosthesis. Orifices of arteries arising in this region are stitched through from within the aneurysmal sac. The distal stump of the tran-

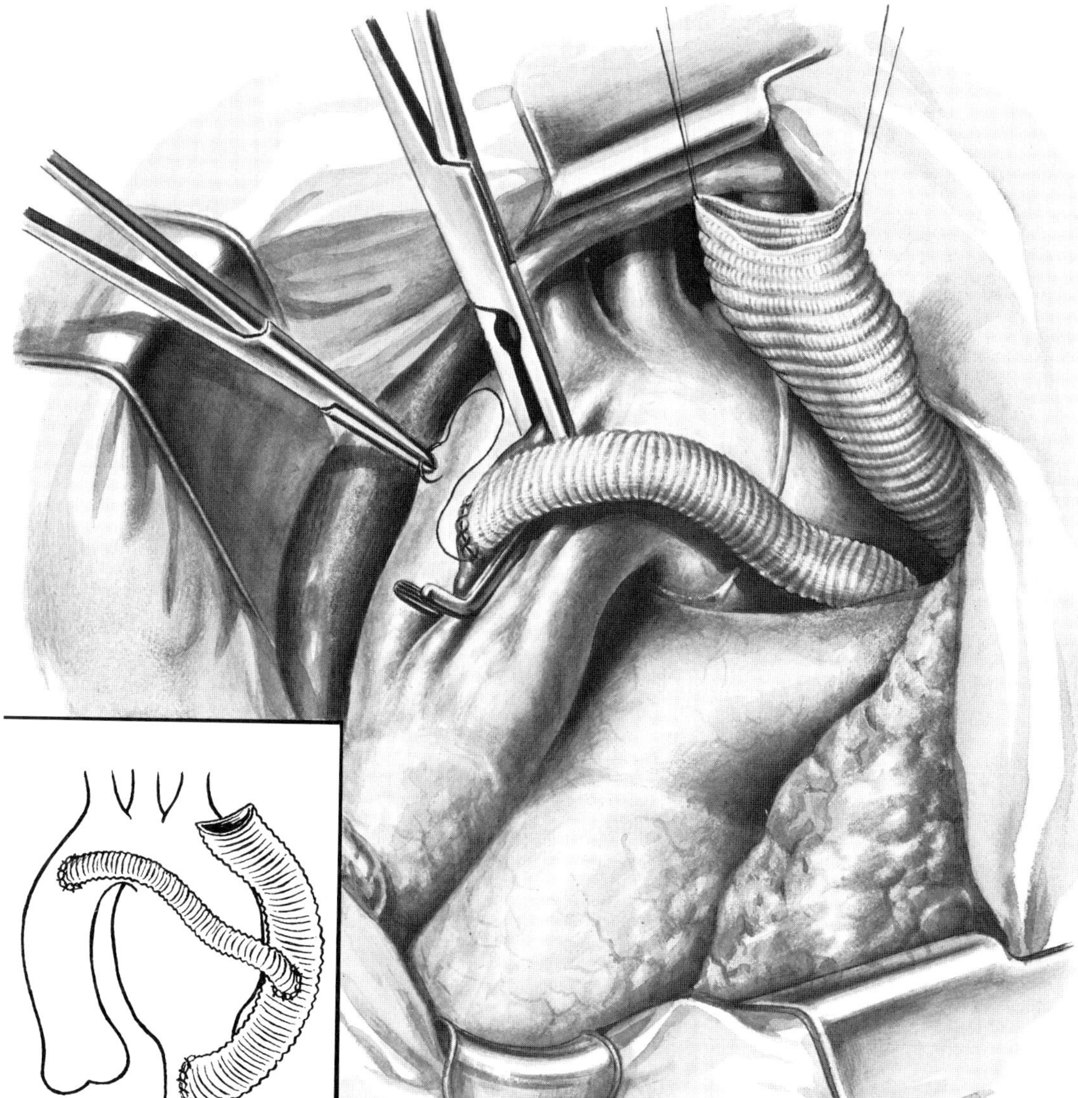

Fig. 524. Clamp is applied along side of ascending aorta, and end-to-side anastomosis is formed between shunt-prosthesis and aorta. *Inset,* schema of temporary shunt.

sected aorta is closed with continuous blanket and Halsted sutures. The proximal anastomosis between the prosthesis and the aorta is formed by the end-to-end techniques with a continuous suture (Fig. 526). The ascending aorta is then clamped along its wall, where it is connected with a temporary shunt; the clamps are removed from the prosthesis of the proximal part of the descending aorta, and blood flow is restored in it (Fig. 527). The shunt prosthesis is disconnected from the ascending aorta, and the defect in its wall is repaired with a continuous suture. The excess part of the shunt prosthesis is cut away, and its proximal end is anastomosed to the

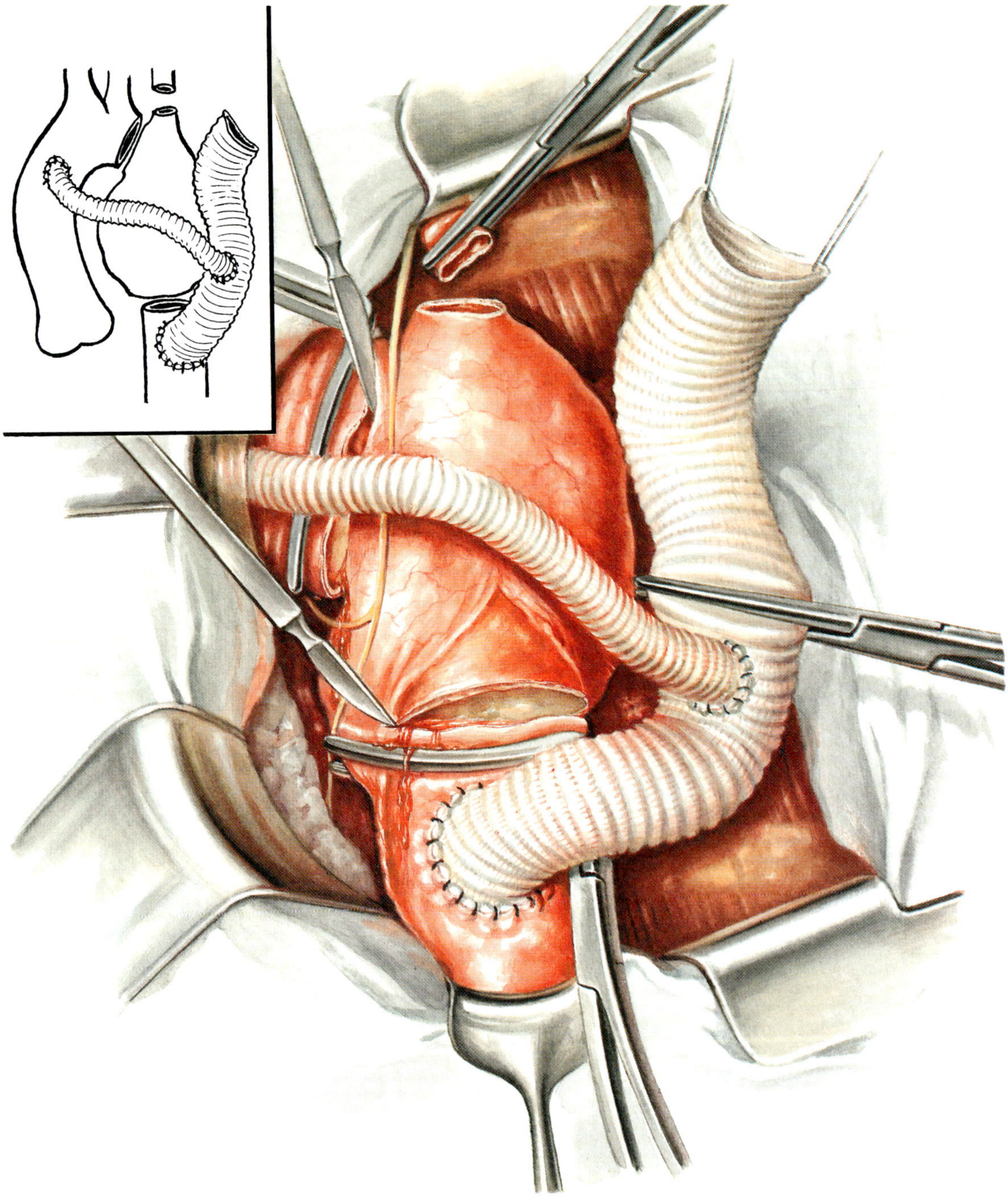

Fig. 525. Aorta is clamped proximal and distal to aneurysm. Clamps are applied to left subclavian artery and to vessel prosthesis proximal to shunt. Blood flow in descending aorta is restored through shunt. Aneurysm is resected. *Inset,* schema of resection of aneurysm and shunting of descending aorta.

end of the left subclavian artery. The clamp is removed from this artery, and the blood flow is restored in it (Fig. 528). To reinforce it, the prosthesis is wrapped as in a cuff with the preserved posterior wall of the aneurysmal sac, the edges of which are stitched with interrupted sutures (Fig. 529).

Hemostasis is carefully performed. Drains are left in the pleural cavity and the anterior mediastinum. The wound is sutured layer by layer in line with the intercostal space. The edges of the transected sternum are drawn together with four wire sutures. Sutures are then applied to the periosteum, the soft tissues, and the skin.

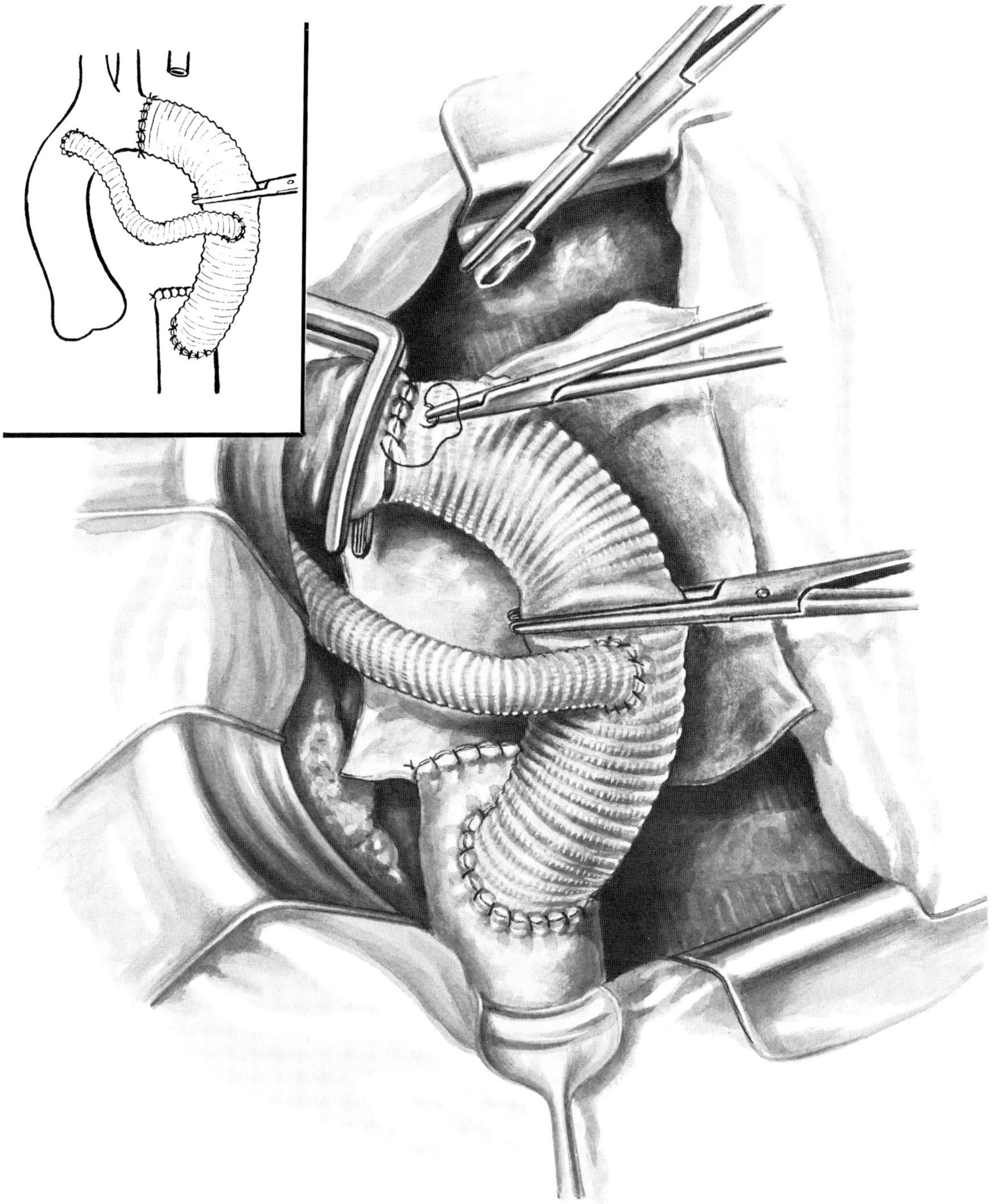

Fig. 526. Distal stump of descending aorta is closed with blanket suture. Proximal anastomosis between aorta and prosthesis is formed by end-to-end technique. Posterior wall of aneurysmal sac has been preserved. *Inset,* schema of prosthetic reconstruction of descending aorta.

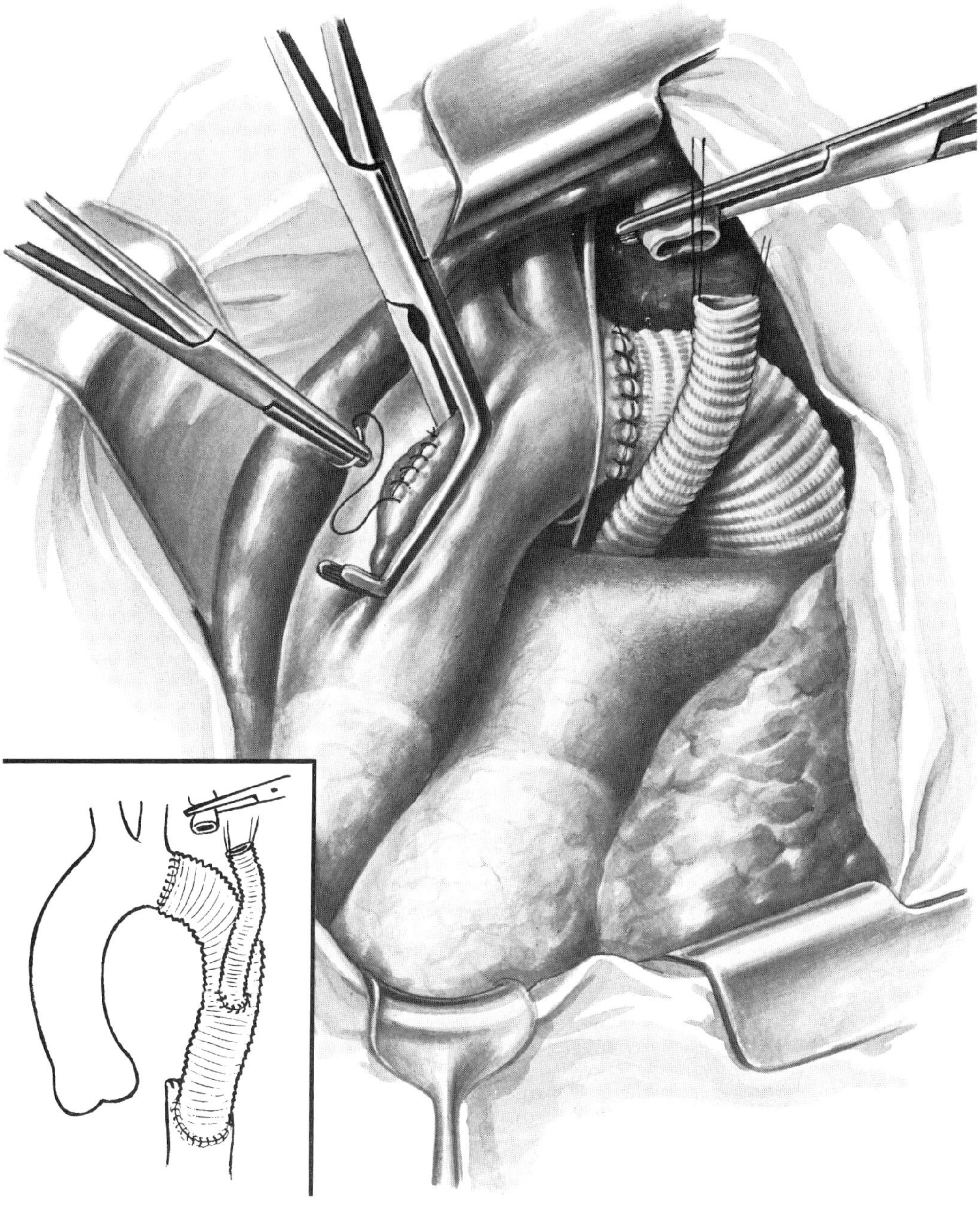

Fig. 527. Shunt-prosthesis is disconnected from ascending aorta. Defect in aortic wall is corrected by continuous vascular suture. Shunt-prosthesis is brought to transected and clamped left subclavian artery. *Inset,* schema of prosthesis of descending aorta with restoration of blood flow in it.

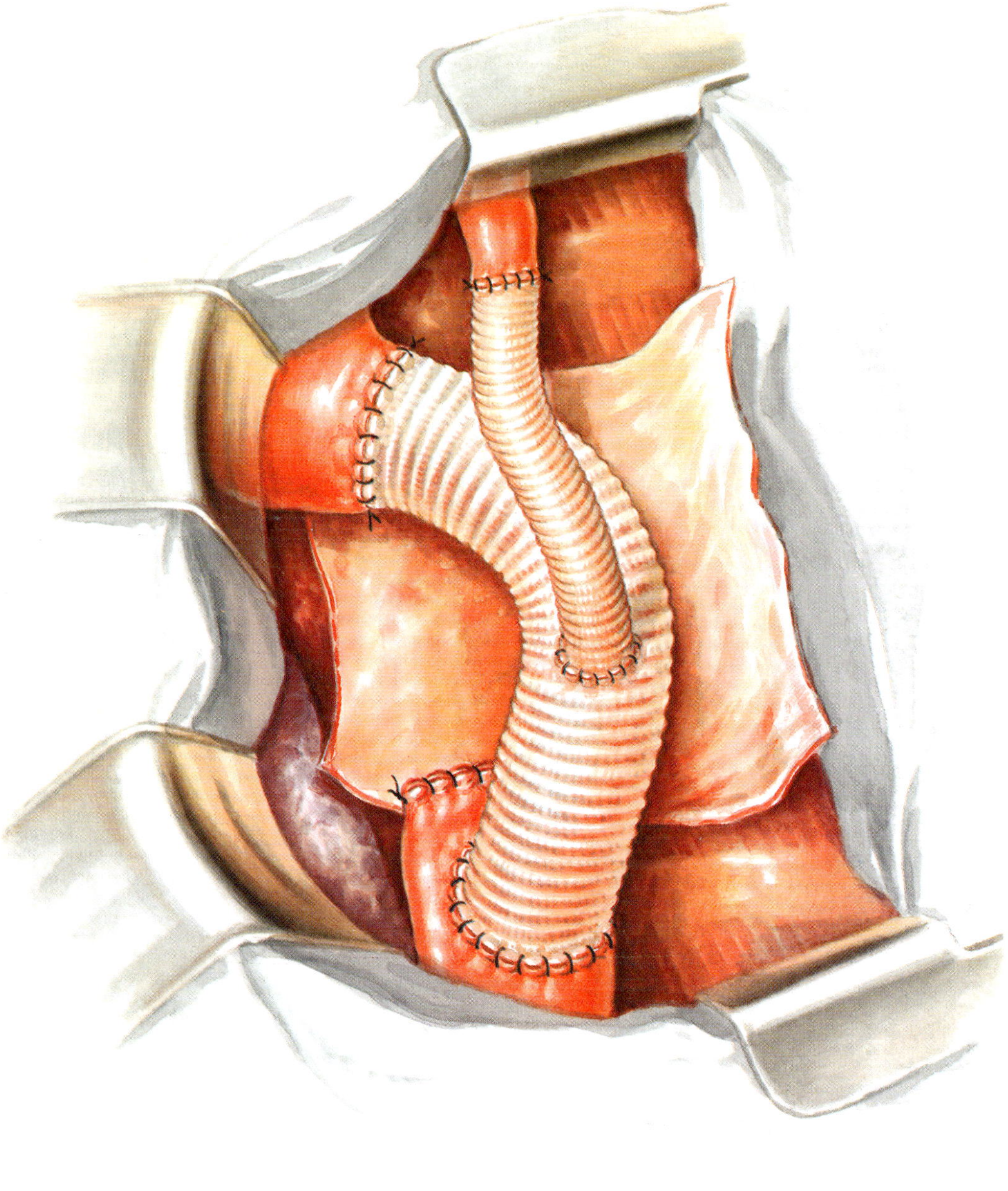

Fig. 528. Subclavian artery reconstructed with prosthesis. Posterior wall of aneurysmal sac is visible.

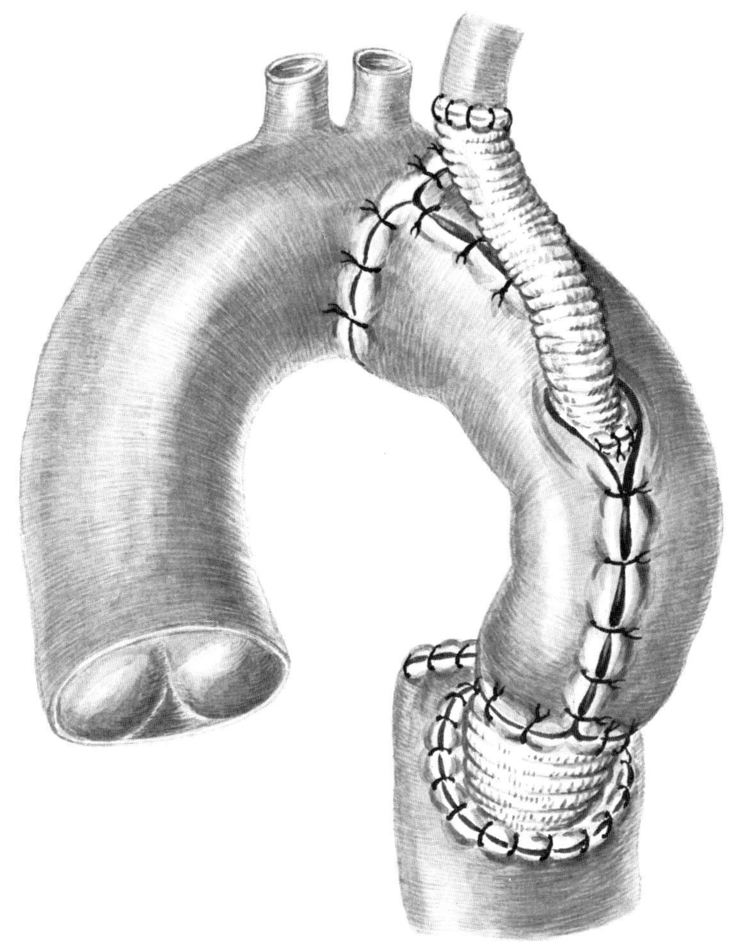

Fig. 529. Schema of descending aorta reconstructed with prosthesis, which is wrapped in posterior wall of aneurysmal sac.

RESECTION OF ANEURYSM OF DESCENDING AORTA AND ITS REPAIR WITH PROSTHESIS IN CONDITIONS OF EXTRACORPOREAL CIRCULATION

Median sternotomy and anterolateral thoracotomy in the left fifth intercostal space are conducted. The pleural cavity and the pericardium are opened. The superior and inferior venae cavae are cannulated through the auricle and the wall of the right atrium and then through the femoral artery. The left lung is pulled medially and caudally, and the descending aorta with the aneurysm is exposed and mobilized. Loops are brought under the aorta,

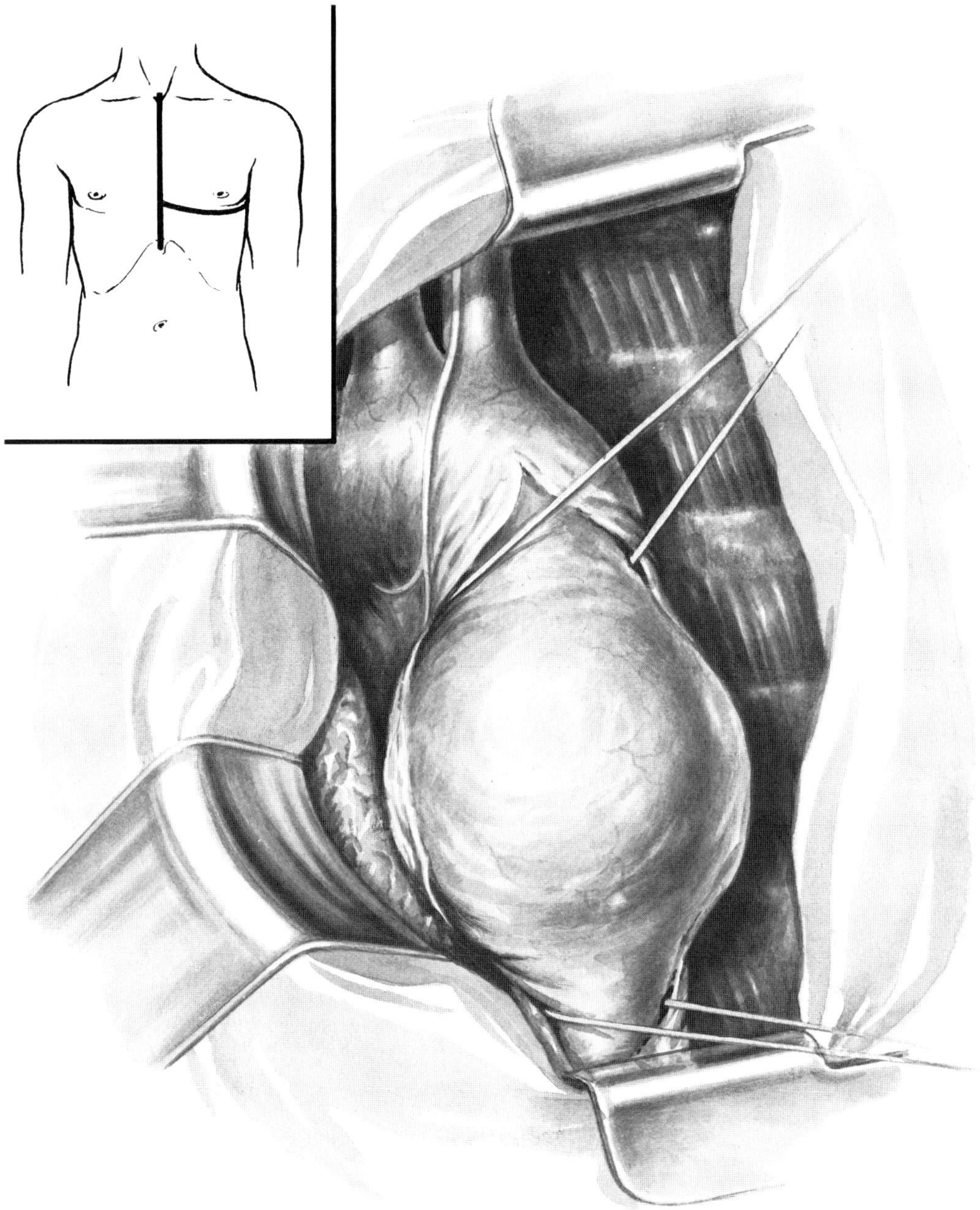

Fig. 530. Left lung is pulled away medially and caudally. Descending aorta with aneurysm has been separated from surrounding structures. Parietal pleura has been cut and aorta raised by loops. *Inset,* schema of operative approach.

which is then raised by them. The parietal pleura and the adventitia overlying the aorta and aneurysm are cut lengthwise (Fig. 530). The heart-lung machine is connected, and the aorta is clamped above and below the aneurysm (Fig. 531). The aneurysm is cut lengthwise and excised except for its posterior wall. The orifices of arteries arising from the descending aorta are sutured from within the aneurysmal sac, after which distal and proximal end-to-end anastomoses are formed between the prosthesis and the ends of the transected aorta (Fig. 532). After the aortic prosthesis has been sutured in place, the heart-lung machine is disconnected, the car-

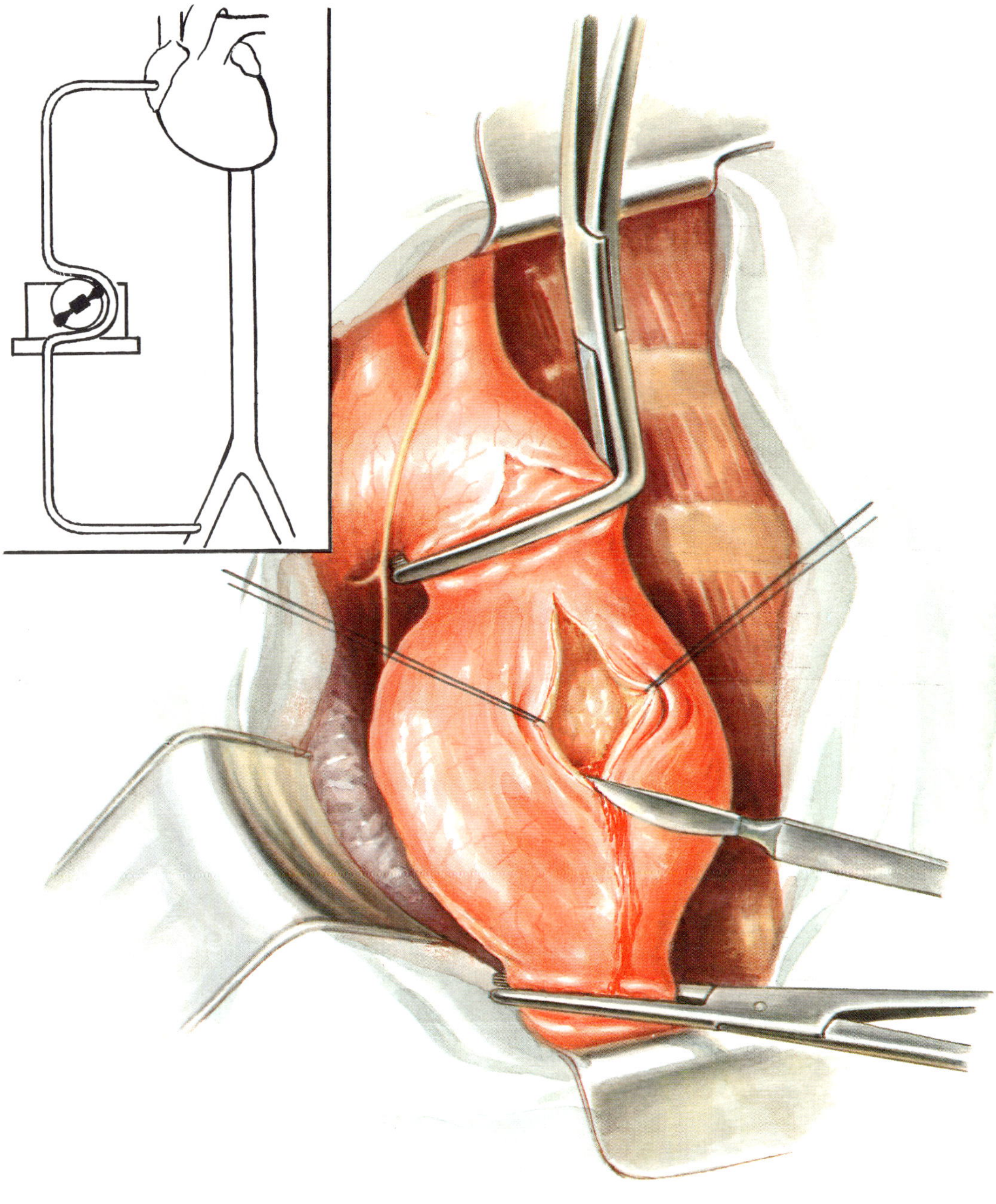

Fig. 531. Extracorporeal circulation is begun *(inset)*. Aorta is clamped above and below aneurysm. Aneurysmal sac is cut lengthwise.

diac sinus rhythm is restored, the clamps are removed from the aorta, and the blood flow is restored in it (Fig. 533).

The prosthesis is wrapped in the posterior wall of the aneurysmal sac as in a cuff, the edges of which are stitched with interrupted sutures over the prosthesis (Fig. 534).

Hemostasis is carefully verified. Drains are introduced into the pleural cavity and the mediastinum. The wound in the thoracic wall is sutured layer by layer. The edges of the transected sternum are drawn together with four wire sutures. Sutures are applied to the periosteum, the soft tissues, and the skin.

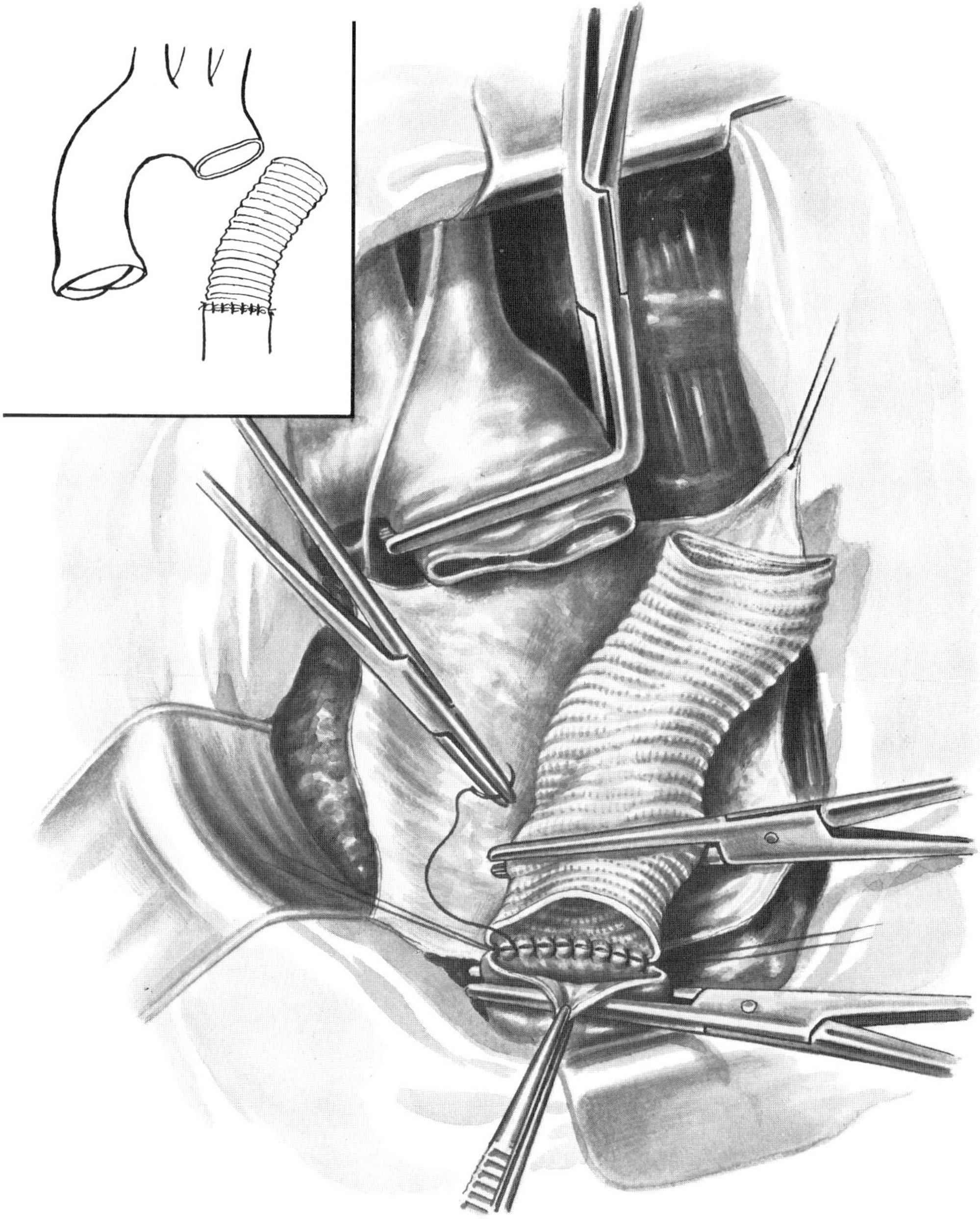

Fig. 532. Prosthetics of descending aorta after resection of aneurysmal sac. Posterior wall of sac is left in place. End-to-end anastomosis of synthetic prosthesis and aorta is formed. *Inset,* schema of completed distal anastomosis.

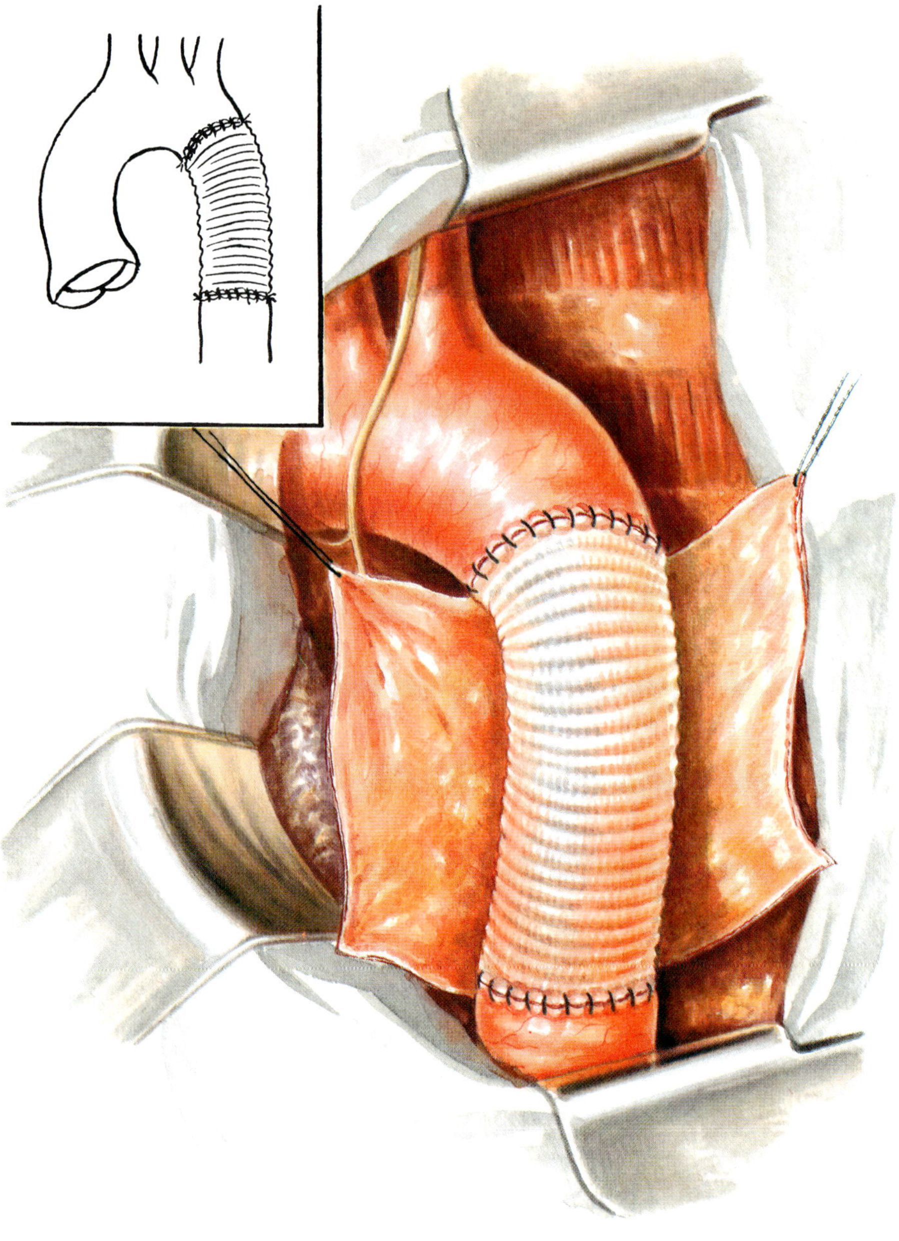

Fig. 533. Prosthetic reconstruction of descending aorta is completed. Flow of blood in aorta is restored. Posterior wall of aneurysmal sac is prepared for reinforcing prosthesis.

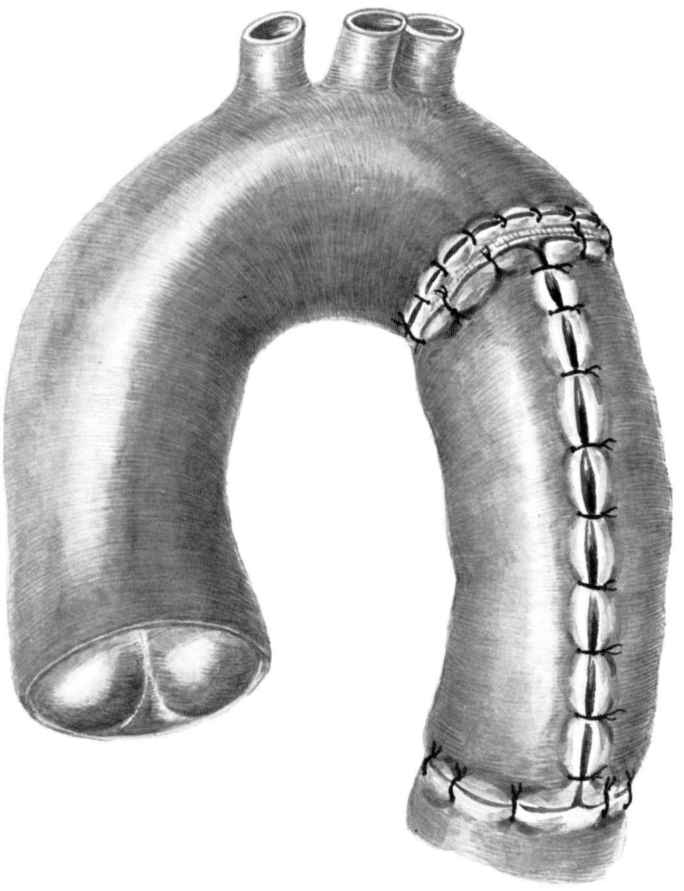

Fig. 534. Schema of descending aorta with applied prosthesis, which is wrapped in posterior wall of aneurysmal sac.

SHUNTING OF ANEURYSM OF AORTIC ARCH IN CONDITIONS OF EXTRACORPOREAL CIRCULATION AND CRANIOCEREBRAL HYPOTHERMIA

Transverse transbipleural throracotomy is carried out in the fourth intercostal space with transection of the sternum. The ascending and descending parts of the aorta and its brachiocephalic branches are separated from the surrounding tissues (Fig. 535). The left lung is alternately moved from right to left during this manipulation. The aneurysm of the aortic arch itself need not be mobilized in the operative method being described Fig. 536).

After the descending part of the thoracic aorta has

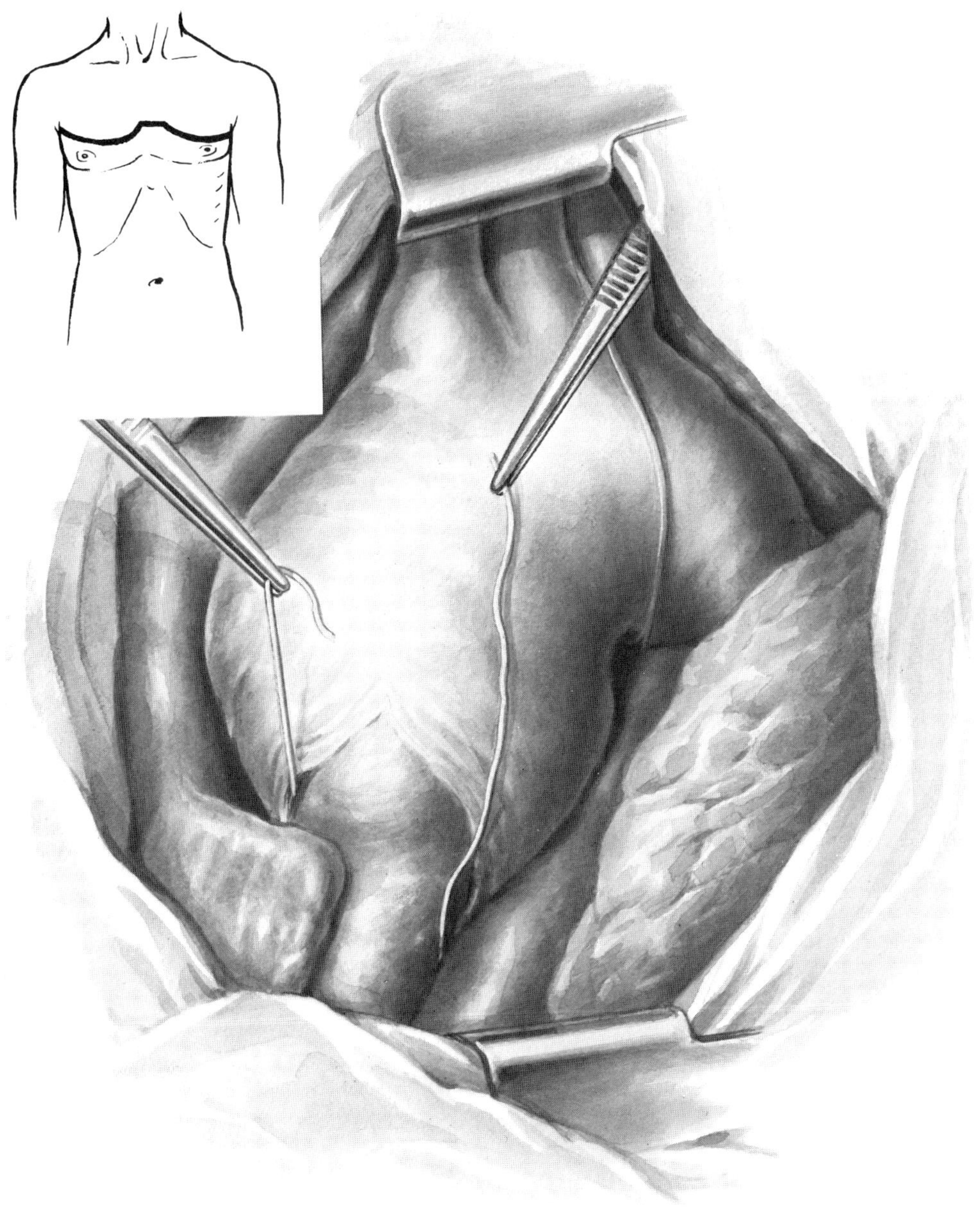

Fig. 535. Aneurysm of aortic arch is separated from surrounding tissues. Loop is brought under ascending aorta. *Inset,* schema of operative approach.

been freed from the surrounding tissues, a clamp is applied along its wall distal to the aneurysm, and an end-to-side anastomosis is formed between the aorta and a branching synthetic prosthesis prepared in advance (Fig. 537). With this anastomosis completed, the clamp is taken off the aorta, and the prosthesis is clamped close to the formed communication. After that the left subclavian artery is clamped and transected (Fig. 538). Its orifice is closed with a blanket suture, and an end-to-end anastomosis is created between the subclavian artery and the corresponding branch of the prosthesis. With this anastomosis established the prosthesis is clamped proximal to the branch corresponding to the left subclavian artery, and the blood flow in this artery is restored (Fig. 539). From this moment on the operation is conducted under conditions of carniocerebral hypothermia. The left carotid artery and the brachiocephalic trunk are successively transected; their orifices are sutured; and these

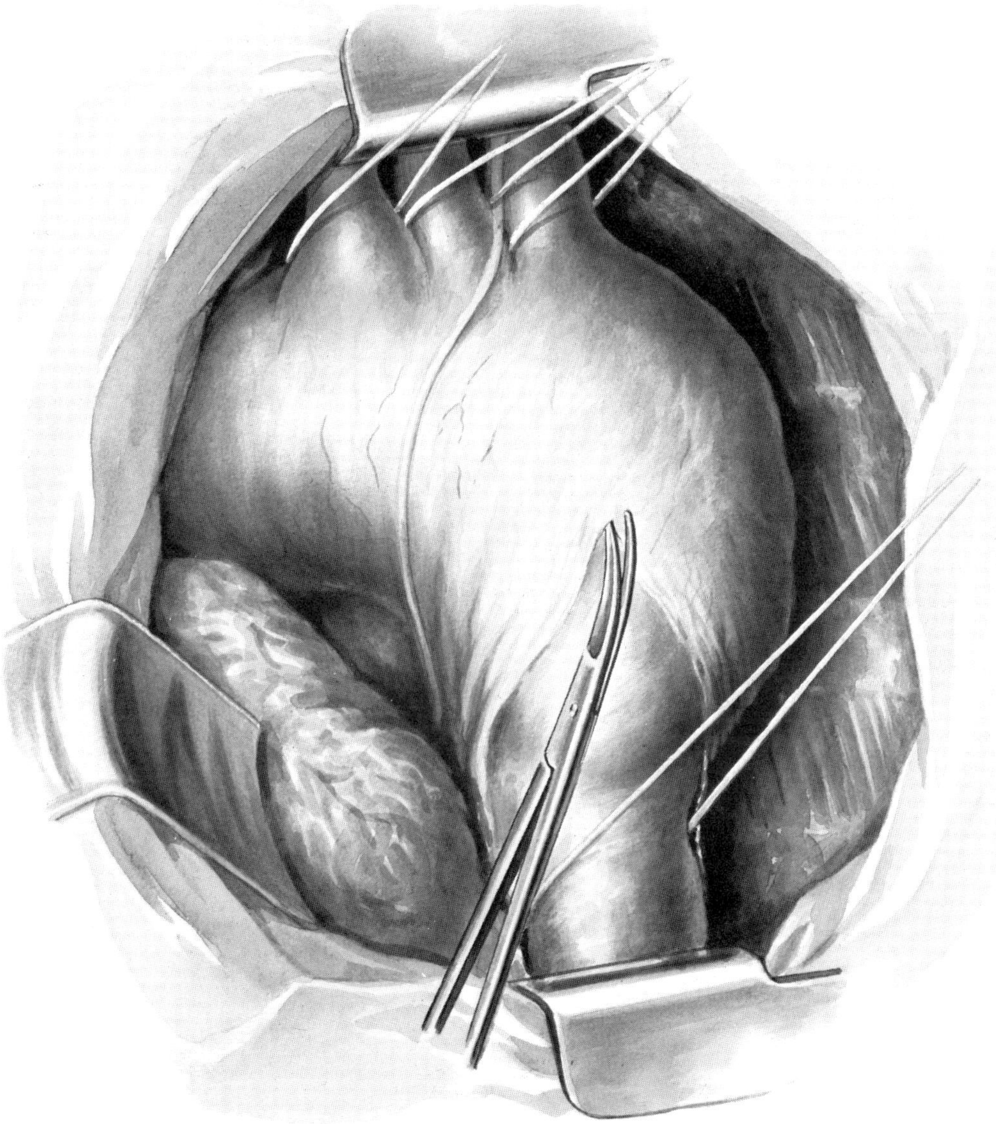

Fig. 536. Left lung is pulled medially and caudally. Pleura is cut over the aneurysm. Loop is brought under descending aorta.

vessels are connected end to end with the corresponding branches of the prosthesis and the blood flow in them is restored (Fig. 540). With circulation in the left carotid artery and the brachiocephalic trunk restored, craniocerebral hypothermia is discontinued. The superior and inferior venae cavae are cannulated through the right auricle and right atrium. The femoral artery is cannulated, and the heart-lung machine connected.

Under extracorporeal circulation the ascending aorta is clamped and transected centrally to the aneurysm (Fig. 541). The peripheral part of the transected aorta is closed completely with a blanket suture, preserving an area of the posterior wall of the aneurysmal sac. End-to-end central anastomosis between the aorta and the prosthesis is created (Fig. 542). The blood flow in the aorta and the prosthesis is restored. The heart-lung machine is disconnected. Cardiac sinus rhythm is restored. The cannulas are removed from the venae cavae and the femoral artery, and the auricle, the wall of the right atrium, and the femoral artery are repaired with sutures. The proximal

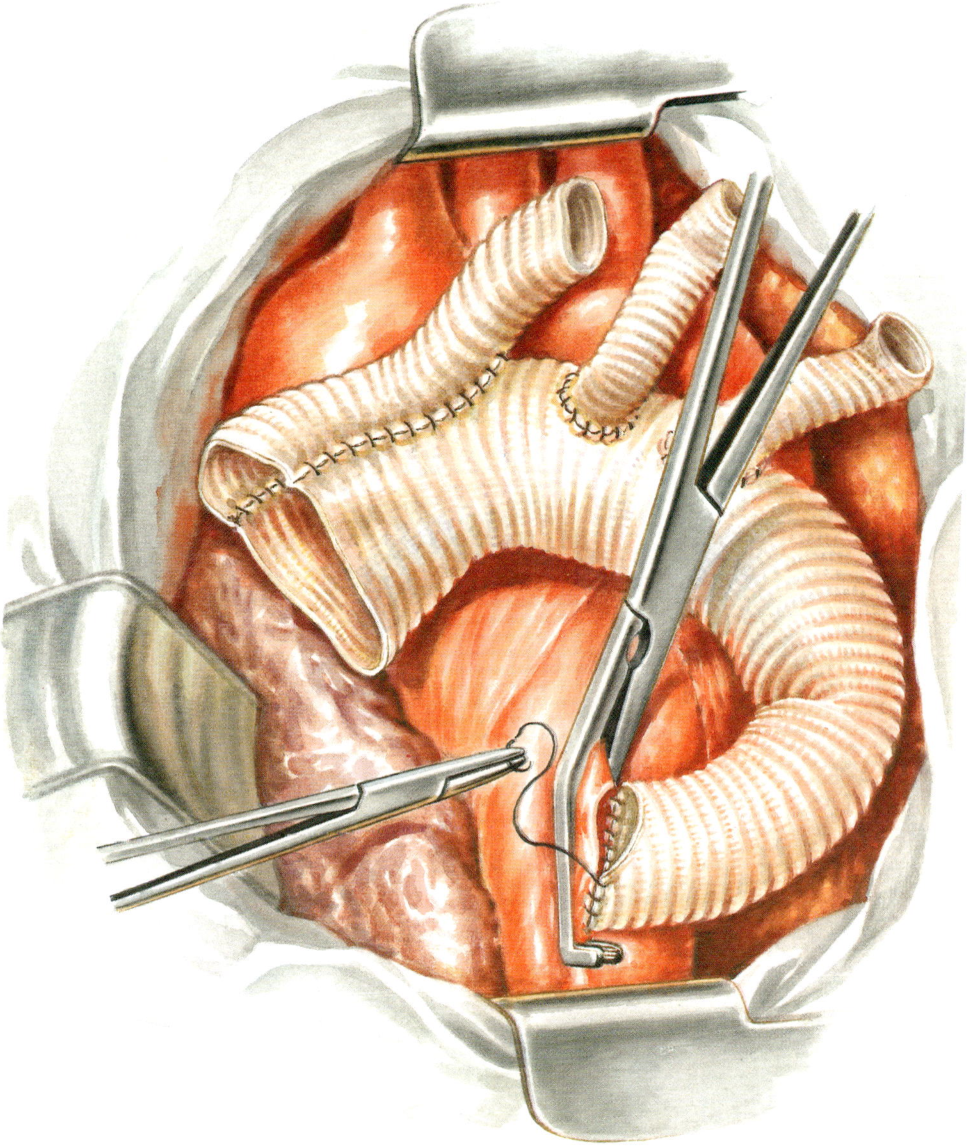

Fig. 537. Clamp is applied along wall in healthy part of descending aorta, and end-to-end anastomosis is formed between synthetic prosthesis and aorta.

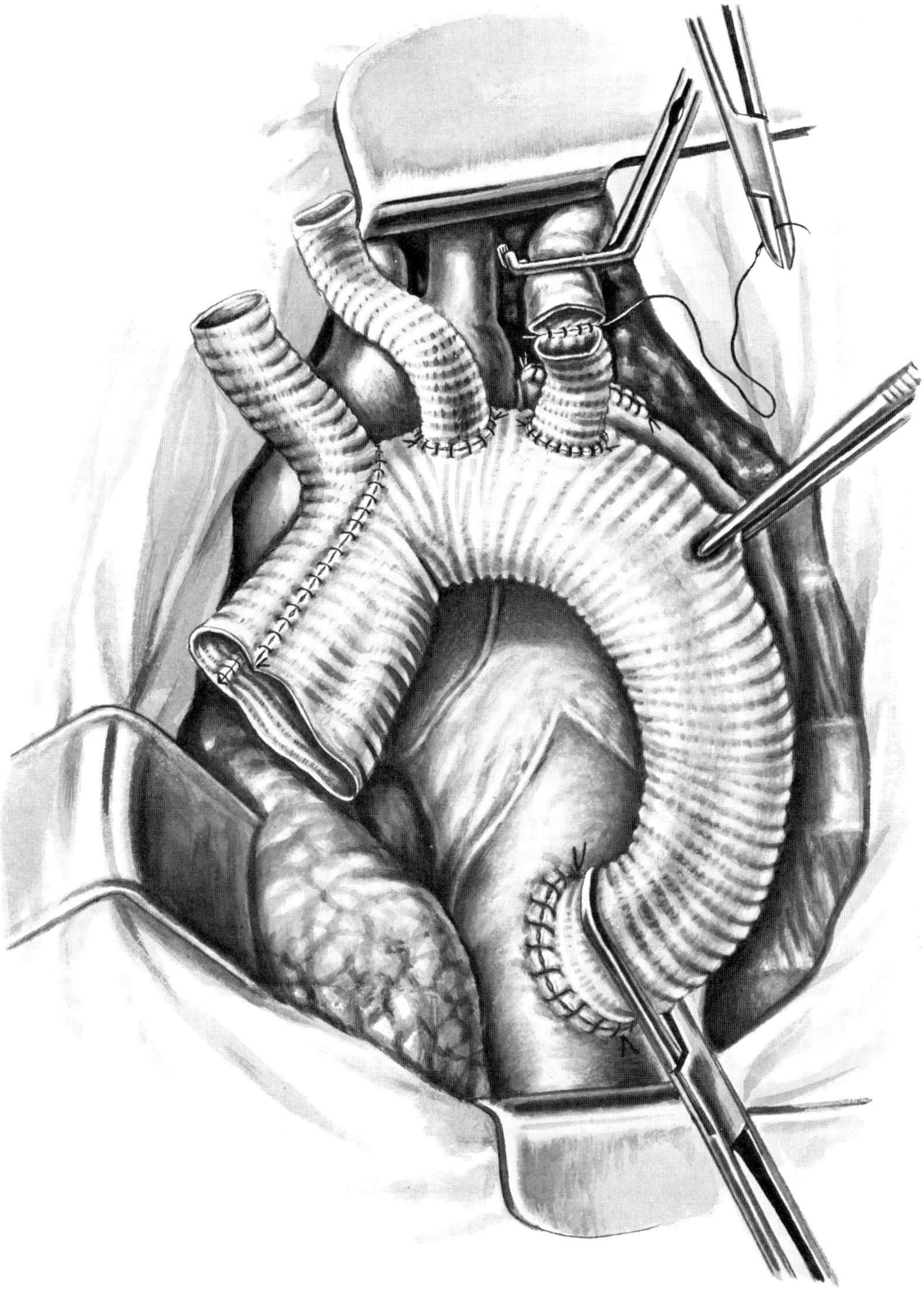

Fig. 538. Prosthesis and aorta are anastomosed. Prosthesis is clamped. Left subclavian artery is transected and its orifice closed with a blanket suture. End-to-end anastomosis is formed between subclavian artery and one branch of prosthesis.

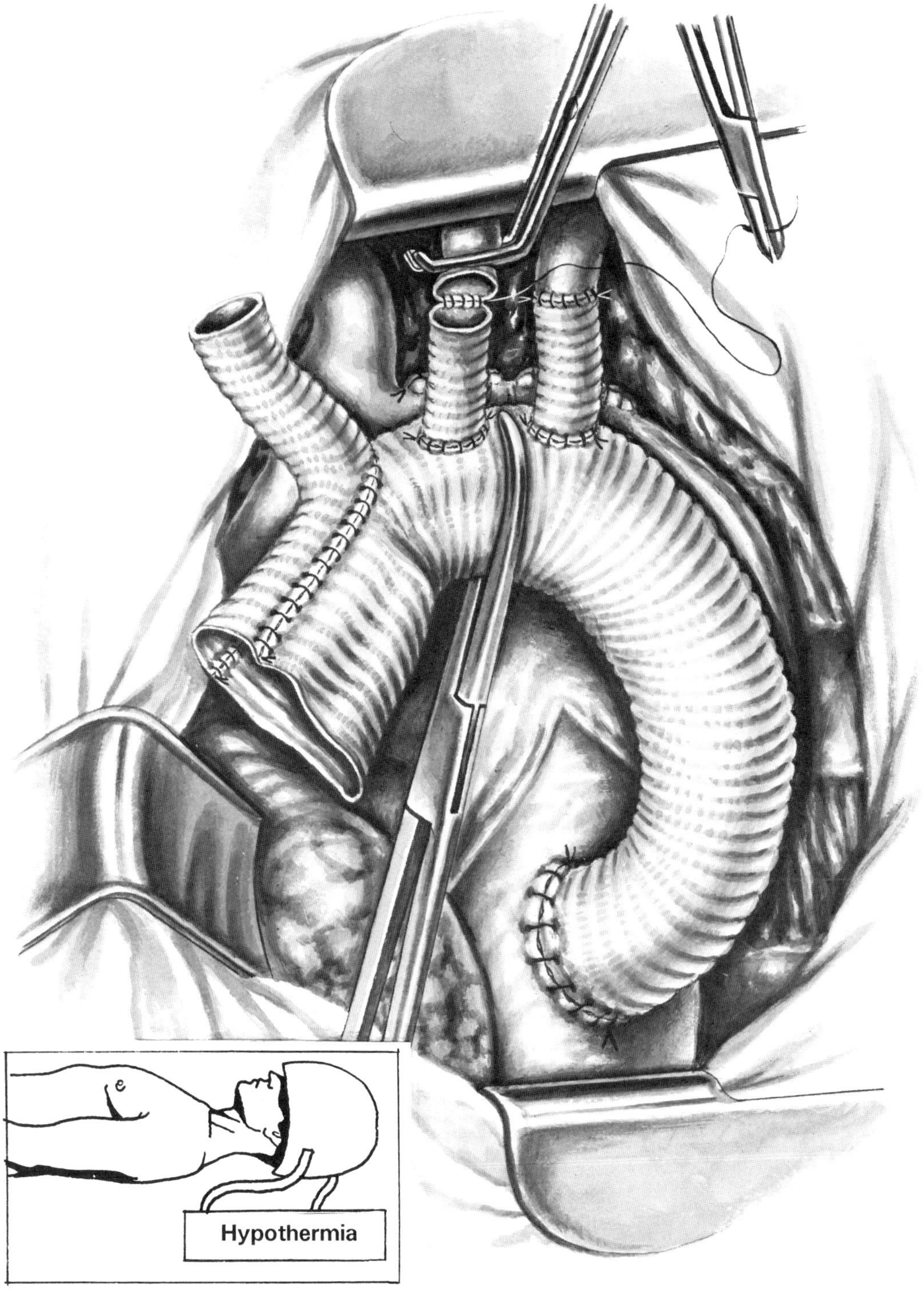

Fig. 539. Prosthetics of left subclavian artery has been completed, and blood flow in it restored. Prosthesis is clamped between its branches to subclavian and left carotid arteries. Left carotid artery is transected and its orifice closed with a blanket suture. Left carotid artery and corresponding branch of prosthesis are anastomosed end to end. *Inset,* schema of craniocerebral hypothermia.

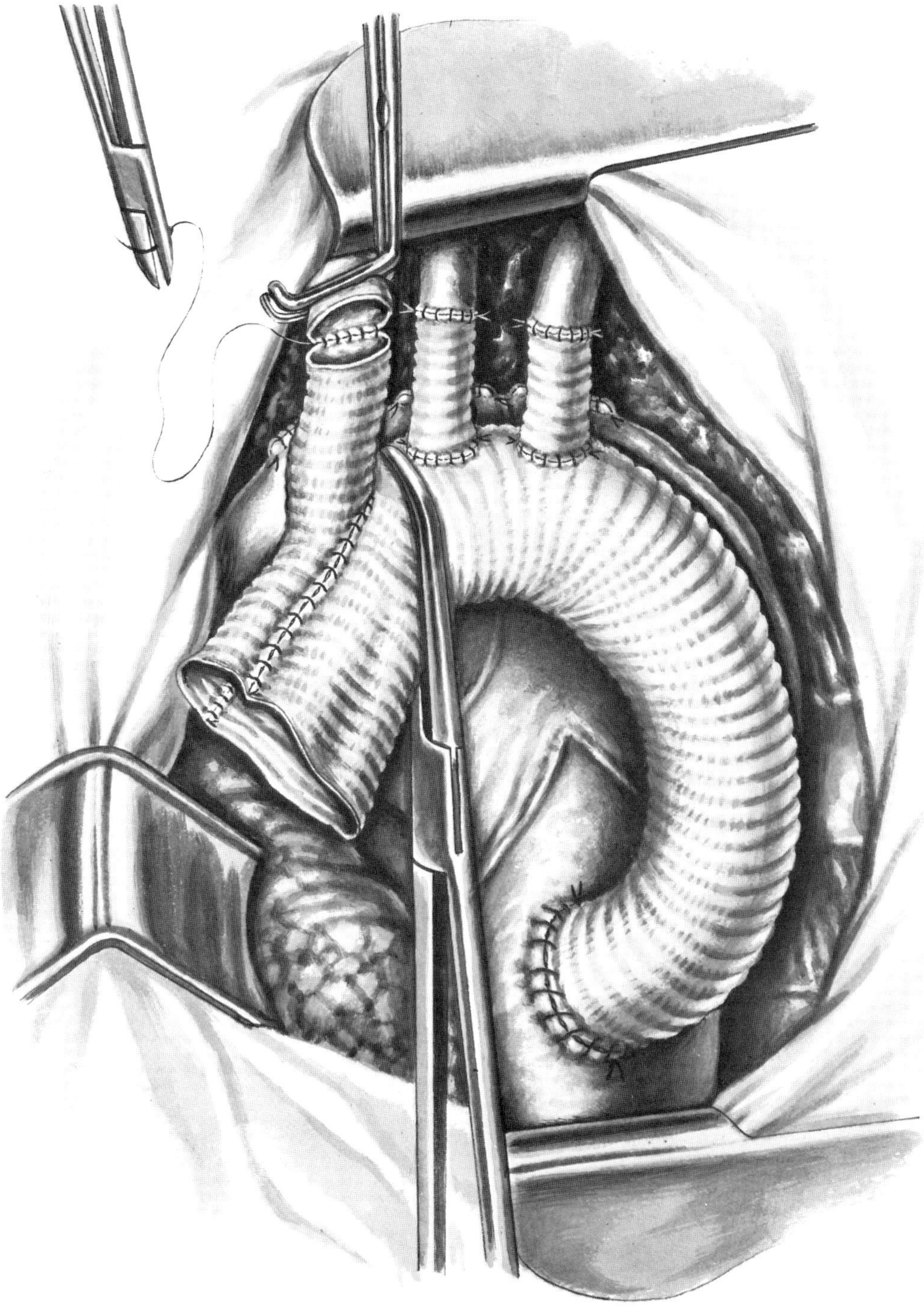

Fig. 540. Left carotid artery is reconstructed with prosthesis. Blood flow in left subclavian and left carotid arteries is restored. Prosthesis is clamped between its branches to left carotid artery and brachiocephalic trunk. Brachiocephalic trunk is transected and its orifice closed with blanket suture. End-to-end anastomosis is formed between transected brachiocephalic trunk and corresponding branch of prosthesis.

anastomosis between the prosthesis and the ascending aorta is covered with the aneurysmal sac as in a cuff (Fig. 543). After clamping the descending aorta, it is transected peripheral to the aneurysm. The stump of the transected aorta and the aneurysmal sac are closed tightly with blanket and Halsted sutures (Fig. 544). Fig. 545 shows the end result of the operation for shunting the aneurysm of the aortic arch.

The wound in the thoracic wall is sutured layer by layer with drains left in both pleural cavities.

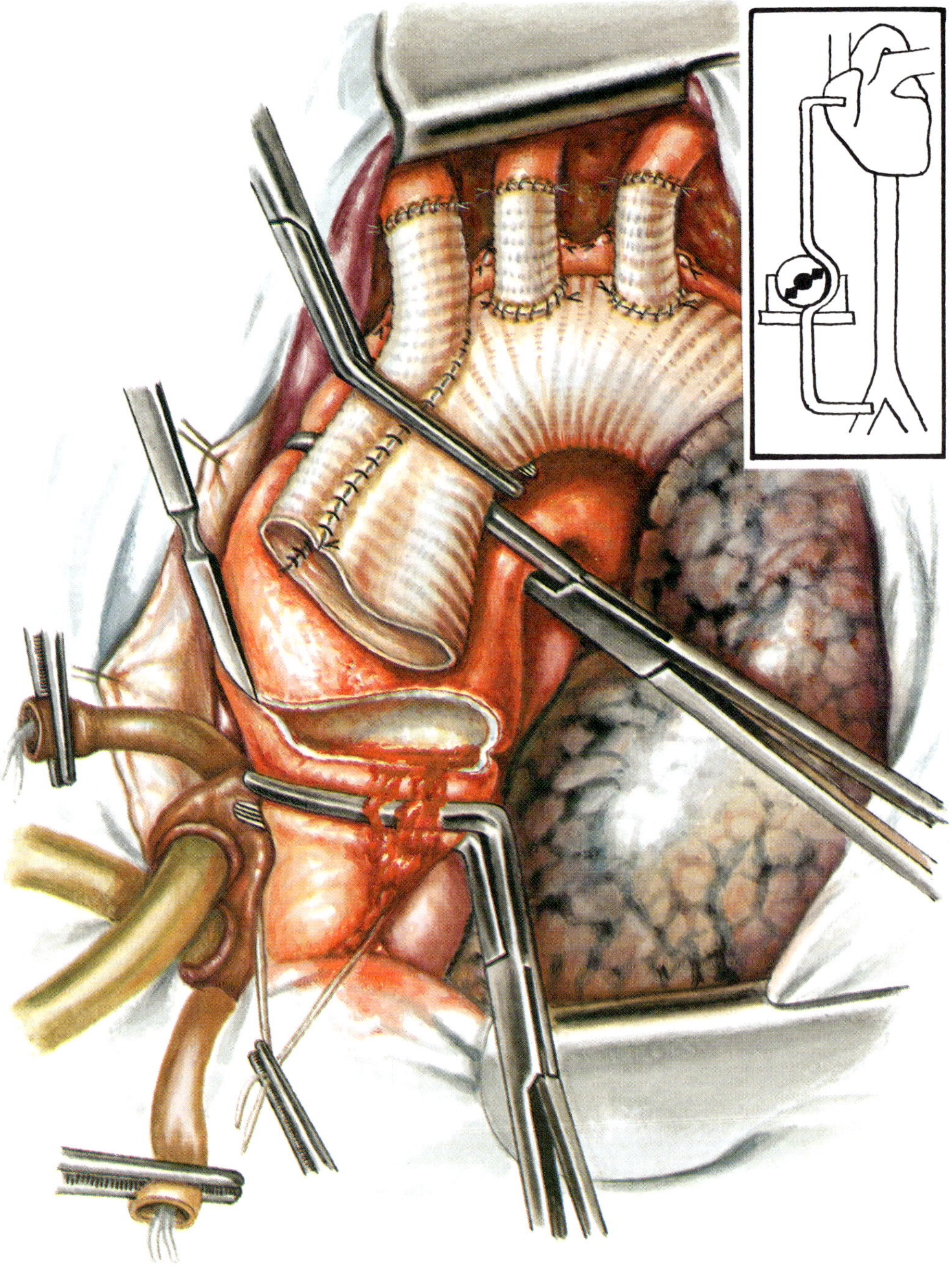

Fig. 541. Blood flow in brachiocephalic branches is restored. Prosthesis is clamped proximal to brachiocephalic trunk. Superior and inferior venae cavae are cannulated through right auricle and wall of right atrium. Ascending aorta is clamped above the orifices of coronary arteries. Ascending aorta is transected proximal to aneurysm. *Inset,* schema of extracorporeal circulation employed in this stage of operation.

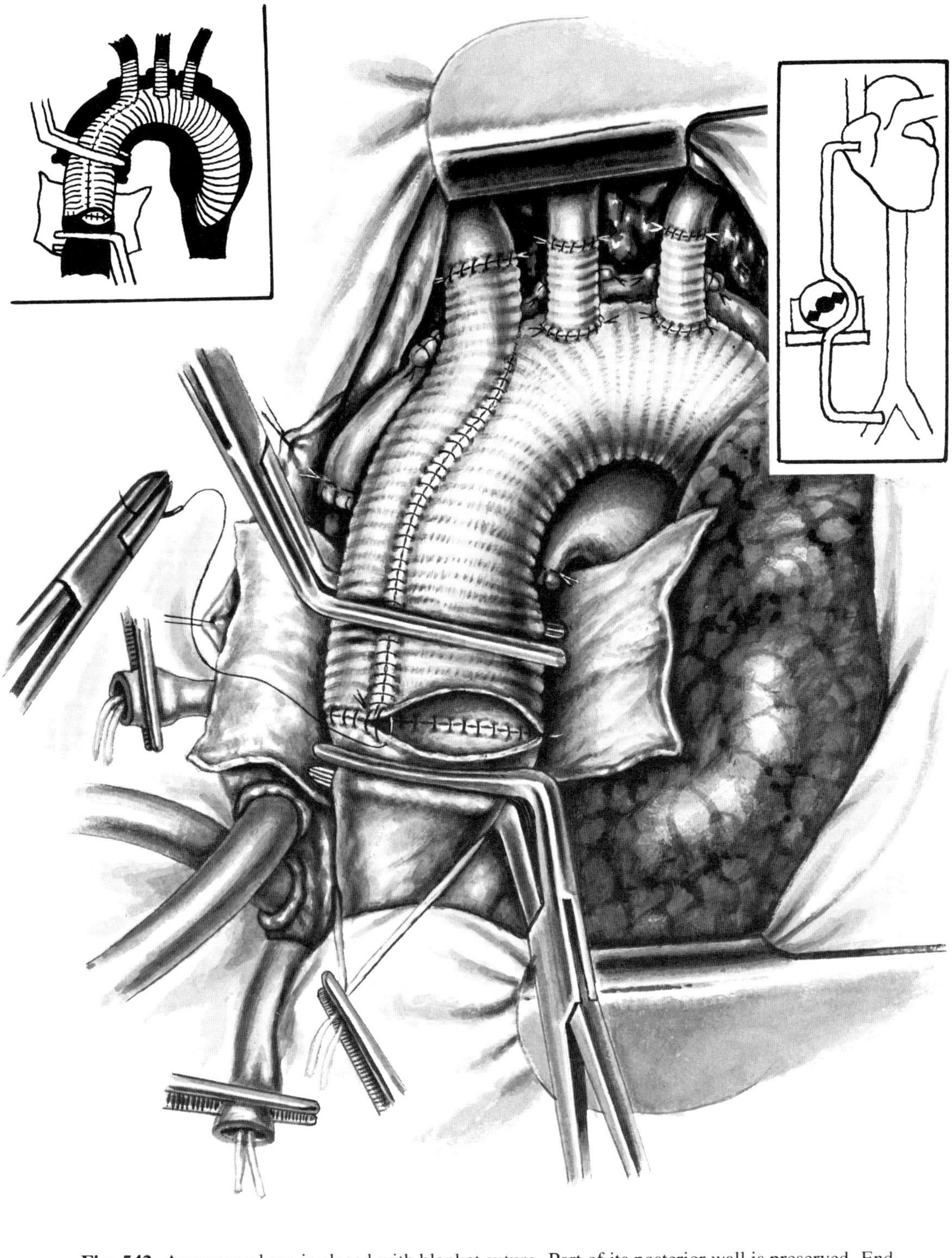

Fig. 542. Aneurysmal sac is closed with blanket suture. Part of its posterior wall is preserved. End-to-end anastomosis is formed between aorta and prosthesis. *Right inset,* schema of stage of operation. *Left inset,* schema of extracorporeal circulation.

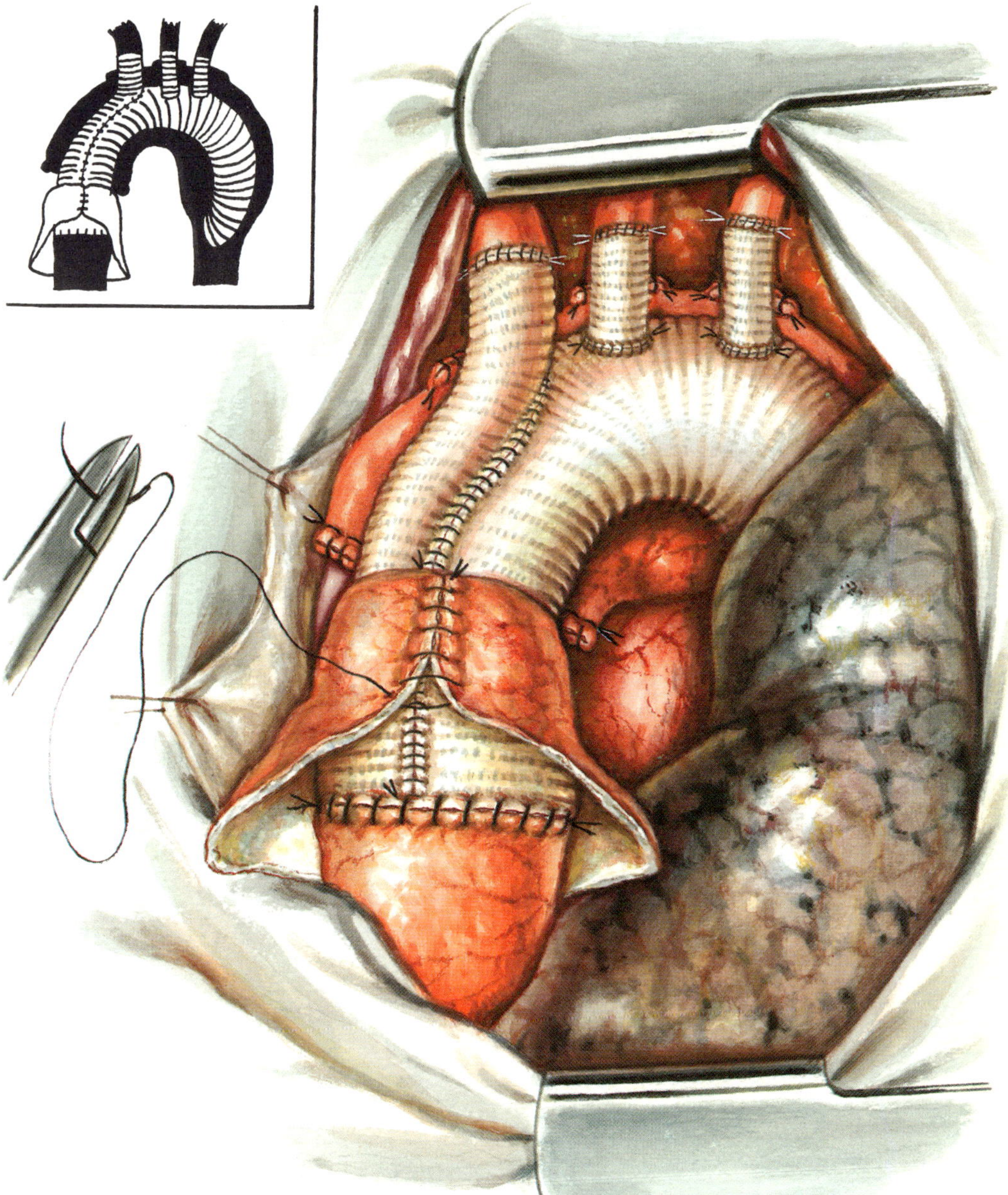

Fig. 543. Anastomosis between prosthesis and ascending aorta is formed. Blood flow in aorta and prosthesis is restored. Cuff is formed from posterior wall of aneurysmal sac for reinforcing anastomosis between aorta and prosthesis.

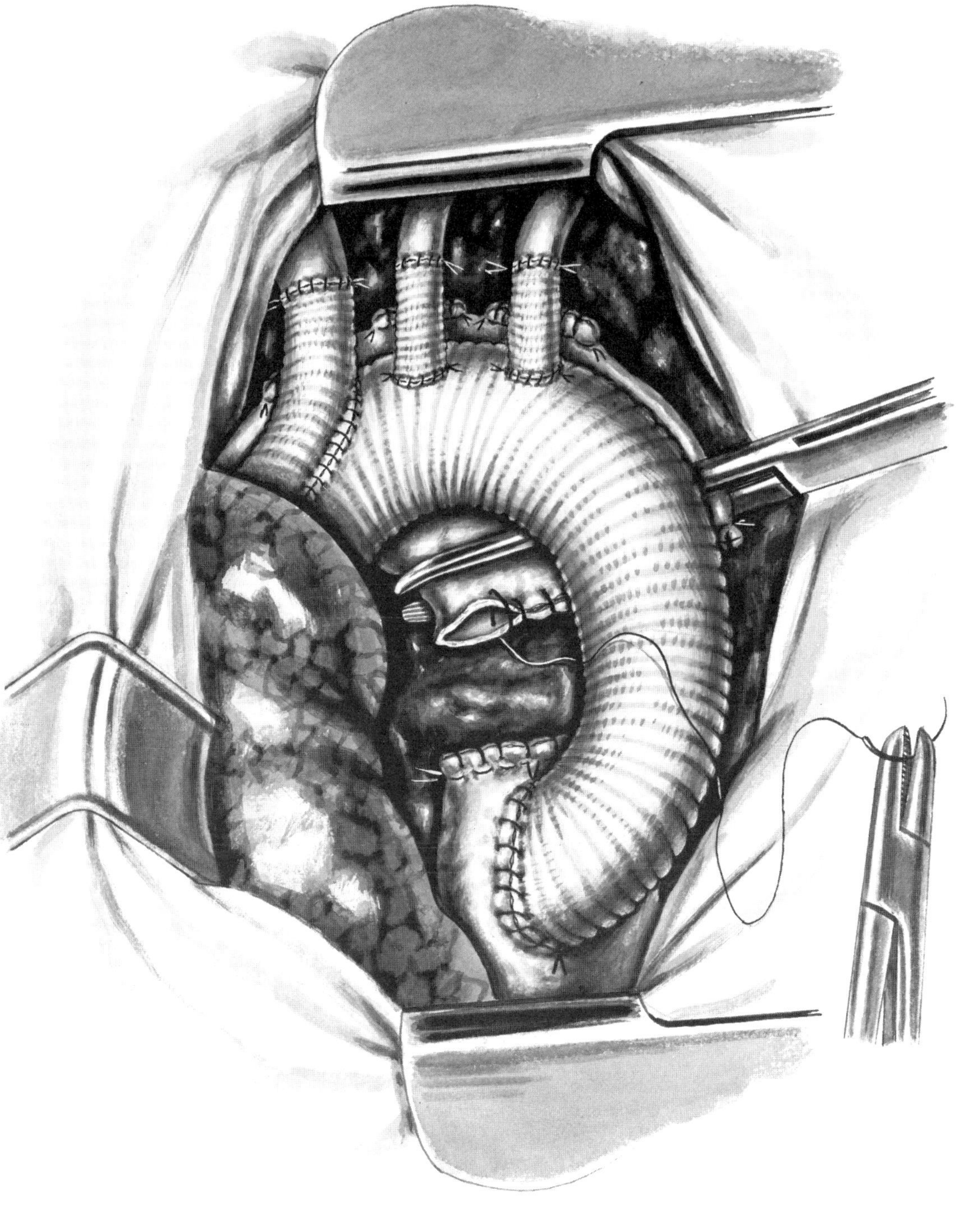

Fig. 544. Descending aorta is transected distal to aneurysm. Blanket suture is applied to proximal stump of transected aorta. Aneurysmal sac is closed with blanket suture.

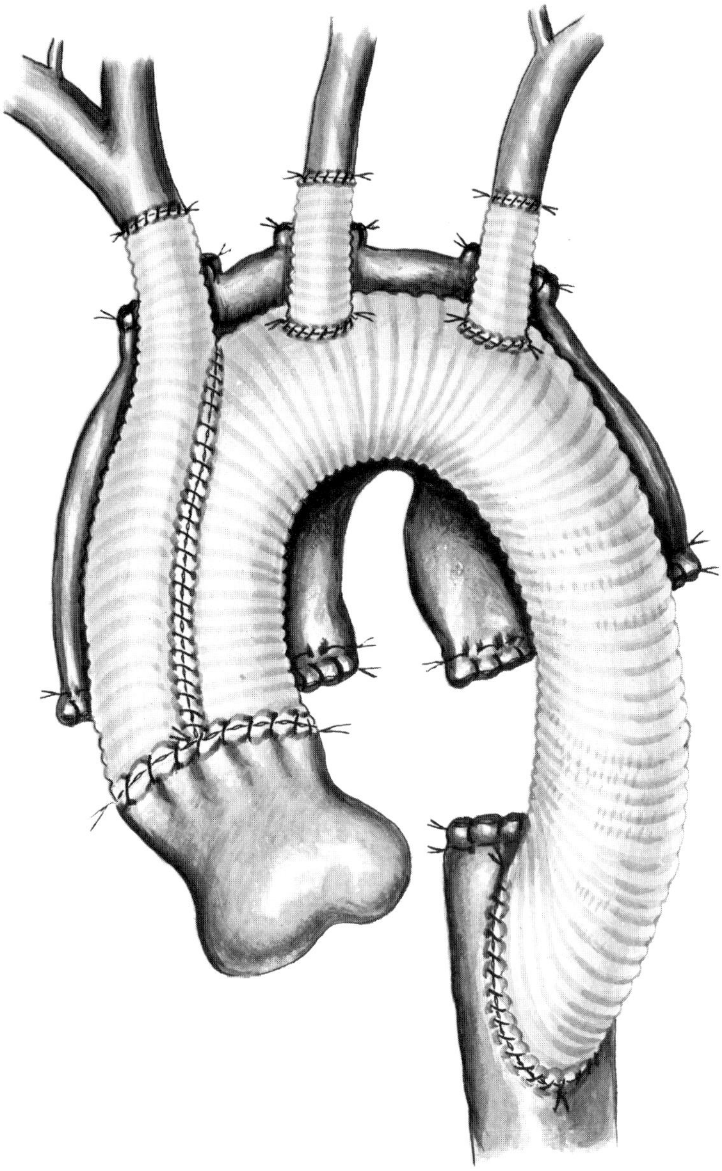

Fig. 545. Schema of shunting of aneurysm of aortic arch.

Operations in aneurysm and occlusion of brachiocephalic branches of aortic arch

RESECTION OF ANEURYSM OF BRACHIOCEPHALIC TRUNK AND ITS PROSTHETICS

The operation is carried out under craniocerebral hypothermia. A transverse incision is made through the soft tissues of the neck, and longitudinal sternotomy is performed. The ascending aorta, the aneurysm, and the right subclavian and right common carotid arteries are freed from the surrounding tissues. The left brachio-

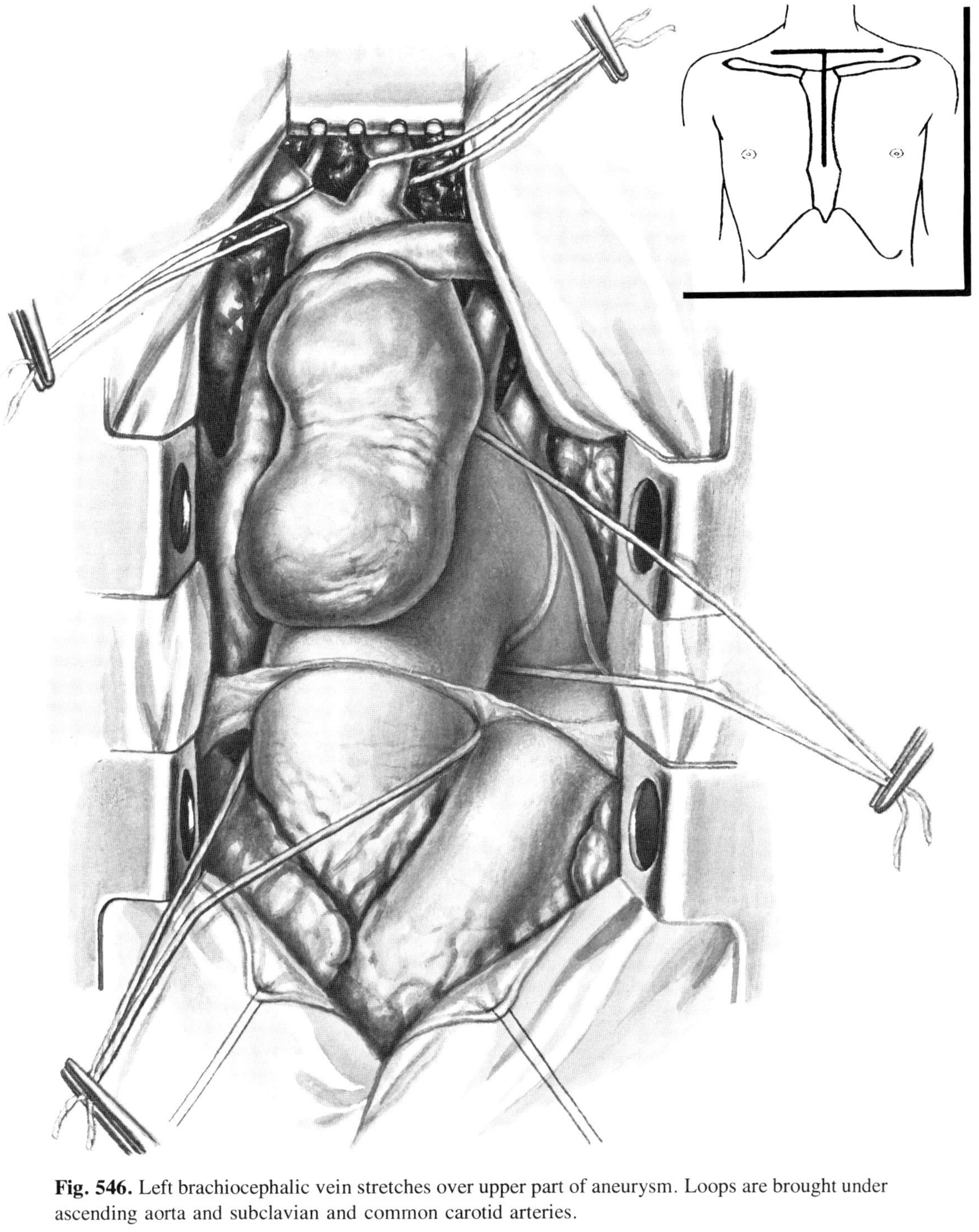

Fig. 546. Left brachiocephalic vein stretches over upper part of aneurysm. Loops are brought under ascending aorta and subclavian and common carotid arteries.

cephalic vein is usually found in front of the aneurysm; it is carefully separated and raised with a loop (Fig. 546). The aorta is clamped laterally at the origin of the brachiocephalic trunk. The apex of the aneurysm is pulled upward and to the right with fenestrated forceps. The blood flow in the right subclavian and common carotid arteries is arrested. The brachiocephalic trunk with the aneurysm is cut away from the aorta and subclavian and

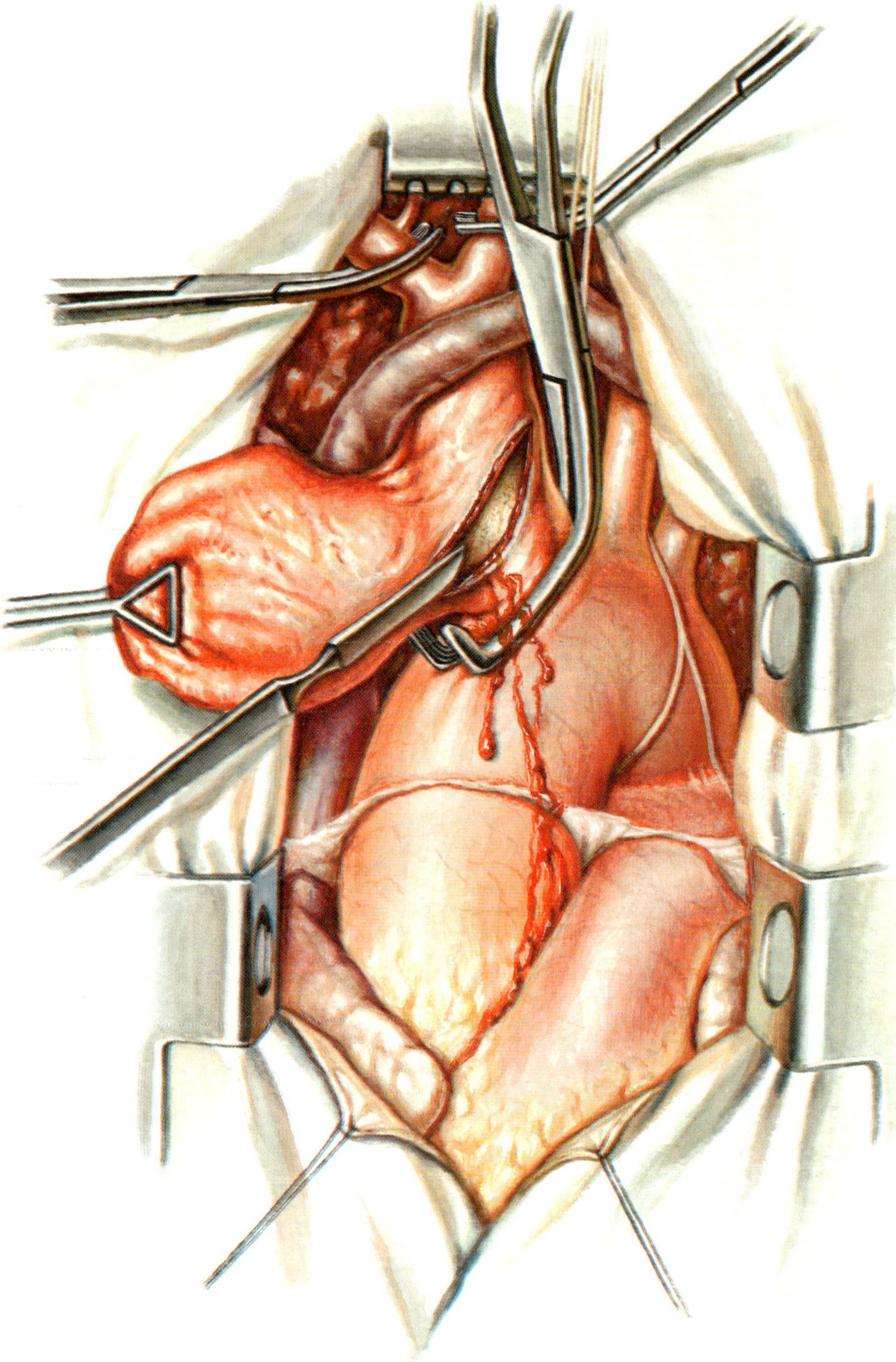

Fig. 547. Apex of aneurysm is raised with fenestrated forceps and pulled to right. Brachiocephalic trunk is clamped at its origin from aorta. Clamps are applied to subclavian and common carotid arteries. Brachiocephalic trunk is transected above clamp.

common carotid arteries (Fig. 547). The defect in the aortic wall is repaired with a continuous blanket suture (Fig. 548). A clamp is applied along the anterior wall of the ascending aorta, and an oval opening is made in it (Fig. 549). The blood flow is restored successively in the common carotid artery and in the subclavian artery by means of a bifurcate prosthesis (Figs. 550 and 551). A drain is left in the anterior mediastinum.

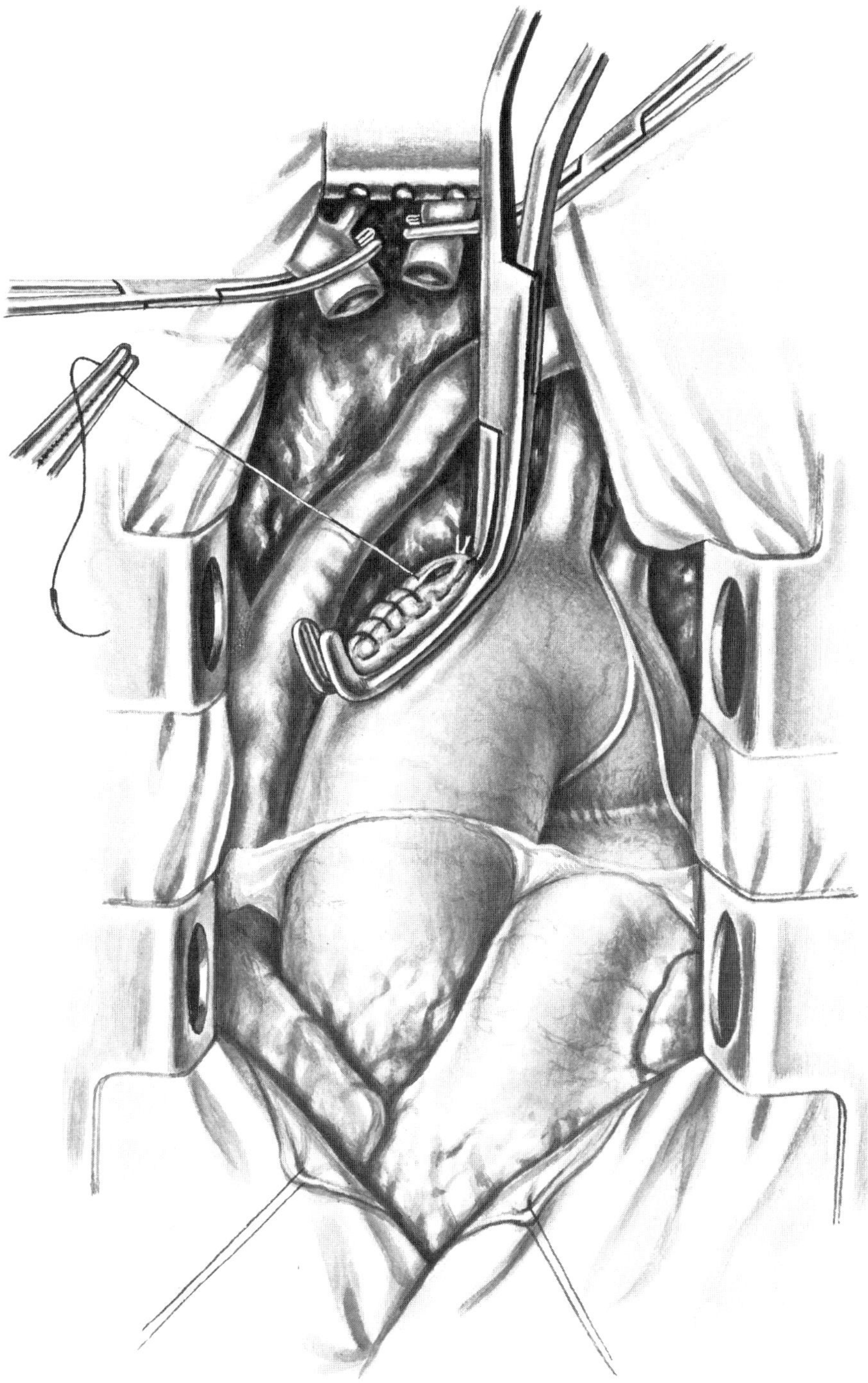

Fig. 548. Continuous suture is applied to aorta.

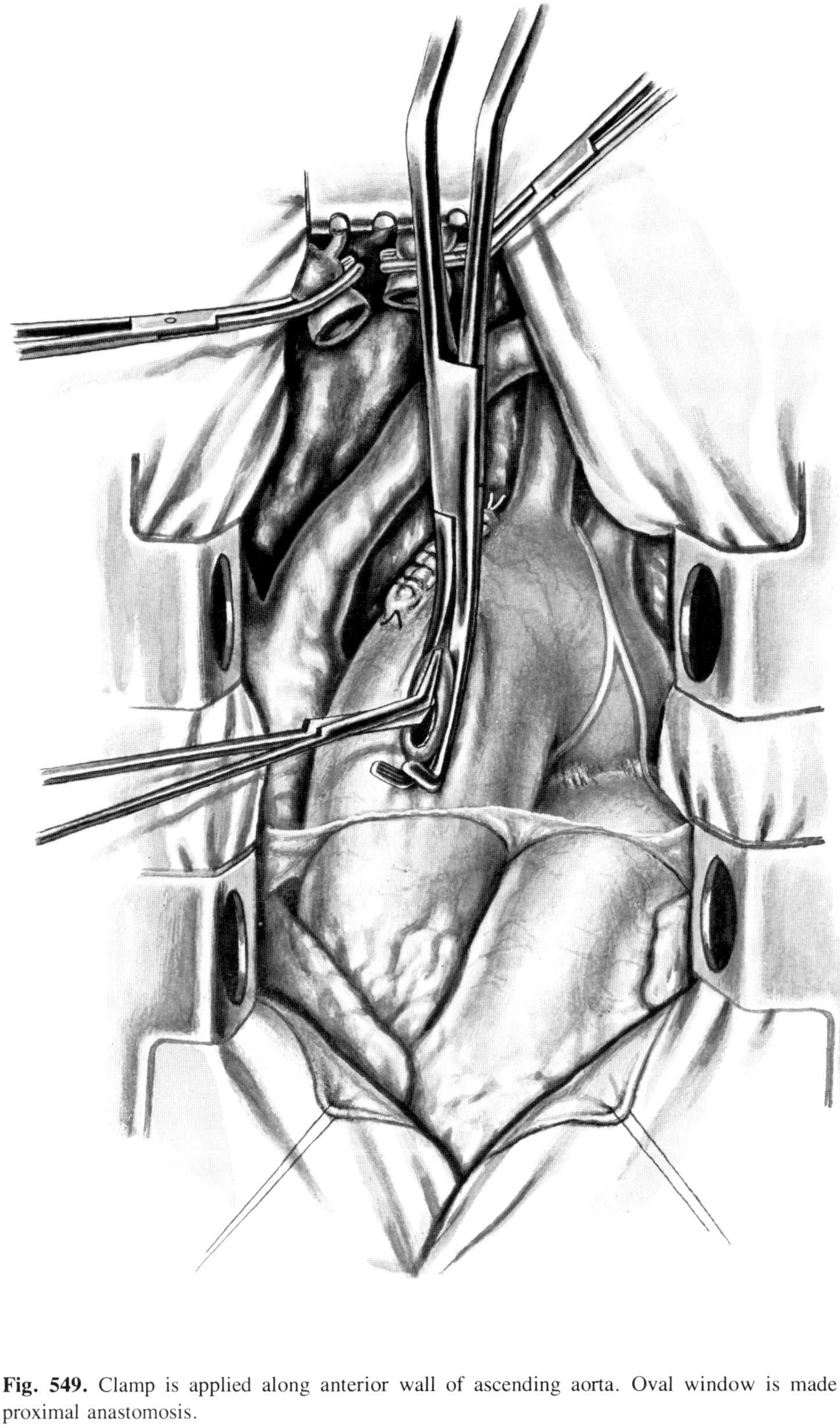

Fig. 549. Clamp is applied along anterior wall of ascending aorta. Oval window is made for proximal anastomosis.

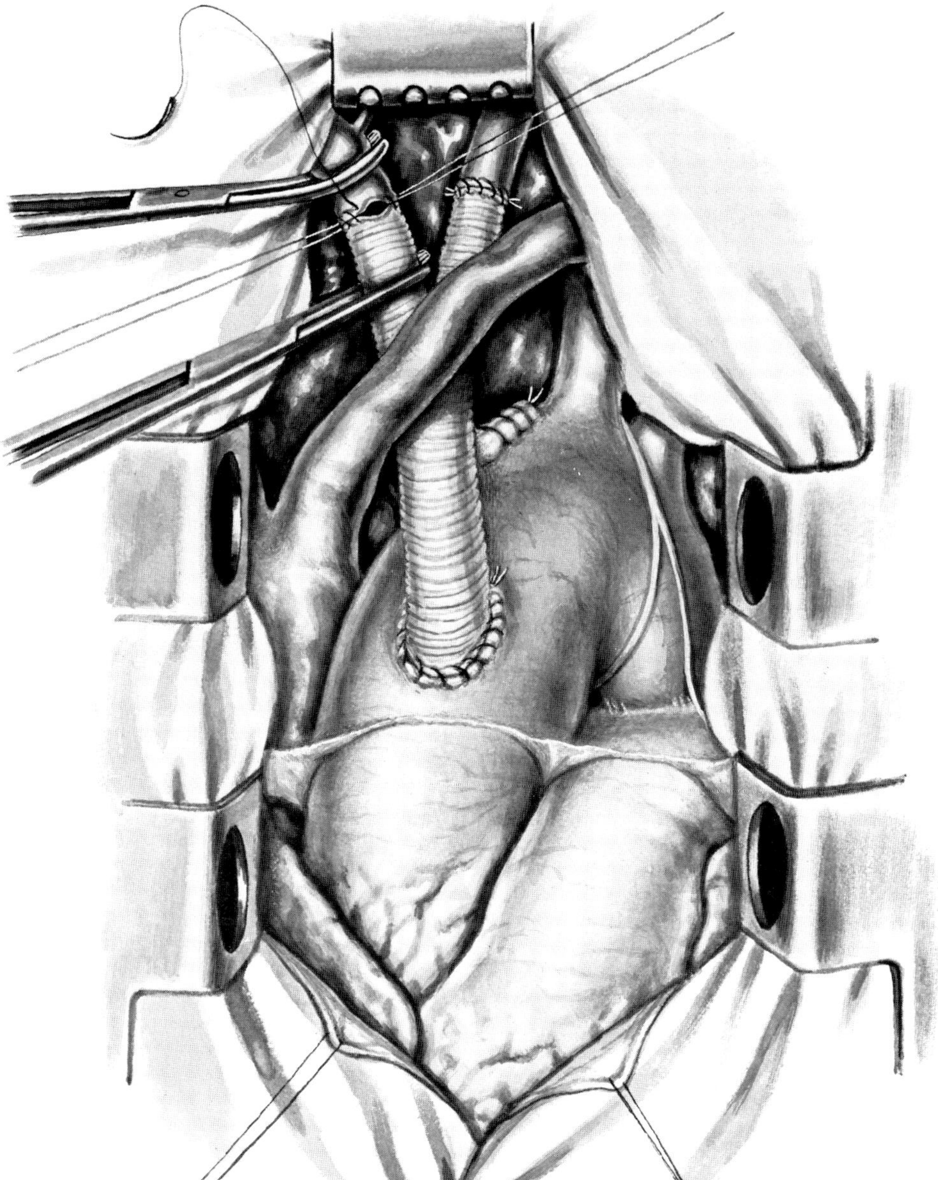

Fig. 550. Replacement of brachiocephalic trunk with bifurcate prosthesis. Prosthesis and subclavian artery are anastomosed. Blood flow in common carotid artery is restored.

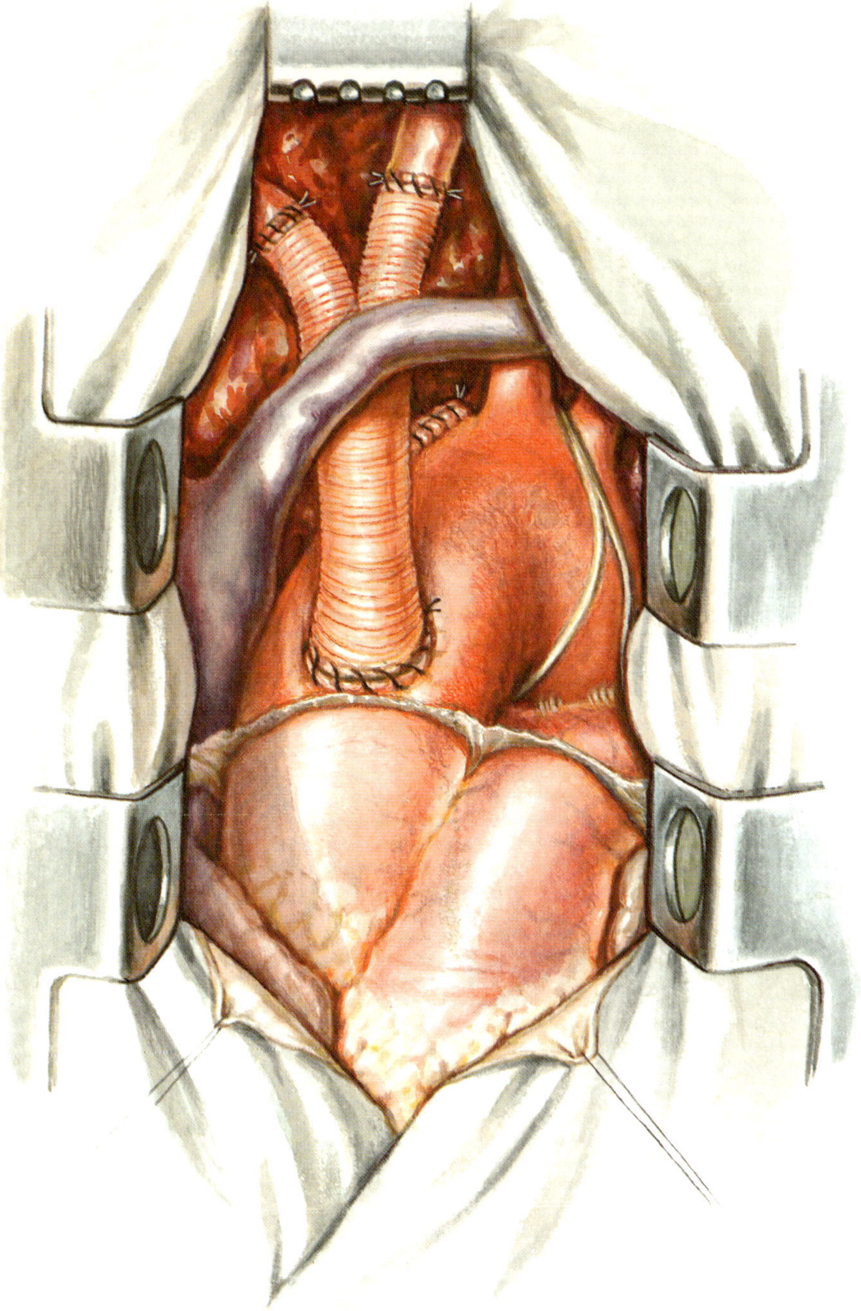

Fig. 551. Circulation in carotid and subclavian arteries is restored.

RESECTION OF ANEURYSM OF LEFT SUBCLAVIAN ARTERY AND ITS PROSTHETICS

In operations for aneurysm of the left subclavian artery a combined approach is employed (Fig. 552). Anterolateral thoracotomy in the left third or fourth intercostal space is carried out with transection of the second and third costal cartilages. The apex of the lung is drawn caudally, and the arch of the aorta and the aneurysm of the subclavian artery are separated from the surrounding tissues (Fig. 553). Then a skin incision is made above the clavicle; the lateral head of the sternocleidomastoid muscle and the anterior scalene muscle are

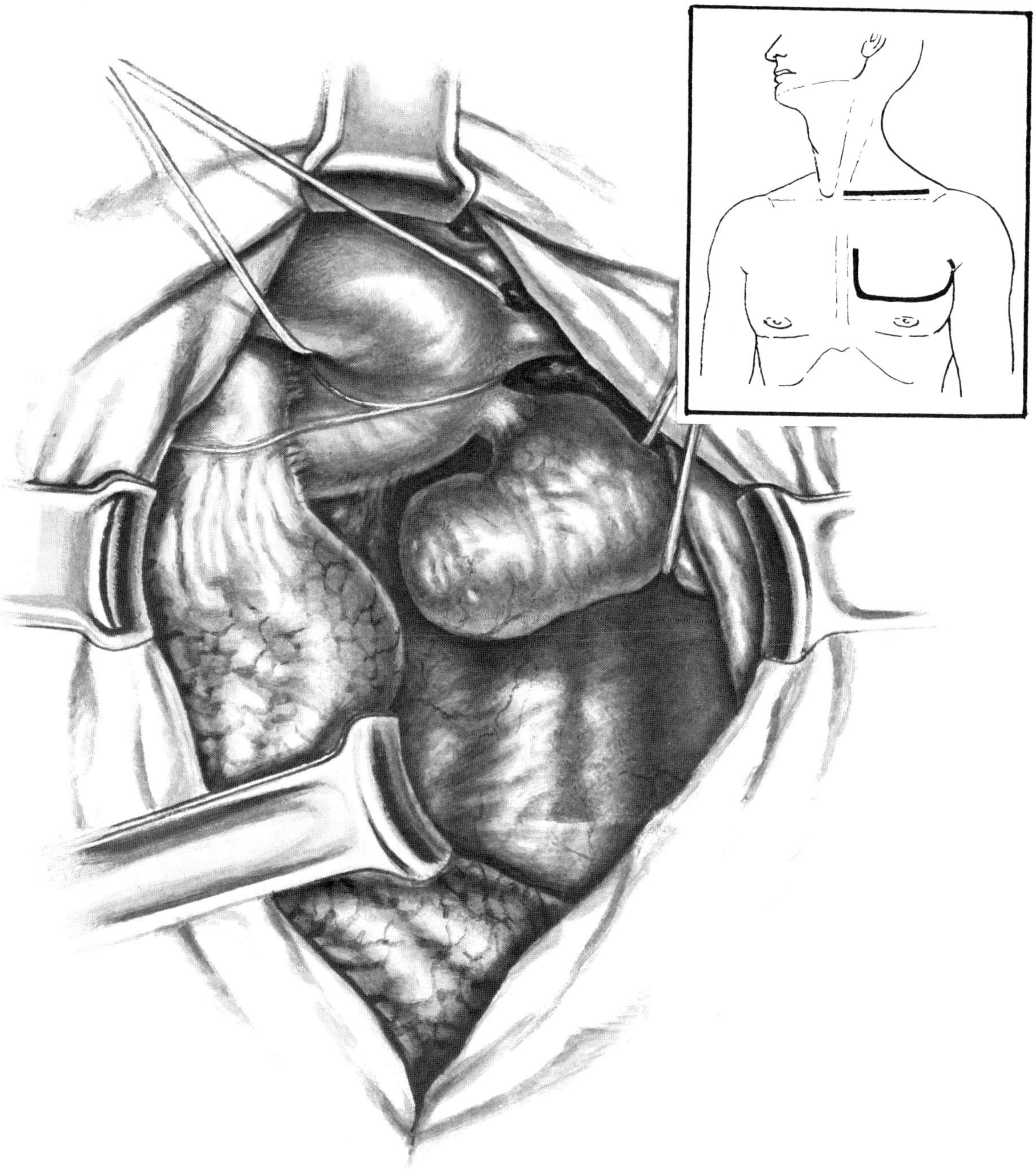

Fig. 552. Loops are brought under arch of aorta and subclavian artery. *Inset,* schema of combined operative approach.

transected; and all three portions of the subclavian artery are separated. The aneurysmal sac is usually located medial to the vertebral artery. To preserve the blood flow in this artery, the subclavian artery is clamped distal to its orifice and the thyrocervical trunk during the operation. Following arteriotomy the synthetic prosthesis and the subclavian artery are anastomosed end to side. The prosthesis is passed into the pleural cavity behind the clavicle. The aortic wall is clamped laterally and cut lengthwise, and an end-to-side anastomosis is formed between the aorta and the prosthesis (Fig. 554). The clamp is taken off the aorta. The subclavian artery is clamped and the aneurysmal sac cut away (Fig. 555). The stump of the subclavian artery is sutured (Fig. 556). The aneurysmal sac is cut away in the supraclavicular region (Fig. 557). The distal stump of the subclavian artery is closed with sutures (Fig. 558). The aneurysm is fully resected. The clamps are removed. A drain is left in the pleural cavity. The wound is sutured layer by layer.

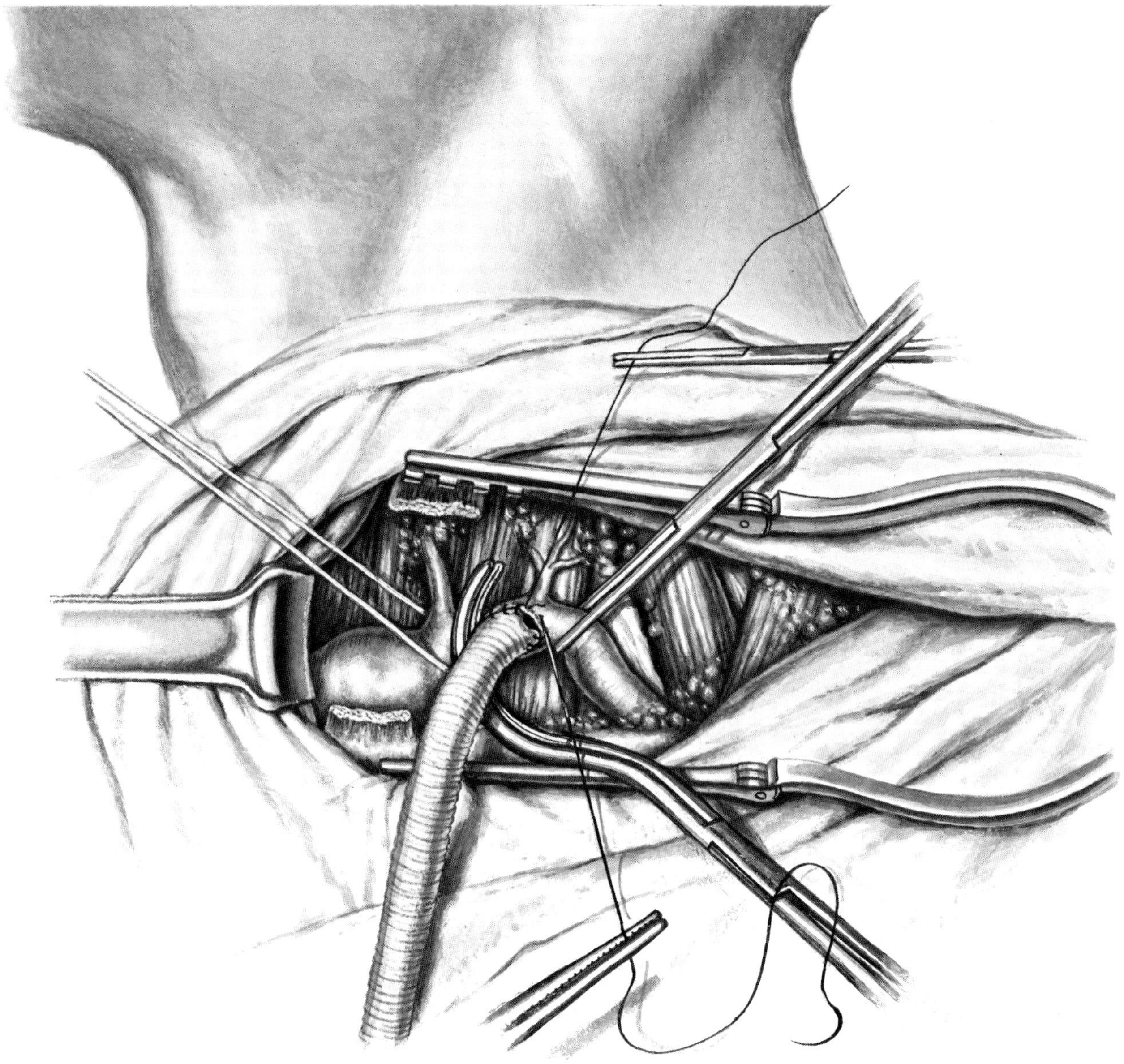

Fig. 553. View of operative wound after transection of anterior scalene muscle. Three portions of subclavian artery are mobilized. Artery is raised by loop and clamped distal to vertebral artery and thyrocervical trunk. End-to-side anastomosis is formed between vessel prosthesis and subclavian artery.

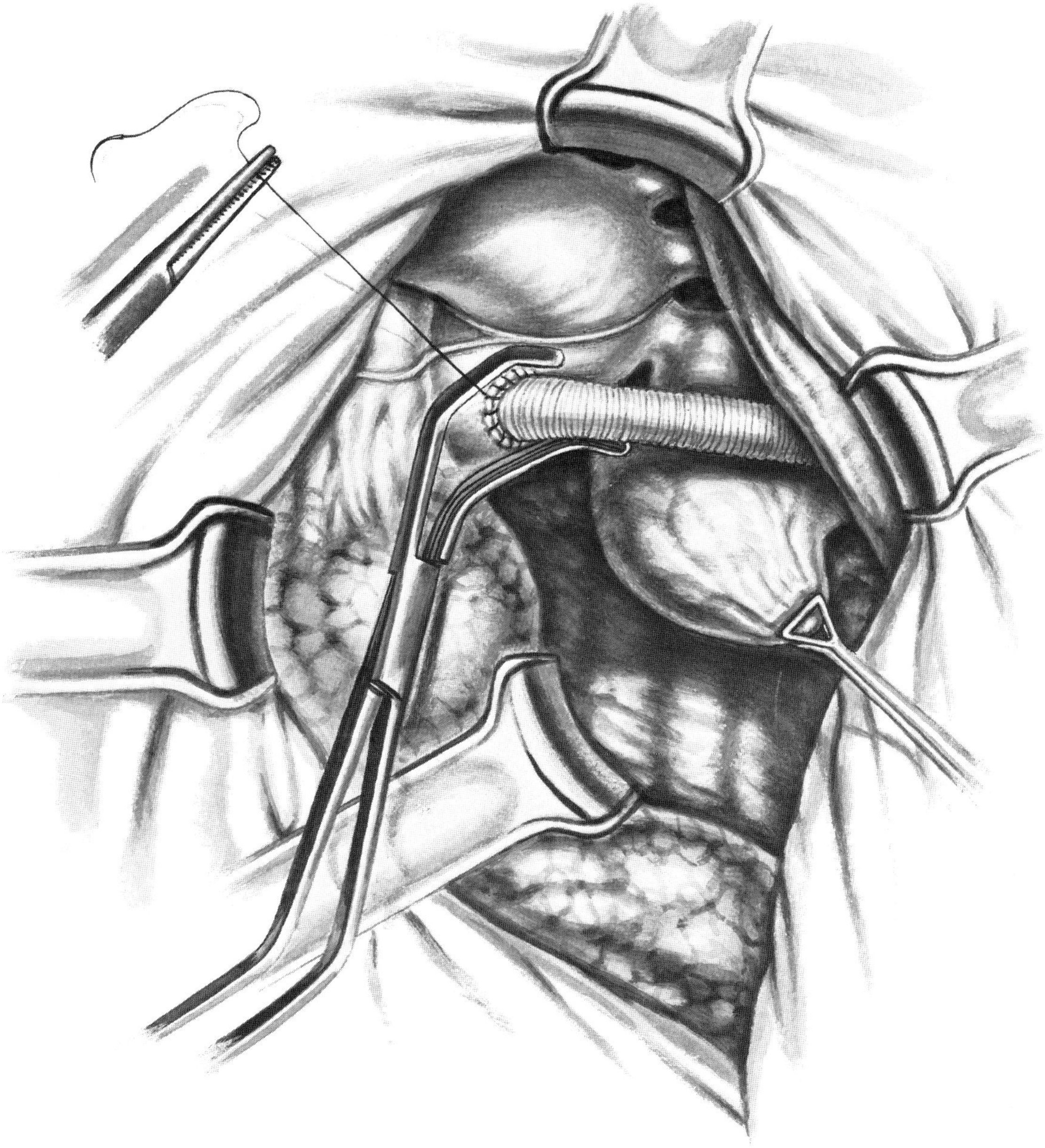

Fig. 554. Synthetic prosthesis is inserted behind clavicle and into pleural cavity. Clamp is applied to aortic wall, and end-to-side anastomosis is formed between prosthesis and aorta. Aneurysmal sac is pulled to left and to back with fenestrated forceps.

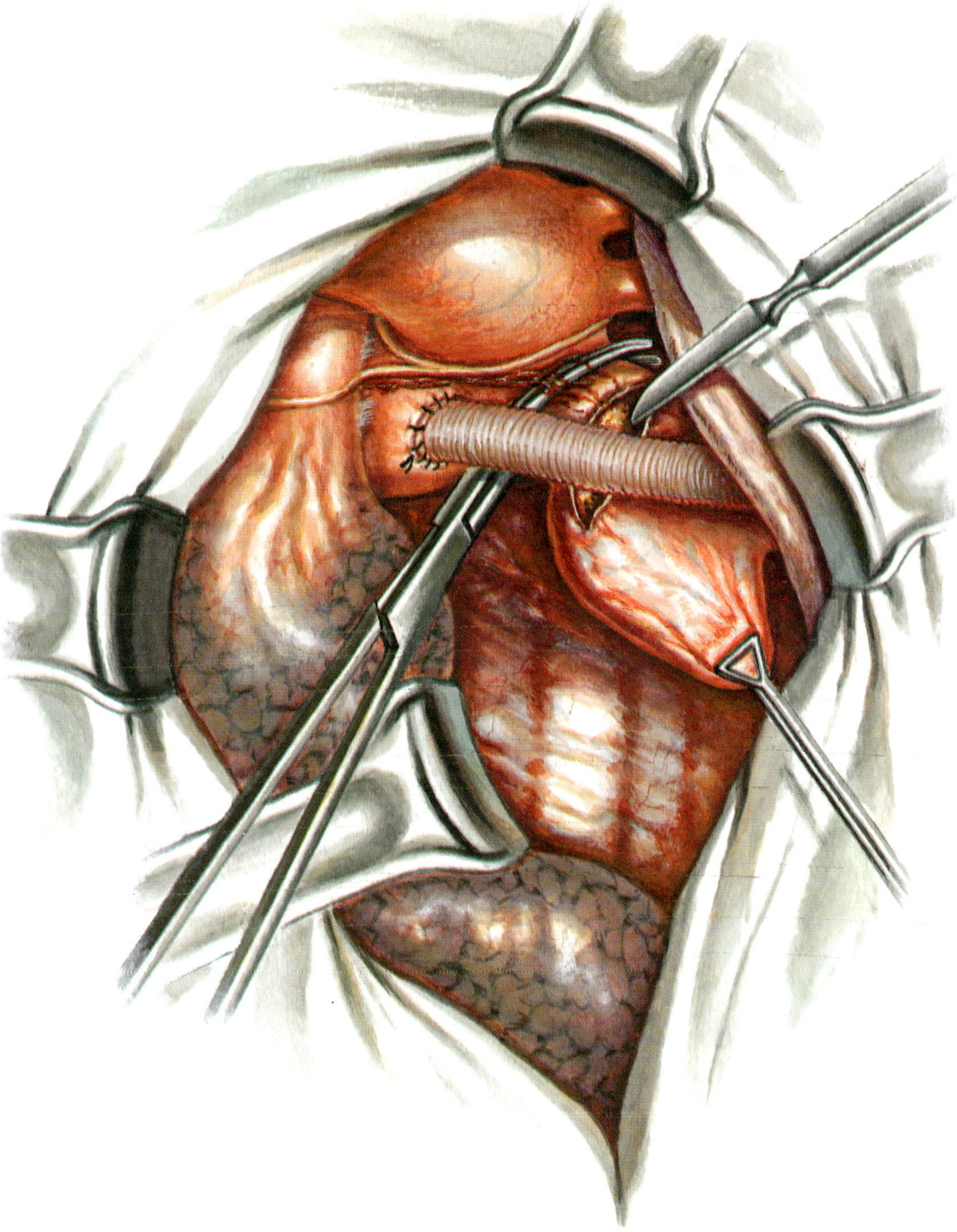

Fig. 555. Subclavian artery is clamped proximal to vertebral artery. Blood flows into vertebral and subclavian arteries from aorta by way of prosthesis. Aneurysmal sac is being resected.

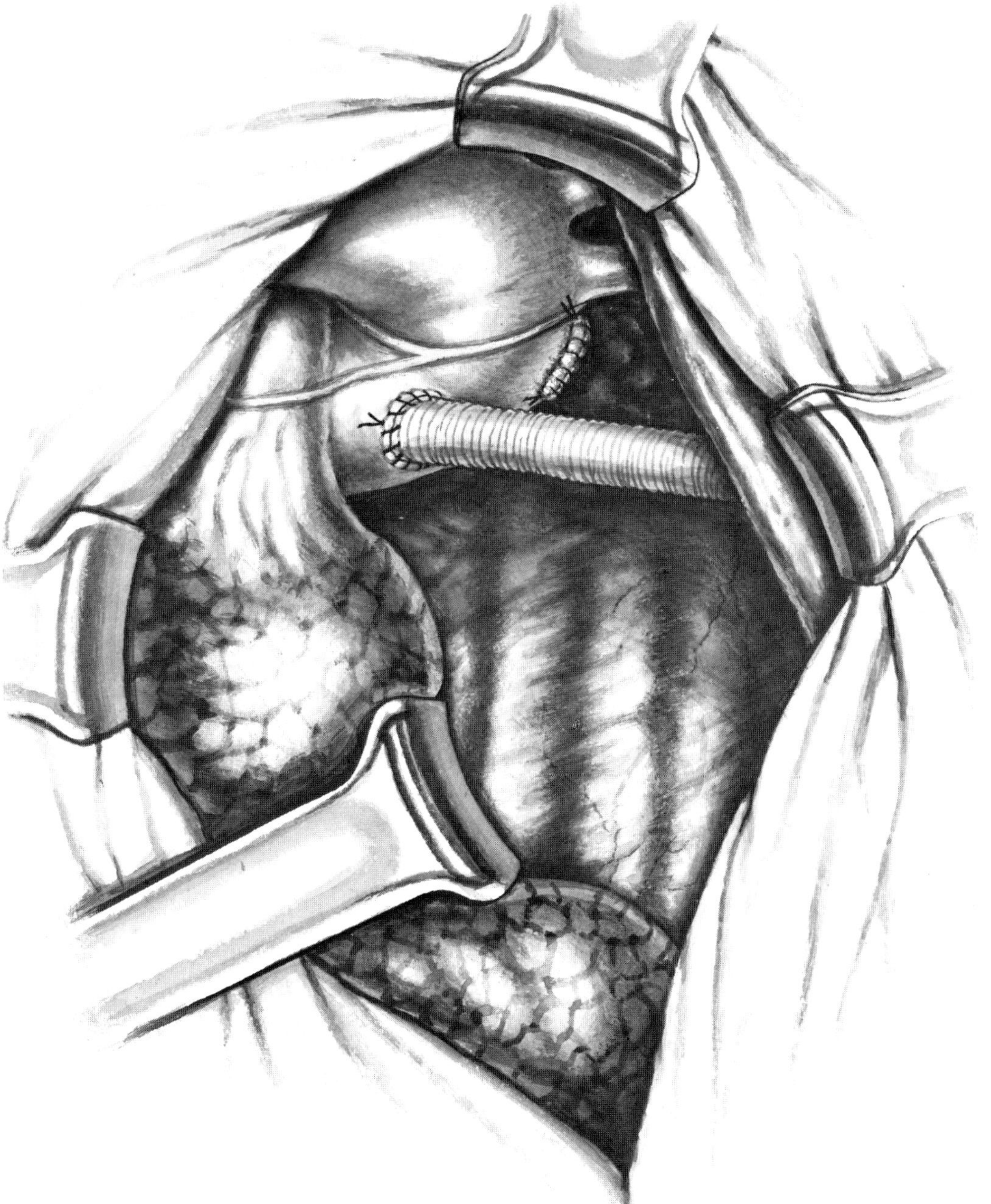

Fig. 556. Orifice of left subclavian artery is closed with sutures.

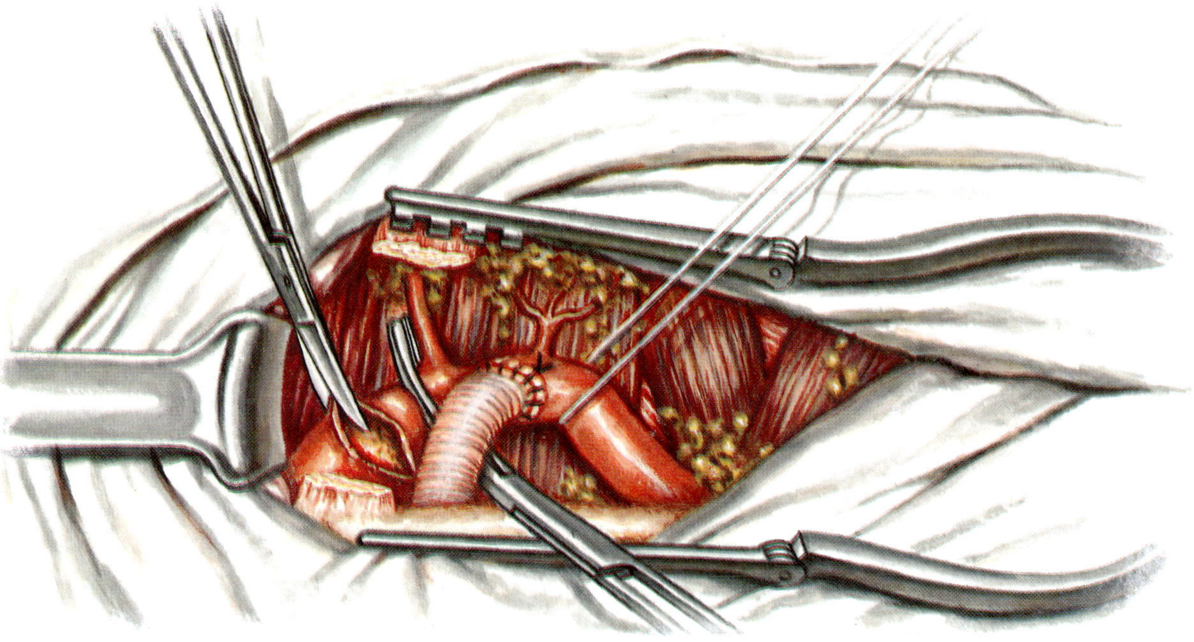

Fig. 557. Aneurysmal sac is cut away in supraclavicular region.

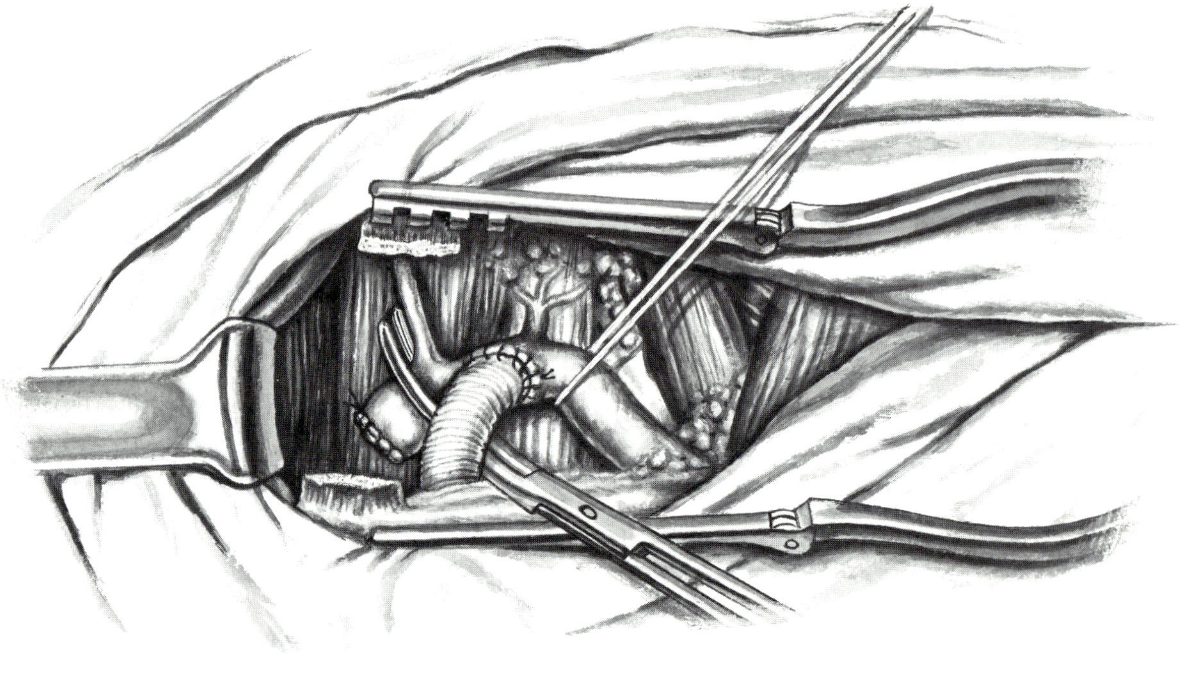

Fig. 558. Peripheral stump of subclavian artery is closed with sutures.

ENDARTERECTOMY FROM BRACHIOCEPHALIC TRUNK WITH LATERAL PLASTIC SURGERY

Partial median sternotomy is performed. The left brachiocephalic vein is freed from the surrounding tissues, held with a loop, and pulled caudally. Loops are also brought under the brachiocephalic trunk and the common carotid and subclavian arteries (Fig. 559). The common carotid and the subclavian arteries are clamped. A clamp is applied along the wall of the aorta at the site of the orifice of the brachiocephalic trunk. The anterior wall of the brachiocephalic trunk is cut lengthwise (Fig. 560), and endarterectomy is performed (Fig. 561). The atherosclerotic intima is detached with a special spade, and the thrombus is removed. The incision in the artery is closed with a graft shaped from the synthetic prosthesis, thus preventing the narrowing of its lumen (Fig. 562). The clamps are removed from the aorta and the common carotid and subclavian arteries, and the flow of blood is restored (Fig. 563). The edges of the sternum are drawn together with two wire sutures. The wound is sutured layer by layer.

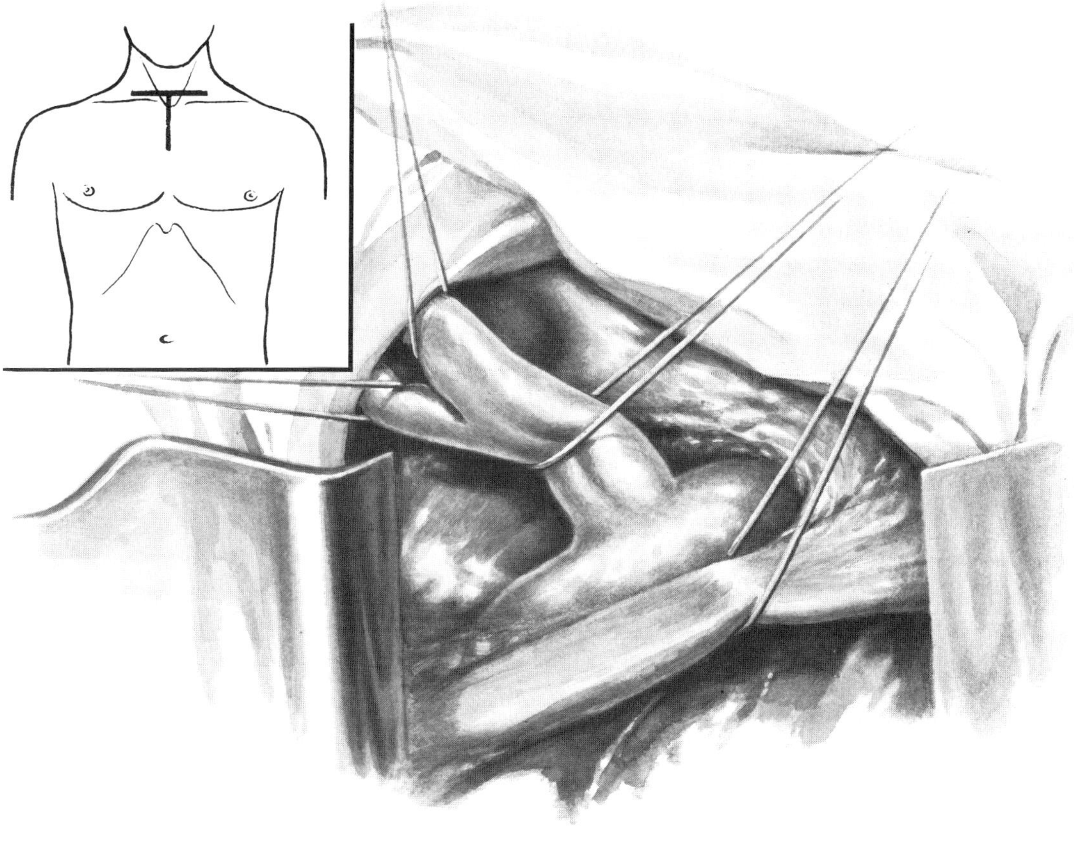

Fig. 559. Left brachiocephalic vein is mobilized and drawn aside by loop; brachiocephalic trunk and common carotid and subclavian arteries are held by loops. *Inset,* schema of operative approach.

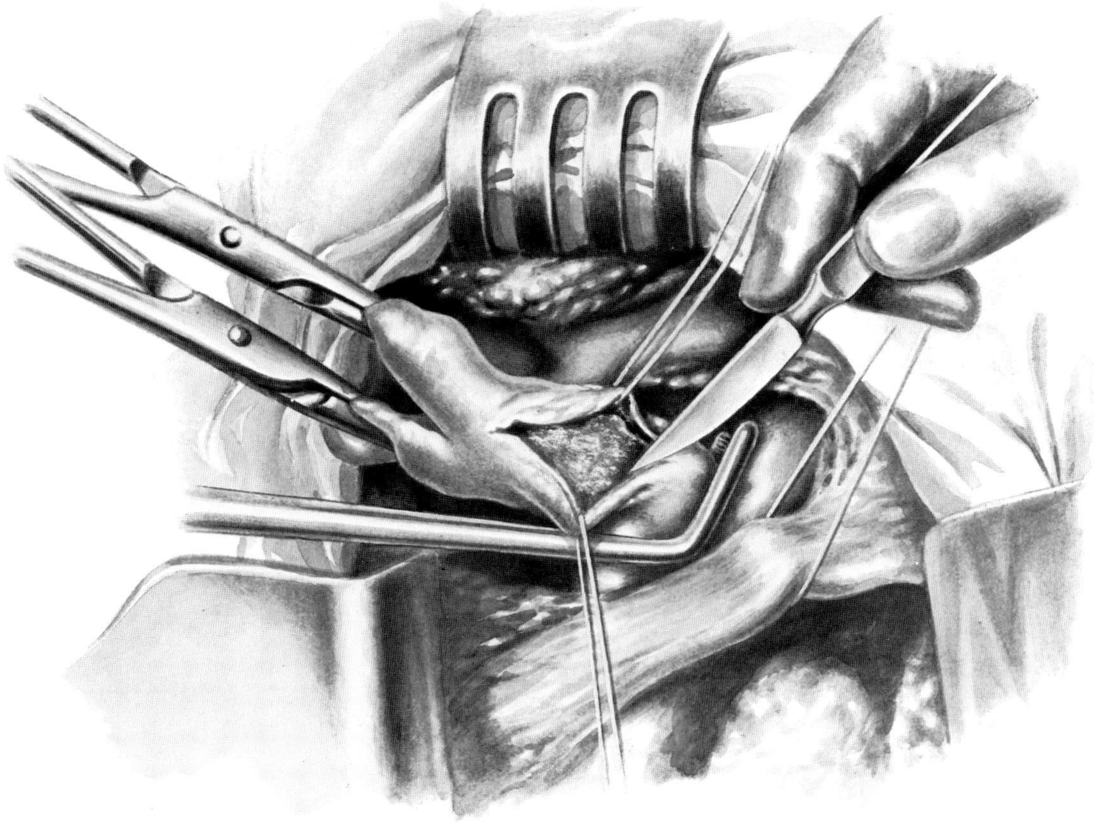

Fig. 560. Common carotid and subclavian arteries are clamped. Clamp is applied along side of aorta. Brachiocephalic trunk is cut lengthwise.

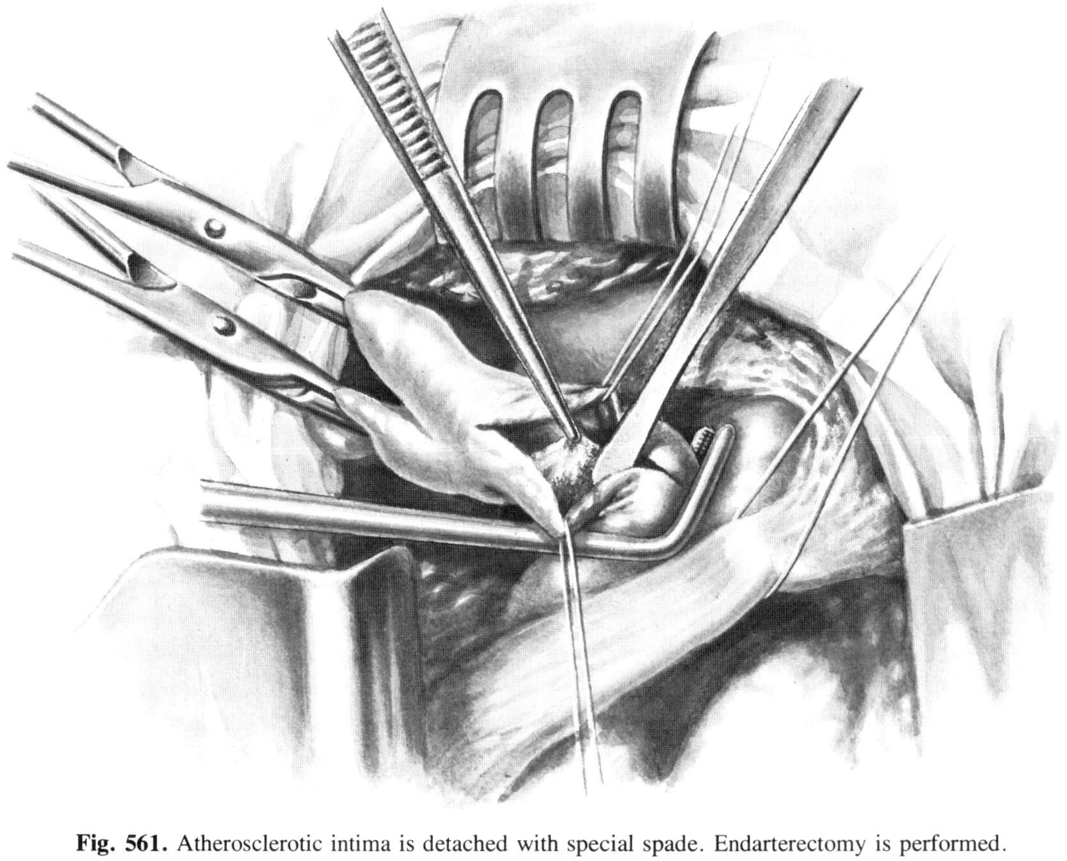

Fig. 561. Atherosclerotic intima is detached with special spade. Endarterectomy is performed.

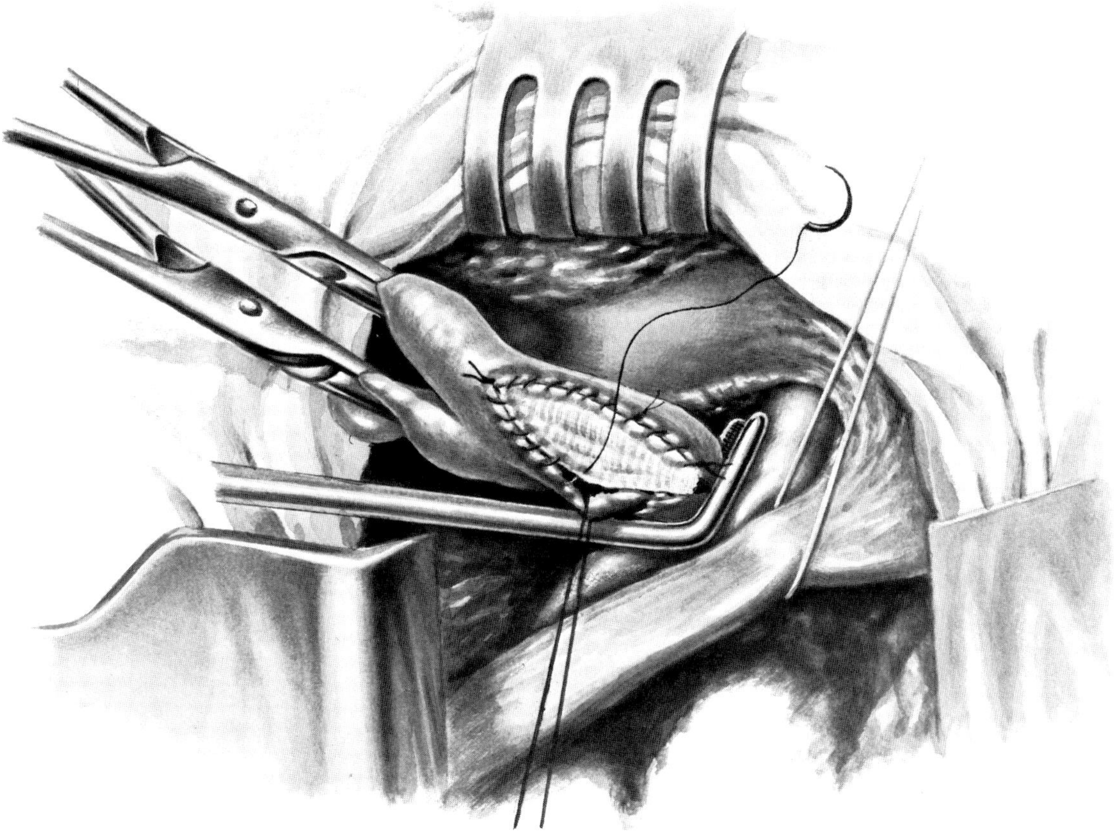

Fig. 562. Defect in brachiocephalic trunk is closed with graft.

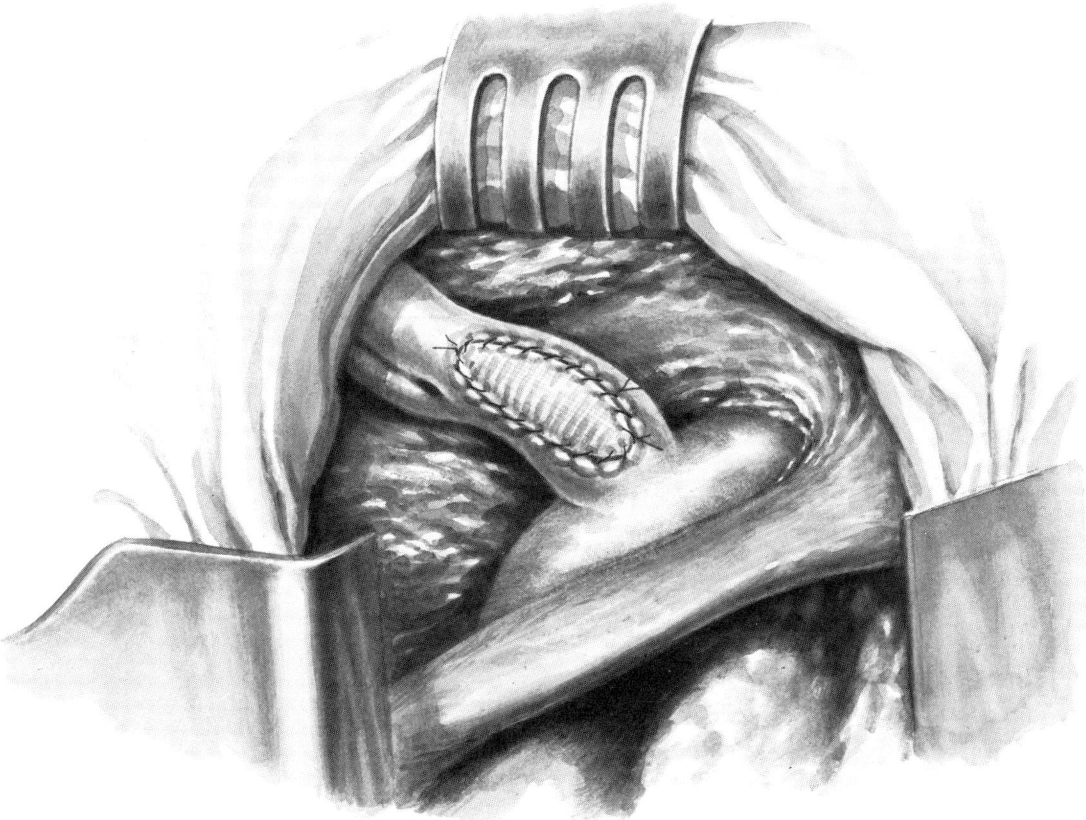

Fig. 563. Brachiocephalic trunk is connected to circulation.

RESECTION OF BRACHIOCEPHALIC TRUNK AND ITS PROSTHETICS

Partial median sternotomy is performed. The brachiocephalic trunk is freed from the surrounding tissues and held with a loop. The left brachiocephalic vein is pulled laterally (Fig. 564). The brachiocephalic trunk is clamped at the orifice and at the bifurcation and transected so that the line of the incision passes centrally to the occlusion (Fig. 565). Endarterectomy from the brachiocephalic trunk is carried out (Fig. 566).

The first stage in prosthetics of the trunk consists in the formation of the central anastomosis by means of a continuous suture (Fig. 567), after which the distal anastomosis is established. The clamps are removed from the reconstructed trunk, and the blood flow is restored (Fig. 568).

The wound is sutured layer by layer.

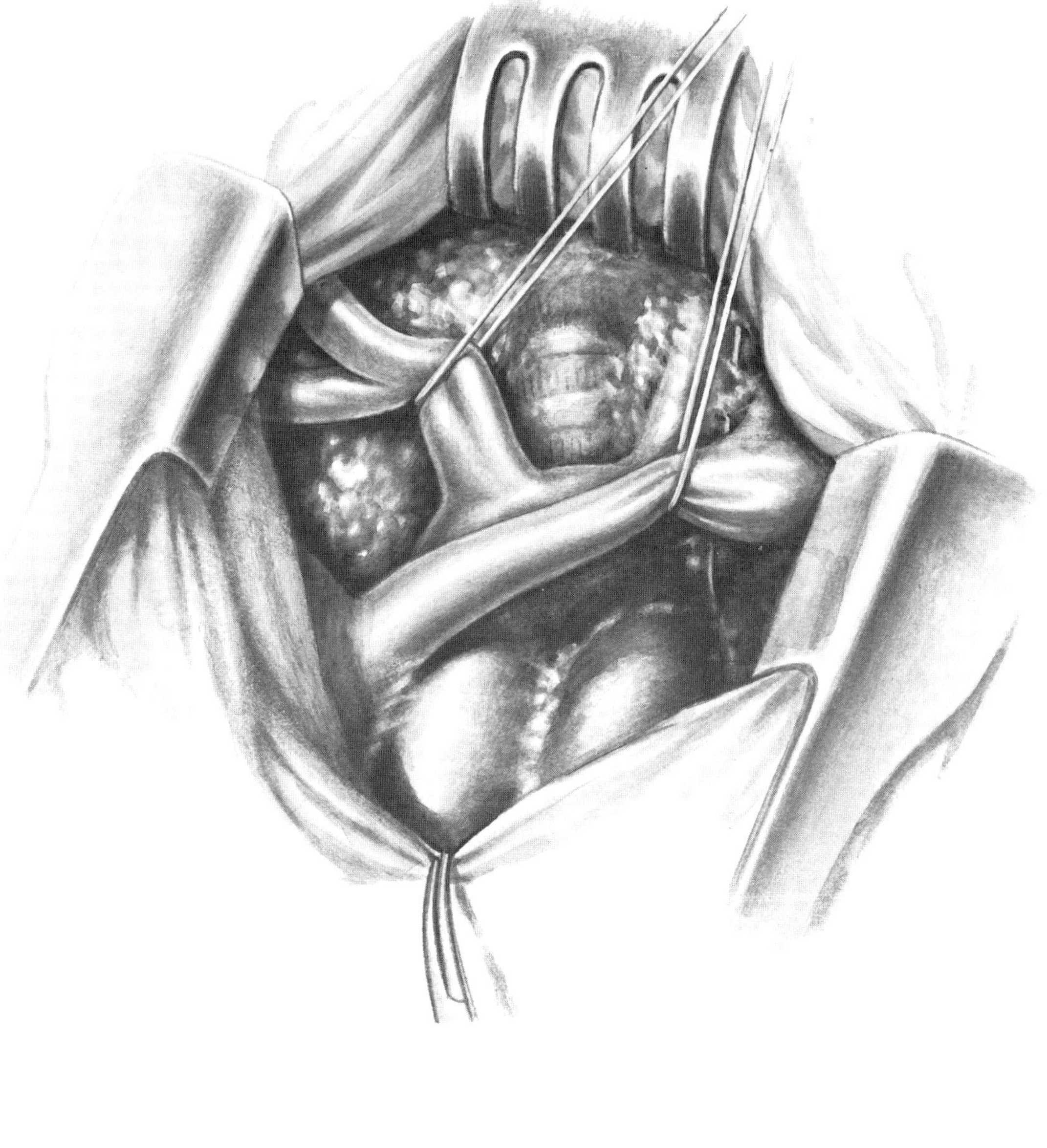

Fig. 564. Left brachiocephalic vein and artery are drawn aside by loops.

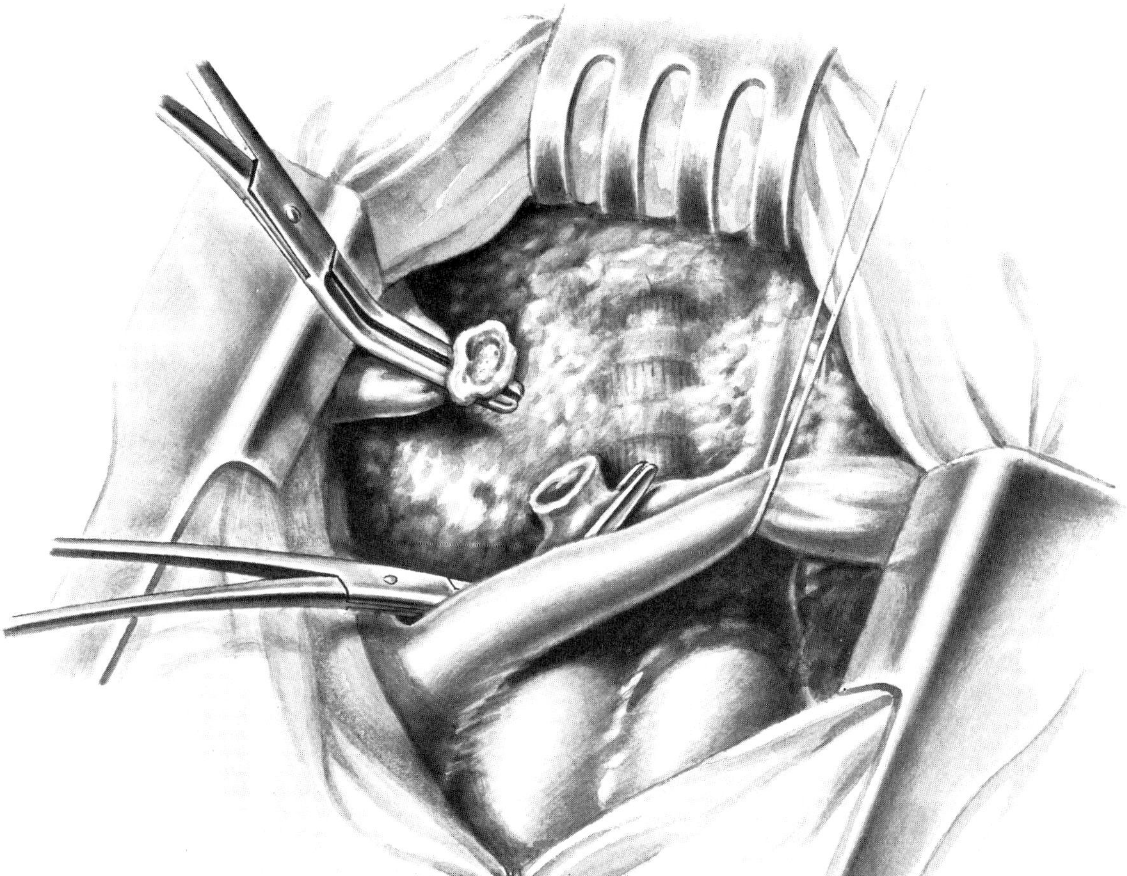

Fig. 565. Brachiocephalic trunk is clamped at its orifice and at bifurcation and transected.

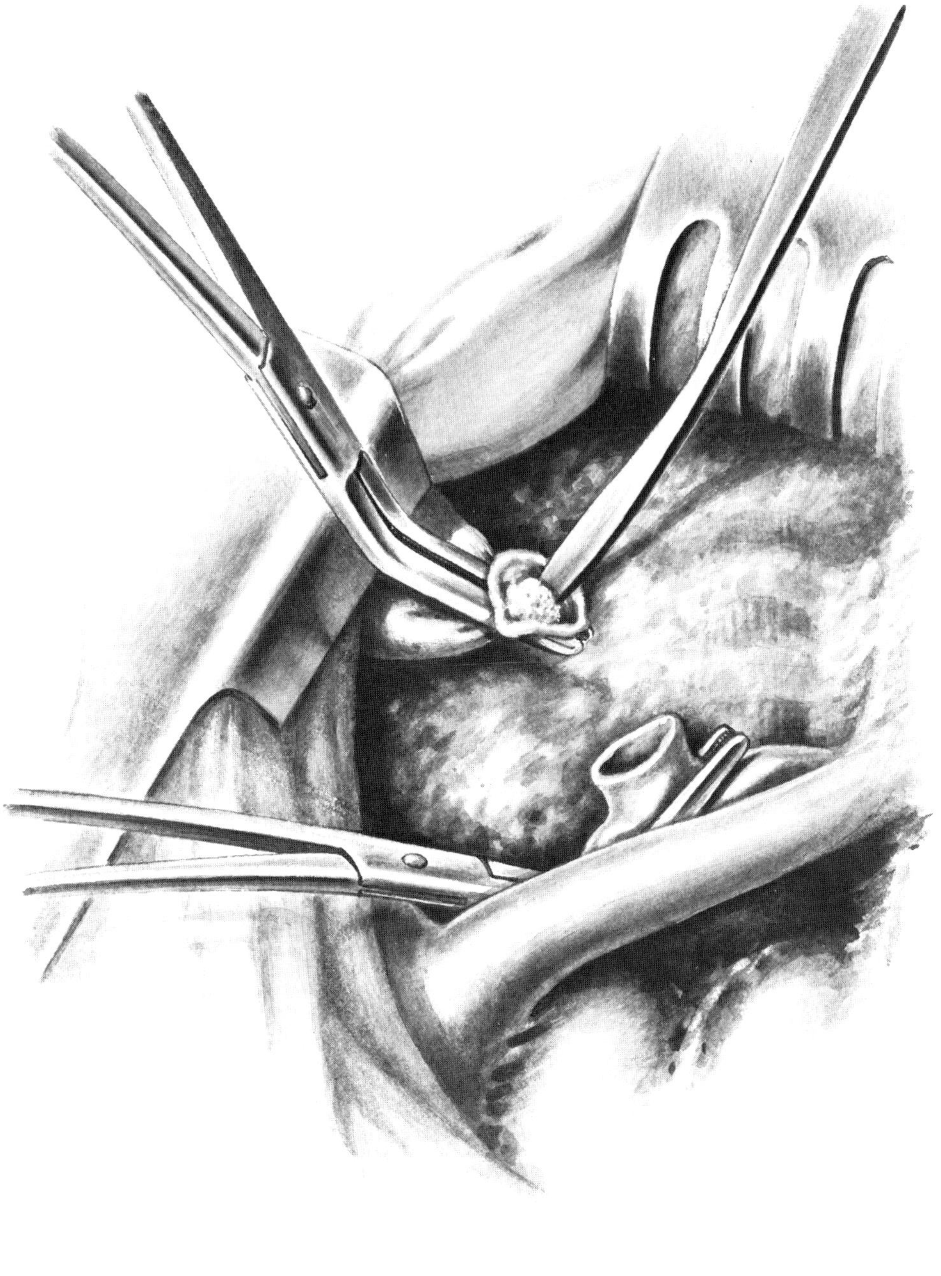

Fig. 566. Endarterectomy from distal segment of brachiocephalic trunk.

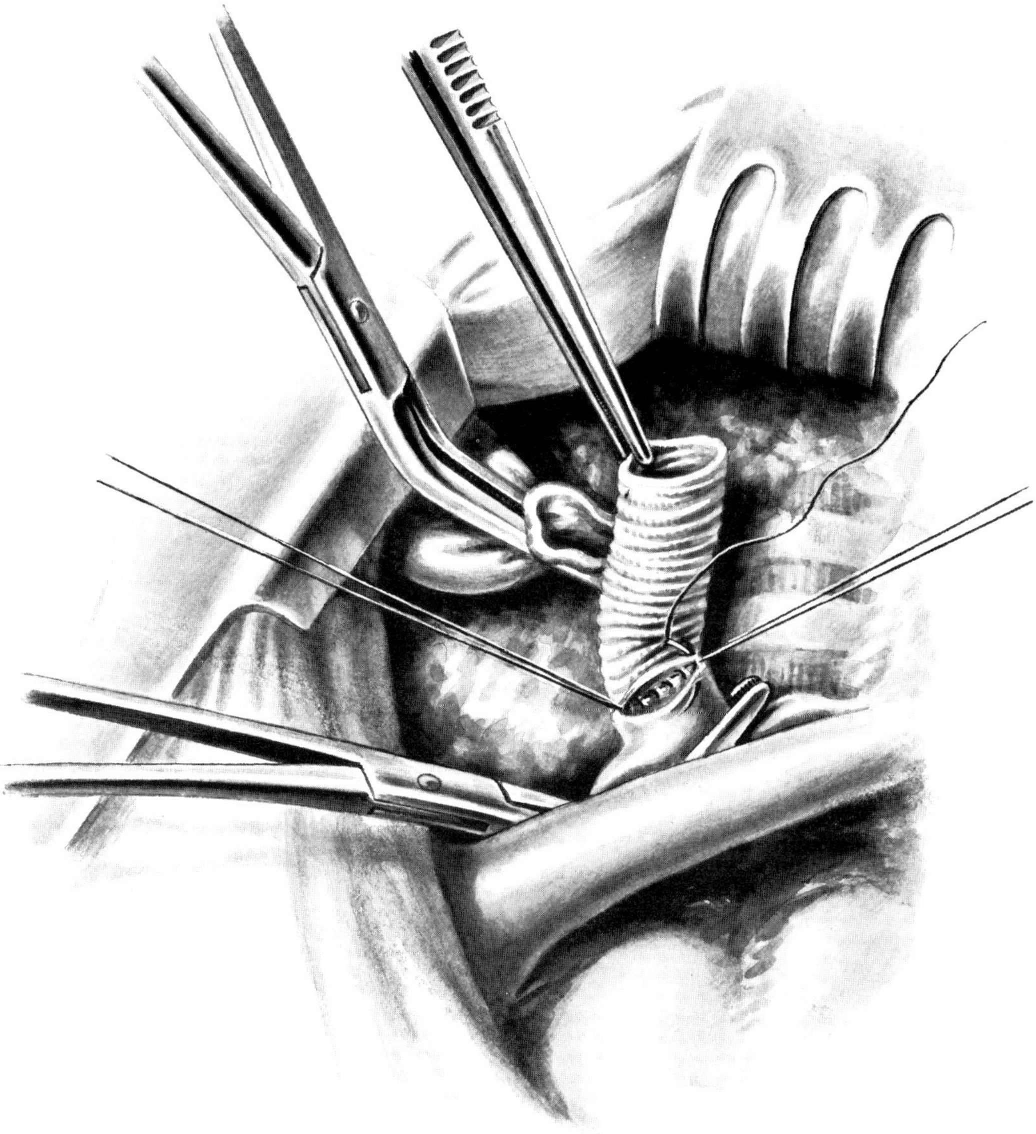

Fig. 567. Proximal anastomosis with prosthesis is formed.

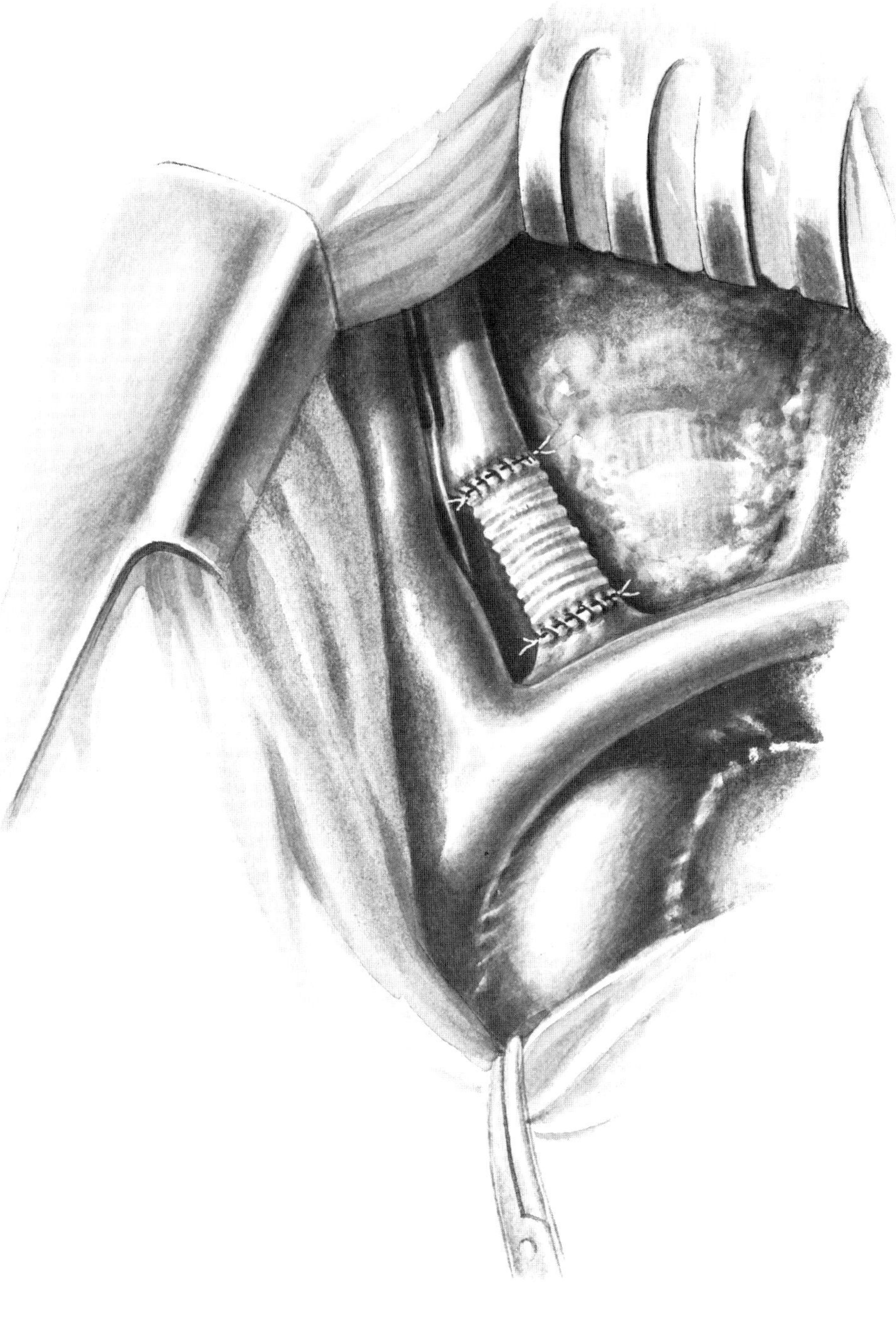

Fig. 568. Artery after reconstruction with prosthesis and restoration of blood flow.

ENDARTERECTOMY FROM ORIFICE OF LEFT VERTEBRAL ARTERY

For operative approach to the vertebral artery a skin incision is made from the jugular notch to the inner border of the lateral third of the trapezius muscle; a combined approach may also be employed (Fig. 569).

The incision is made through the skin, the superficial fascia, and the platysma, and the sternocleidomastoid muscle or its lateral head is transected. The posterior wall of the sheath of the sternocleidomastoid muscle is cut, and the neurovascular bundle of the neck is exposed (Fig. 570); the bundle is drawn medially; the phrenic nerve is freed above the anterior scalene muscle and moved laterally. The anterior scalene muscle is transected (Fig. 571) and the subclavian artery exposed; a loop is brought under it. The artery is raised, and its wall with the orifice of the vertebral artery in it is clamped laterally. A clamp is applied to the vertebral artery distal to the occlusion (Fig. 572). The vertebral vein is ligated and transected. The subclavian artery is opened with a semioval incision where the vertebral artery arises from it (Fig. 573). Endarterectomy from the orifice of the vertebral artery is carried out by the eversion method (Fig. 574). After the pathologically changed intima has been removed together with the atherosclerotic plaque or thrombus, the subclavian artery is repaired with a continuous suture (Fig. 575), the clamps are removed, and the blood flow in the vertebral artery is restored.

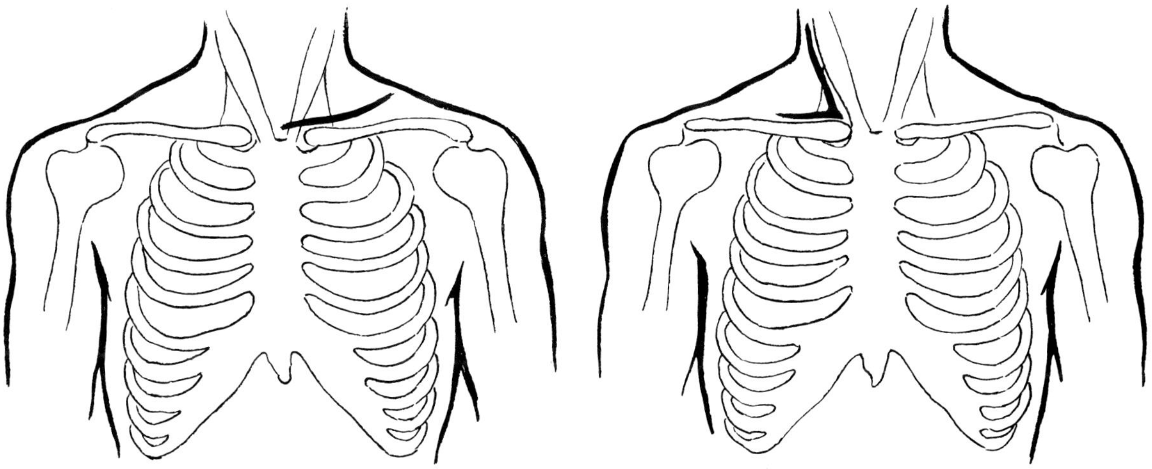

Fig. 569. Schema of operative approaches to vertebral artery.

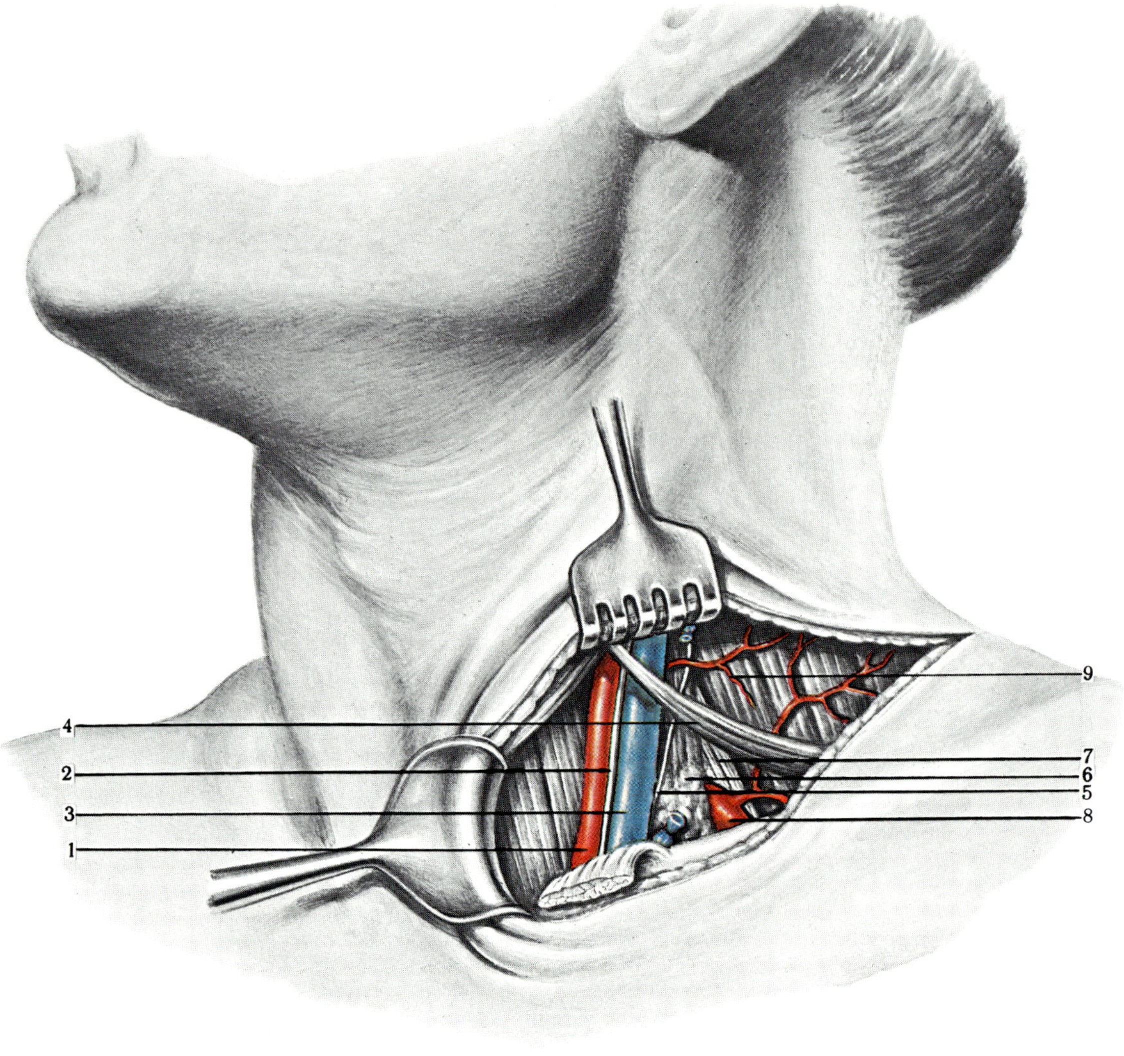

Fig. 570. Topographoanatomical relationships in operative wound after transection of sternocleidomastoid muscle.

1 Common carotid artery
2 Vagus nerve
3 Internal jugular vein
4 Omohyoid muscle
5 Phrenic nerve
6 Anterior scalene muscle
7 Middle scalene muscle
8 Subclavian artery, third portion
9 Transverse cervical artery

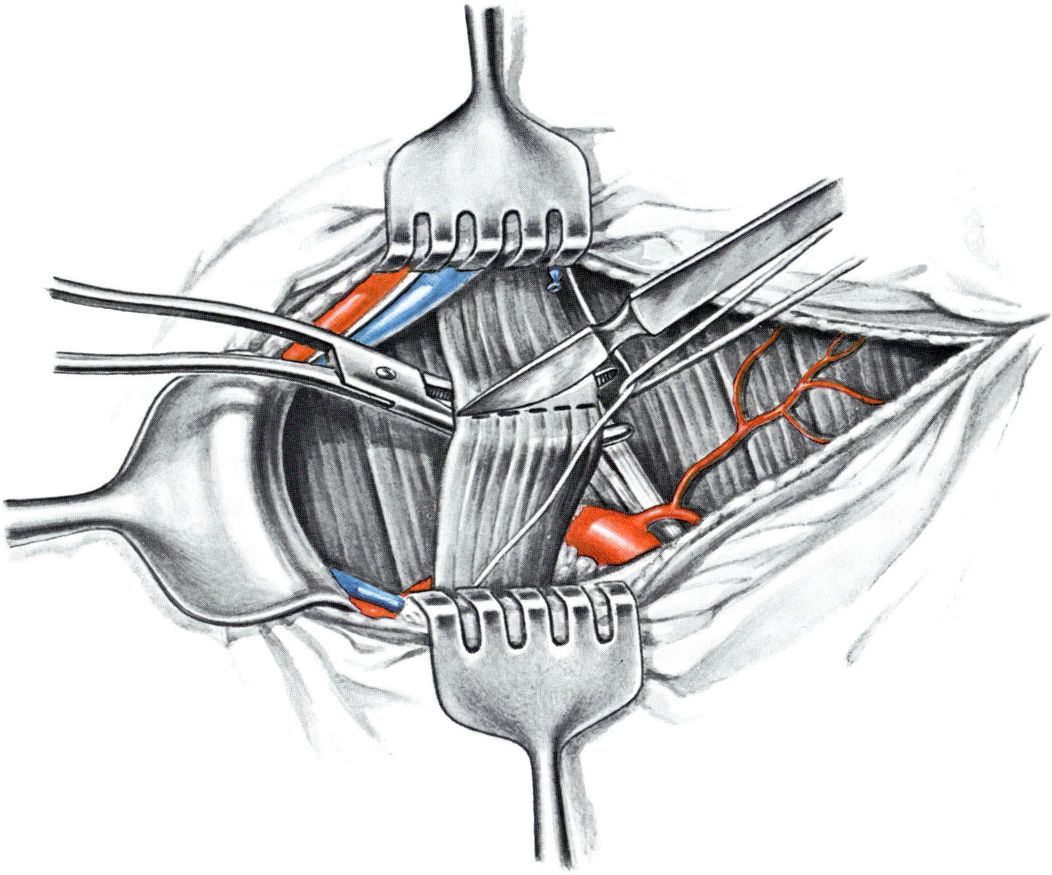

Fig. 571. Transection of anterior scalene muscle. Neurovascular bundle of neck is drawn medially; phrenic nerve is raised by loop and drawn laterally.

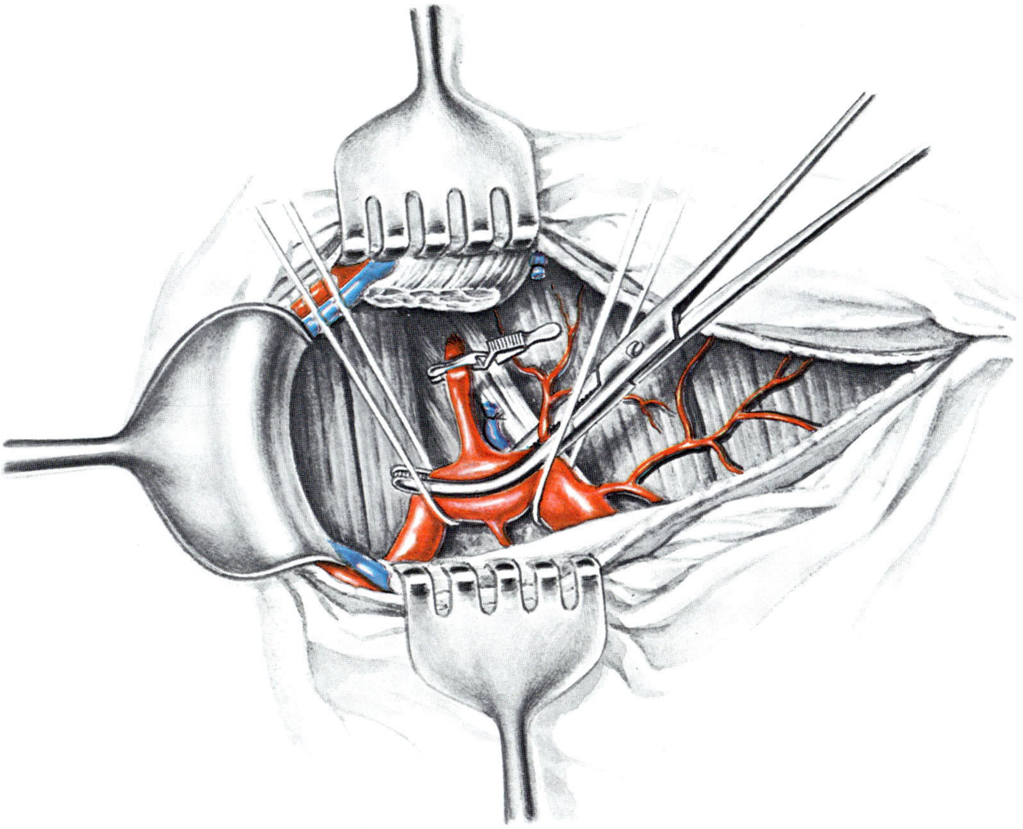

Fig. 572. Subclavian artery is raised on loops. Clamp is placed along its wall where the orifice of vertebral artery is located. Vertebral artery is clamped distal to occlusion.

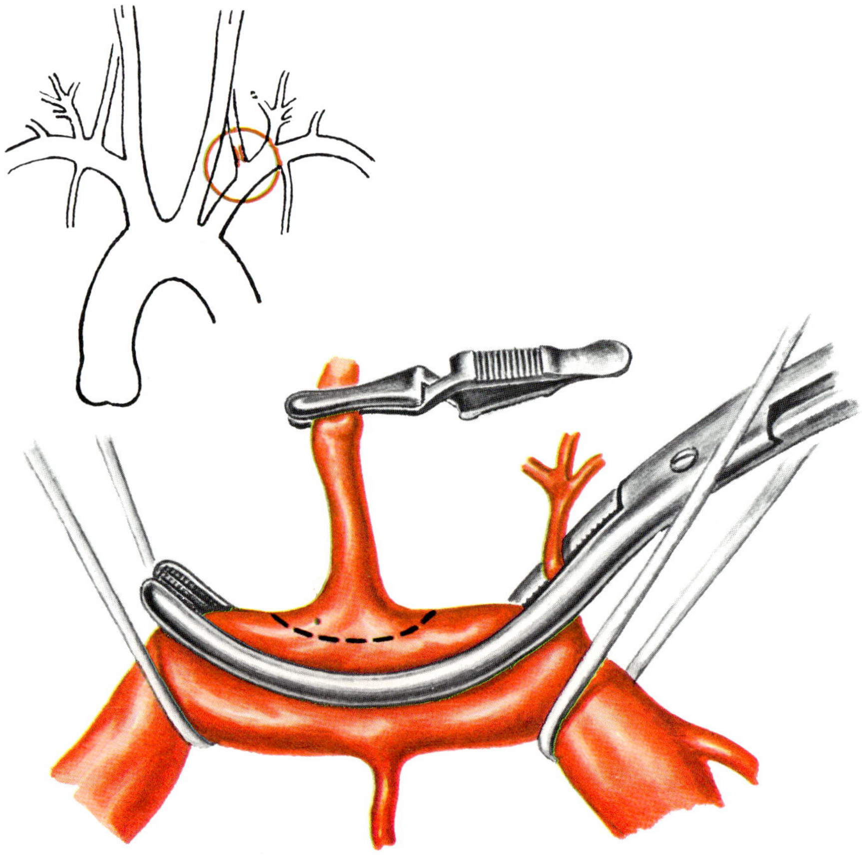

Fig. 573. Site of incision of subclavian artery at orifice of vertebral artery is indicated by dashed line. *Inset,* stenosis of orifice of vertebral artery.

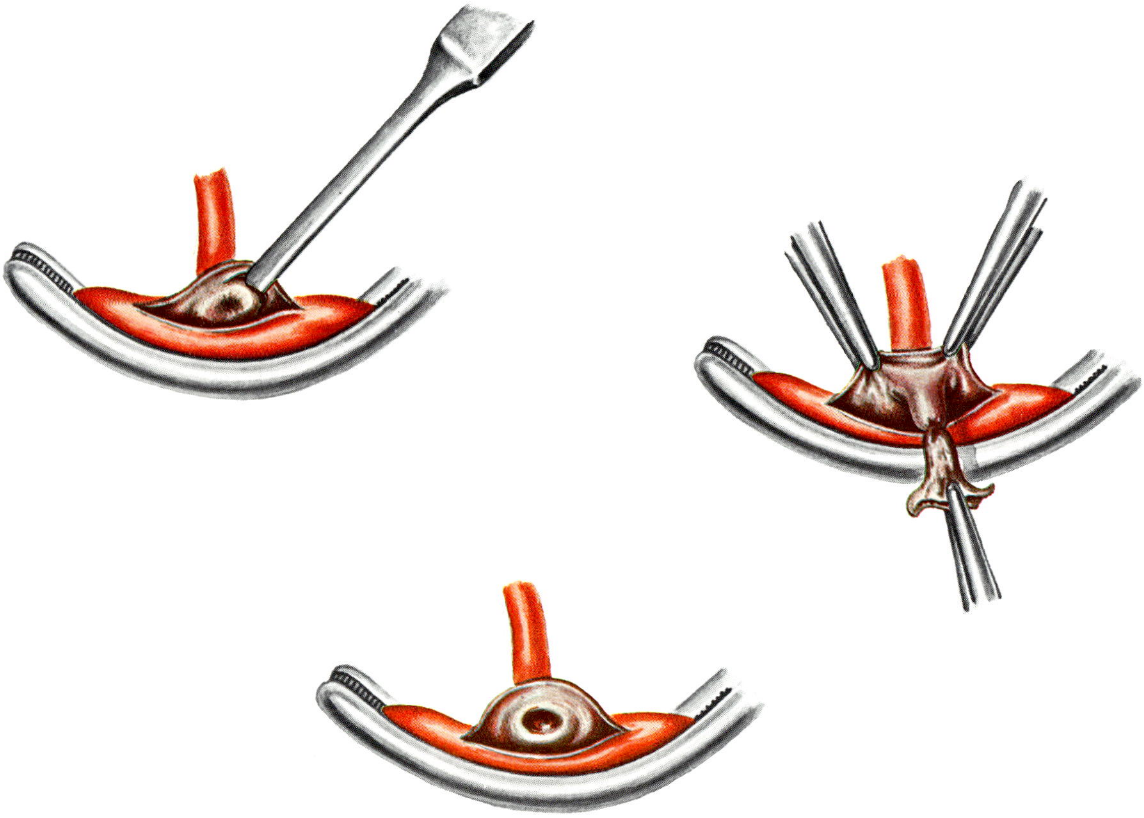

Fig. 574. Eversion endarterectomy from orifice of vertebral artery through lumen of subclavian artery.

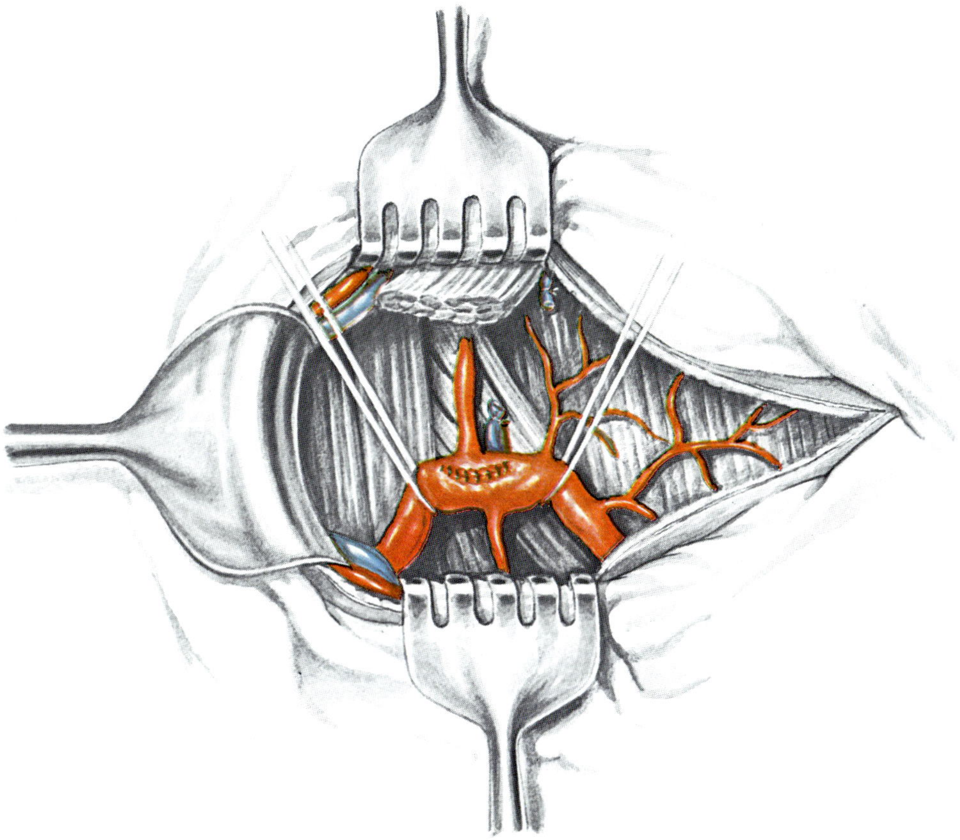

Fig. 575. Incision in subclavian artery is closed with continuous suture, clamps are removed, and blood flow is restored.

RESECTION OF ABNORMALLY TORTUOUS CAROTID AND SUBCLAVIAN ARTERIES

In affection of the carotid artery the skin incision is made along the lateral border of the sternocleidomastoid muscle from the mandibular angle to the jugular notch. When the subclavian artery is affected, the incision is made 1 to 2 cm above the clavicle from the sternoclavicular articulation to the inner border of the trapezius muscle. In tortuosity of both arteries the combined approach is employed (Fig. 576).

The lateral head of the sternocleidomastoid muscle is transected, and the dorsal wall of its sheath and the anterior scalene muscle are cut. The internal jugular vein and the phrenic nerve are drawn medially (Fig. 577). The common carotid and the subclavian arteries are freed from the surrounding tissues, and loops are brought under them. The common carotid artery is clamped peripheral and central to the pathological segment and resected (Fig. 578). The length of the resection

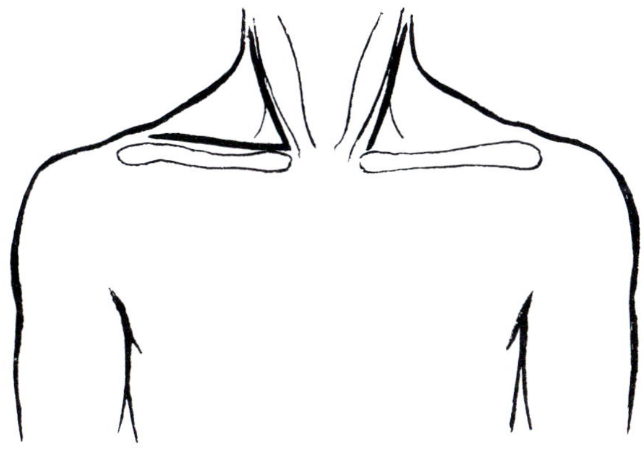

Fig. 576. Schema of operative approaches.

is determined so that in reconstruction of the common carotid and the subclavian arteries the anastomoses will be created without stretching. The use of a prosthesis or an autograft makes the operation more difficult. The common carotid and subclavian arteries are reconstructed by end-to-end anastomoses. The technique of establishing such an anastomosis with Halsted sutures is represented in Fig. 579.

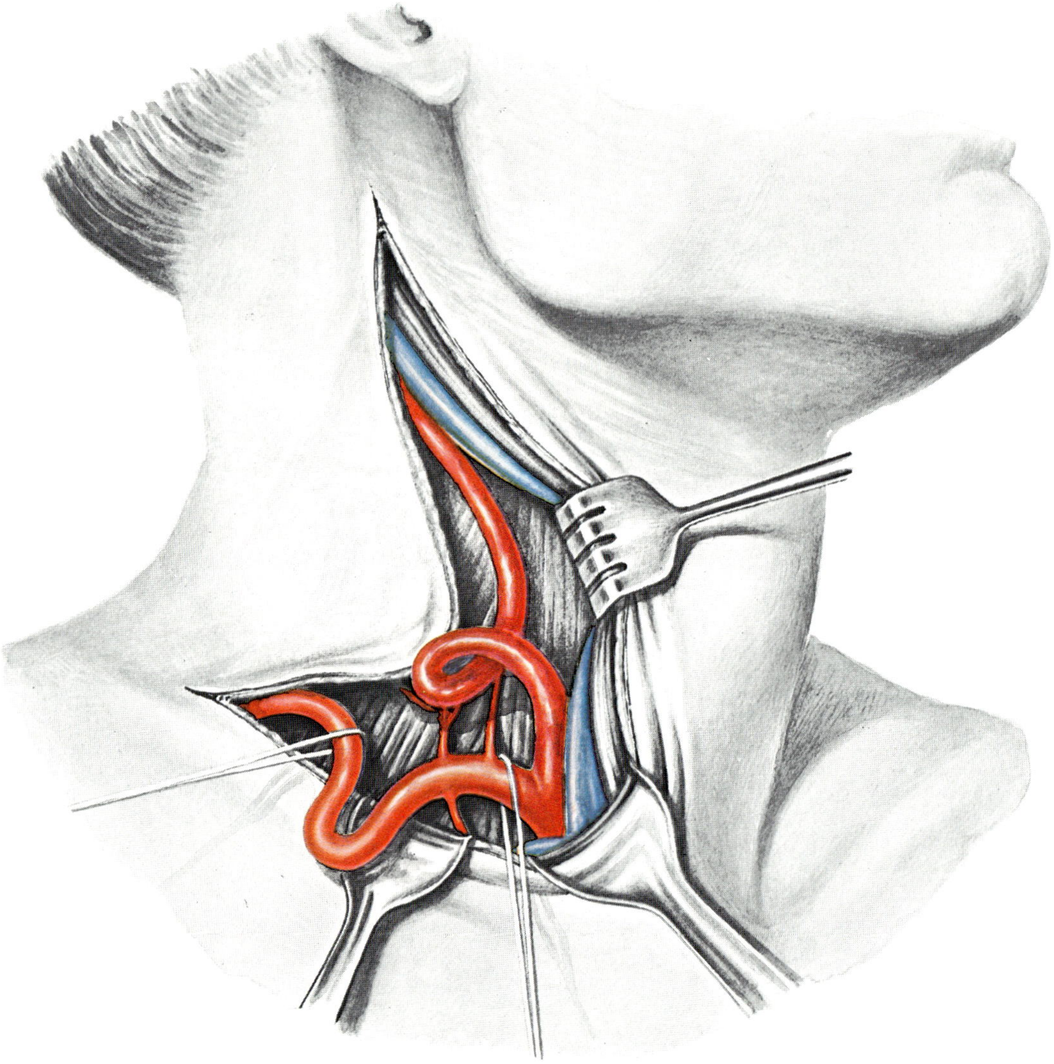

Fig. 577. View of operative wound after subclavian and common carotid arteries have been mobilized. Subclavian artery is held by loops.

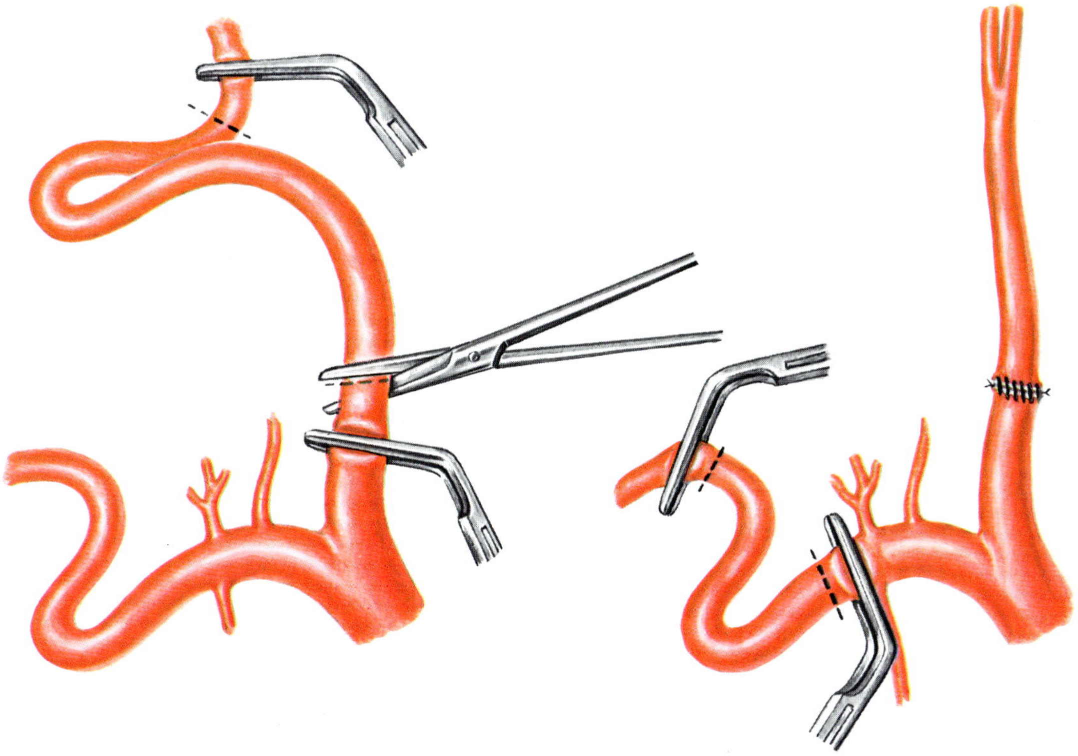

Fig. 578. Common carotid artery is clamped. Diseased segment of common carotid artery is resected.

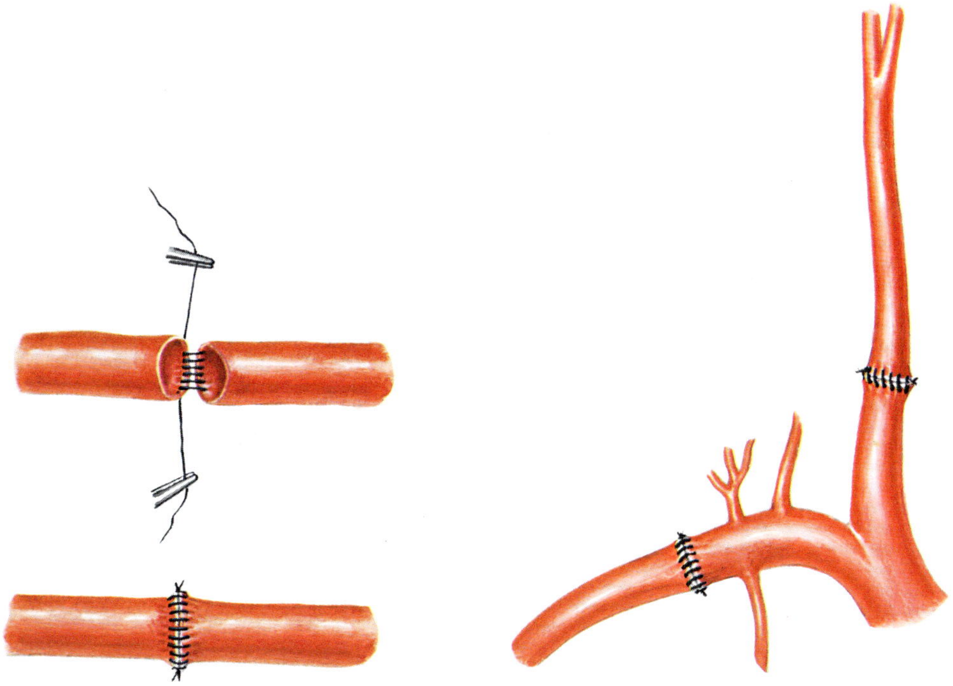

Fig. 579. Techniques of end-to-end anastomosis by means of Halsted sutures. View of reconstructed subclavian and common carotid arteries.

SHUNTING OF SUPERIOR VENA CAVA IN ITS OCCLUSION

A shunt is created in thrombosis or cicatricial stricture of the superior vena cava (''the superior vena cava syndrome'') (Fig. 580). The intervention is performed through a right anterolateral approach in the fourth intercostal space. The pericardium is opened wide, ventral and parallel to the phrenic nerve. The superior vena cava is freed from the surrounding tissues cranial to the lesion; whenever necessary, both brachiocephalic veins are also freed (Fig. 581).

The brachiocephalic veins are clamped, and a round

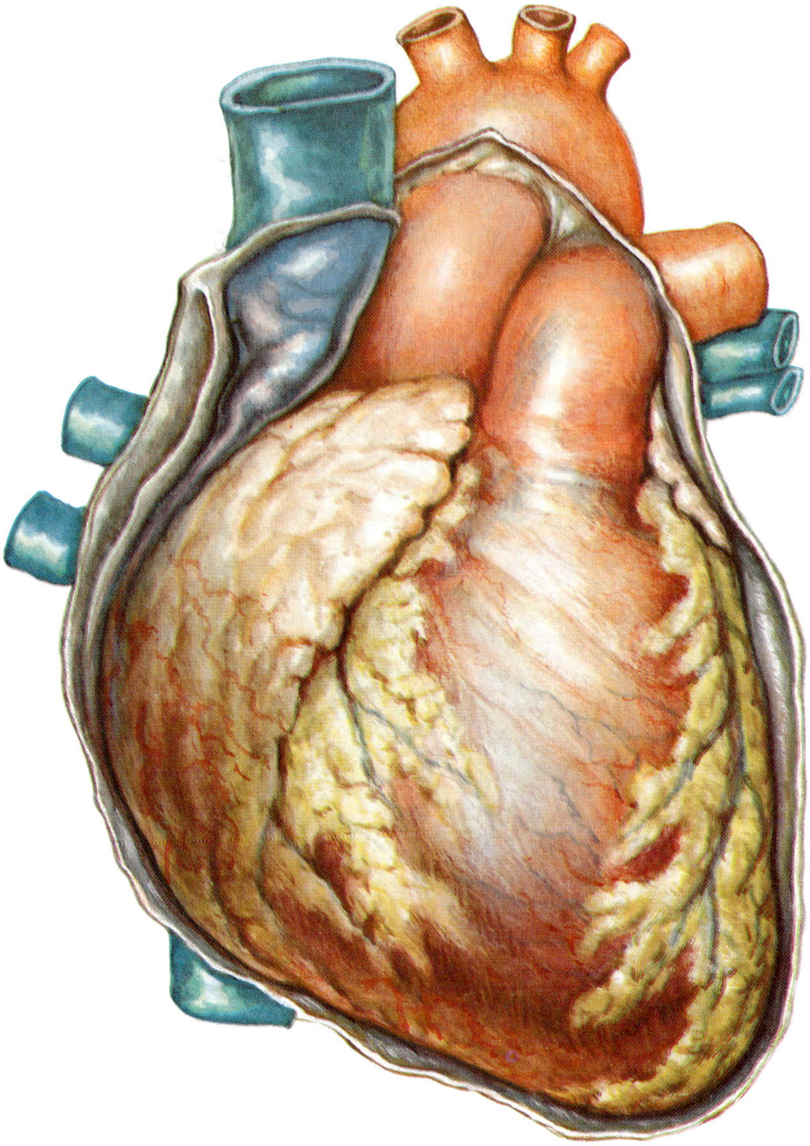

Fig. 580. View of superior vena cava in thrombosis.

opening is formed in the anterior wall of the superior vena cava for anastomosing (Fig. 582). A plastic prosthesis of an appropriate diameter is grafted (Fig. 583). The posterior wall of the anastomosis is formed by means of a continuous Halsted suture. The ends of this continuous suture are secured by tying them with the interrupted sutures. The anterior wall of the anastomosis is formed with blanket or Halsted sutures. With the upper anastomosis established, the anastomosis between the right atrial auricle and the prosthesis is begun. Satinsky's clamp is applied to the base of the auricle, and a round opening is formed on its lateral wall (Fig. 584). The anastomosis between the auricle and the prosthesis is formed in the same manner as the upper anastomosis (Fig. 585). After the clamps are removed, drainage of venous blood from the system of the vena cava into the right atrium is restored (Fig. 586).

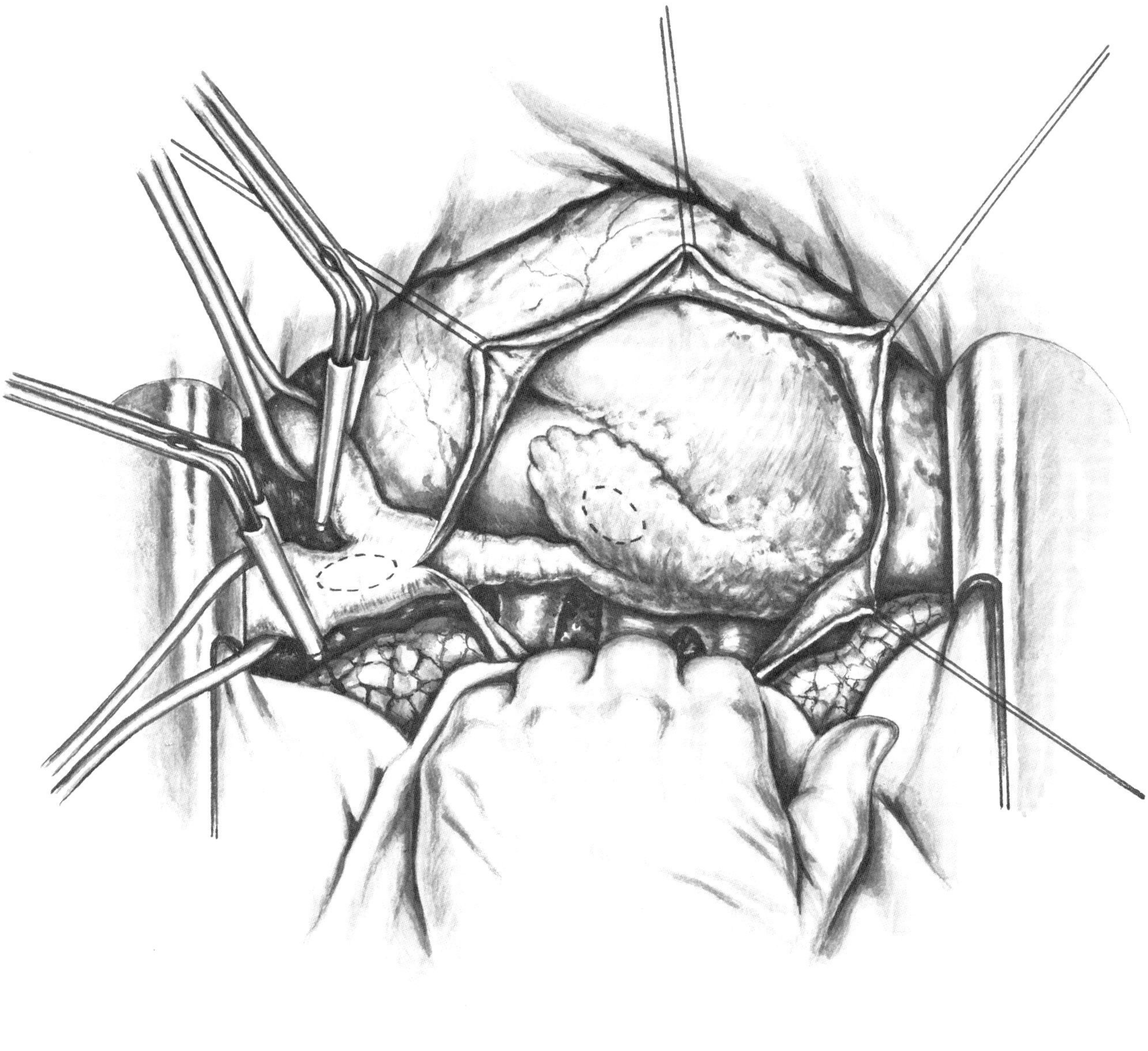

Fig. 581. Pericardium is opened. Clamps are applied to cerebrobrachial veins.

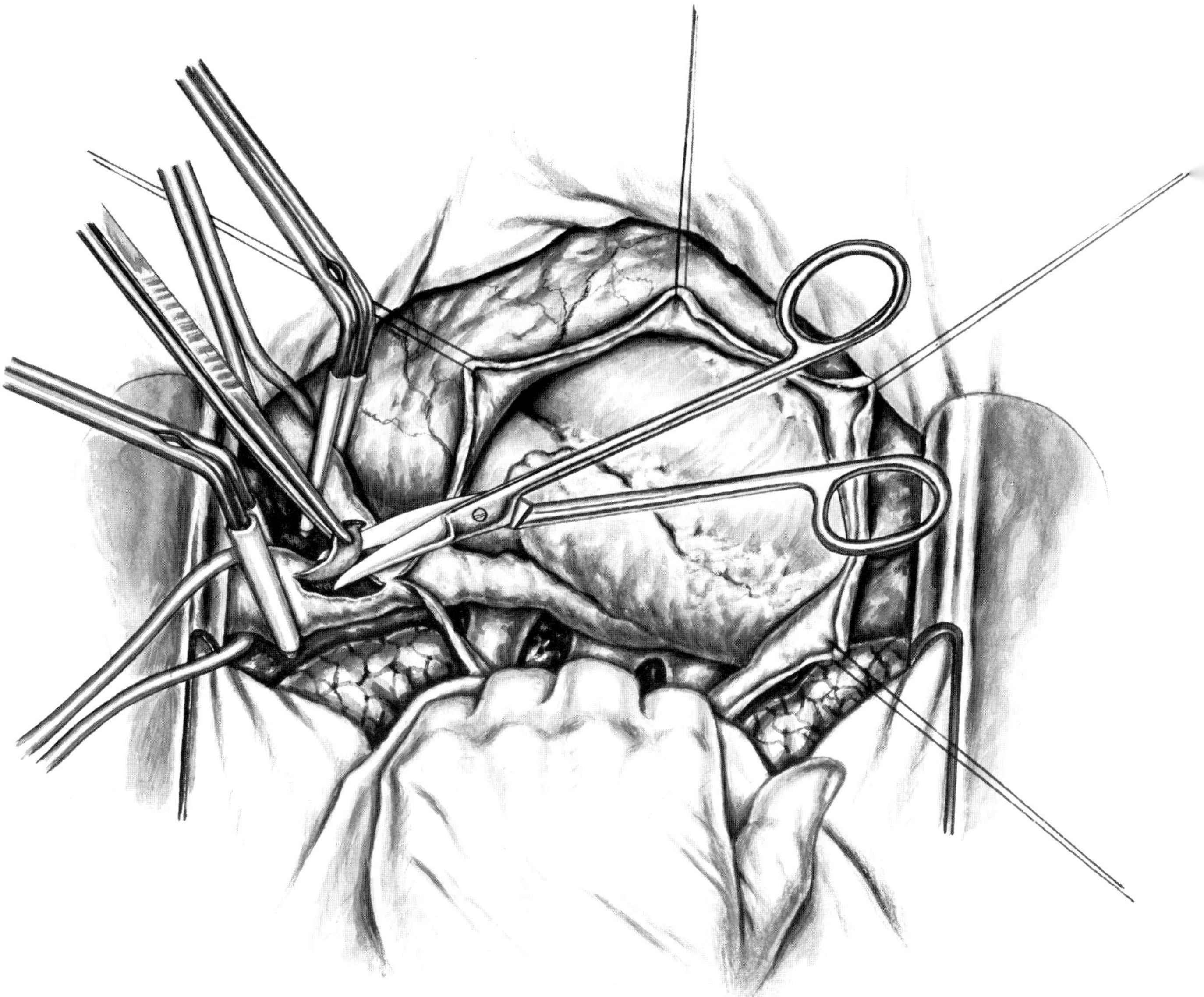

Fig. 582. Opening is formed in wall of vena cava for anastomosis.

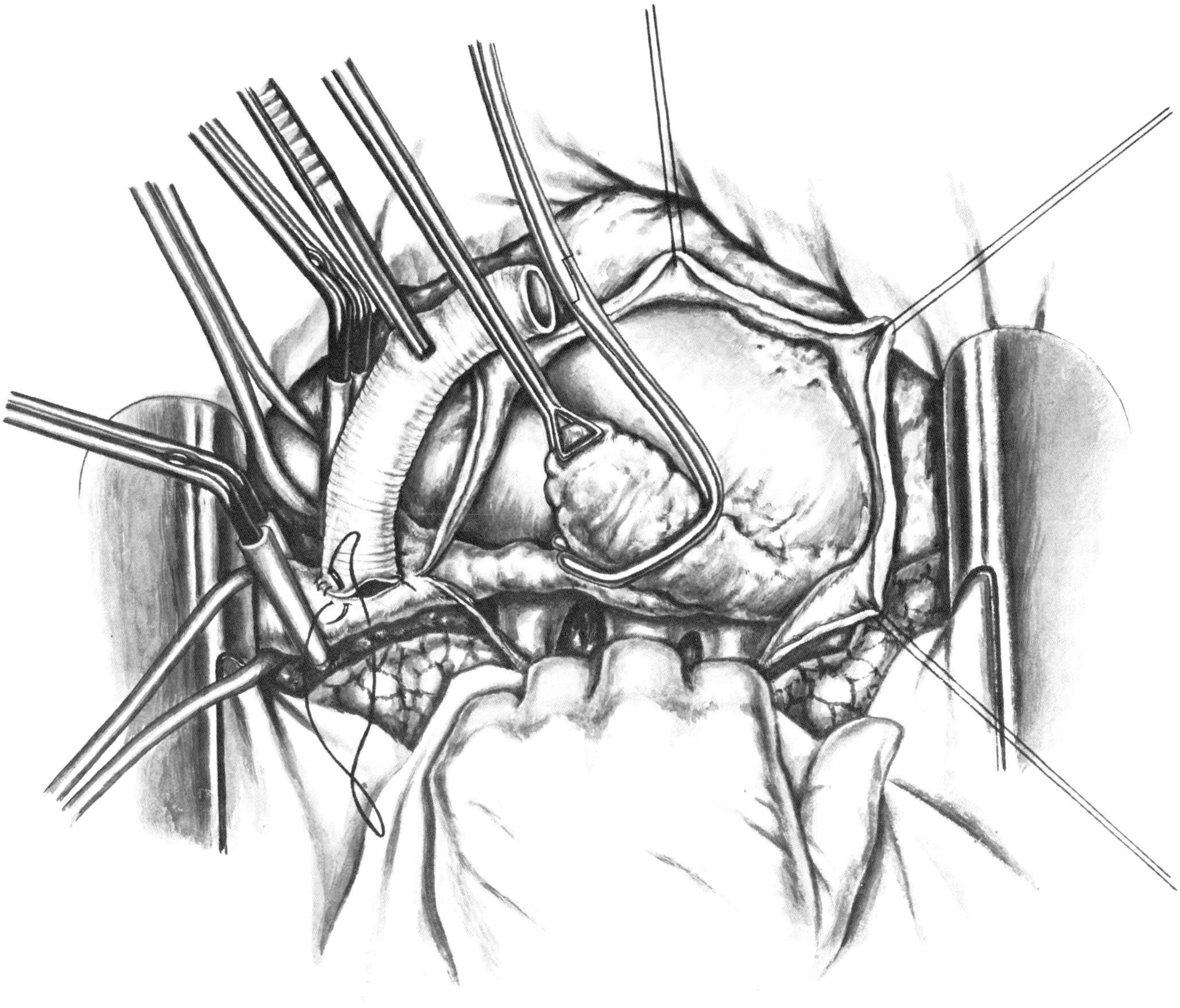

Fig. 583. Formation of anastomosis between vena cava and prosthesis.

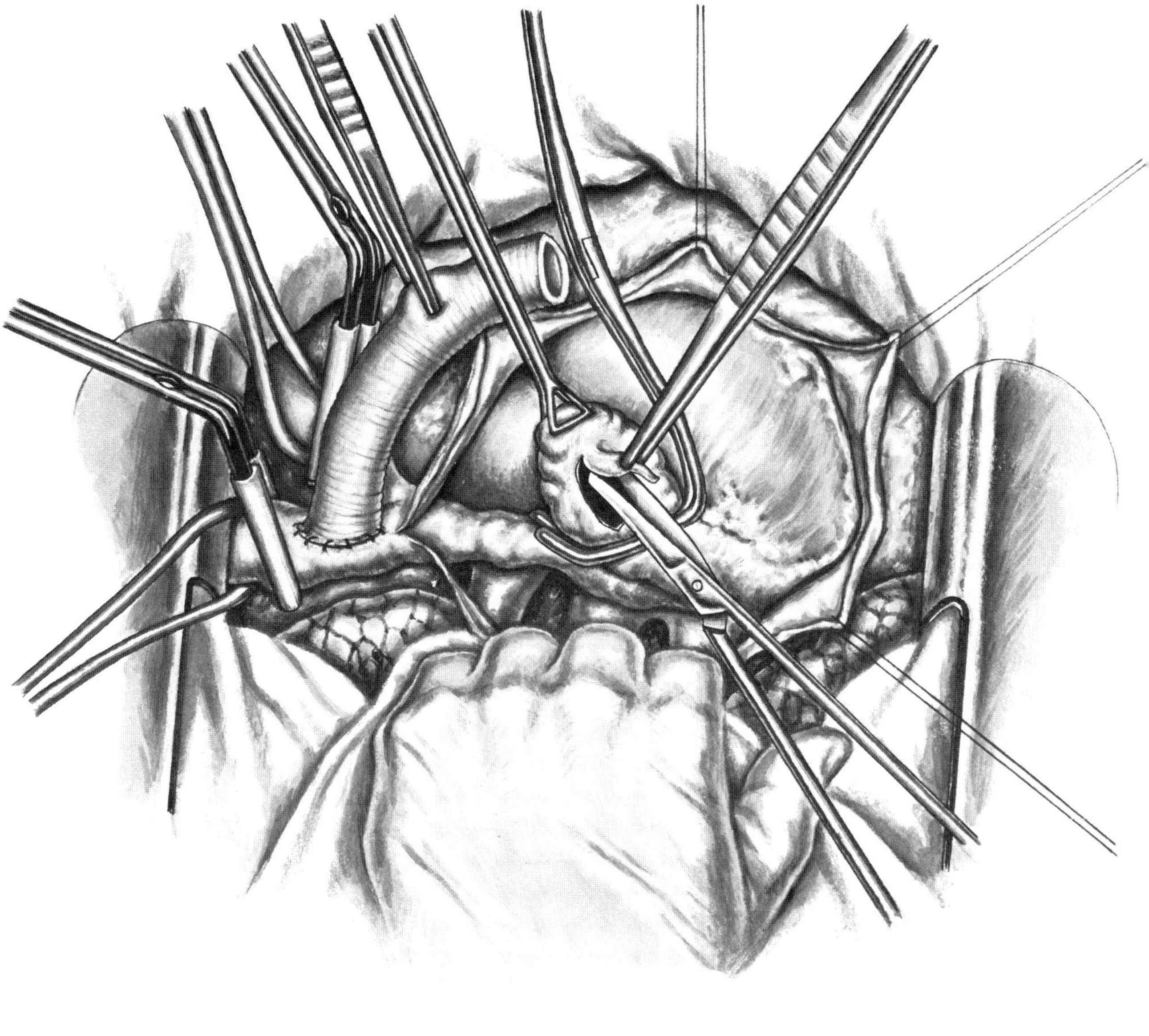

Fig. 584. Opening is formed in right atrial auricle for anastomosis.

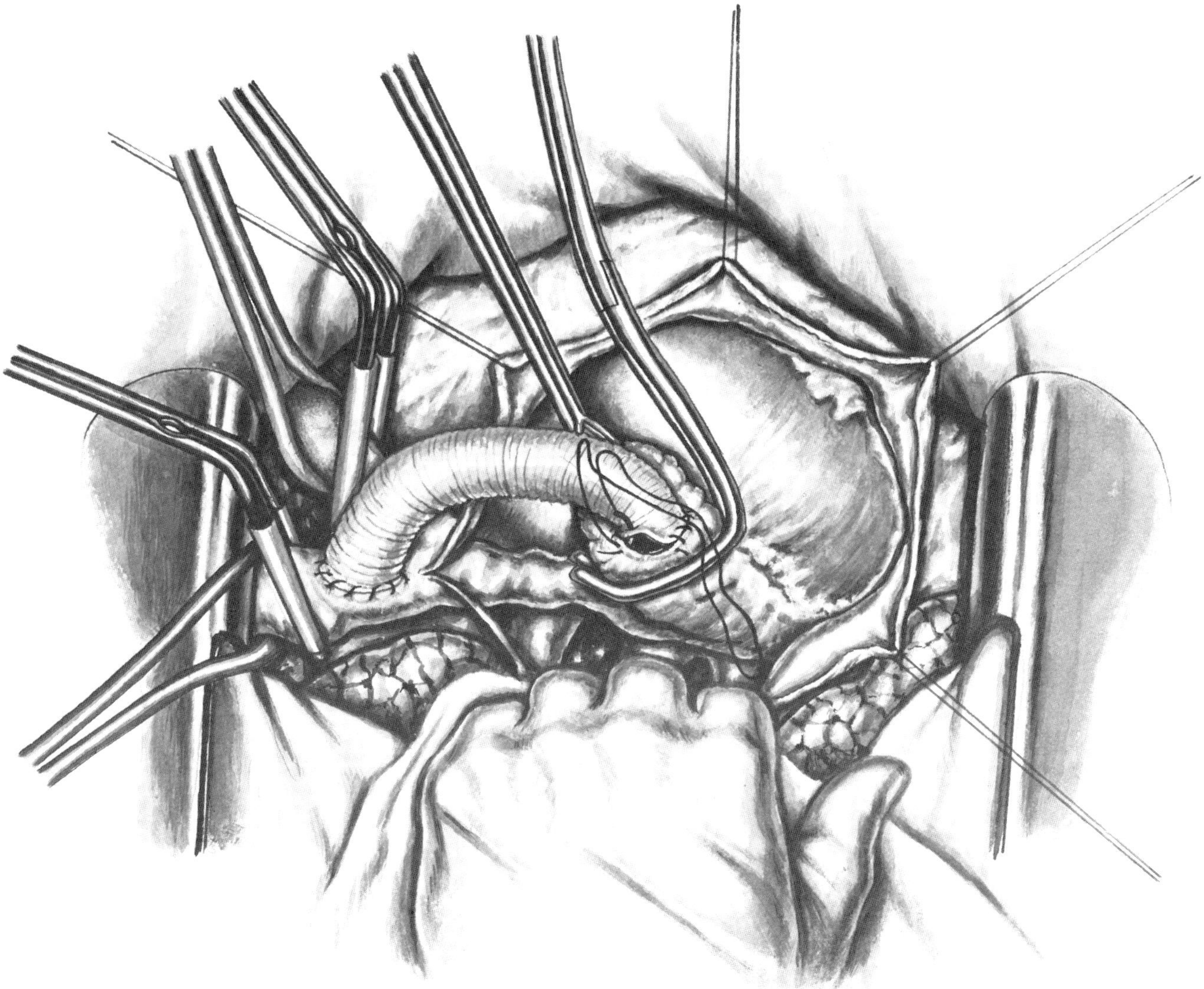

Fig. 585. Formation of anastomosis with auricle.

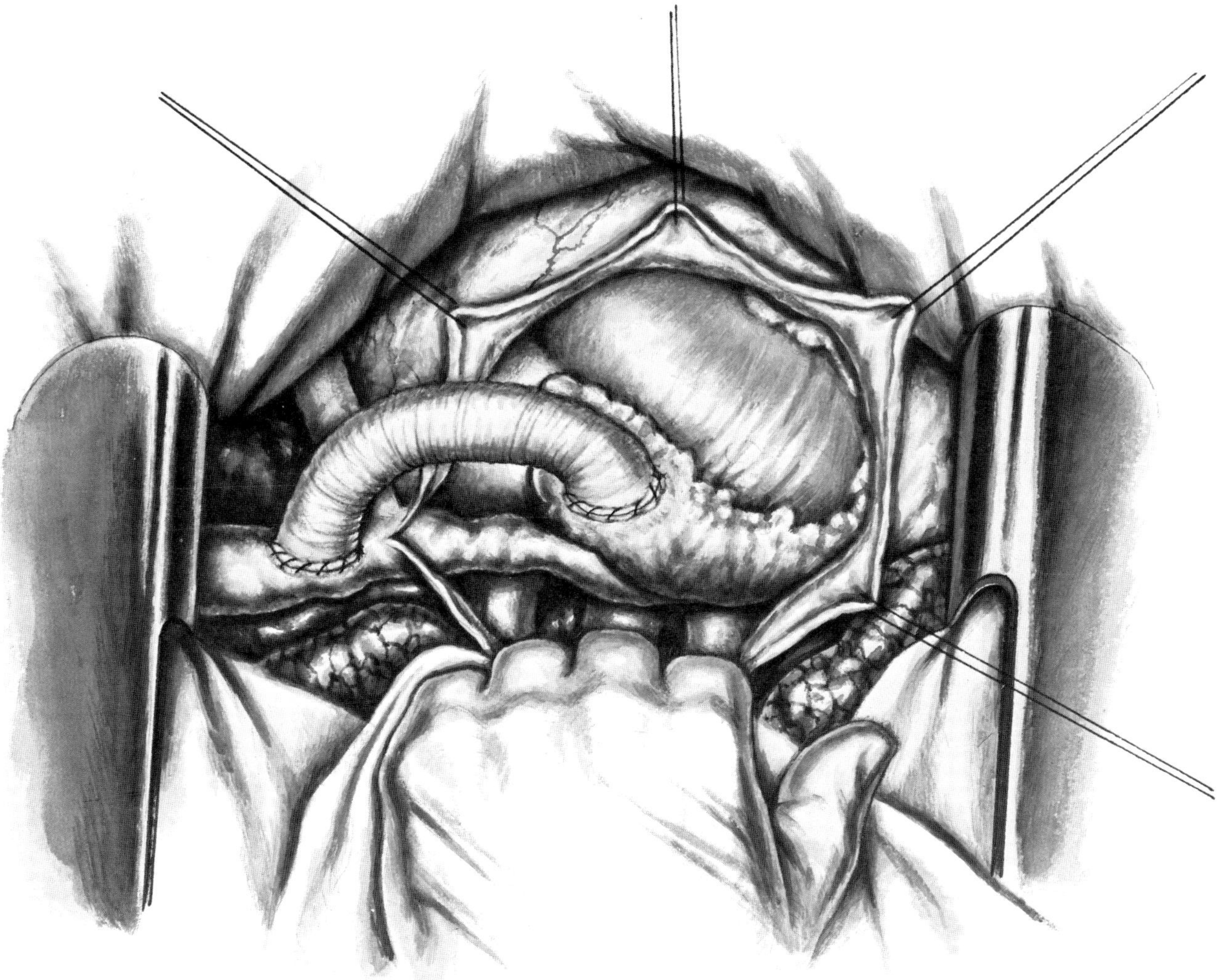

Fig. 586. View of superior vena cava to right atrium shunt.

EMBOLECTOMY FROM PULMONARY ARTERY (TRENDELENBURG'S OPERATION)

Embolectomy is indicated in massive embolism of the pulmonary artery, which may be carried out by Trendelenburg's method (Fig. 587). Left anterolateral approach in the fourth intercostal space is employed. The pericardium is opened wide, ventrally and parallel to the phrenic nerve. It is important to cut the pericardium at a high level, so that the pulmonary trunk might be sufficiently exposed. Two traction sutures are applied to the wall of the pulmonary trunk. The pulmonary trunk is clamped at the base, and its wall is cut lengthwise between the traction sutures for a distance of 1.5 to 2 cm. The tip of a powerful aspirator is alternately introduced into the right and left pulmonary arteries, and the thrombotic masses are aspirated. Once it is assured that all thrombi have been removed, the site of the incision in the pulmonary trunk is clamped with a soft-vessel clamp. The clamp is removed from the base of the pulmonary trunk. The arrest of blood flow into the pulmonary

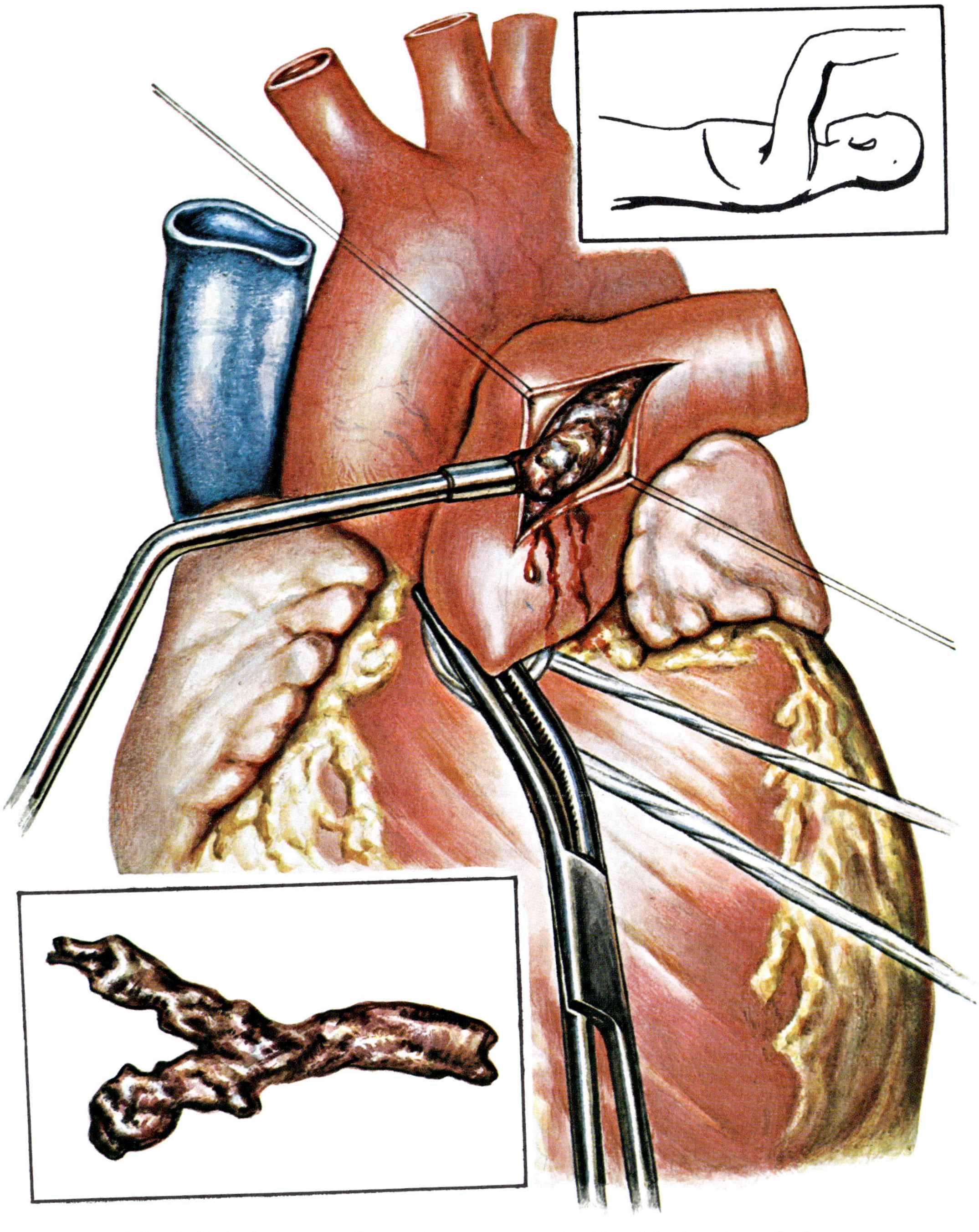

Fig. 587. Embolectomy from pulmonary artery by Trendelenburg's method.

arteries should not exceed two minutes. The opening in the wall of the pulmonary trunk is closed with a continuous suture.

Trendelenburg's embolectomy is currently rarely resorted to. Emboli are usually removed from the pulmonary artery under conditions of extracorporeal circulation (Fig. 588).

A transsternal approach is employed. The pericardium is opened wide.

Extracorporeal circulation* is connected, and the pulmonary trunk is cut lengthwise closer to the bifurcation. The thrombotic masses are removed from the right and left pulmonary arteries by means of an aspirator. To remove thrombi from small branches of the pulmonary artery, masmage of the lungs is performed through widely opened pleural cavities. The wall of the pulmonary trunk is repaired with double-row Halsted and blanket sutures. Drains are introduced into both pleural cavities and the mediastinum. The wound in the thoracic cage is closed with sutures.

*The techniques of connecting the heart-lung machine are described in Volume I, pp. 312-320.

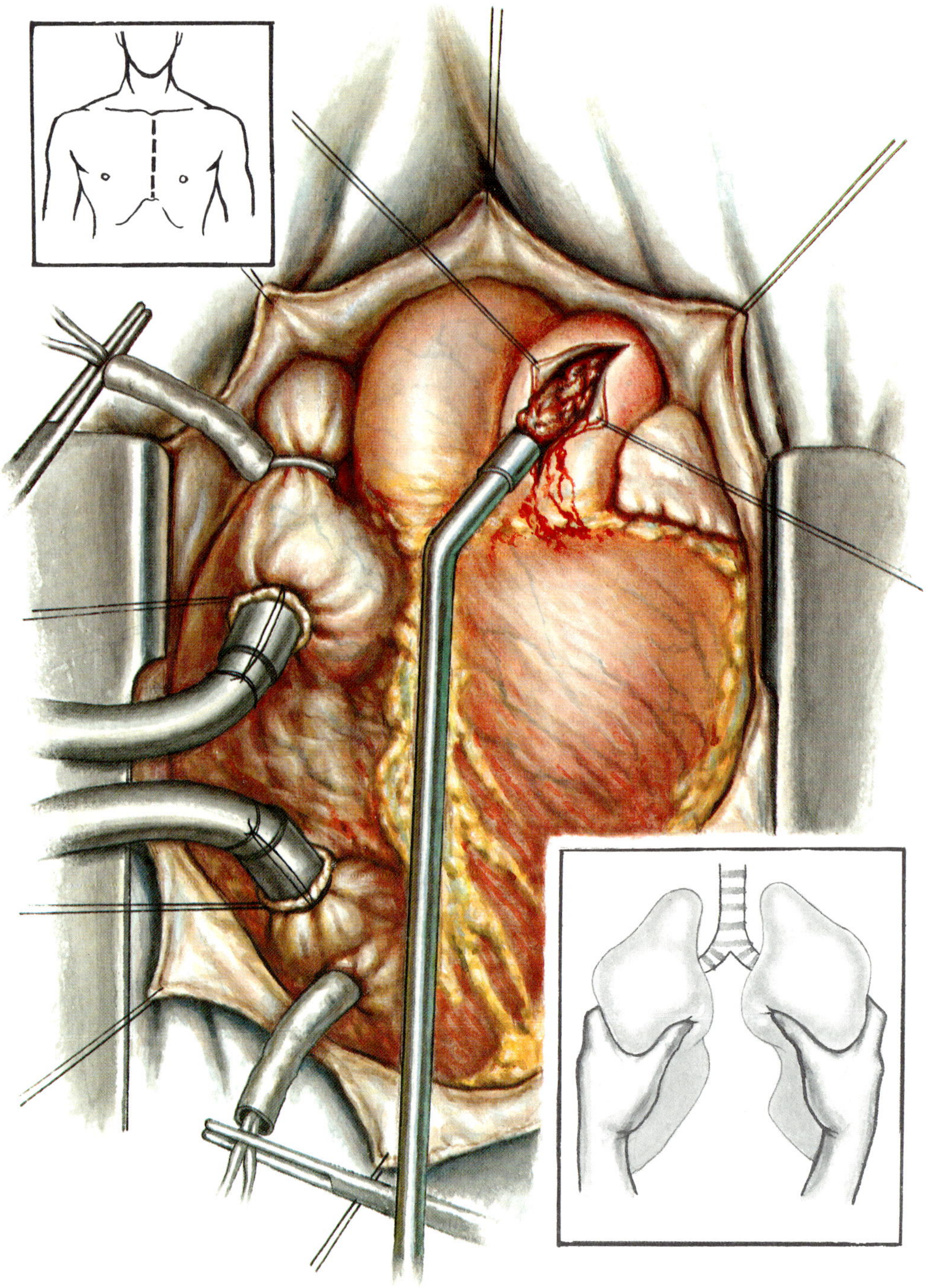

Fig. 588. Embolectomy from pulmonary artery under extracorporeal circulation.

OPERATIONS ON THE ESOPHAGUS

Operations in tumors of the esophagus

EXTIRPATION OF THORACIC ESOPHAGUS IN CANCER (DOBROMYSLOV-TOREK OPERATION)

The esophagus is usually approached through right thoracotomy in the fourth or seventh intercostal space. The patient is placed on his left side with a small bolster under the middle part of the thoracic cage. When the tumor is localized in the supradiaphragmatic part of the esophagus, a left approach in the seventh intercostal space is used.

After the thoracic cavity is opened, the lung is moved ventrally. The mediastinal pleura is cut with scissors from the diaphragm to the upper thoracic aperture. In cases with a tumor in the middle or upper part of the thoracic esophagus it is necessary to transect the arch of the azygos vein between two ligatures.

The cranial and caudal segments of the esophagus are freed from the cellular tissue, and gauze strips or rubber tubes are brought under them. While the esophagus is held on them, its affected portion is freed from the mediastinal tissues along its entire length (Fig. 589). Bleeding from the small esophageal vessels is arrested by ligation, coagulation, or tamponade.

The esophagus is ligated twice with a stitched-through ligature 4 to 5 cm caudal to the tumor and transected. A mechanical organ stitcher (the УО-40 instrument) may be employed instead of ligatures; the esophagus is also stitched through twice with it (Fig. 590). The caudal esophageal stump is buried in a purse-string suture,

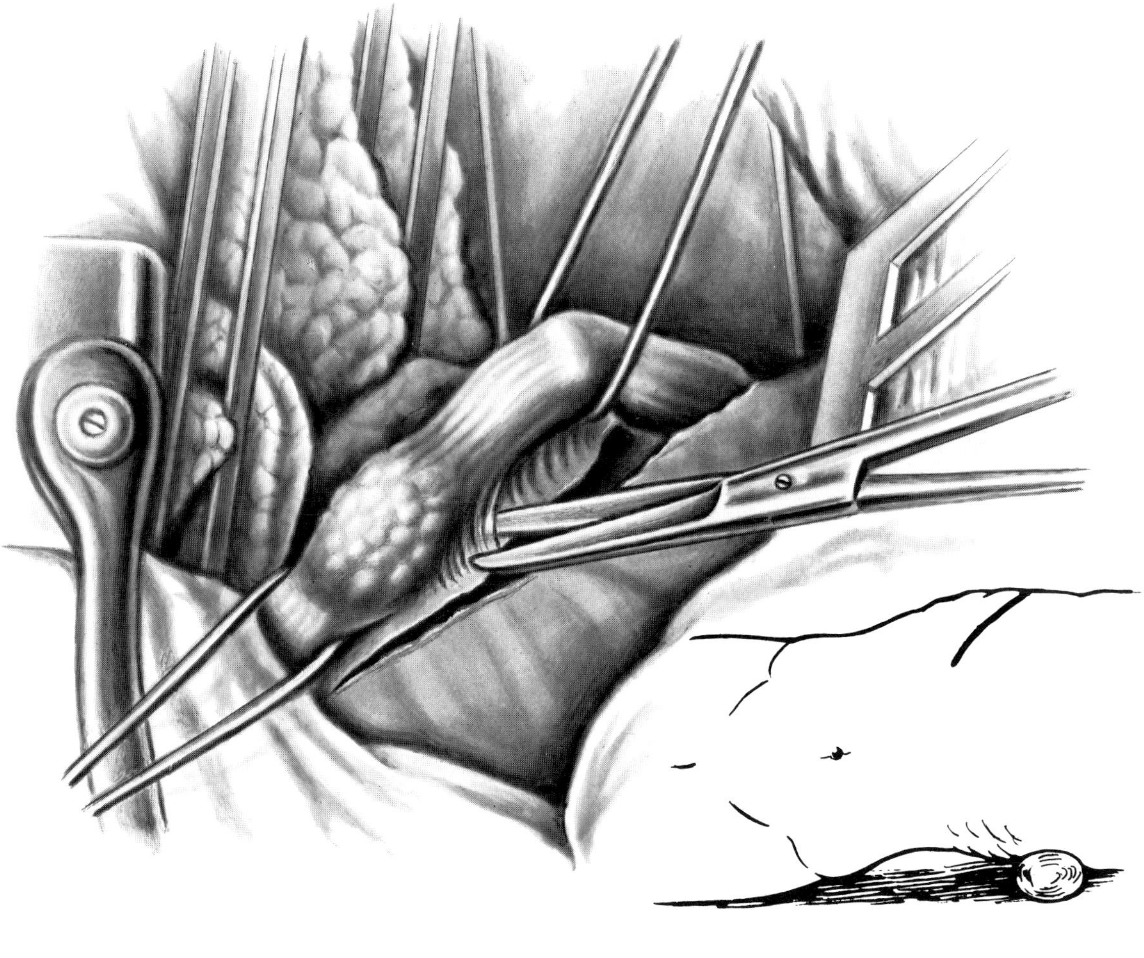

Fig. 589. Esophagus with tumor is mobilized from mediastinal cellular tissue.

above which interrupted sutures are applied (Fig. 591). The esophagus is then transected cranial to the tumor, also after being stitched through with two ligatures or twice with the YO-40 instrument. The resected esophageal segment with the tumor is removed. When the tumor is small, the esophagus is resected after the cranial stump with the tumor has been transposed to the neck. To prevent contamination of the mediastinum, a rubber cap is fitted to the cranial esophageal stump and fastened over the tumor with a circular ligature (Fig. 592). This ligature is used for drawing out the esophageal stump to the neck.

The patient is then placed on his back with a small bolster under his shoulder blades so that his head is thrown back and turned to the left or right depending on whether the stump will be drawn out to the right or left of the trachea. An incision about 3 to 4 cm long is made along the lower third of the medial border of the sternocleidomastoid muscle. The esophagus is approached by blunt and sharp dissection, and its stump is

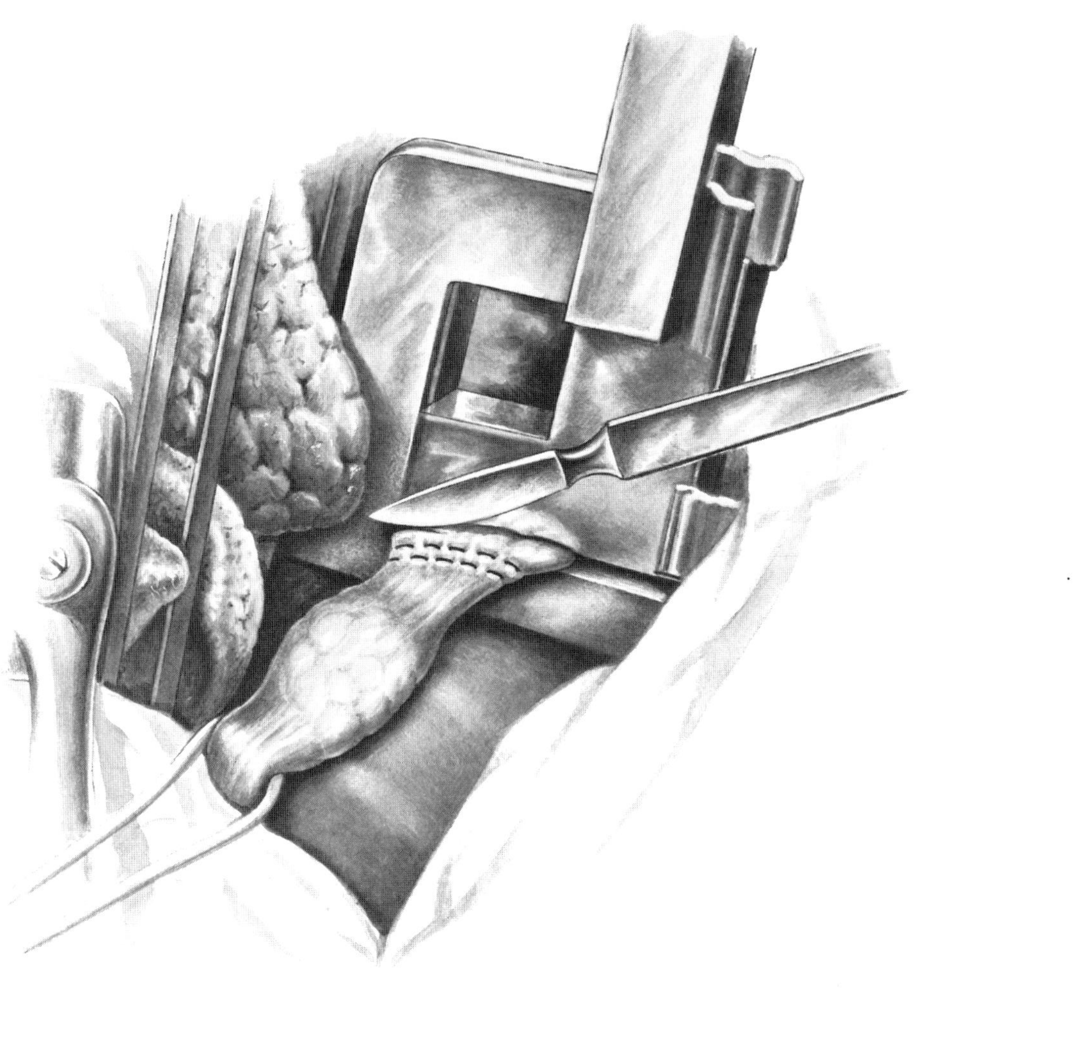

Fig. 590. Esophagus is stitched through twice by means of YO-40 instrument and transected between rows of metal staples.

grasped with the finger and brought out through the wound in the neck.

The esophageal stump may also be transposed to the neck by a combined method. In this case the surgeon advances his right index finger from the thoracic cavity through the superior mediastinum to the neck. A small skin incision is made on the neck over the protruding finger. A narrow tunnel is formed between the muscles of the neck by the blunt and sharp techniques; the ends of the ligature are held with the finger or an instrument; and the cranial esophageal stump attached to the ligature is brought out to the neck.

The esophageal stump drawn out of the thoracic cavity is placed on the anterior thoracic wall; the site where the esophagostoma will be formed is chosen; and a 2.5 to 3 cm skin incision is made. A tunnel is formed under the skin through this incision by means of dressing forceps, which communicates with the wound on the neck. The ends of the ligature on the esophageal stump are grasped with an instrument, pulled through the tunnel

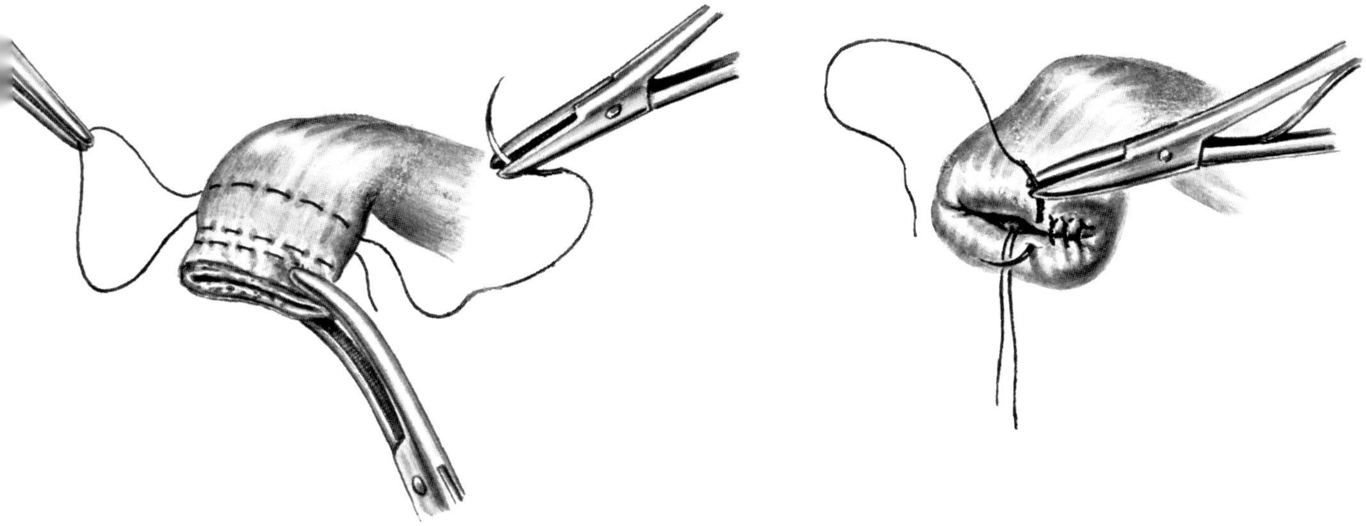

Fig. 591. Lower esophageal stump is closed with sutures.

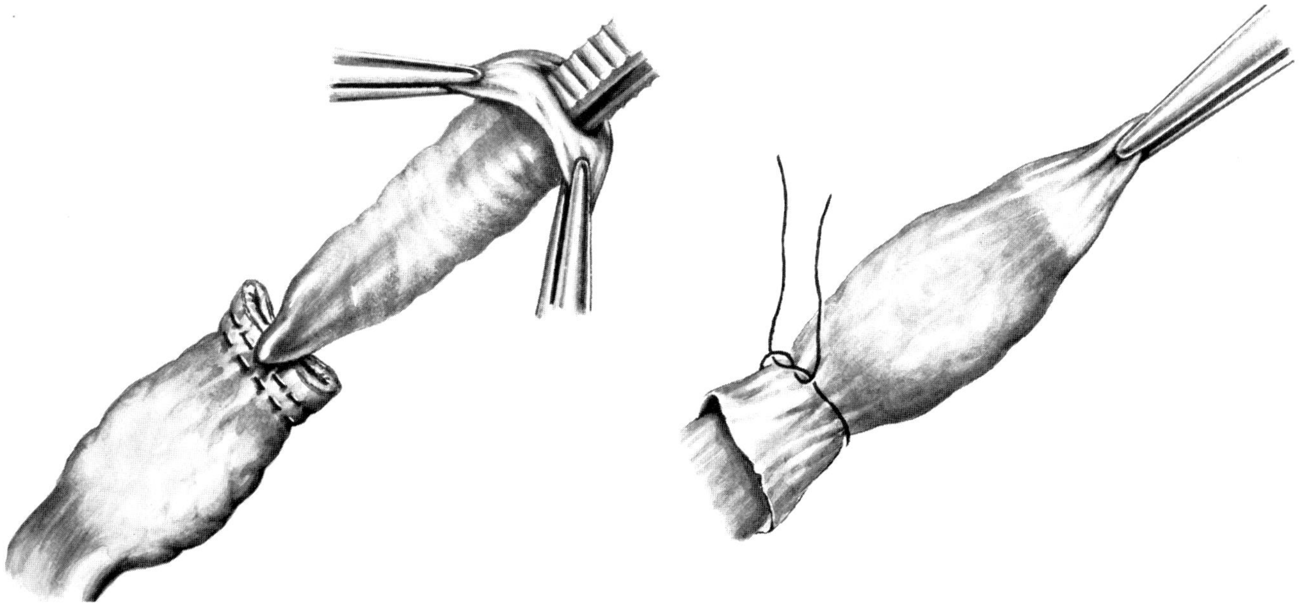

Fig. 592. Upper esophageal stump together with tumor is covered with isolating rubber cap.

(Fig. 593), and drawn out through the lower skin incision. The esophagus is cut away 4 to 5 cm from the border of the tumor (Fig. 594). An esophagostoma is established with interrupted sutures placed through all the esophageal coats. Stitches are applied to the edges of the skin incision on the neck (Fig. 595), and the wound on the neck is sutured. A drain is left in the pleural cavity. The wound in the thoracic cage is sutured completely.

Witzel's gastrostoma is formed after the superior esophagostoma has been established and the thoracic wound sutured.

The patient lies on his back with a bolster under him at the level of the sternal xiphoid process. Superior

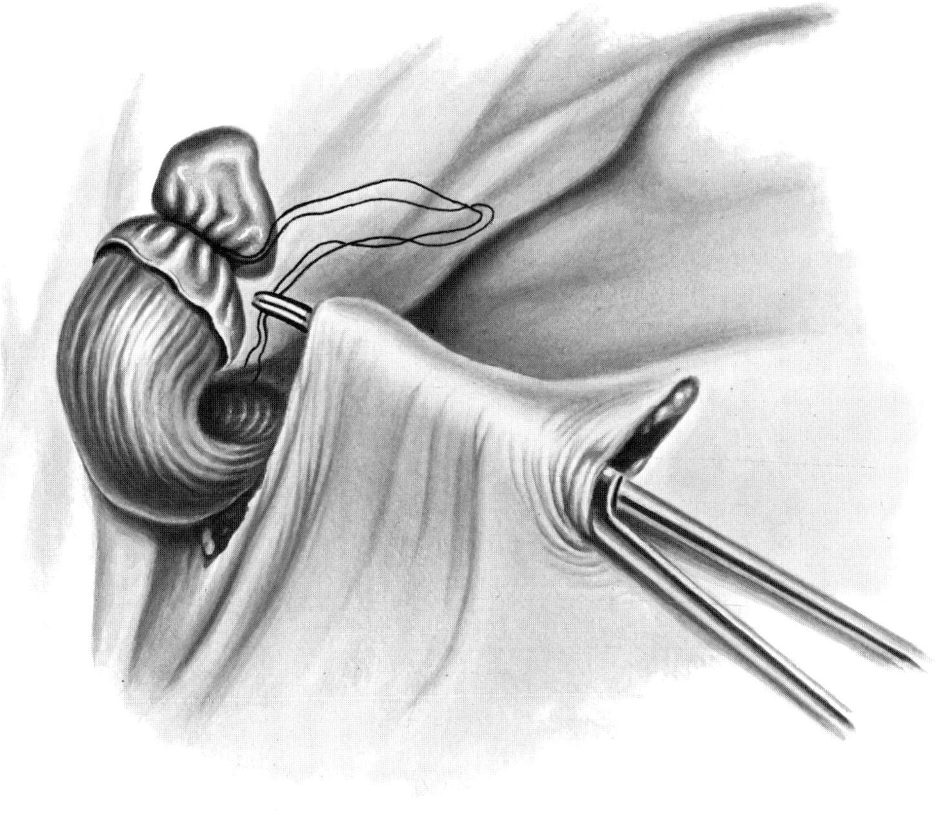

Fig. 593. Upper esophageal stump is drawn along tunnel under skin and brought out to anterior thoracic wall through incision in neck.

median laparotomy is performed or the rectus abdominis muscle is transected. The abdominal cavity is examined for cancer metastases to the lymph nodes of the subdiaphragmatic region. This is essential for making a decision in regard to subsequent esophagoplasty.

A rubber tube about 1.5 cm in diameter is placed on the anterior gastric wall and, by means of interrupted seromuscular sutures, sunk into a tunnel formed by two folds of the gastric wall (Fig. 596). It is advisable to place the tube in such a way that its bevelled upper end is in the region of the air bubble in the fundus of the stomach, which prevents the escape of gastric contents.

A purse-string suture is applied to the gastric wall around the end of the tube emerging from the tunnel.

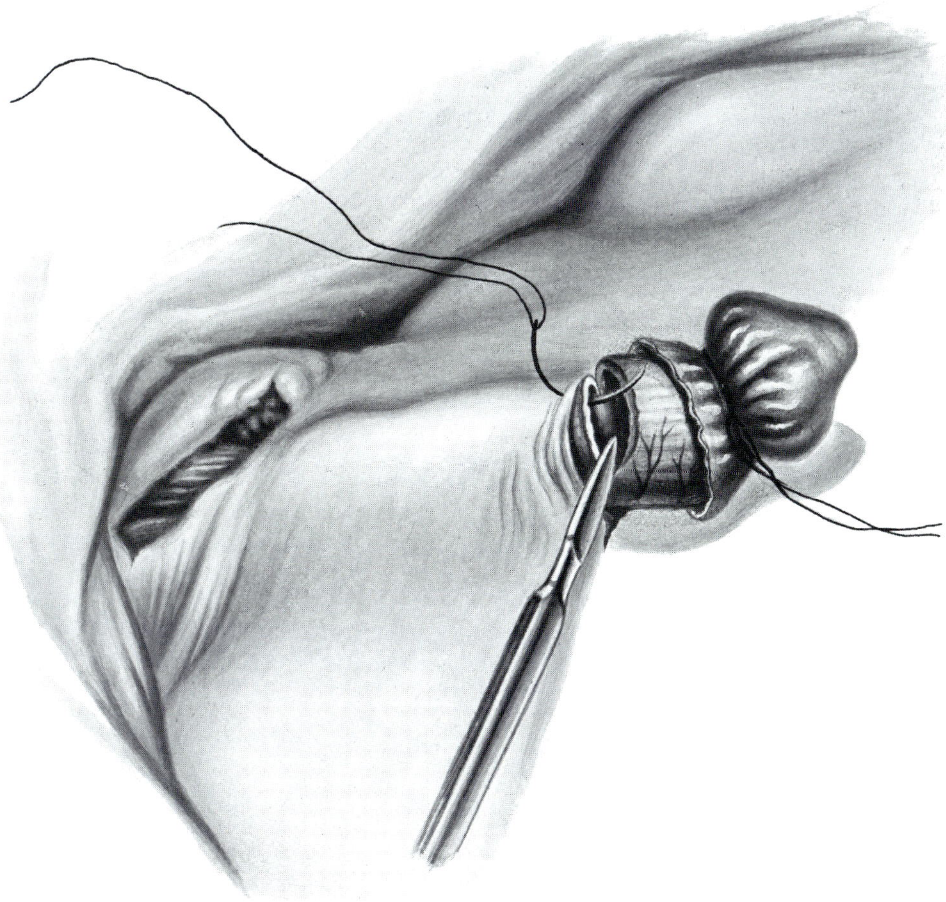

Fig. 594. Diseased portion of upper esophageal stump is cut away.

The end of the tube is pulled caudally with forceps, and an incision about 1 to 1.5 cm long is made with a scalpel in the gastric wall inside the purse-string suture (Fig. 597). The end of the tube is introduced into the stomach through this incision (Fig. 598), and the purse-string suture is tied over it. A second row of interrupted sutures is applied over the purse-string suture and the first row of stitches forming the tunnel (Fig. 599).

Two threads are stitched through the muscular coat of the stomach at the lower margin of the canal (Fig. 600), and then a cut about 3.5 cm long is made in the anterior abdominal wall 4 to 5 cm to the left of the midline and slightly below the left costal arch. The free end of the gastrostomy tube and both threads are brought out through this opening (Fig. 601).

The ends of the threads previously applied to the

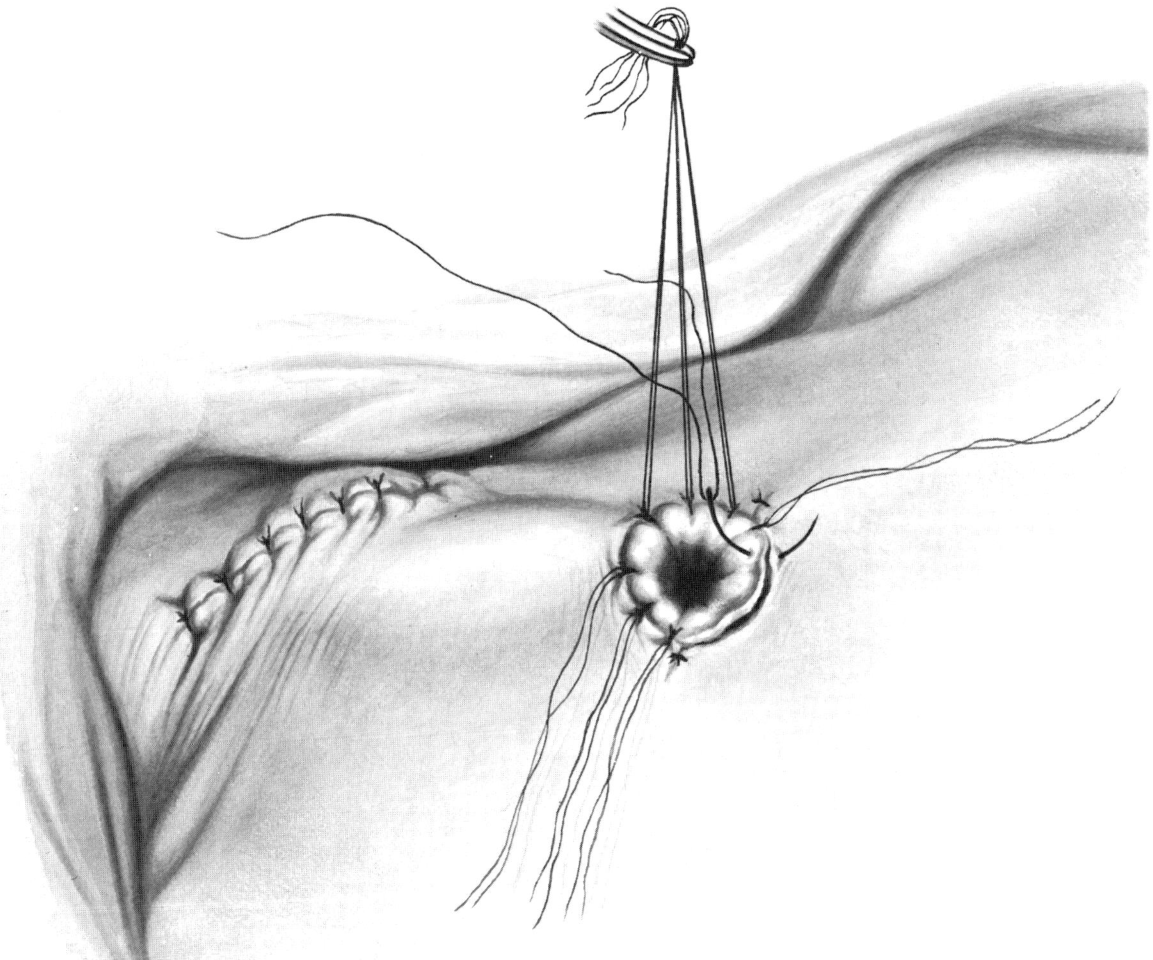

Fig. 595. Esophagostoma is formed on anterior thoracic wall.

gastric wall are stitched through the edges of the incision in the peritoneum, aponeurosis, and skin; the anterior pair of threads ends at the cranial end of the wound, and the posterior pair at the caudal end. When the ends of these threads are pulled, the lower edge of the tunnel on the gastric wall is pressed tightly to the peritoneum, thus isolating the rubber tube from the free abdominal cavity. As the ends of each pair of threads are tied, they tighten the edges of the abdominal wound around the tube. The anterior wall of the stomach near to the tube may be additionally secured to the parietal pleura from the side of the median wound with two or three interrupted sutures. The median abdominal wound is completely sutured.

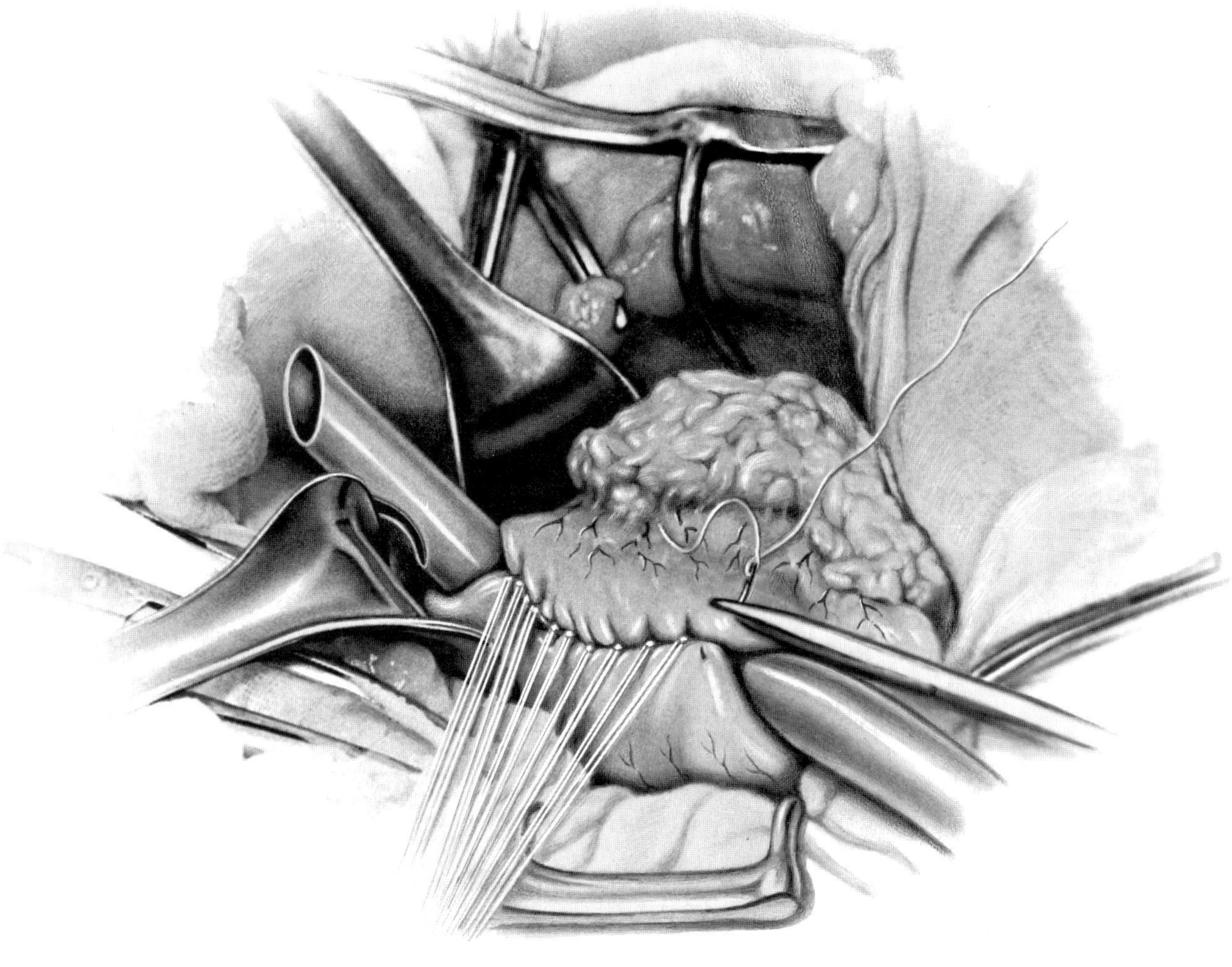

Fig. 596. Tunnel of gastrostoma is formed on anterior gastric wall. Interrupted seromuscular sutures are applied over rubber tube.

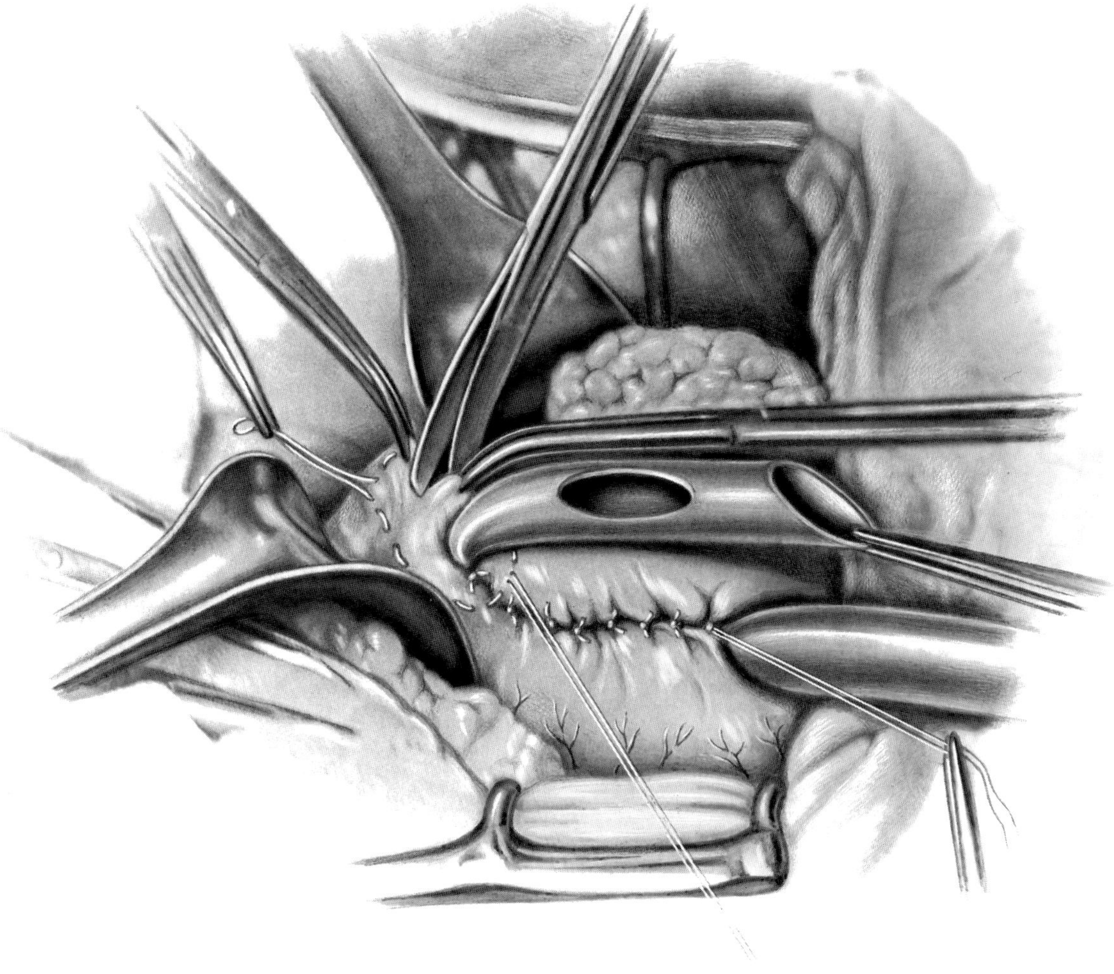

Fig. 597. Gastric wall is cut in center of purse-string suture at upper canal of gastrostoma.

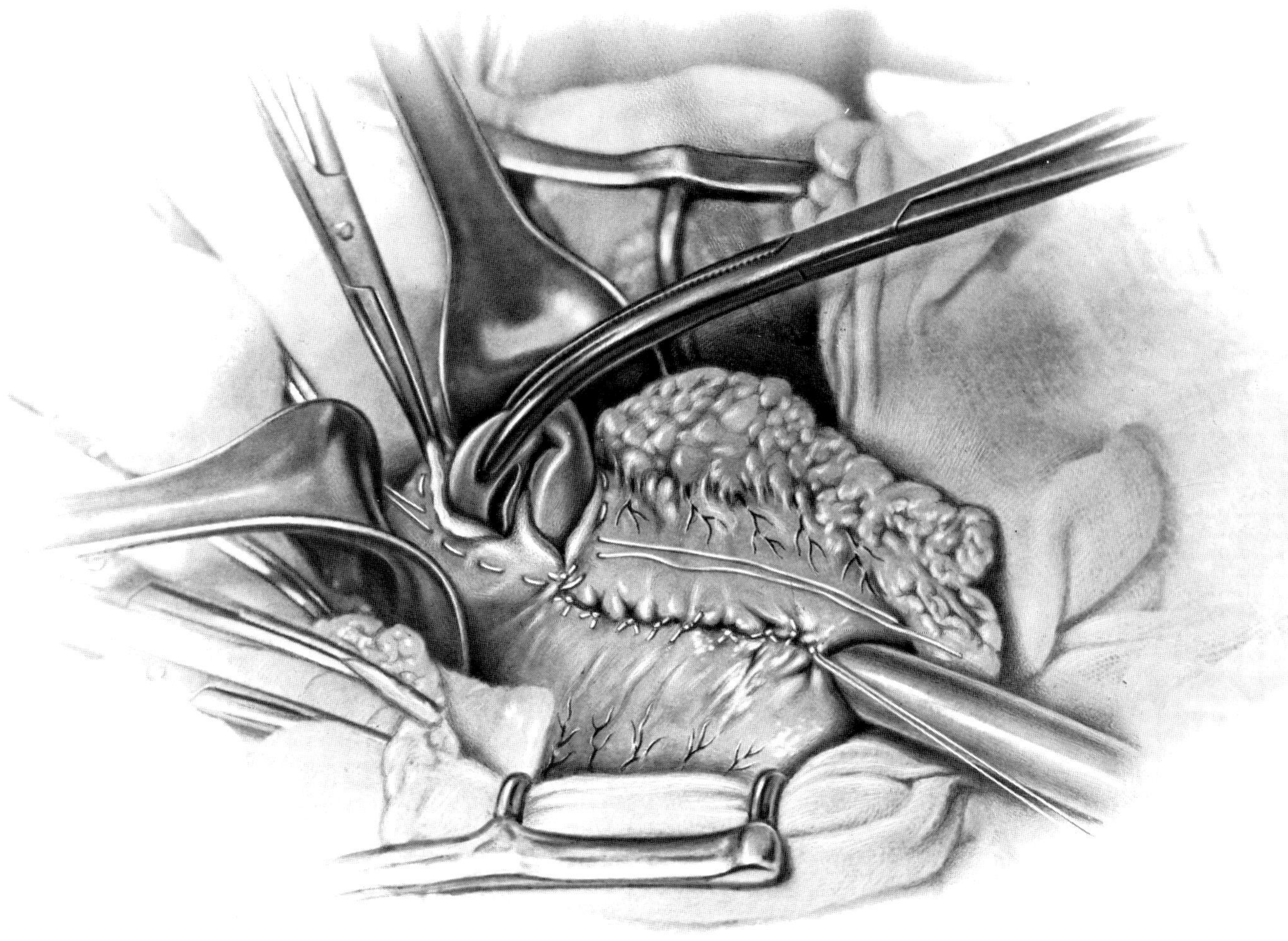

Fig. 598. End of rubber tube is introduced into cavity of stomach.

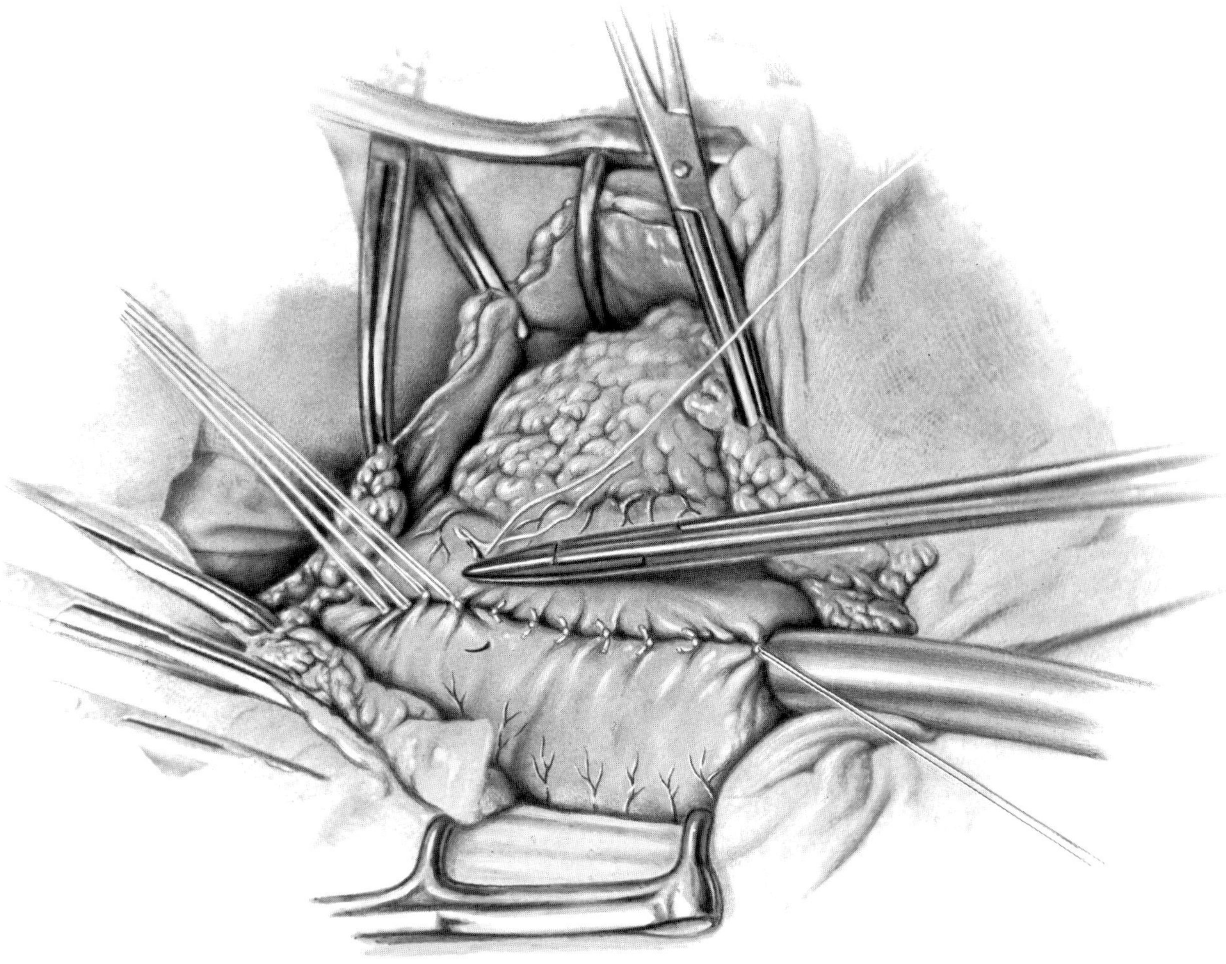

Fig. 599. Second row of interrupted sutures is applied over purse-string suture and rubber tube.

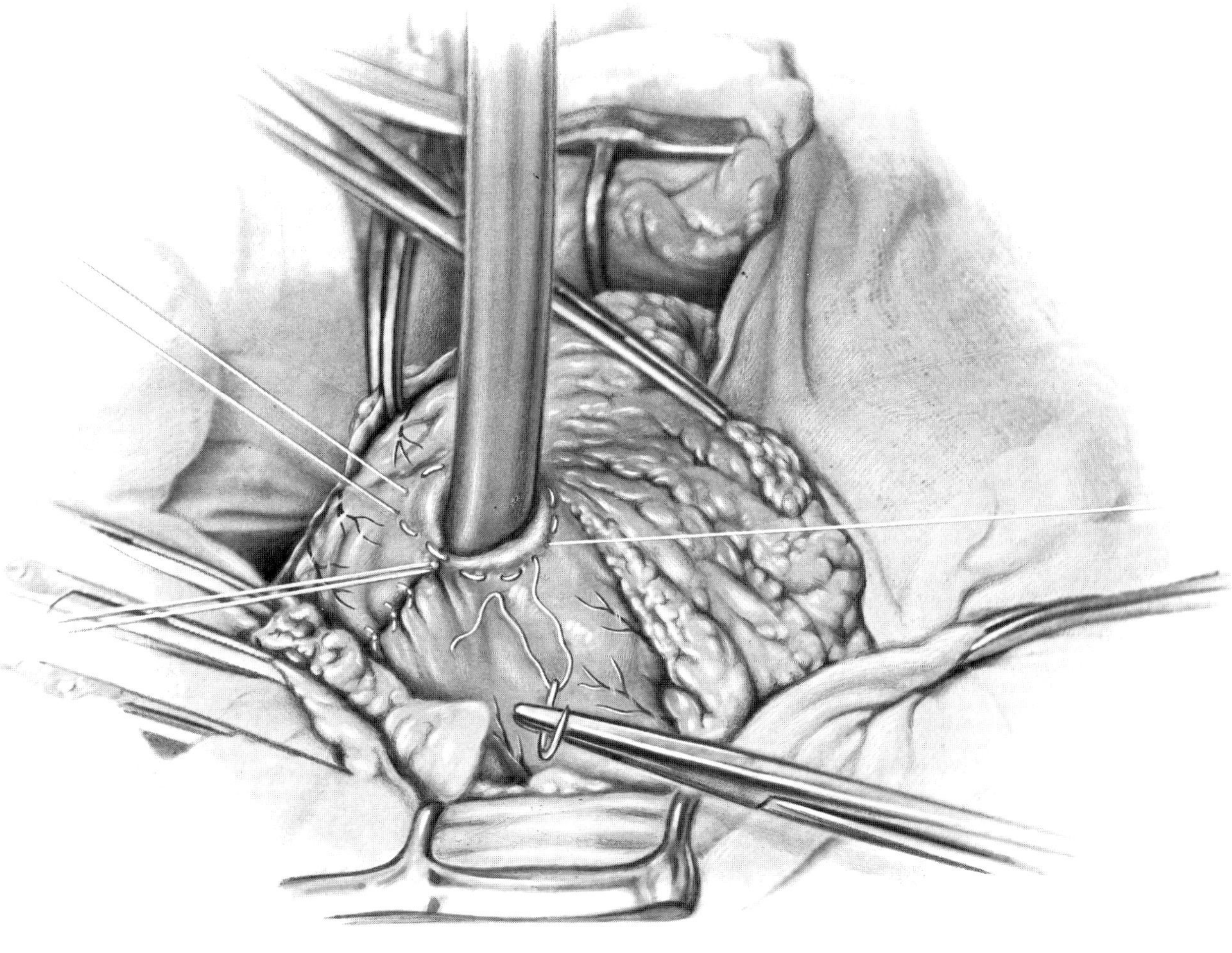

Fig. 600. Two ligatures are stitched through lower edge of gastrostoma tunnel.

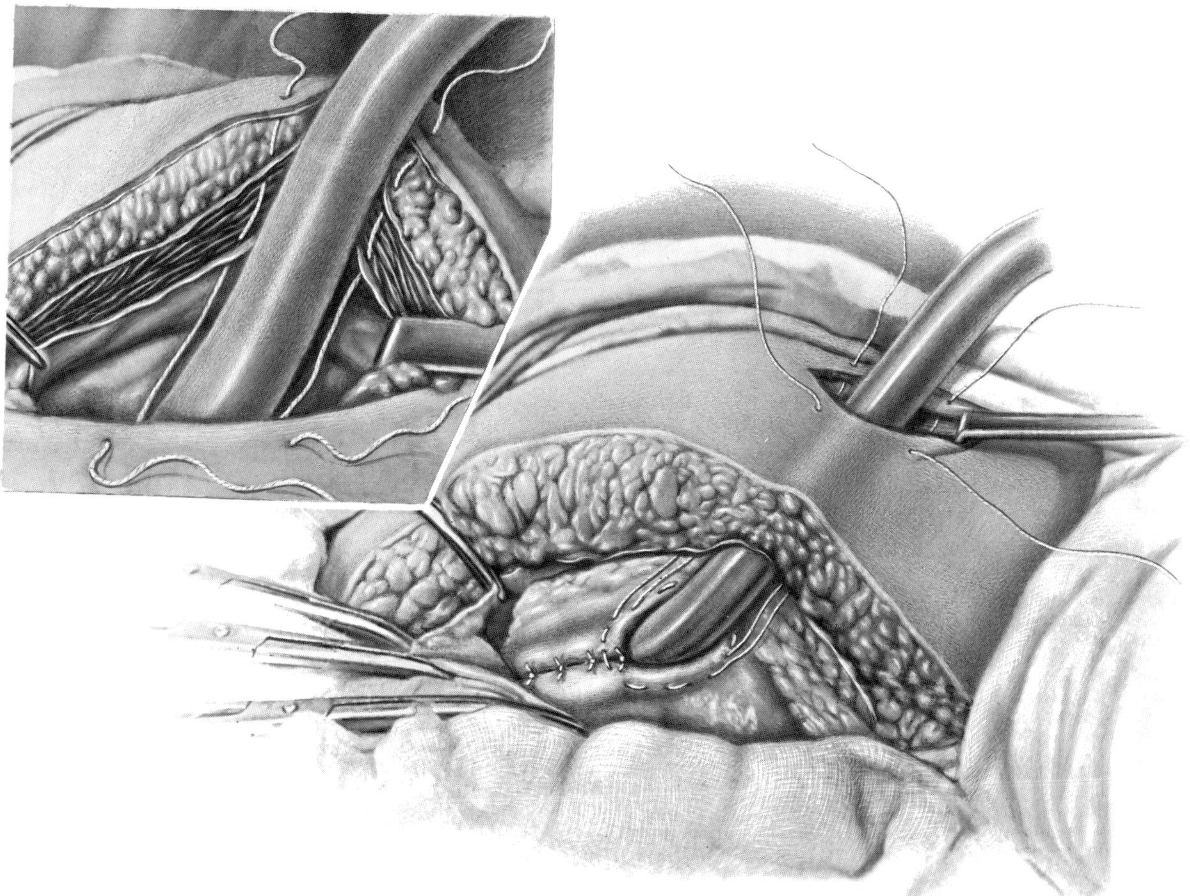

Fig. 601. Gastrostoma tube is fastened in separate incision made in anterior abdominal wall.

RESECTION OF CARDIA AND LOWER THIRD OF ESOPHAGUS

Access is gained through seventh or eighth intercostal space. For a wider approach the costal arch is transected in the cartilaginous part, which is resected for a distance of 1.5 to 2 cm for better adaptation of the tissues of the thoracic wall in closure of the wound.

After the edges of the wound have been drawn apart, the lung is moved cranially, and the pulmonary ligament stretched during this manipulation is transected (Fig. 602), as the result of which the mediastinum is opened. The diaphragm is cut between clamps in the direction of the esophagus (Fig. 603). Areas of the diaphragm involved in the tumor are resected.

The lower part of the esophagus is freed from the mediastinum by blunt dissection and held with a gauze

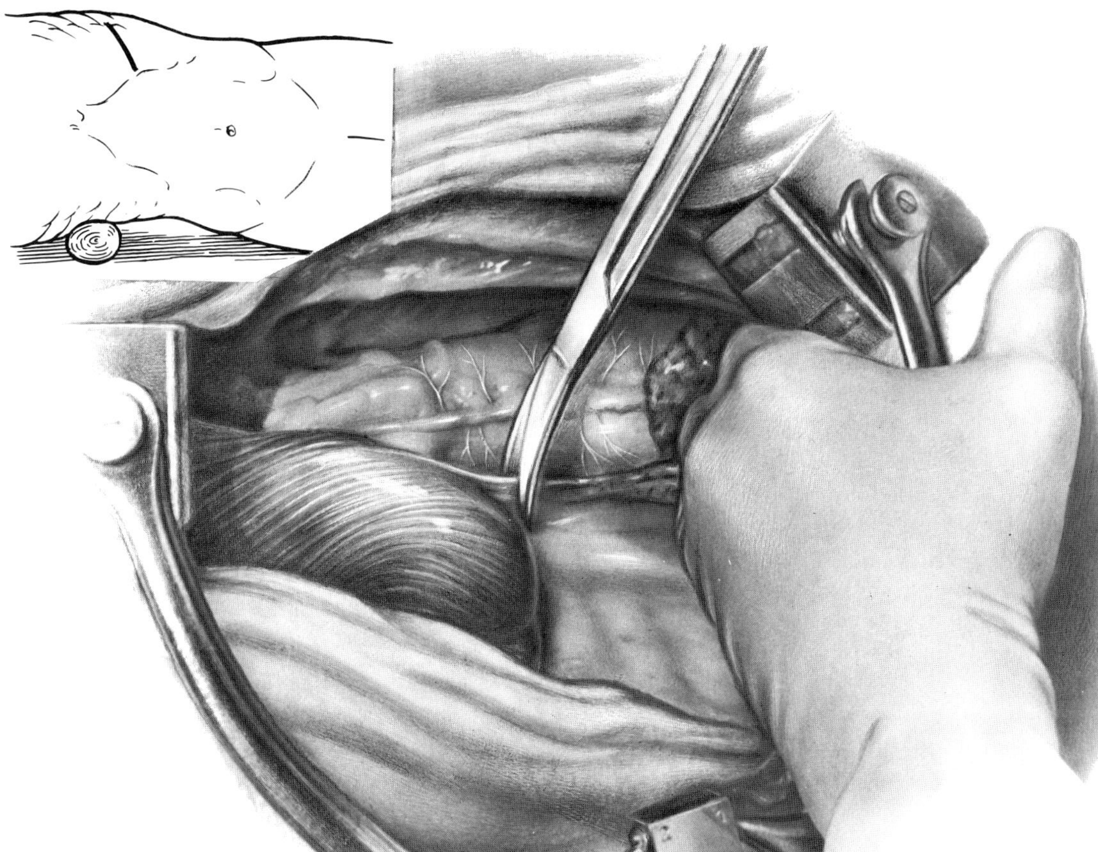

Fig. 602. Pulmonary ligament is transected.

strip or rubber tube (Fig. 604). Each vagus nerve is separately transected with scissors cranial to the tumor. The edges of the diaphragmatic wound are stitched through with double blanket stitches at each large transected vessel (Fig. 605).

The gastrosplenic ligament with the short gastric arteries (Fig. 606) and the gastrohepatic ligament (lesser omentum) with the superior branches of the left gastric artery (Fig. 607) are successively transected between two clamps and ligated. The stomach is pulled ventrally and slightly to the right. As a result the gastropancreatic ligament with the left gastric artery and vein in its thickness is well outlined; these vessels are transected between two clamps and ligated with ligatures stitched through them (Fig. 608).

The proximal portion of the stomach is mobilized, and after two crushing clamps are applied, the esophagus is transected cranially and the stomach caudally to the tumor (Fig. 609), and the resected part is removed. The caudal gastric stump is closed with a continuous hemo-

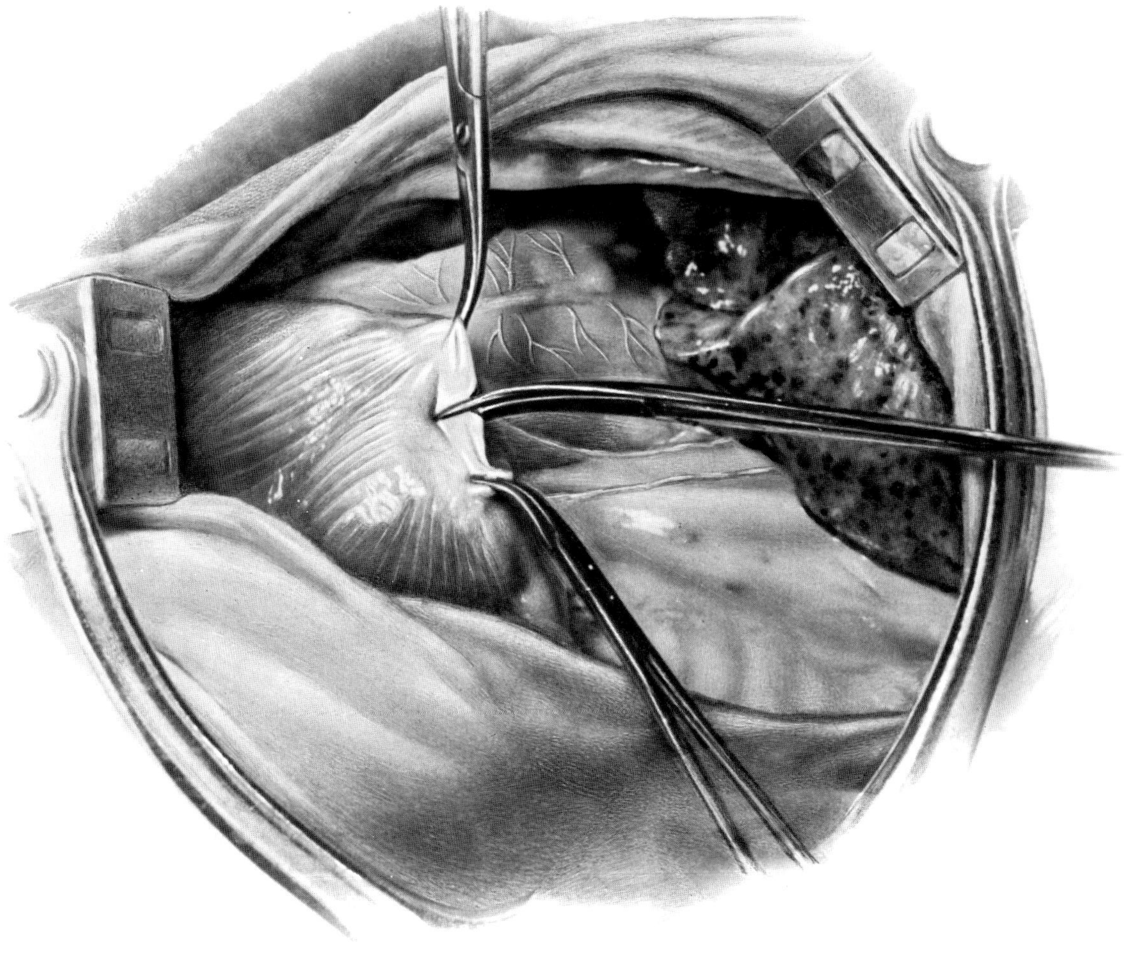

Fig. 603. Diaphragm is cut between two clamps.

static catgut suture over which a second row of interrupted silk seroserous sutures is applied (Fig. 610). An incision 2 to 2.5 cm long is made in the ventral wall of the stomach for anastomosing with the esophagus.

The stumps of the esophagus and stomach are brought closer to each other, and the formation of an anastomosis is begun; interrupted posterior seromuscular ("suspending") sutures are first applied (Fig. 611, *A*), and then a row of interrupted sutures are passed through all the coats of the posterior lip of the anastomosis (Fig. 138, *B, C*). Similar double-row sutures are applied to the anterior wall of the anastomosis (Fig. 611, *D*). In some instances the line of the anastomosis is strengthened with a third row of reinforcing widely spaced interrupted seromuscular sutures.

The edges of the diaphragm are sutured to each other and to the walls of the stomach with interrupted sutures (Fig. 612). Drains are left in the pleural cavity. The wound in the thoracic cage is completely sutured.

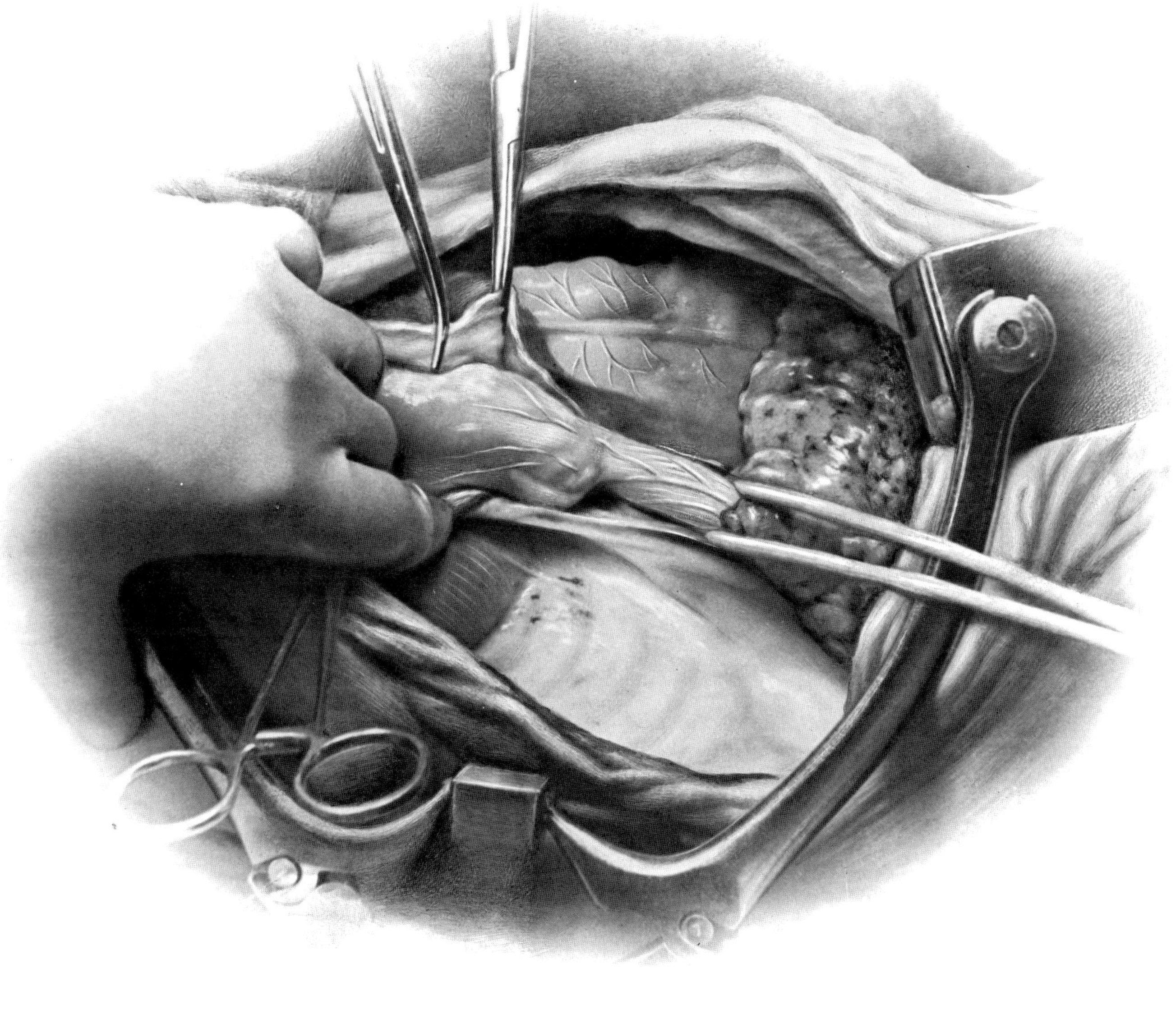

Fig. 604. Lower part of esophagus freed from mediastinum is held on rubber tube.

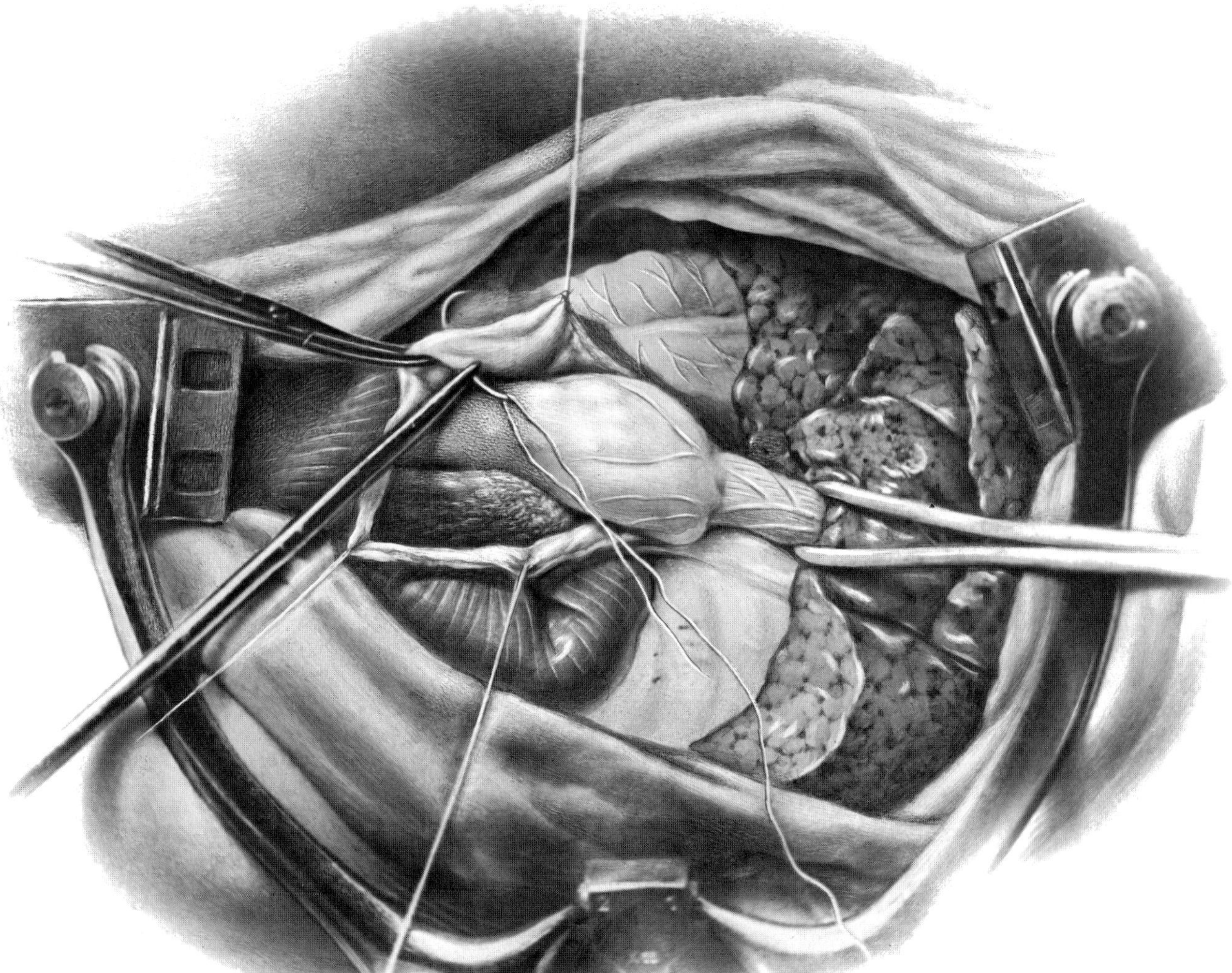

Fig. 605. Arrest of bleeding from transected vessels of diaphragm and fixation of edges of diaphragmatic incision with stitched catgut ligatures.

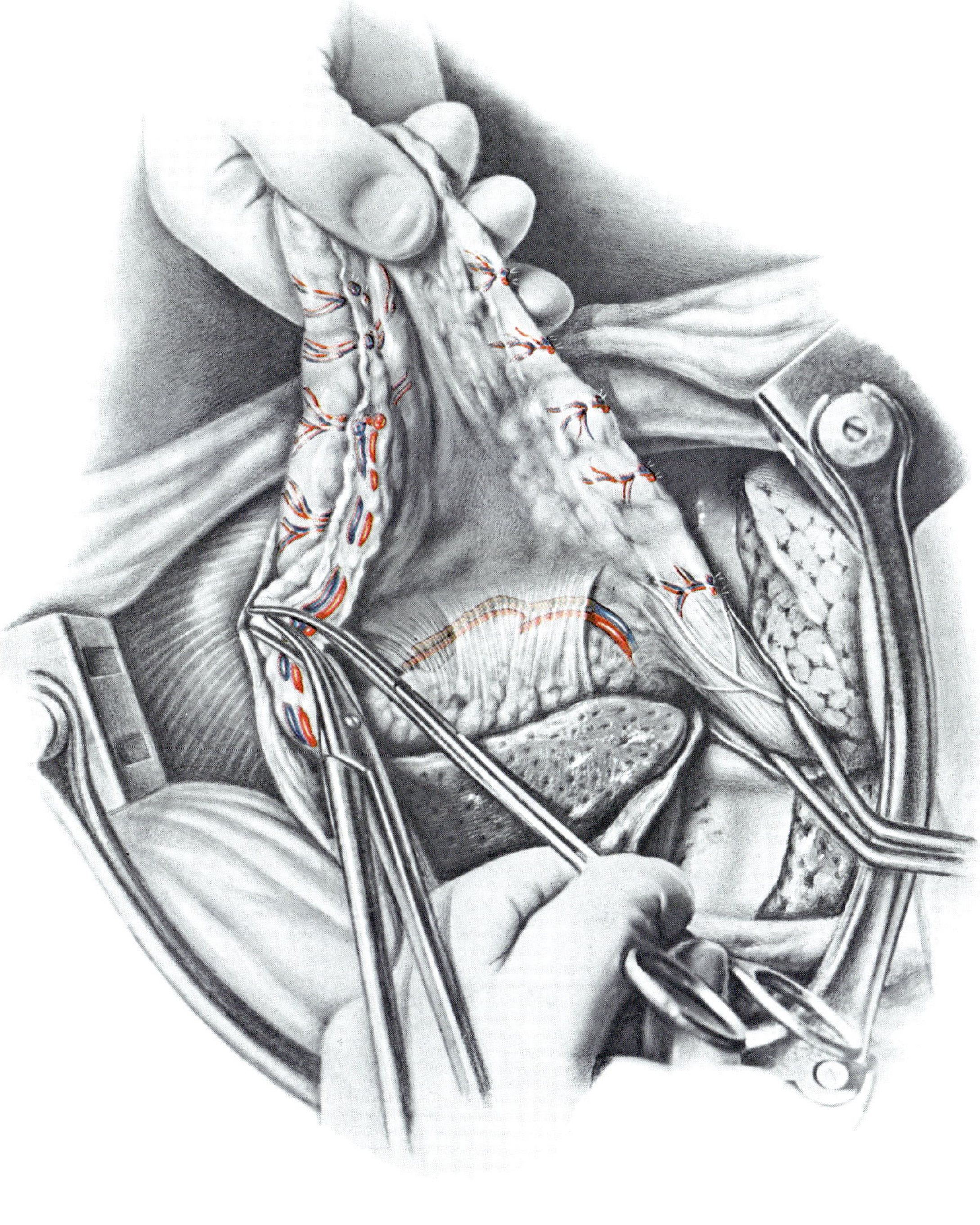

Fig. 606. Proximal part of stomach is mobilized along greater curvature. Gastropancreatic ligament is seen in center.

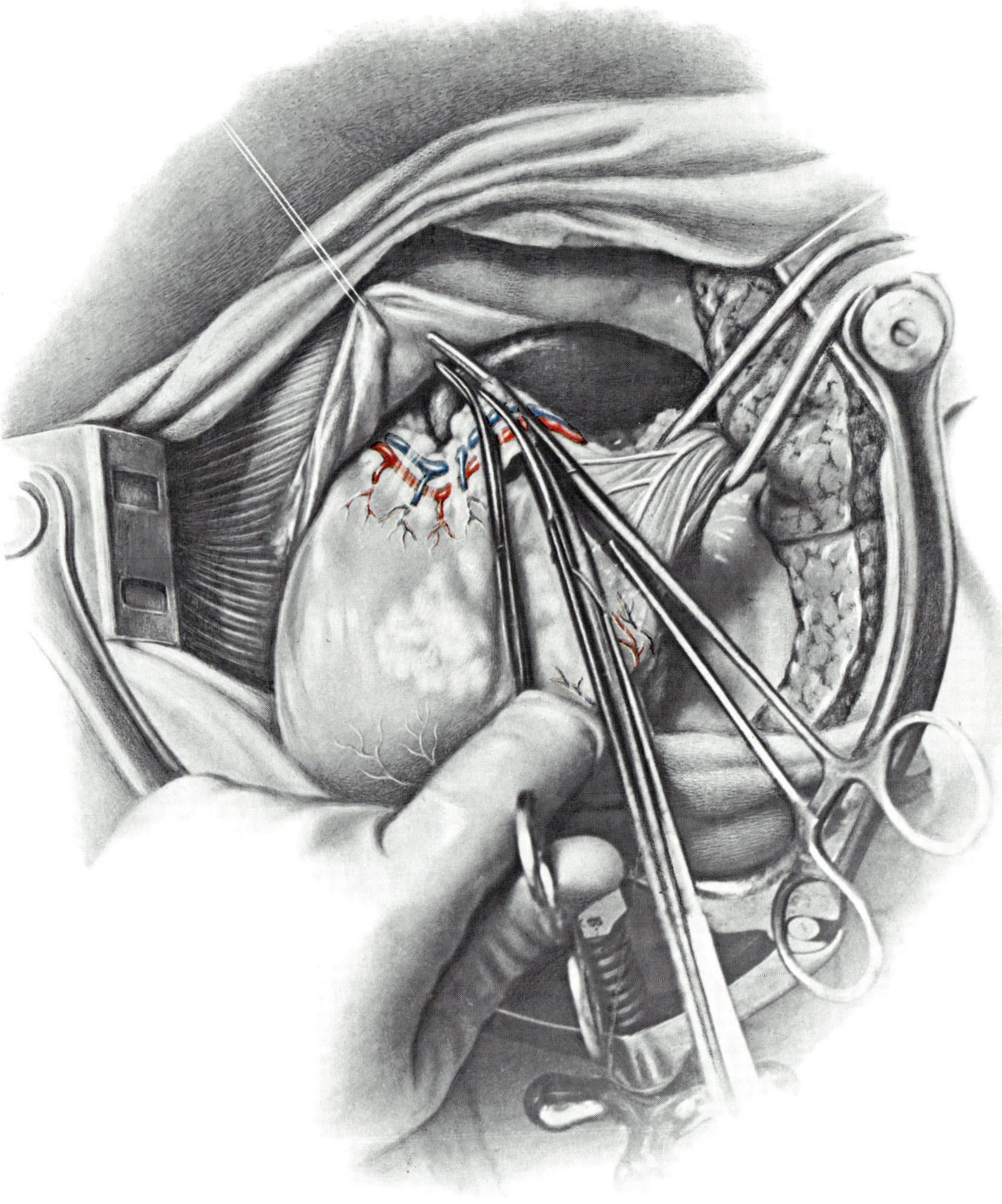

Fig. 607. Proximal part of stomach is mobilized along lesser curvature. Large branches of left gastric artery are transected.

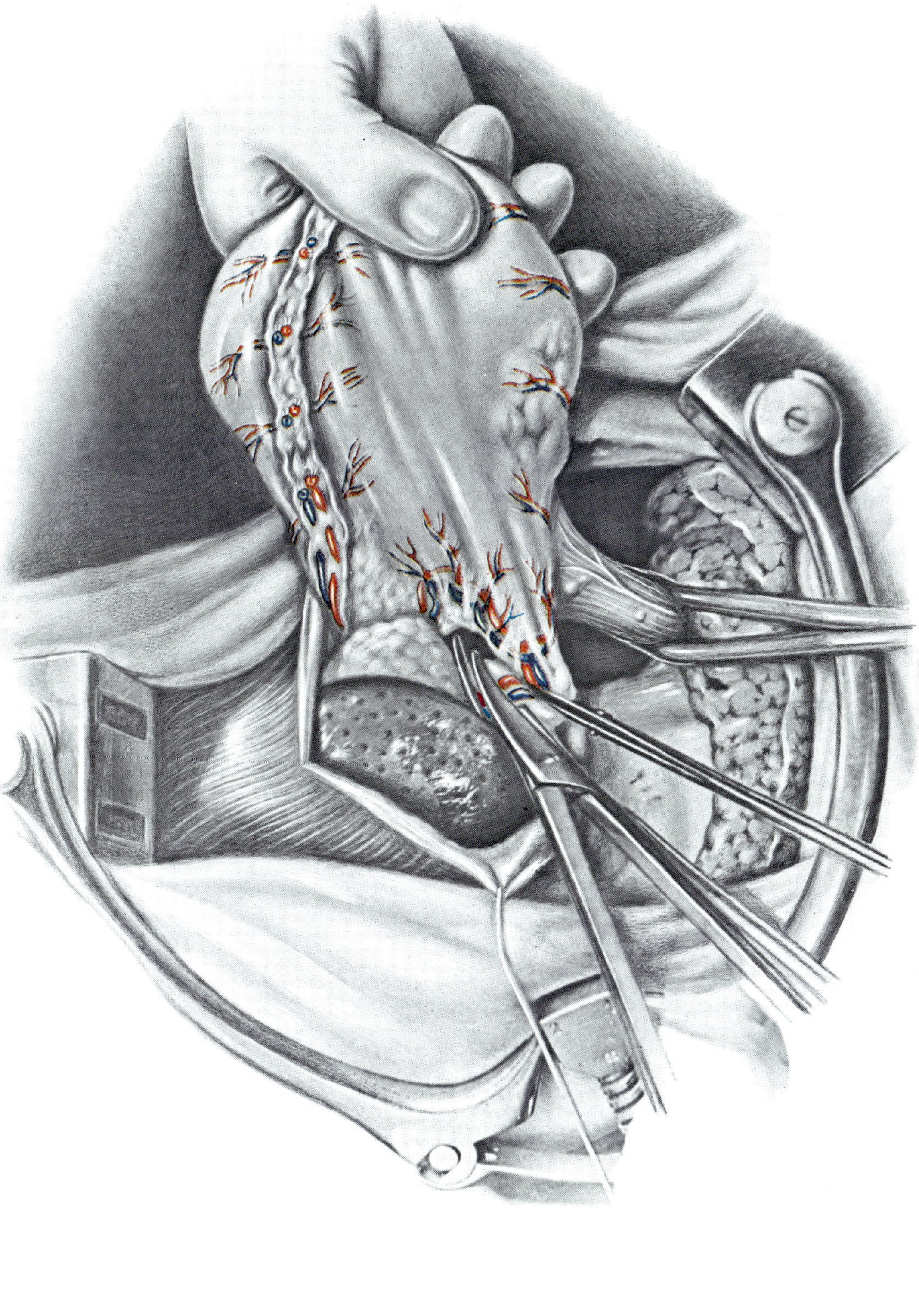

Fig. 608. Left gastric artery and veins are transected in gastropancreatic ligament.

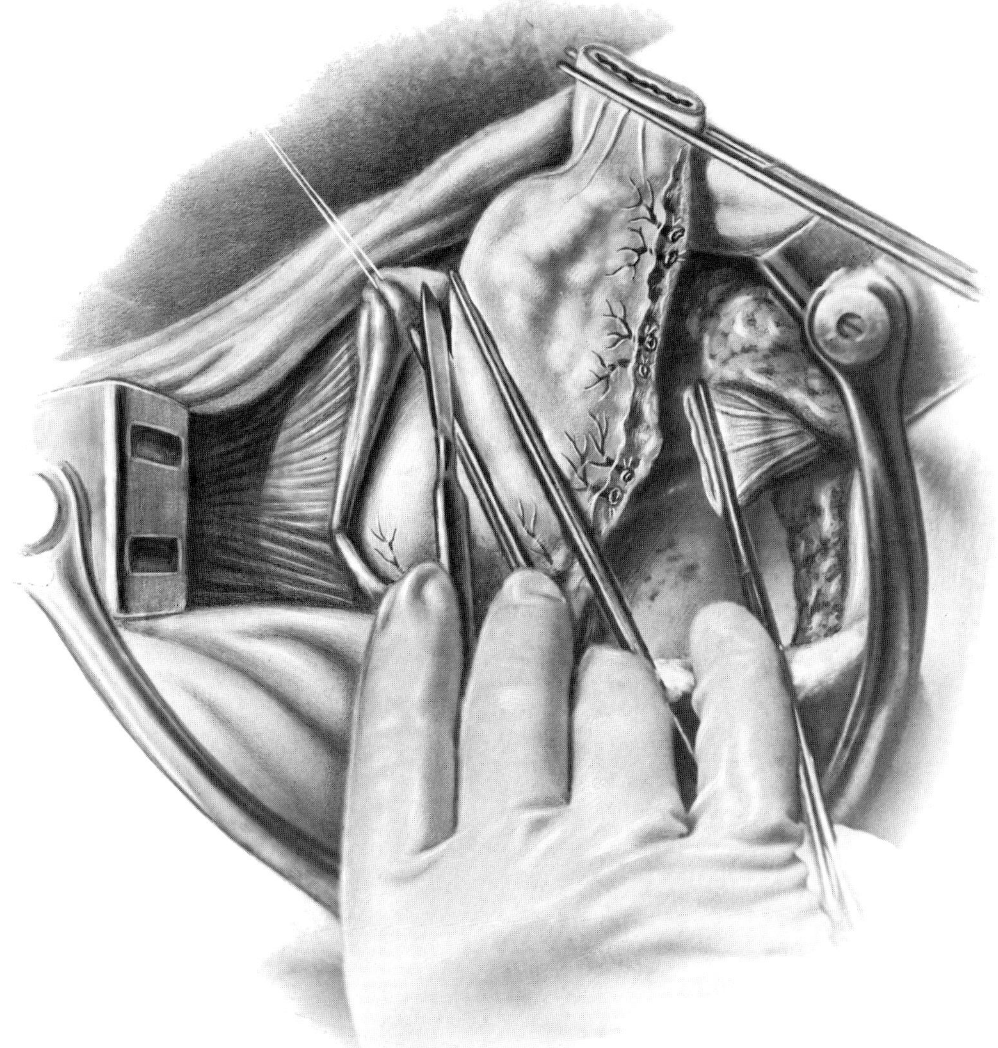

Fig. 609. Esophagus is transected above tumor. Stomach is divided between two crushing clamps in subcardiac portion below tumor.

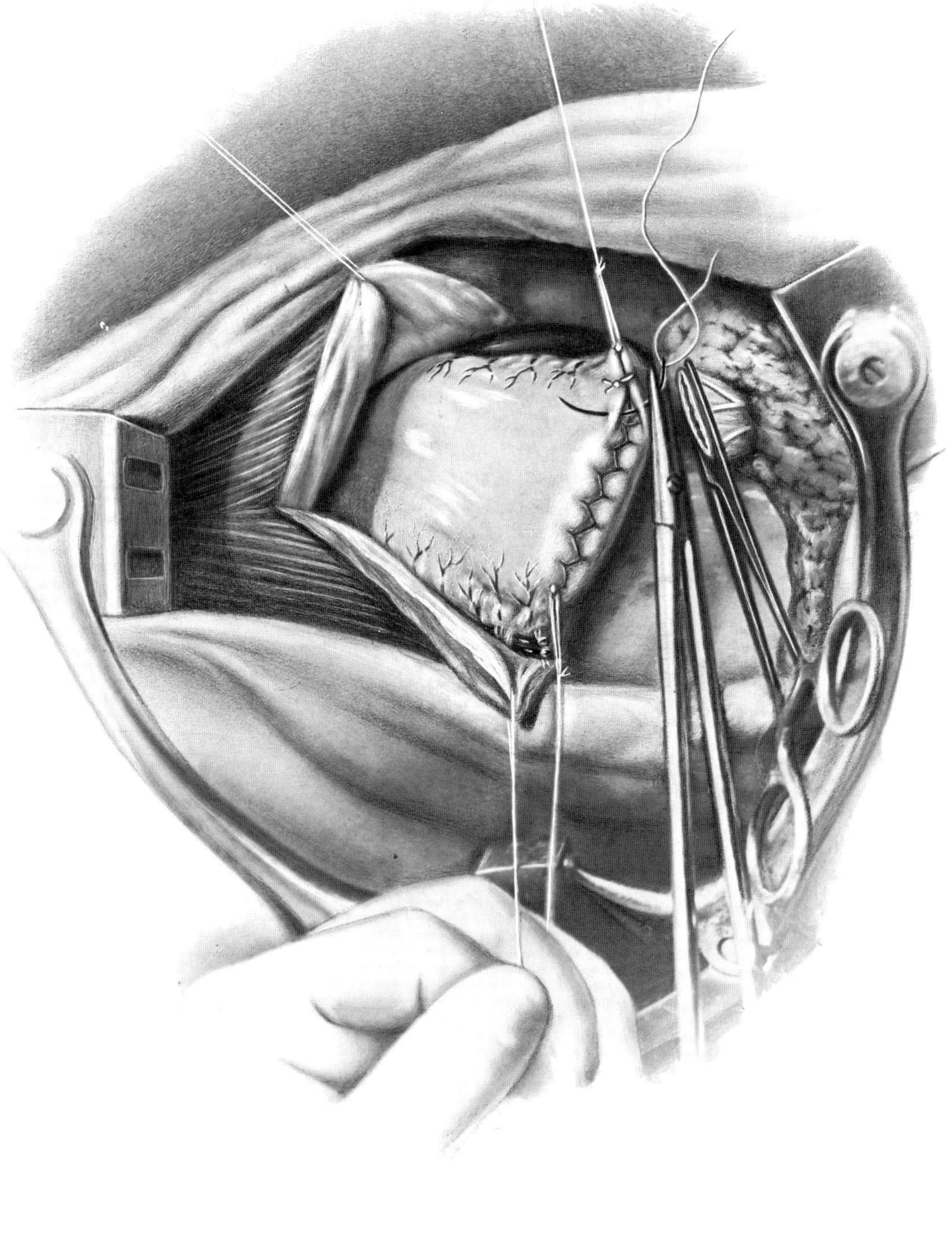

Fig. 610. Application of second row of interrupted seromuscular sutures to gastric stump.

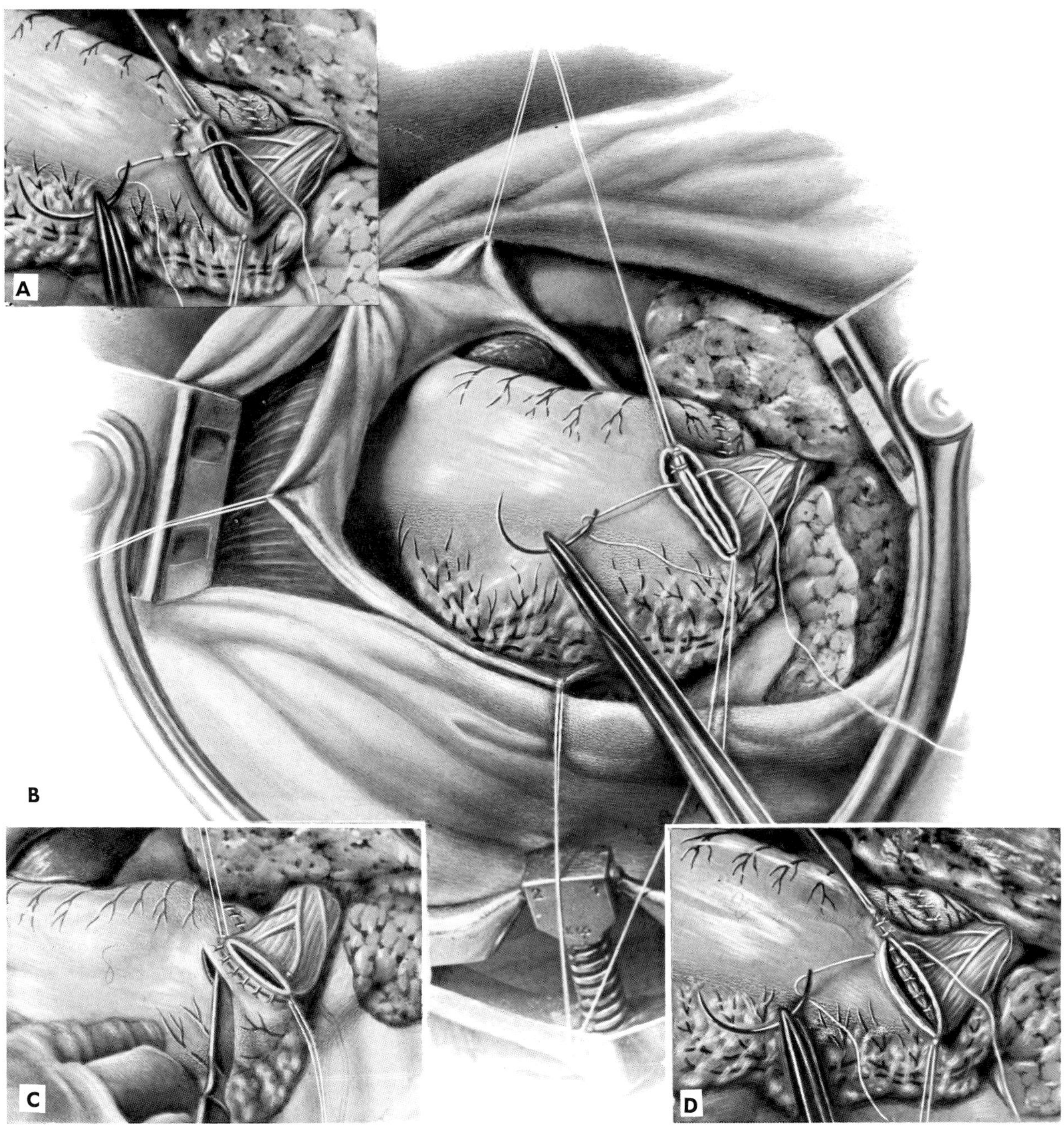

Fig. 611. Techniques of esophagogastric anastomosis. **A,** Application of dorsal seromuscular sutures to anastomosis between gastric stump and esophagus. **B,** Formation of opening in gastric stump for esophagogastric anastomosis. **C,** Application of internal sutures to dorsal lip of esophagogastric anastomosis. **D,** Application of sutures to ventral lip of esophagogastric anastomosis.

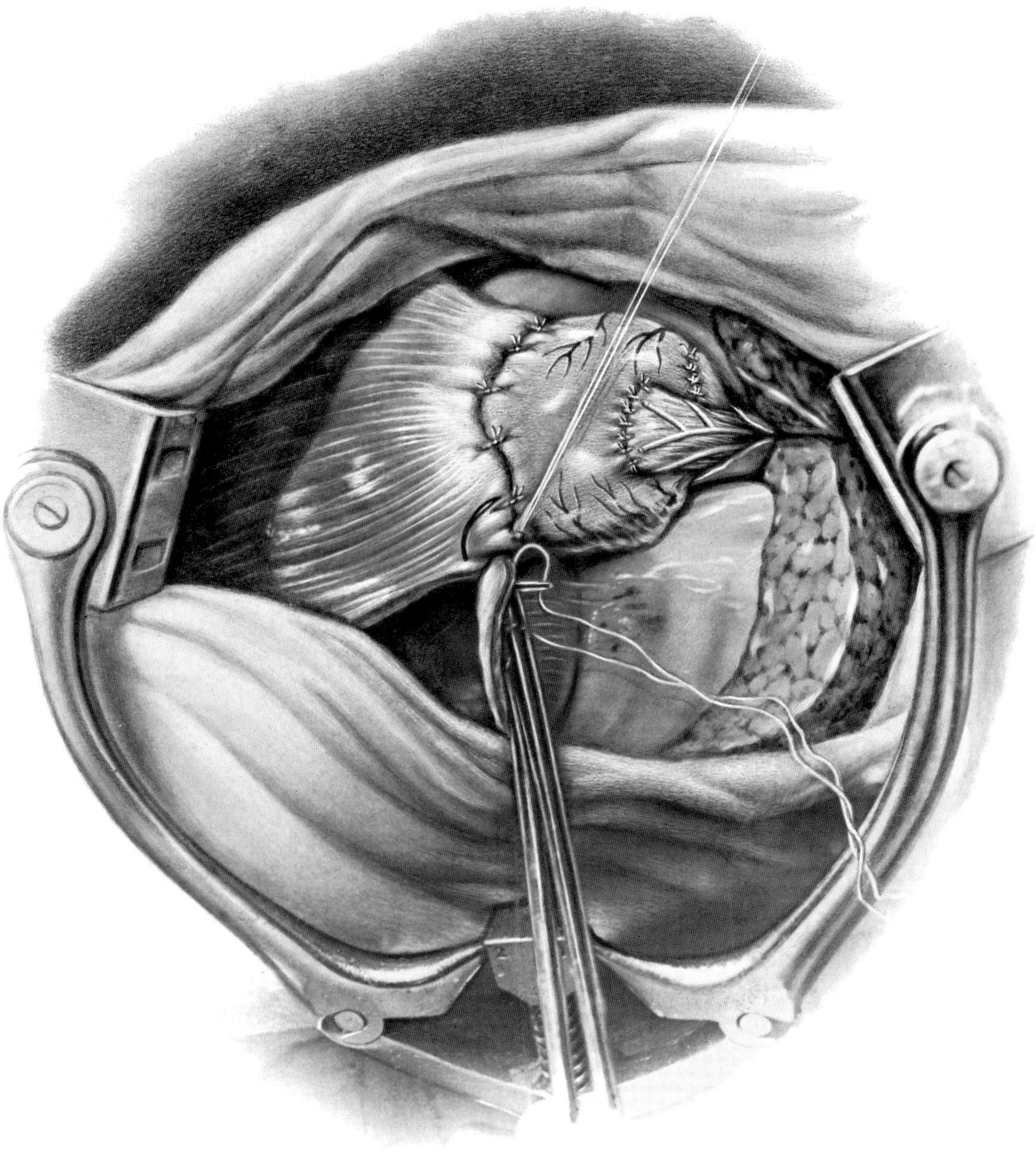

Fig. 612. Stomach is fastened with interrupted sutures to opening in diaphragm. Edges of diaphragmatic wound are being sutured.

RECANALIZATION AND PROSTHETIC REPLACEMENT OF LOWER PART OF ESOPHAGUS AND CARDIA IN CANCER

This palliative operation may be used in inoperable cancer of the thoracic esophagus and cardia. Endoprosthetics of the esophagus is accomplished by means of a mesh Lavsan prosthesis.

The prosthesis is a crimped tube 1.5 to 2 cm in diameter and up to 15 to 20 cm long. It has a semirigid rim at one of its ends for fixation above the upper pole of the tumor. If the esophageal lumen in the region of the tumor is sufficiently preserved, a steel string with a spring guide is introduced in the anterograde direction under esophagoscopic control, along which bougienage is accomplished. The endoprosthesis is fitted onto a bougie of the corresponding diameter and introduced into the esophagus so that its rim is positioned above the tumor.

In cases in which the string guide cannot be advanced

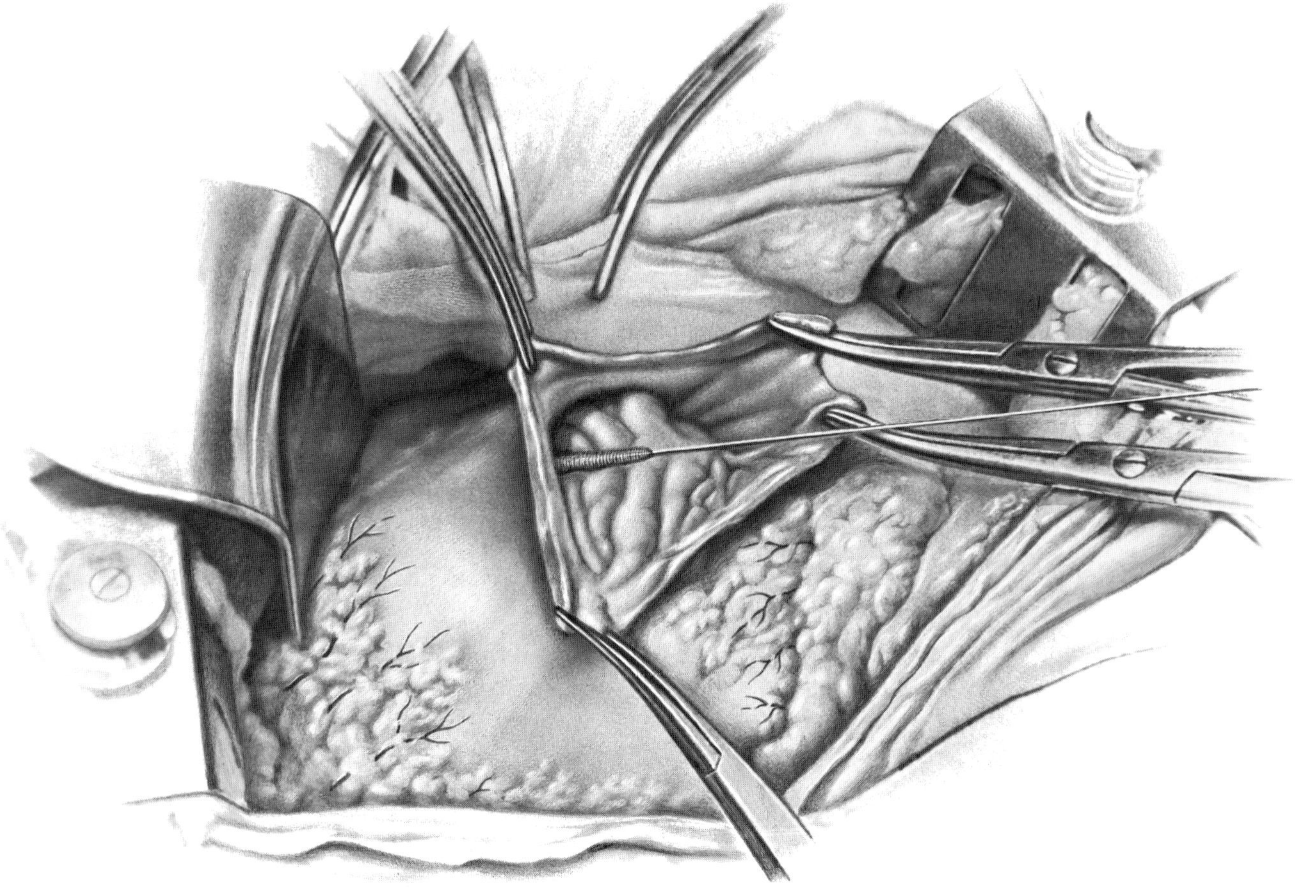

Fig. 613. Steel string with spring guide is introduced into esophagus through incision in anterior gastric wall.

beyond the tumor by means of the esophagoscope, retrograde bougienage of the esophageal tumor is carried out with hollow bougies along the string guide, which excludes the possibility of the esophagus's being perforated by the tip of the bougie (Fig. 613).

The largest bougie (No. 34-40) with four long, strong threads fastened to its end is advanced beyond the tumor from the stomach (Fig. 614). As soon as the threads emerge into the mouth, the assistant cuts them off the end of the bougie and stitches them through the end of the prosthesis. By pulling the ends of the threads from the abdominal cavity, the surgeon draws the prosthesis down along the bougie into the esophagus and stomach (Fig. 615). As soon as the "rim" of the prosthesis reaches the cranial border of the tumor, which may be determined by the resistance to the further descent of the prosthesis, the bougie and string are removed from the cavity of the prosthesis (Fig. 616, *A*). Should the prosthesis be too long and its lower end in the stomach is considerably below the tumor, it is cut (Fig. 616, *B*). The gastric wall is repaired with double-row sutures (Fig. 616, *C*). The wound in the abdominal wall is sutured tightly.

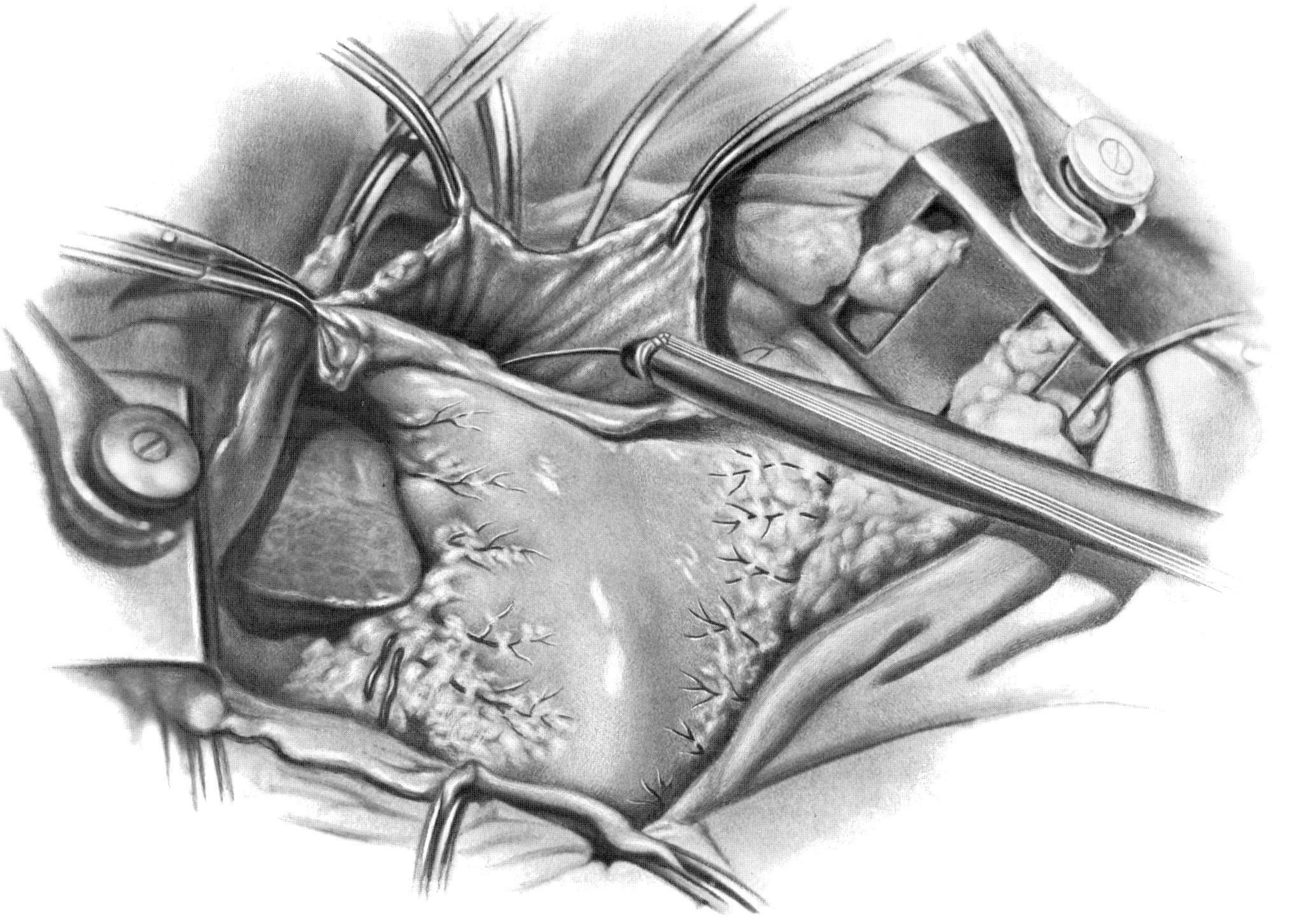

Fig. 614. Retrograde bougienage of tumor of esophagus with hollow bougie on steel string with spring guide. Four thick Lavsan threads are attached to tip of guide for drawing prosthesis from cavity of mouth down into esophagus.

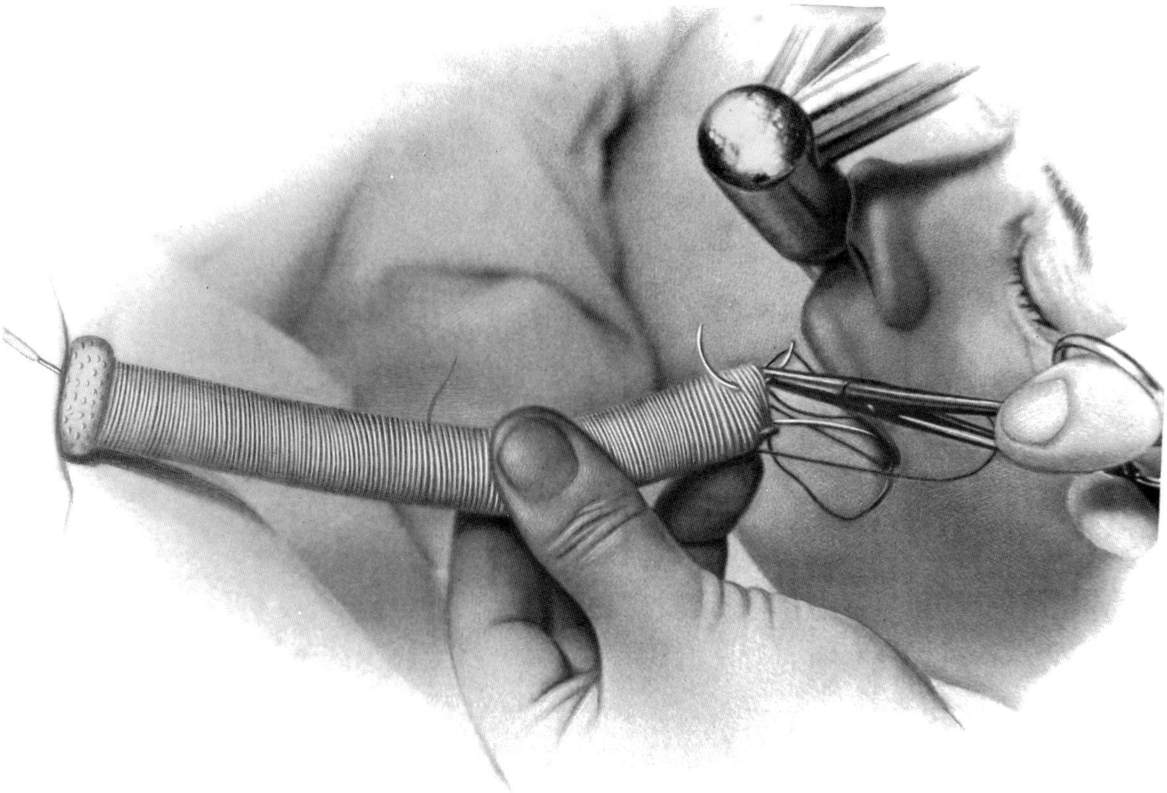

Fig. 615. Four Lavsan threads brought out through esophagus in retrograde direction are stitched to lower rim of Lavsan endoprosthesis for bringing it down. String with spring guide passes through cavity of prosthesis.

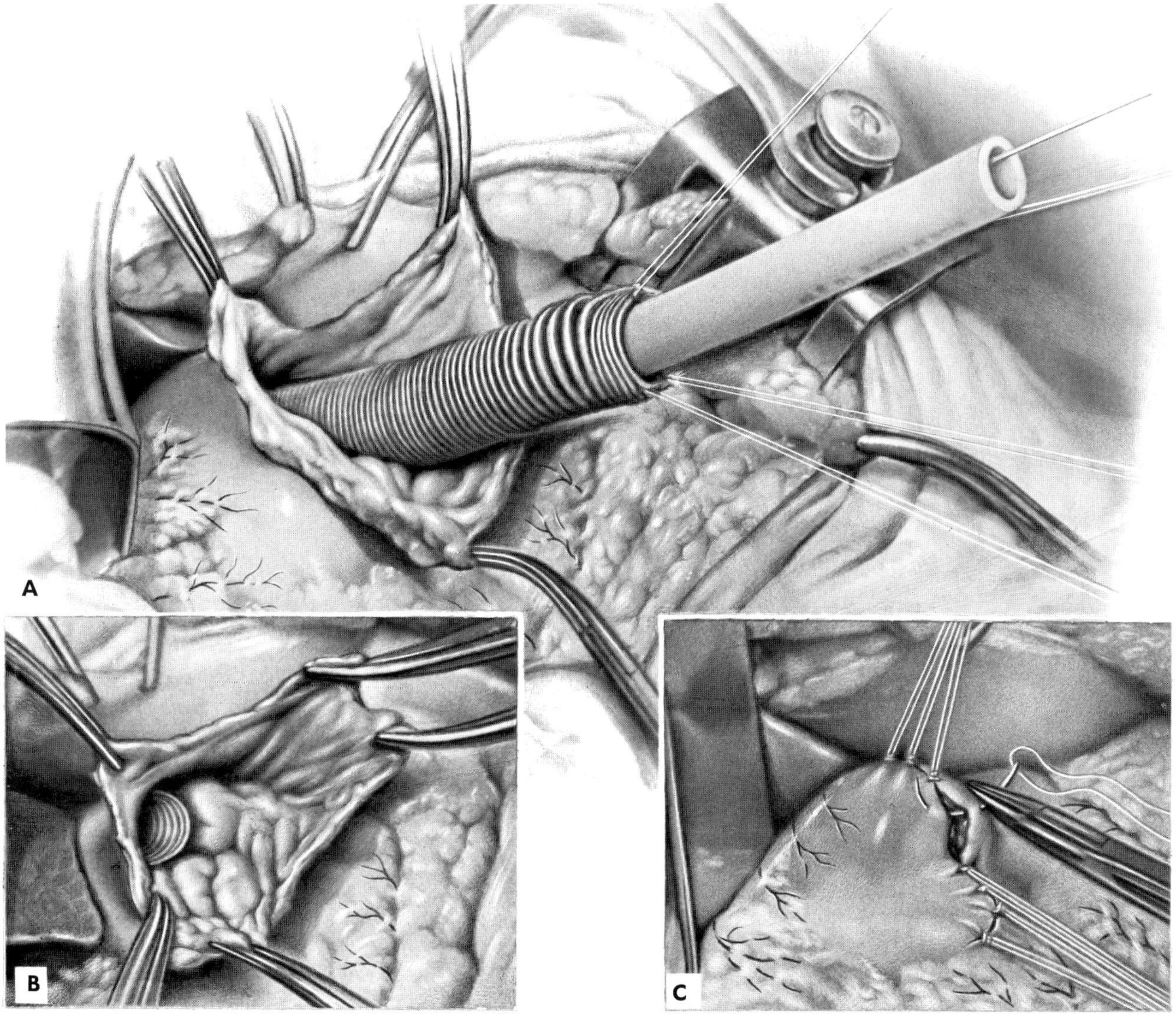

Fig. 616. Stages of introduction of endoprosthesis into esophagus. **A,** Crimped Lavsan prosthesis is drawn down along bougie and fitted into canal of esophageal and cardiac tumor. **B,** Excess part of endoprosthesis in stomach is cut away. **C,** Gastric wound is closed with sutures.

ENUCLEATION OF LEIOMYOMA OF ESOPHAGUS

Depending on the location of the tumor, the approach may be transthoracic (most commonly) or transabdominal (less frequently).

In a transthoracic approach the mediastinal pleura is cut at the level of the tumor, and the esophagus is freed from the mediastinum.

The esophageal muscular coat overlying the leiomyoma is cut lengthwise. The muscular fibers are pushed off the tumor with a tampon, and a traction ligature is stitched through the new growth. In some cases when the tumor is not covered by the muscular layer, the ligature is stitched through it immediately after the esophagus has been separated from the mediastinum. While the tumor is being pulled by the traction ligature, it is separated from the submucous layer with scissors (Fig. 617) and a tampon (Fig. 618) and removed. Enucleation should be performed with caution to avoid injury to the esophageal mucous coat.

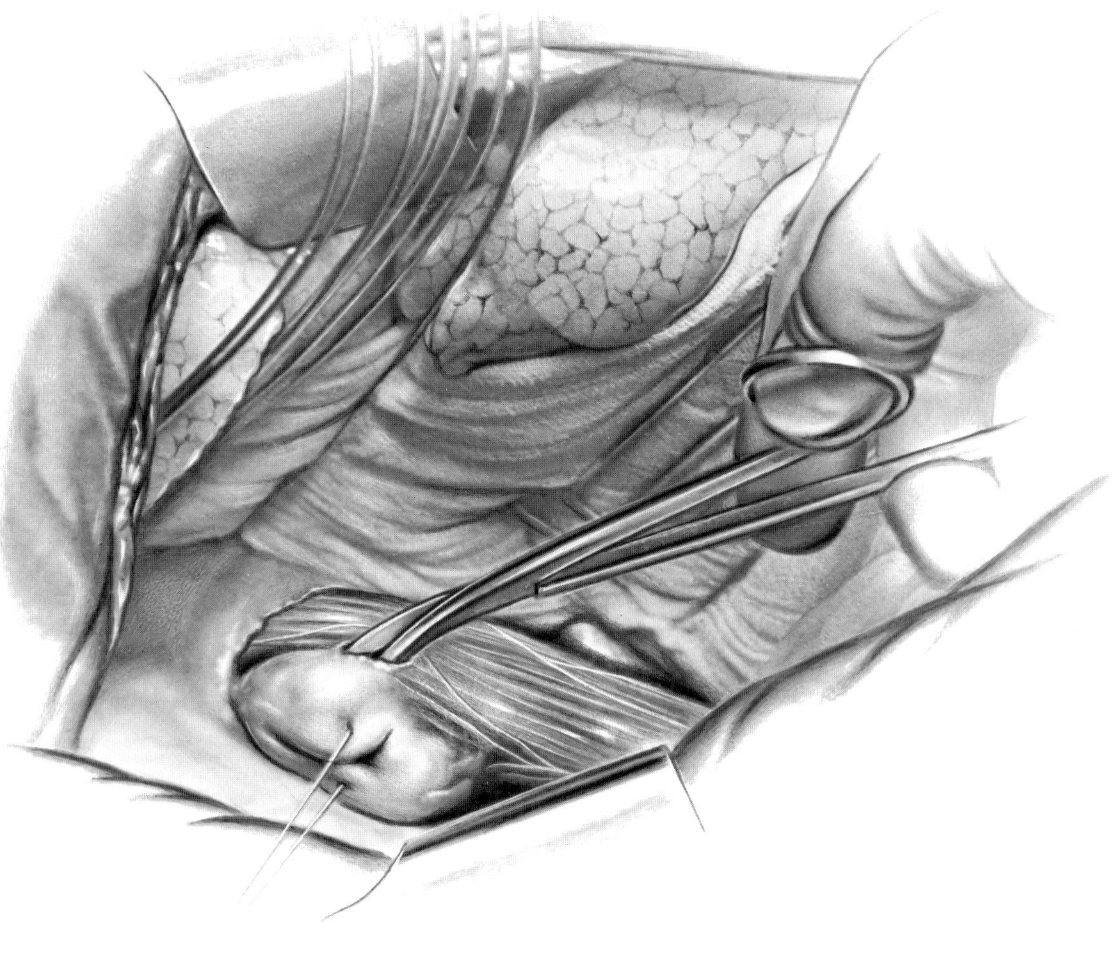

Fig. 617. Leiomyoma of esophagus is held with stitched ligature. Border of tumor is freed from under muscular coat with scissors.

With the tumor removed, interrupted sutures are applied to the muscular coat of the esophagus (Fig. 619) and then widely spaced sutures to the edges of the mediastinal pleura. In some cases damage to the mucous coat cannot be avoided because the tumor is fused with it. If the inflicted wound is relatively small, it is sutured lengthwise. A continuous catgut suture is first applied to the mucous coat (Fig. 620) and then interrupted nonabsorbable sutures to the muscular coat of the esophagus (Fig. 621). To avoid constriction of the esophagus, the sutures are applied to its wall over a thick gastric tube. The mediastinal pleura is closed with interrupted sutures placed over the line of the esophageal suture. The pleura directly overlying the caudal corner of the esophageal wound is either not sutured or repaired with rarely spaced sutures. A drain is introduced into the pleural cavity with its end set caudal to the level of the sutured esophageal wound. The wound in the thoracic wall is closed completely.

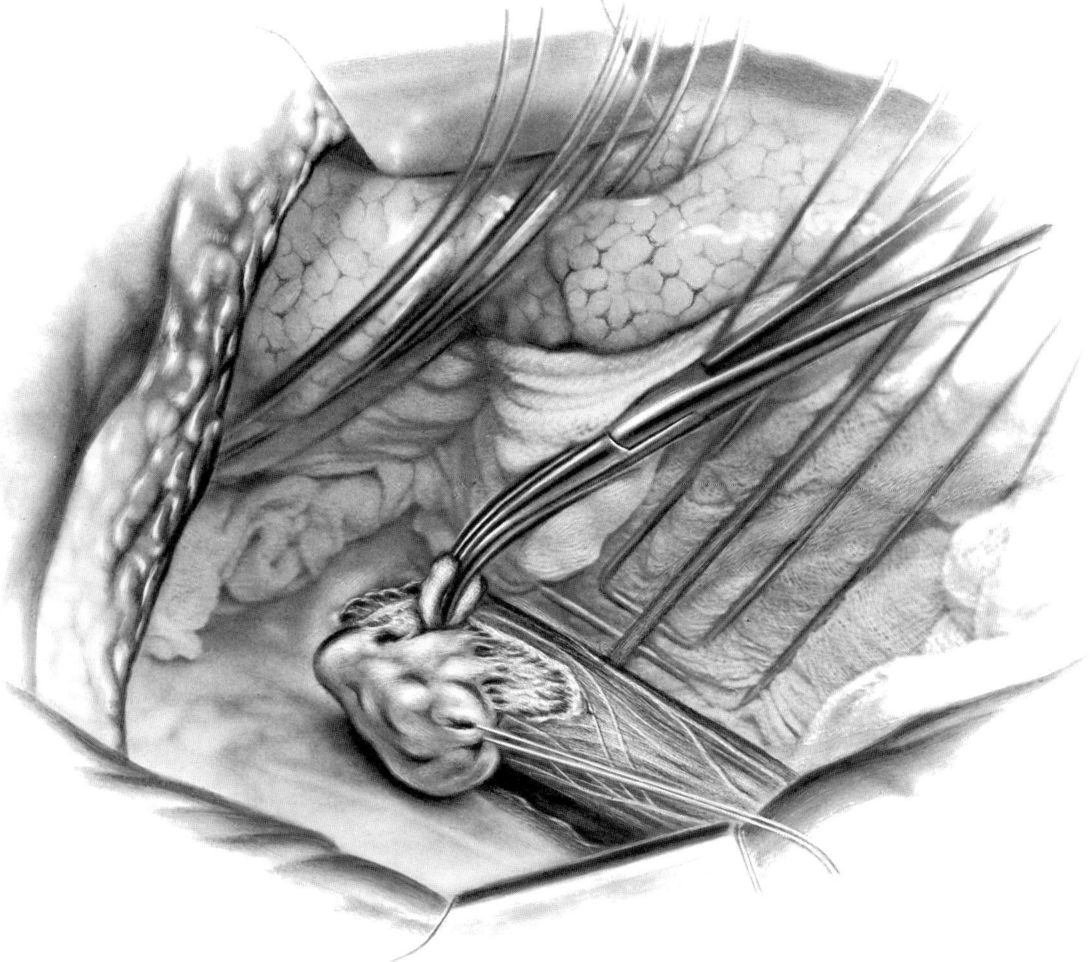

Fig. 618. Leiomyoma is separated from esophageal submucous layer with tampon.

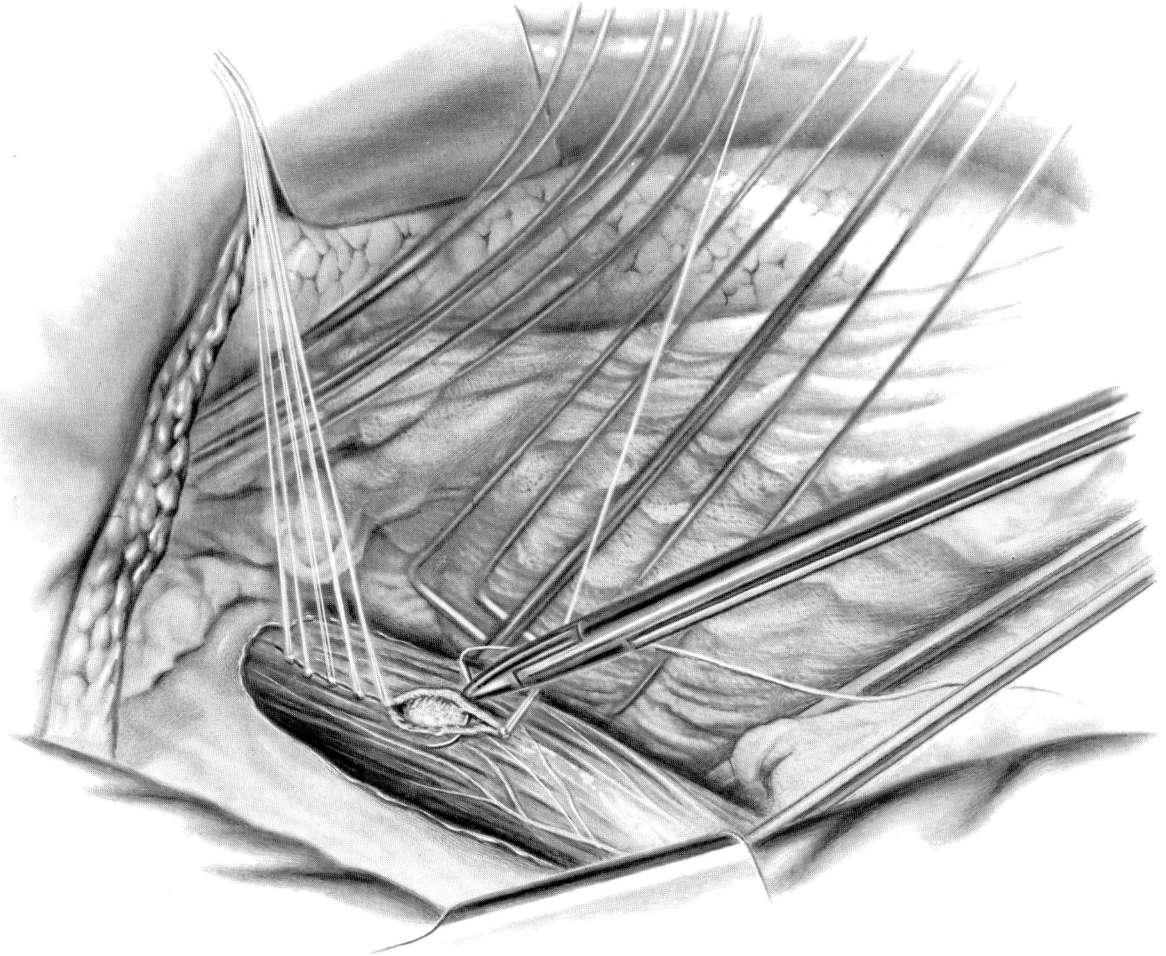

Fig. 619. Defect in esophageal muscular coat is repaired with interrupted sutures.

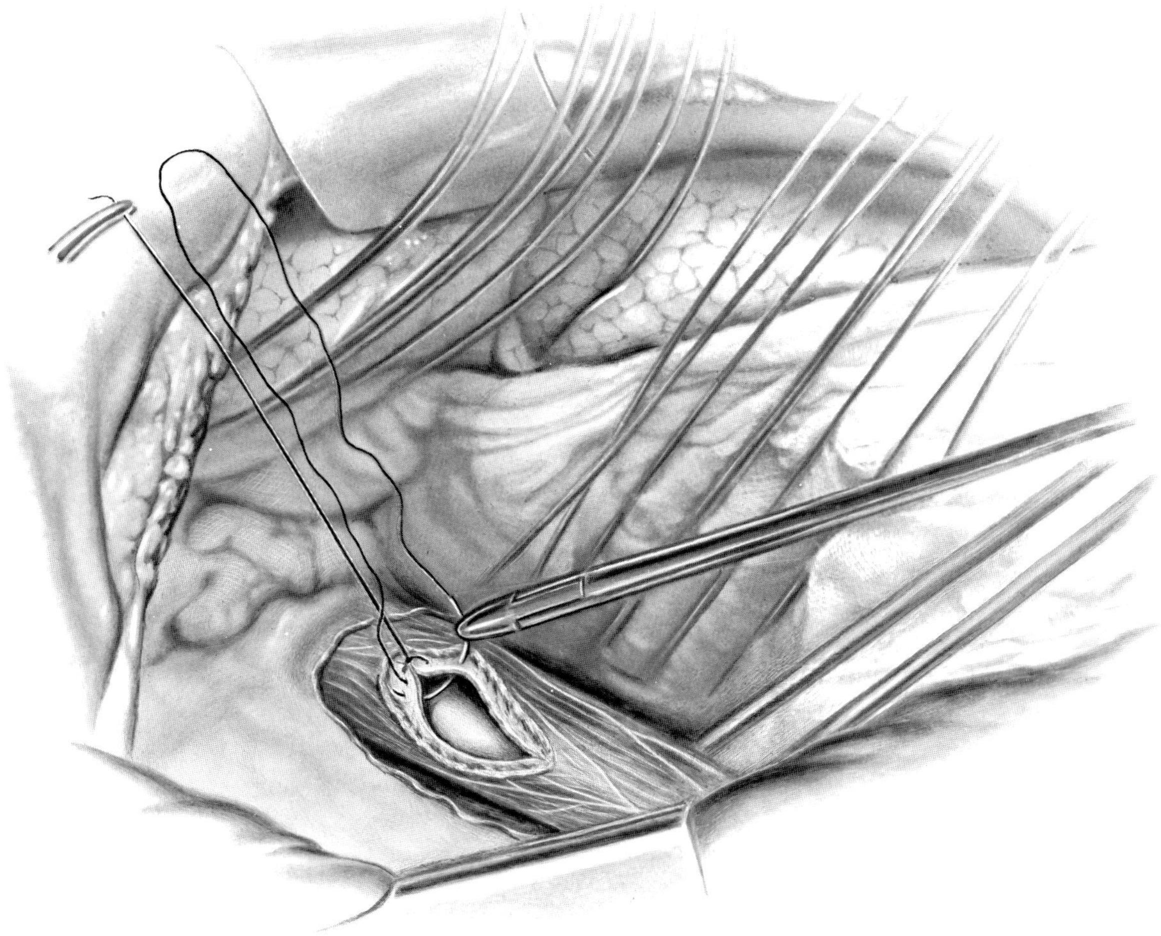

Fig. 620. Continuous catgut suture is applied to wound in esophageal mucous coat.

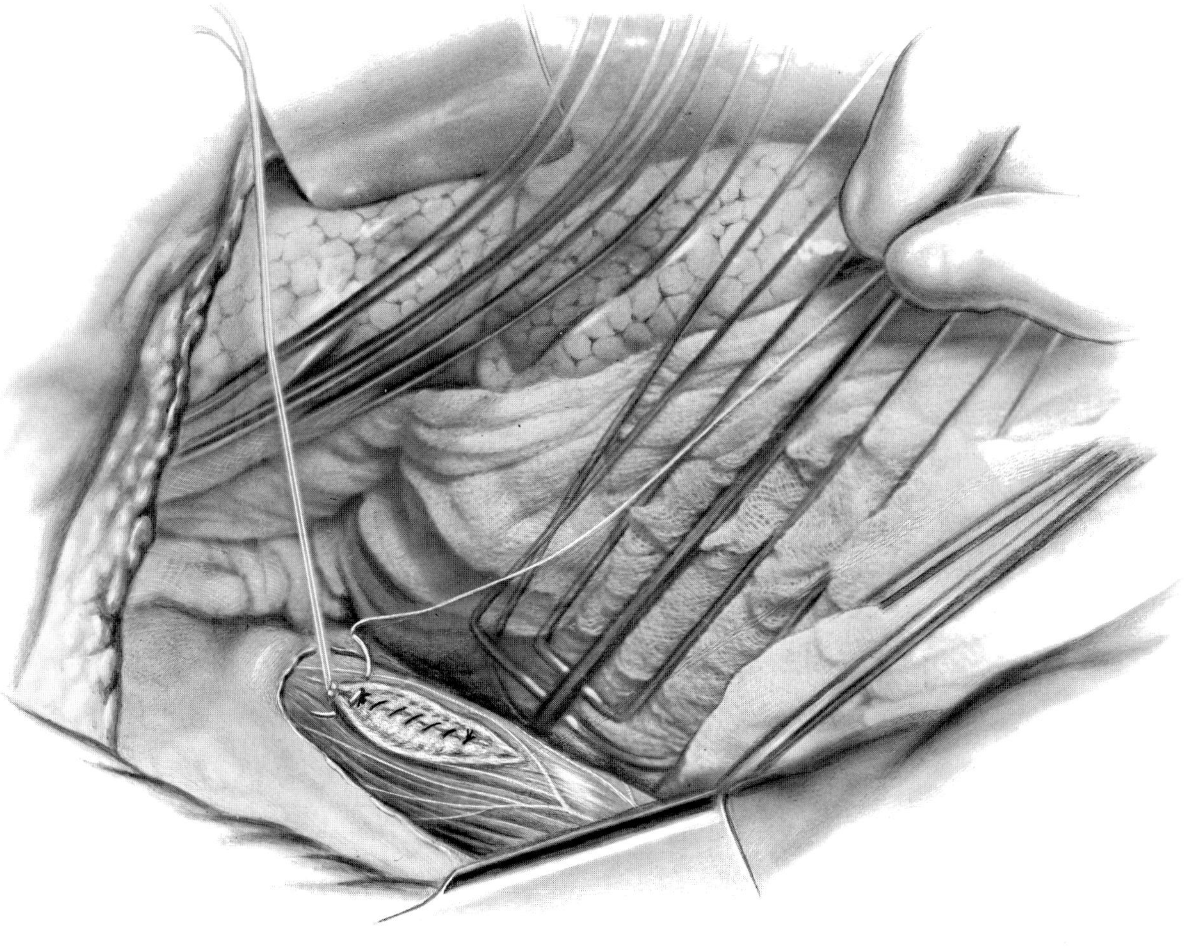

Fig. 621. Interrupted sutures are applied to esophageal muscular coat.

Restorative and reconstructive operations

TOTAL ESOPHAGOPLASTY

The small intestine, the large intestine, and the stomach are used as grafts in plastic surgery of the esophagus. The peculiarity of total plastics consists in the replacement of the entire thoracic and abdominal parts of the esophagus, and also part or the whole of the cervical portion, with these organs.

Total esophagoplasty may be antethoracic, retrosternal, retrocostal, or retromediastinal depending on the placement of the graft. At present the most commonly used methods for transposition of the graft onto the neck in total esophagoplasty are the antethoracic and the retrosternal techniques.

Total esophagoplasty is used for replacing the esophagus that has been extirpated for any among a variety of diseases (mainly for malignant tumors of the esophagus), as well as in cicatricial stenoses of the cervical esophagus or pharynx, the superior thoracic portion or along the entire length of the esophagus. In some cases (usually when thoracotomy is contraindicated) antethoracic and retrosternal esophagoplasty may be employed in a localized cicatricial stenosis of the middle and inferior thoracic portions of the esophagus.

Median laparotomy is the best approach for examination of the abdominal organs and the choice of one of them (the small or large intestine or the stomach) for mobilizing as the graft. We should strive to choose a graft from that part of the gastrointestinal tract whose vascularization in each individual case would most adequately meet the tasks of total esophagoplasty; that is, a very long graft has to be mobilized. When intestinal grafts are used, preference should be given to isoperistaltic loops over antiperistaltic loops, although the latter may be employed when it proves difficult to separate an isoperistaltic intestinal segment with a sufficiently reliable blood supply.

PLASTIC SURGERY WITH THE SMALL INTESTINE

TECHNIQUES FOR SHAPING THE GRAFT FOR ESOPHAGOPLASTY AFTER ROU-HERTZEN AND YUDIN

The best conditions for separating a graft of the small intestine are to be found in its cranial portion, where the caliber of the intestinal arteries and arcades between them is usually the largest, the length of the intestinal arteries is sufficient, and the avascular fields of the mesentery bounded by two pairs of intestinal arteries and veins and the arcades between them are well developed. The operation is begun with median laparotomy. The initial portion of the jejunum is brought out into the wound, and 10 to 15 cm from the Treitz ligament the arcade between the first and second pairs of arteries and veins of the small intestine is ligated and transected (Fig. 622).

The mesentery is cut in the avascular field between the second, third, and fourth radial arteries and veins; the trunks of these vessels are exposed by blunt and sharp dissection 2 to 3 cm below the bifurcation (Fig. 623), ligated, and transected (Fig. 624). After the vessels are transected, the incisions in the mesenteric avascular fields are made slightly deeper with scissors

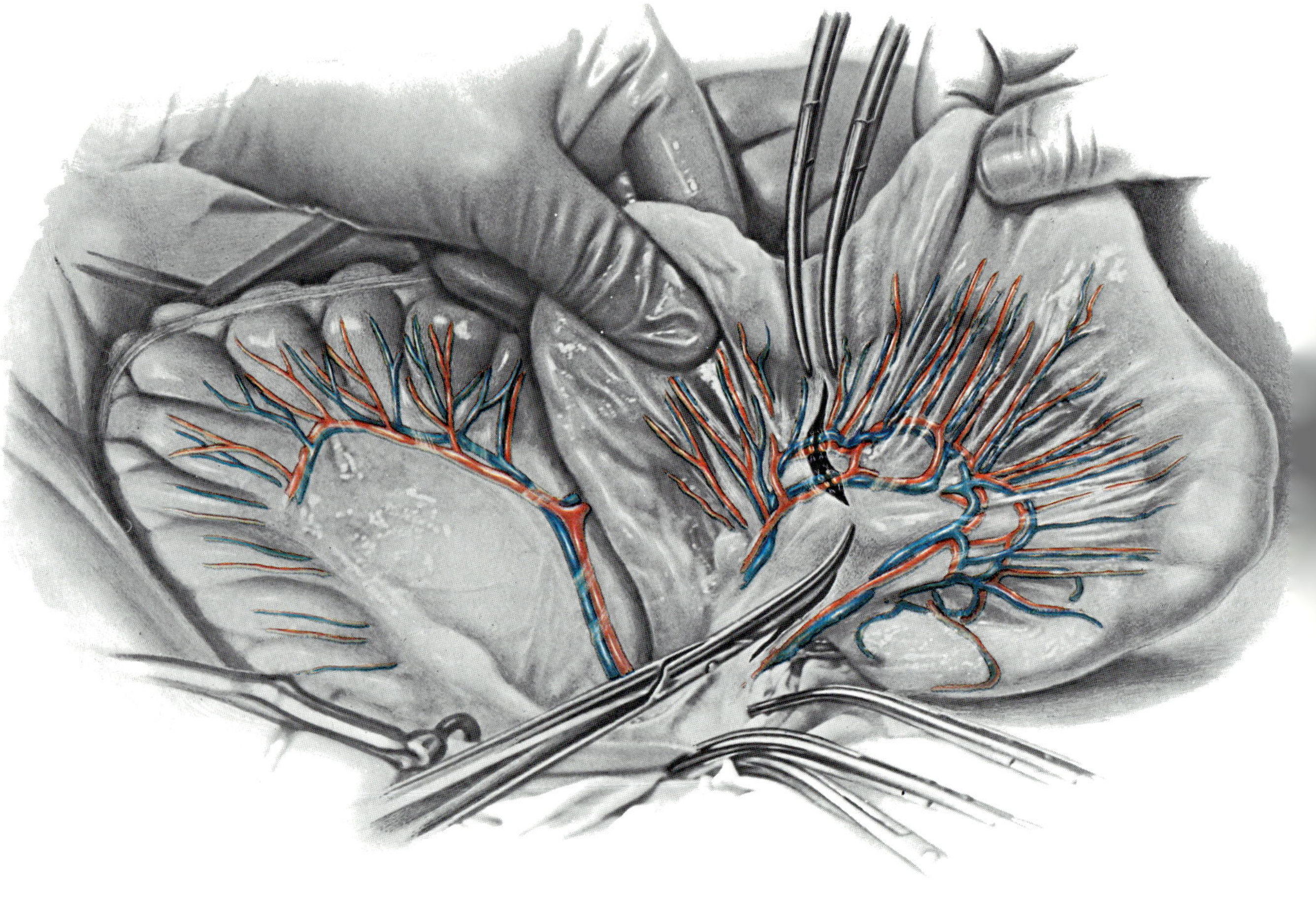

Fig. 622. Vascular arcades between first and second pairs of arteries and veins of small intestine are ligated and transected near Treitz's ligament. First avascular field of mesentery of small intestine is cut.

to draw out the vascular arcades under the mobilized intestine into almost a straight line, thus elongating the graft (Fig. 625). The intestine is transected directly above the divided vascular arcade between the first and second radial arteries (Fig. 626). Its oral stump is covered with a gauze napkin to prevent contamination of the abdominal cavity, while the aboral stump is sutured and buried in a purse-string suture (Fig. 627). If it is intended to anastomose the intestinal stump with the esophagus a few days after the mobilization of the graft, single seroserous sutures are applied to the stump over the purse-string sutures. The ligatures on the aboral stump are not cut away until the transplant is transposed to the neck.

The small intestine is again transected between two crushing clamps above the vascular arcades close to the fifth radial artery supplying the graft (Fig. 628). The caudal stump of the intestinal graft is transposed to the ventral wall of the stomach and anastomosed with it end to side (Fig. 629). After a tunnel is formed under the skin in front of the sternum or in the anterior mediastinum, the superior stump is transposed to the neck and fastened with a stitched ligature or anastomosed with the esophagus. The continuity of the intestine is restored by creating end-to-end or end-to-side anastomosis between its clamped stumps. The abdominal cavity is closed completely. In some instances (in severe ciciatricial shrinking of the stomach after chemical burn, in

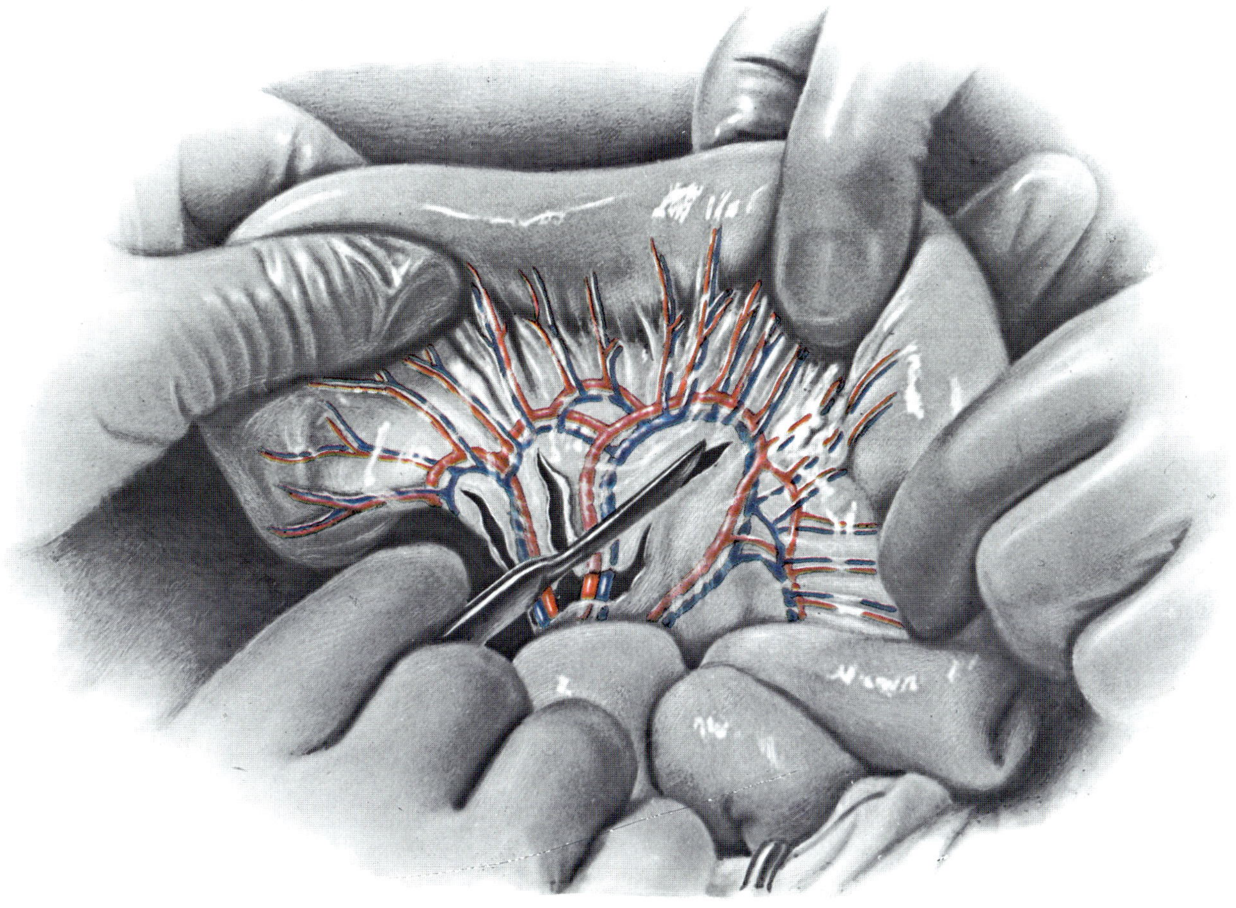

Fig. 623. Mesentery of small intestine is cut in avascular fields between second, third, and fourth pairs of arteries and veins of small intestine.

considerable adhesions in the upper abdominal cavity, etc.) it is inexpedient to establish an anastomosis between the graft and the stomach. Under these circumstances, after the cranial stump of the graft has been formed, the mobilized intestine is not clamped a second time, but the continuity of the small intestine is restored by means of a Y-shaped enteroenterostomy close to the base of the graft (Yudin's modification) (Fig. 630). The cranial stump of the graft is transposed to the neck. The abdominal cavity is closed.

In both instances three radial arteries and veins are transected in forming the graft. In practice, however, it is sometimes necessary to ligate four and even five radial vessels to obtain a graft of the required length, which may cause serious disorders in the blood supply to the intestine.

The graft may be elongated 10 cm without additional ligation of the vessels by mobilizing the root of the mesentery of the small intestine after Petrov-Khundadze's method.

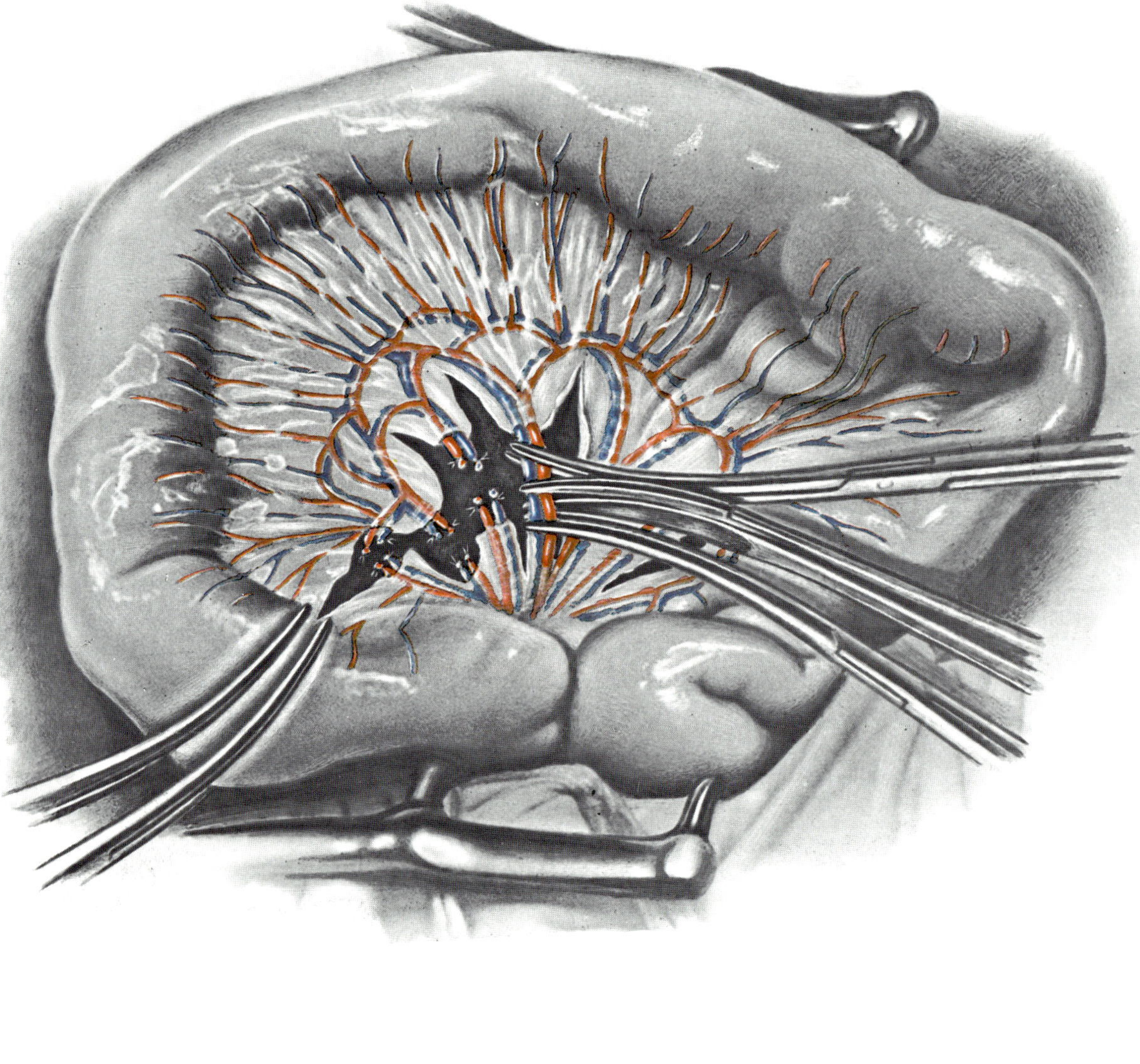

Fig. 624. Arteries and veins of small intestine are transected below site of their division into branches.

Its technique is as follows. The assistant grasps the ileocecal portion of the intestine with his hand and moves it medially and cranially, as a result of which the posterolateral sheet of the peritoneum is tightened behind the cecum and below the ileal mesentery. This peritoneal sheet is cut laterally caudal to the ascending colon and cecum and transversely under the root of the mesentery of the small intestine (Fig. 631).

While the assistant continues to pull the cecum and terminal part of the ileum, the root of the mesentery of the small intestine together with the vessels is detached from the posterior abdominal wall by the blunt method with a tampon or gauze napkin and is transposed cranially (Fig. 632). Separation of the root of the mesentery should be continued until the lower horizontal part of the duodenum becomes visible in the wound (Fig. 633). The root of the mesentery thus mobilized may be fastened to the upper corner of the wound in the anterior abdominal wall with two or three sutures.

The effectiveness of this manipulation to a great

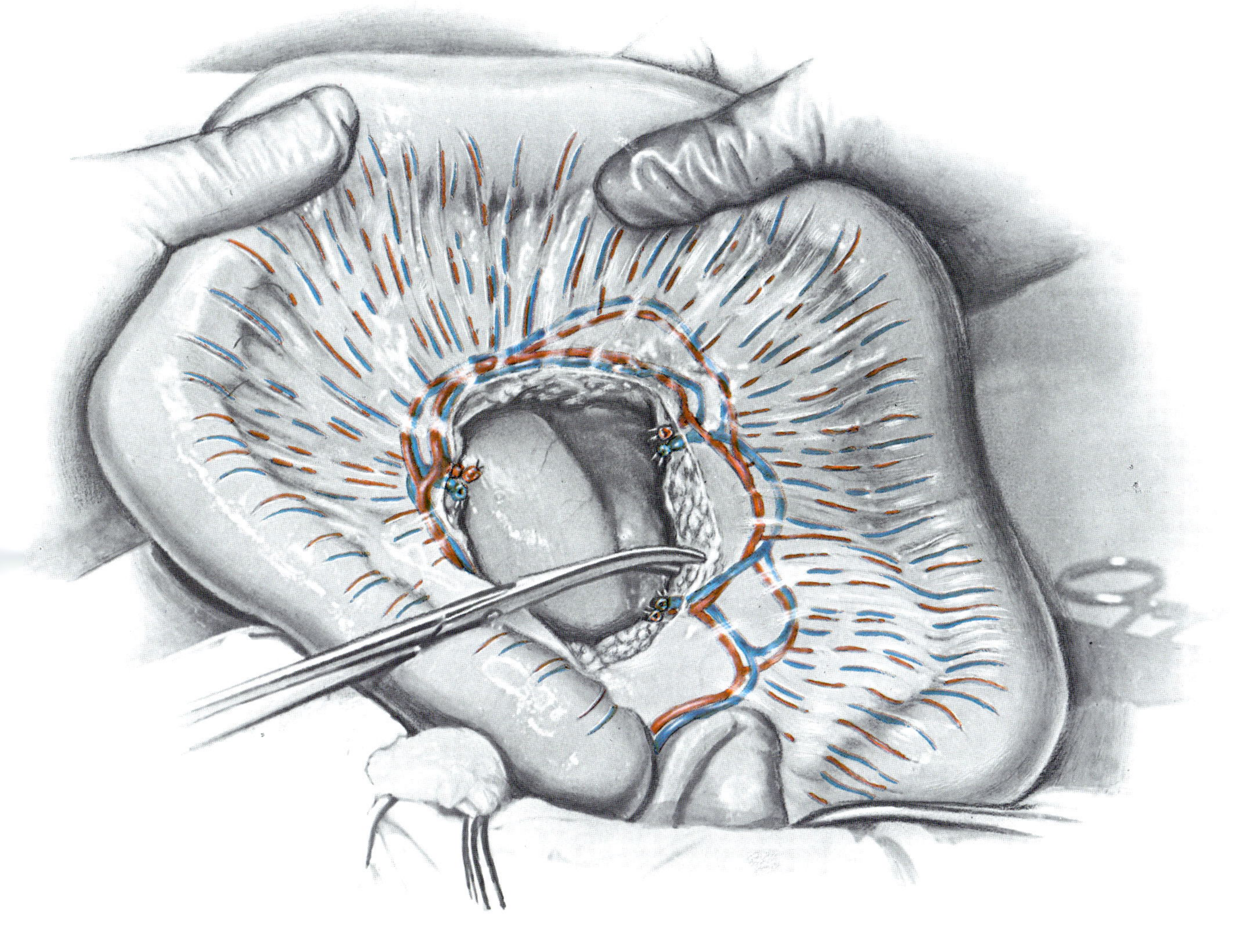

Fig. 625. Incisions in avascular fields of mesentery are made deeper to straighten out chain of vascular arcades.

extent depends on the length of the mesenteric root and the use of proper techniques. When the root of the small intestine is short and the intestinal vessels to be ligated in mobilization of the graft divide at a low level, the length of the graft may be increased by ligating and transecting secondary vascular arcades in their crotch (Fig. 634). This straightens out the chain of vascular arcades, increasing the length of the graft 4 to 7 cm whenever the main intestinal arteries to be ligated form a sharp or right angle at their division into two branches.

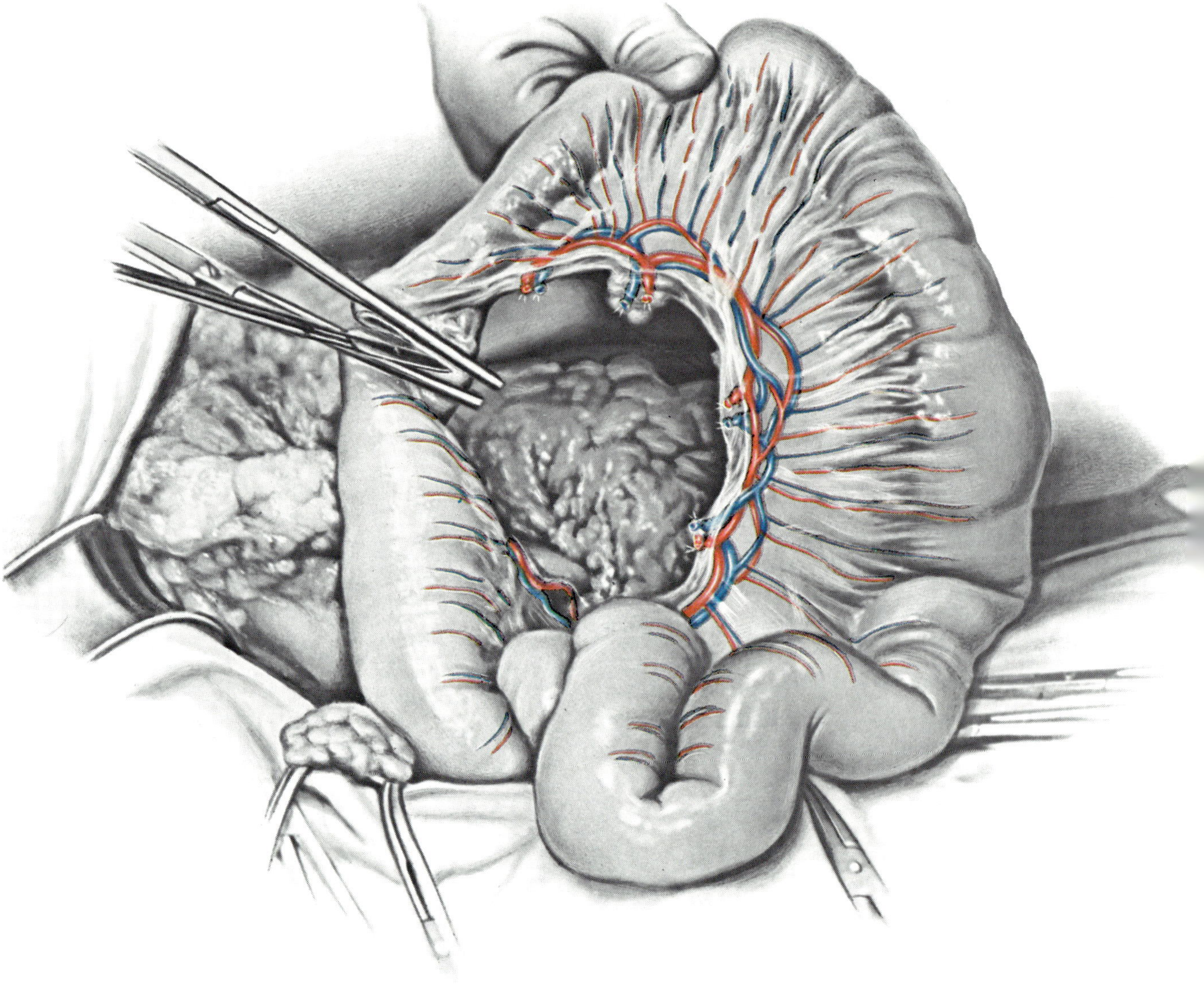

Fig. 626. Mobilized loop of small intestine is transected 10 to 15 cm from Treitz's ligament.

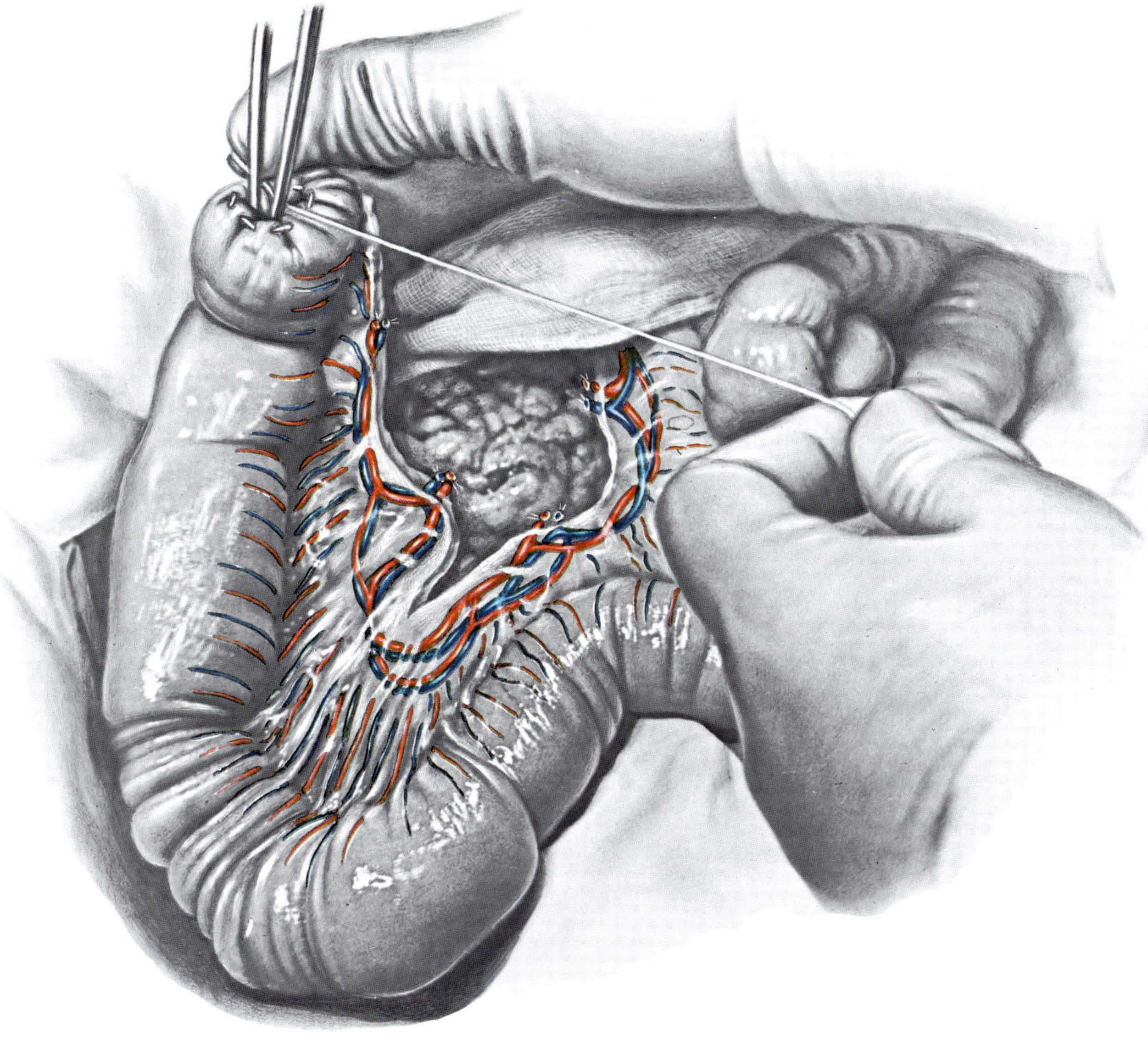

Fig. 627. Superior stump of graft is closed with continuous blanket suture and then buried in purse-string suture.

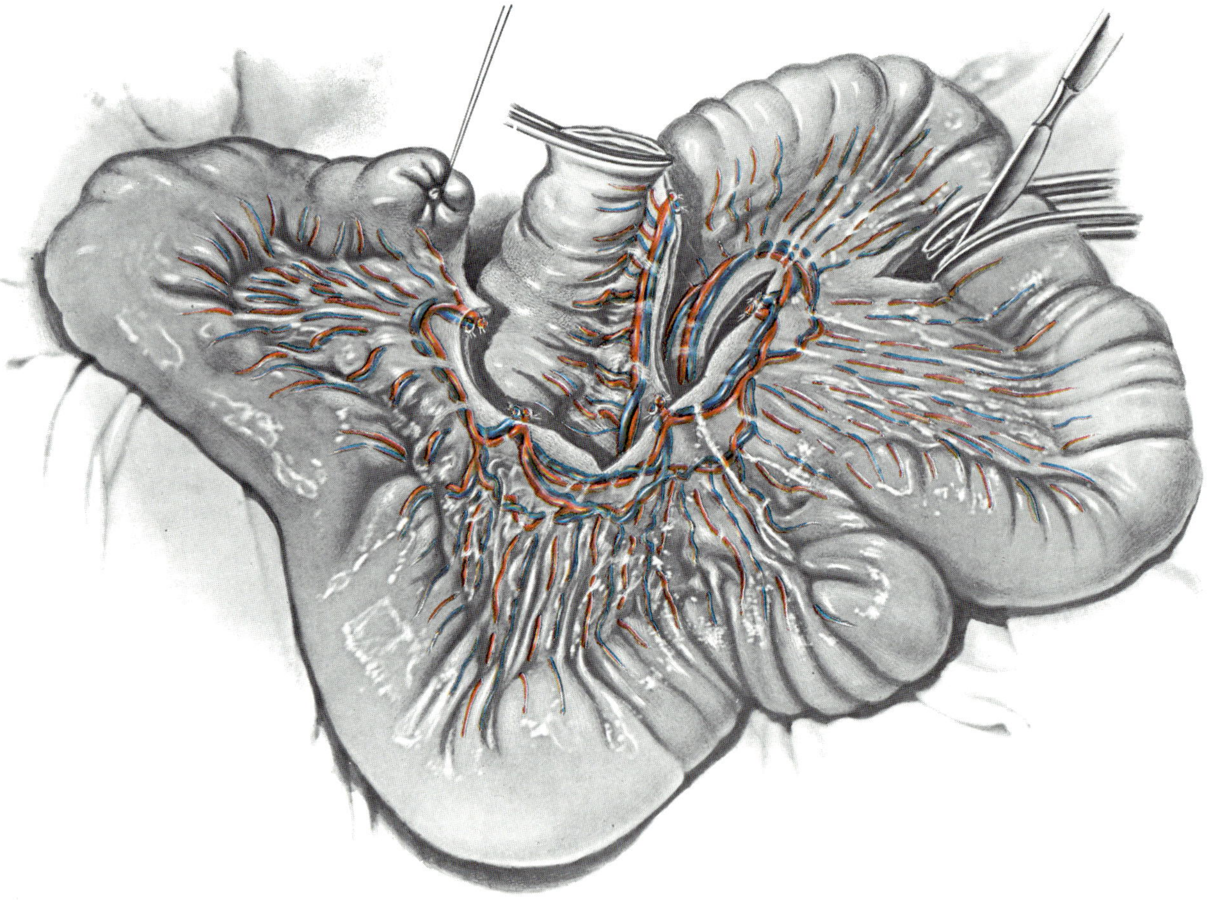

Fig. 628. Second transection of mobilized loop of small intestine at base of graft near its vascular pedicle.

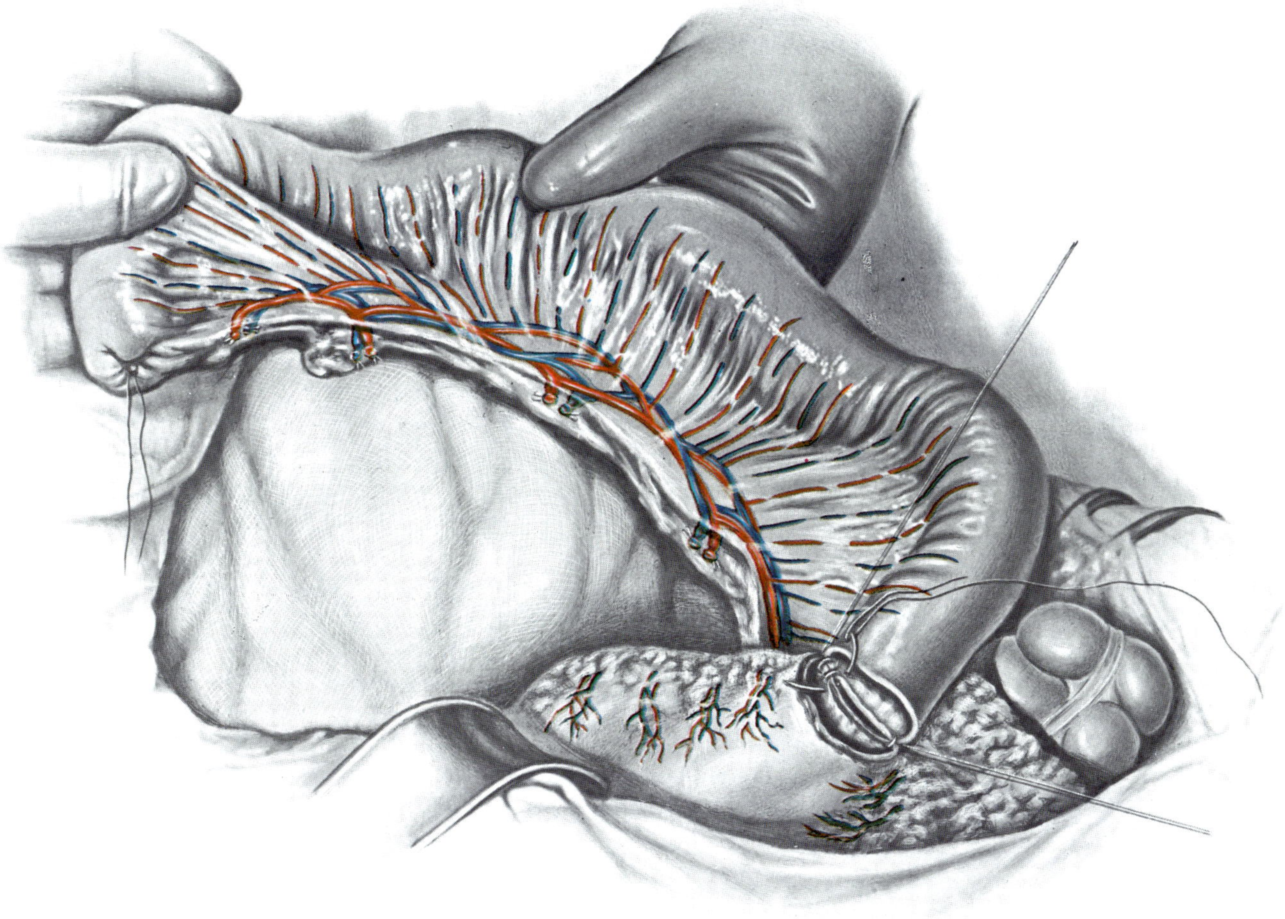

Fig. 629. Formation of anastomosis between lower stump of graft and stomach.

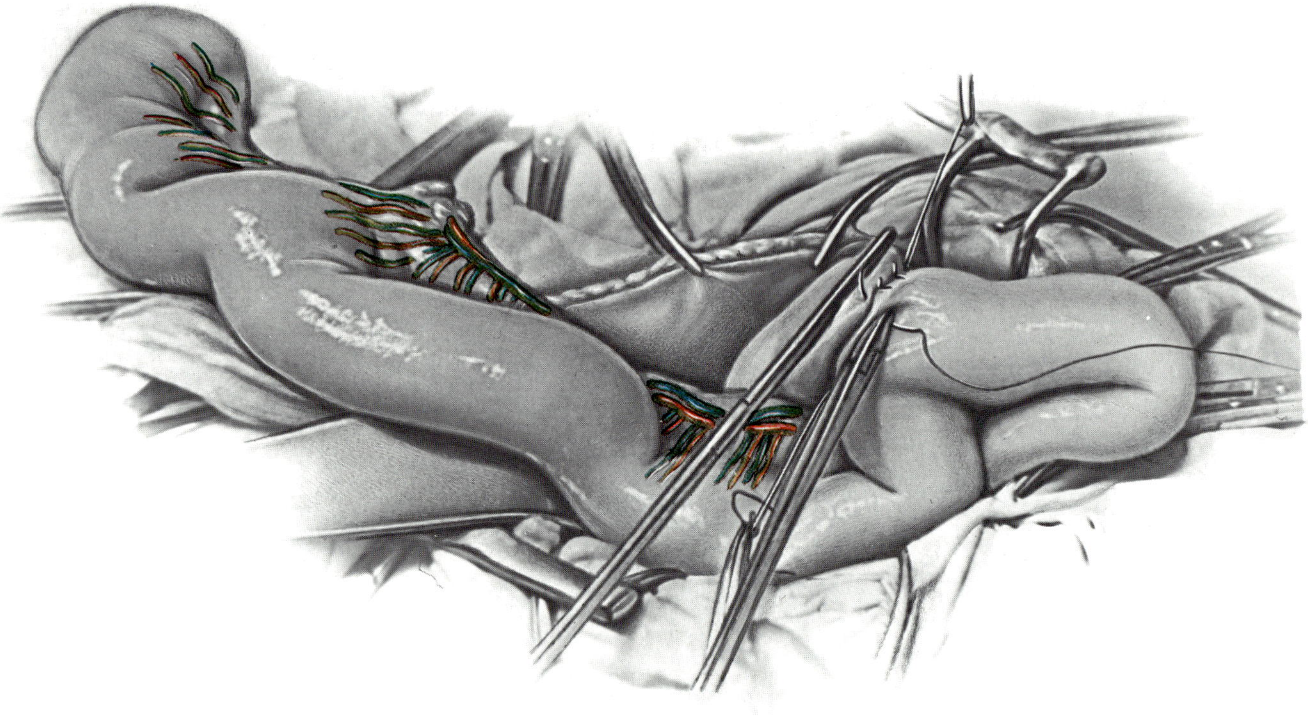

Fig. 630. Y-shaped enteroenterostomy in esophagoplasty after Yudin.

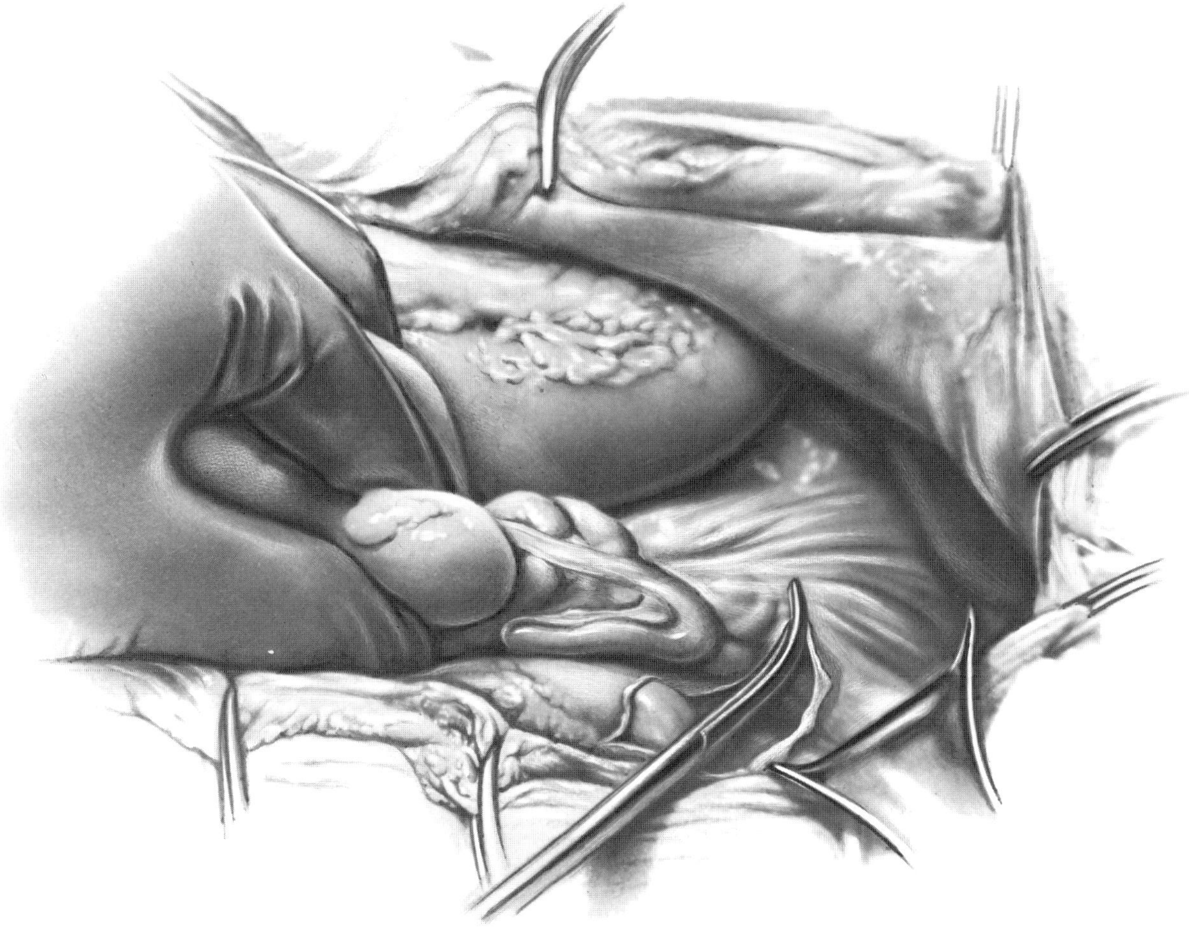

Fig. 631. Parietal peritoneum is cut in right lateral canal under dome of cecum.

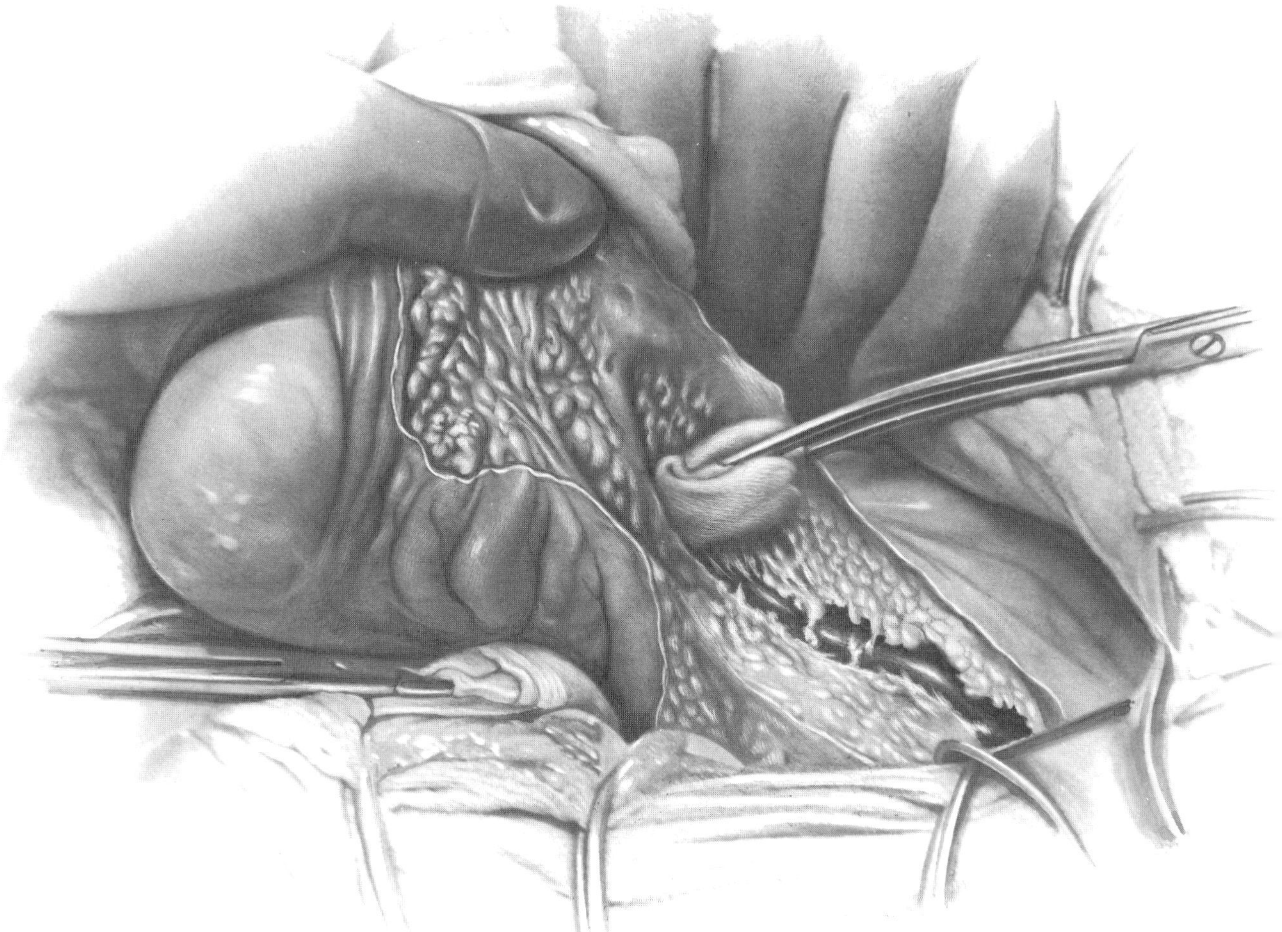

Fig. 632. Dome of cecum and mesentery of small intestine are separated from posterior abdominal wall.

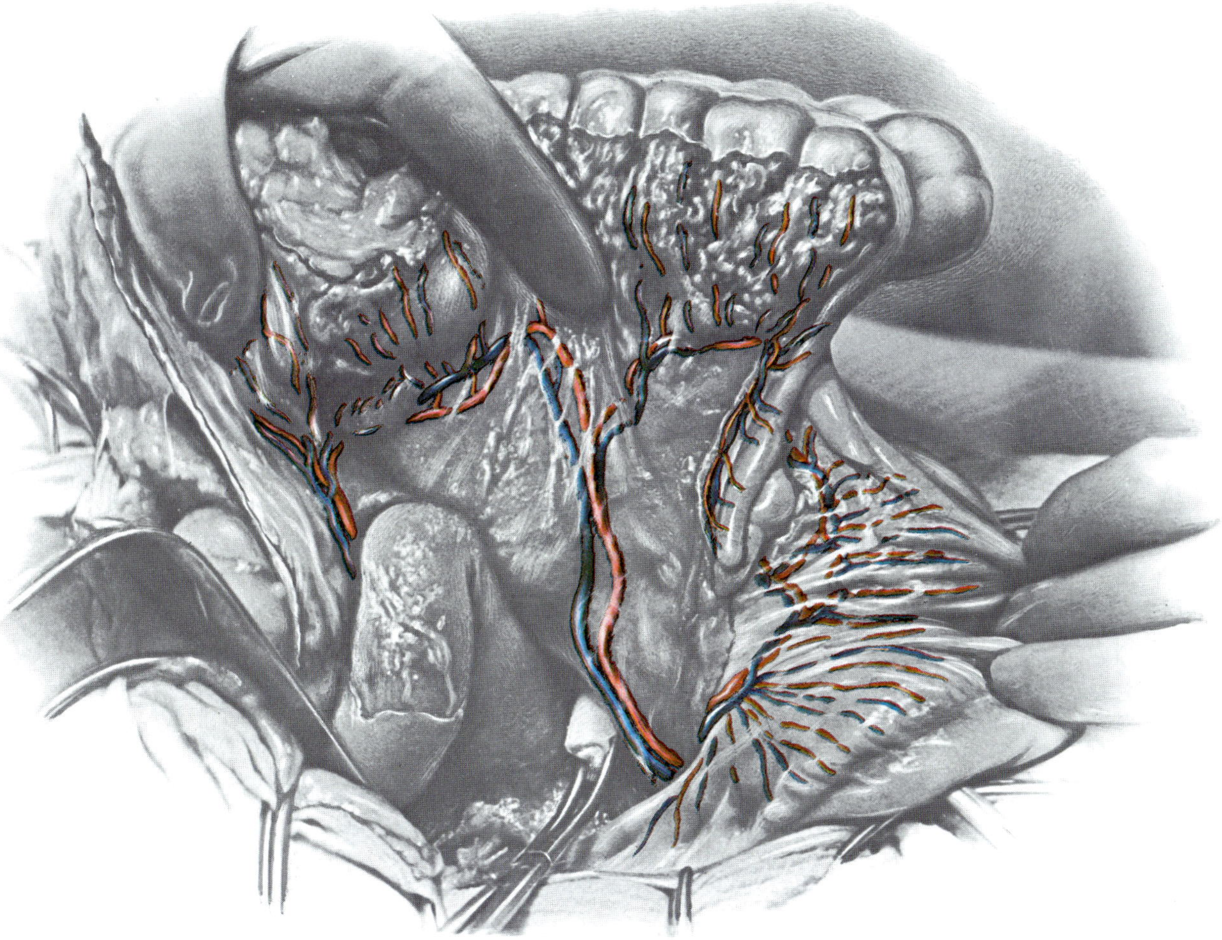

Fig. 633. Separated cecum, ascending colon, and lower part of root of mesentery of small intestine are raised. Lower horizontal portion of duodenum is visible deep in wound.

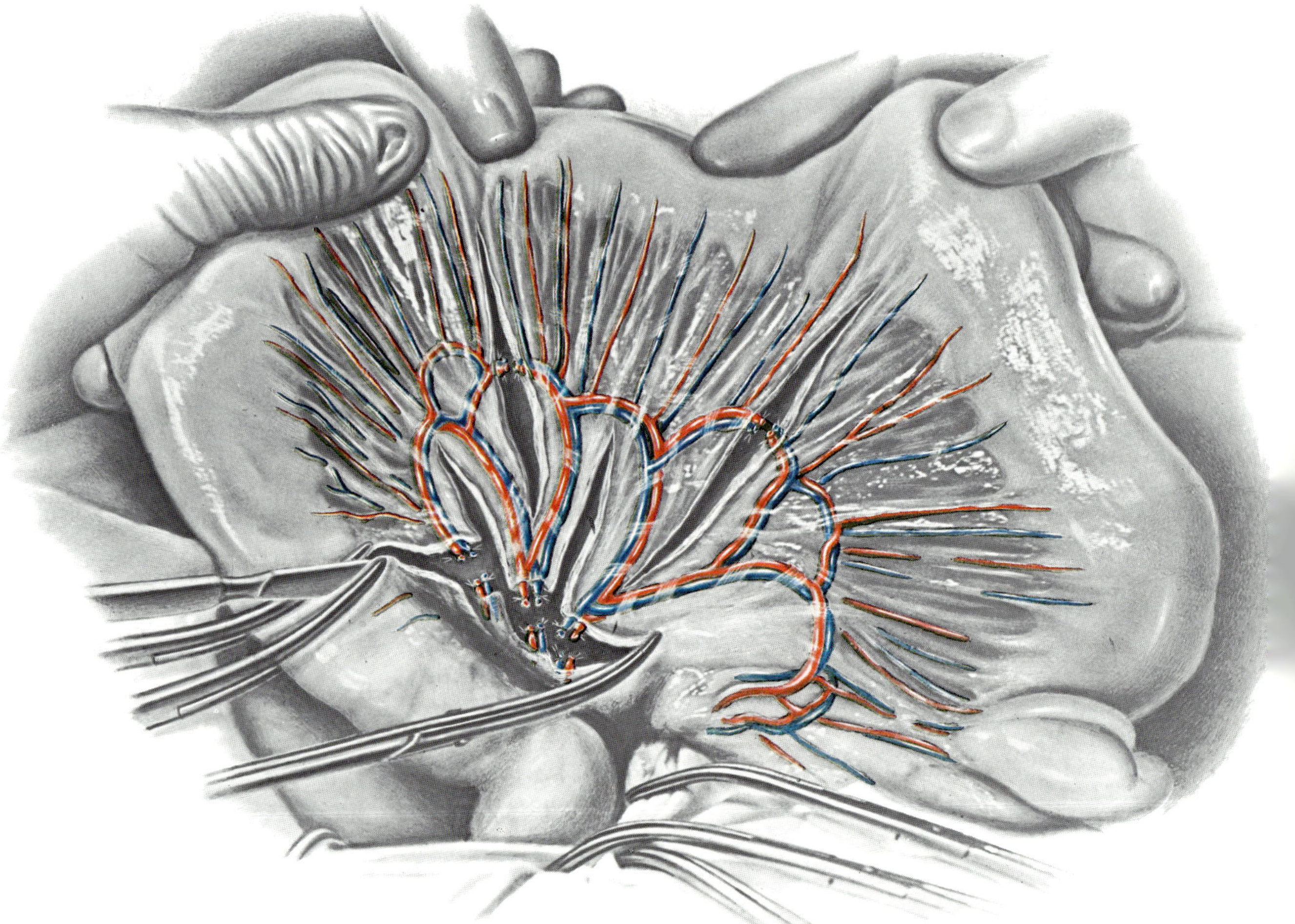

Fig. 634. Method for elongating graft of small intestine. Mesentery is cut in crotch of arteries and veins of small intestine, which divide at low level.

PLASTIC SURGERY WITH THE LARGE INTESTINE

RETROSTERNAL PLASTICS WITH RIGHT COLON AND TERMINAL ILEUM

The abdominal cavity is opened by an incision made from the sternal xiphoid process to the midpoint between the navel and the pubis.

The omentum is cut away from the right half of the transverse colon in the avascular zone, and the right phrenicocolic ligament holding the hepatic flexure of the colon is transected.

The surgeon or assistant grasps the cecum with his hand and pulls the ileocecal angle medially and cranially. The peritoneum is cut with scissors or a scalpel along its reflection in the right lateral canal from the hepatic flexure of the colon to the level of the cecum, and then, passing around the cecum, the incision in the peritoneum is continued transversely below the terminal portion of

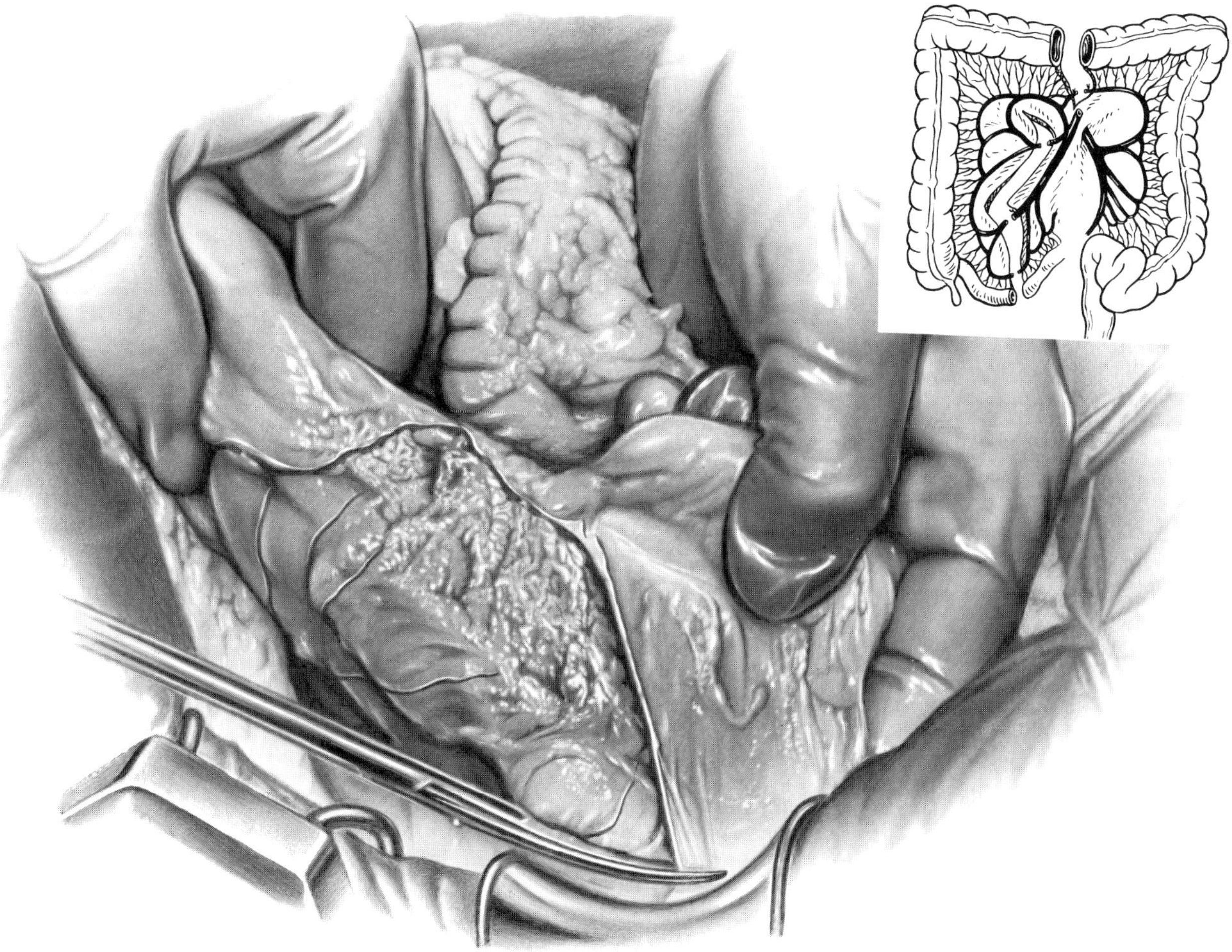

Fig. 635. Parietal peritoneum is cut in right lateral canal and below dome of cecum.

the ileum to the level of the spine (Fig. 635). The ileocecal angle, the ascending colon, and the right part of the transverse colon are detached by the sharp and blunt techniques from the posterior abdominal wall medially until the sites of the branching of the ileocolic and right colic arteries and the veins of the same name become visible.

The assistant holds the part of the ileum that is 15 to 20 cm from the dome of the cecum firmly while the surgeon ligates and transects the arterial and venous arcades between the ileocecal and the last artery of the small intestine at this level (Fig. 636).

The medial peritoneal sheet of the mesentery of the cecum and ascending colon is cut, and the main trunks of the ileocecal and those of the right cecal artieries, if such exist, and the veins are exposed. Soft-vessel clamps

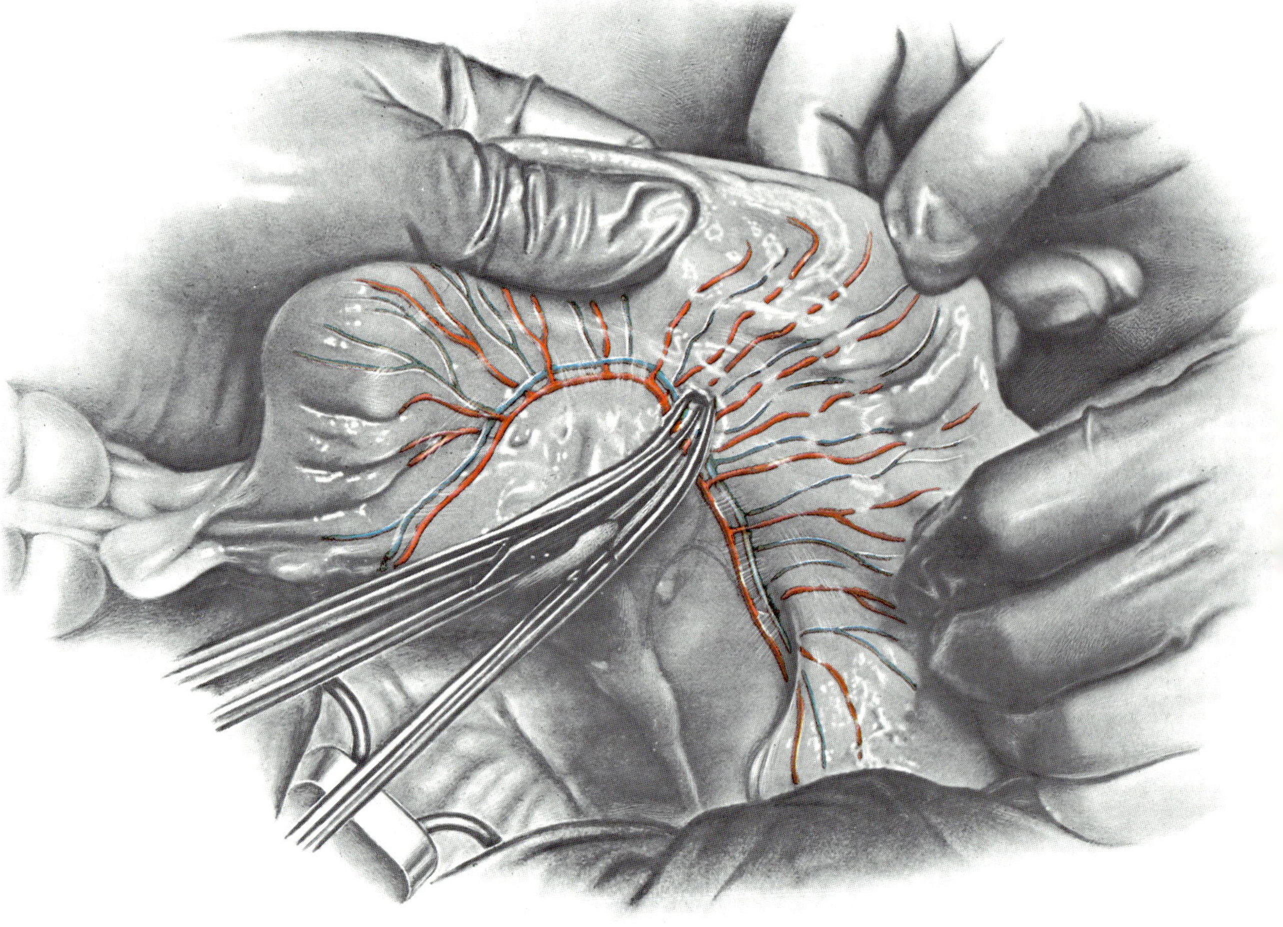

Fig. 636. Transection of vascular arcade under terminal part of ileum.

are applied to them so as to study the blood supply to the future graft. If there are no signs of deficiency of the arterial and venous systems in the right parts of the large intestine, the main trunks of the ileocecal and right cecal arteries and the veins are transected between two clamps (Fig. 637), and their stumps are tied.

The mobilized parts of the colon and ileum are cut away from the posterior abdominal wall along the avascular fields of the mesentery (Fig. 638). The incision in the mesentery terminates between the ligated stumps of the vascular arcades under the ileum and close to the main trunk of the middle colic artery. The ileum and the transverse colon are then transected: the first above the ligated vascular arcade and the second slightly to the left of the level of the middle colic artery (Fig. 639). The left branch of the middle colic artery forming Riolan's

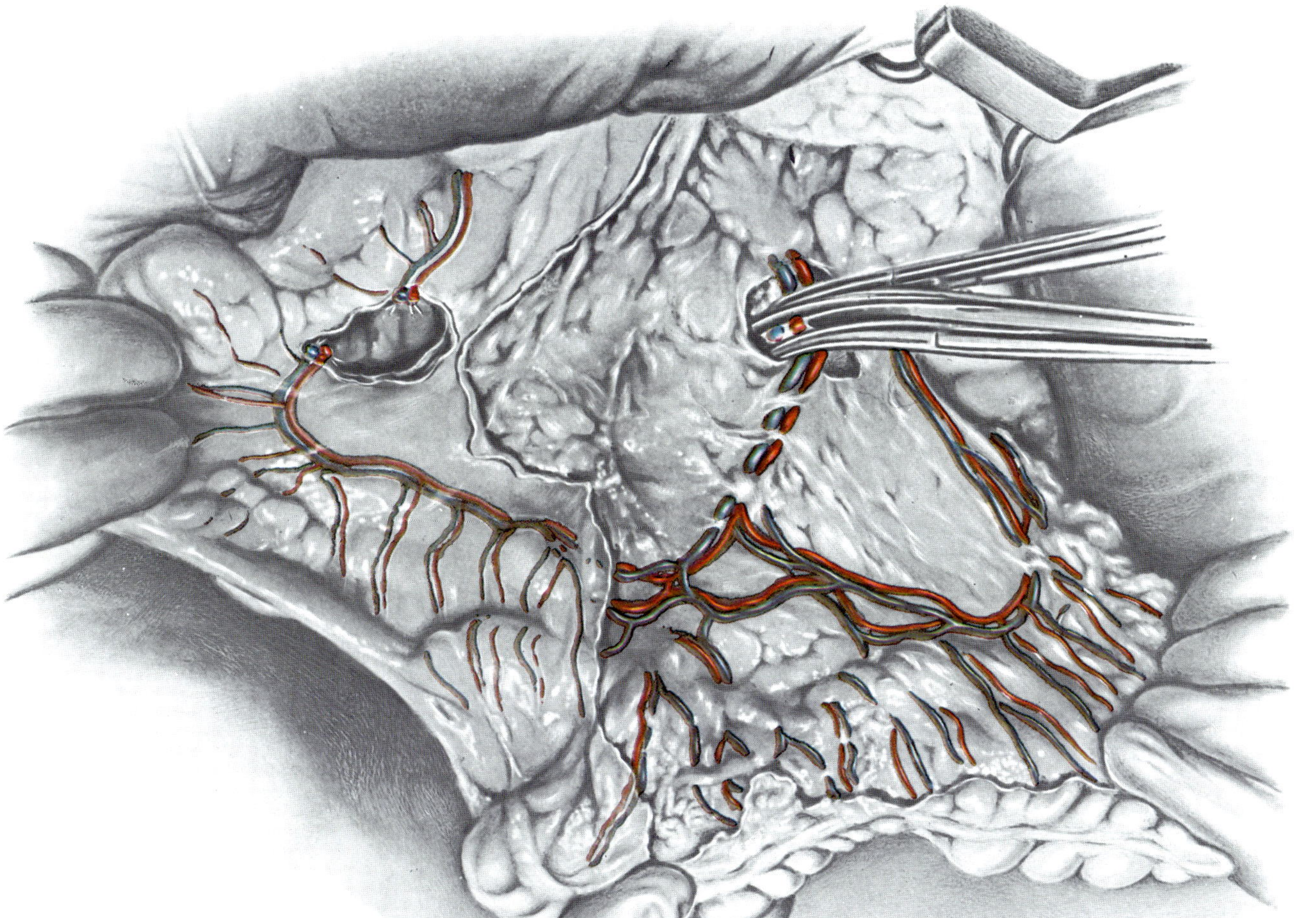

Fig. 637. Ileocolic arteries and veins are transected proximally to site of their division into branches.

arch may be transected when there is confidence that the blood supply to the left half of the transverse colon will not be impaired. If there is no such assurance, the transverse colon is transected above the vascular arch, which is left intact.

Both ends of the transected ileum and the end of the remaining portion of the transverse colon are closed with double-row sutures. The proximal stump of the transverse colon is anastomosed end to side with the stomach, preferably with its middle part closer to the lesser curvature (Fig. 640). The graft is lowered into the abdominal cavity until the anastomosis between the ileum and the transverse colon, which is usually created side to side, has been completed.

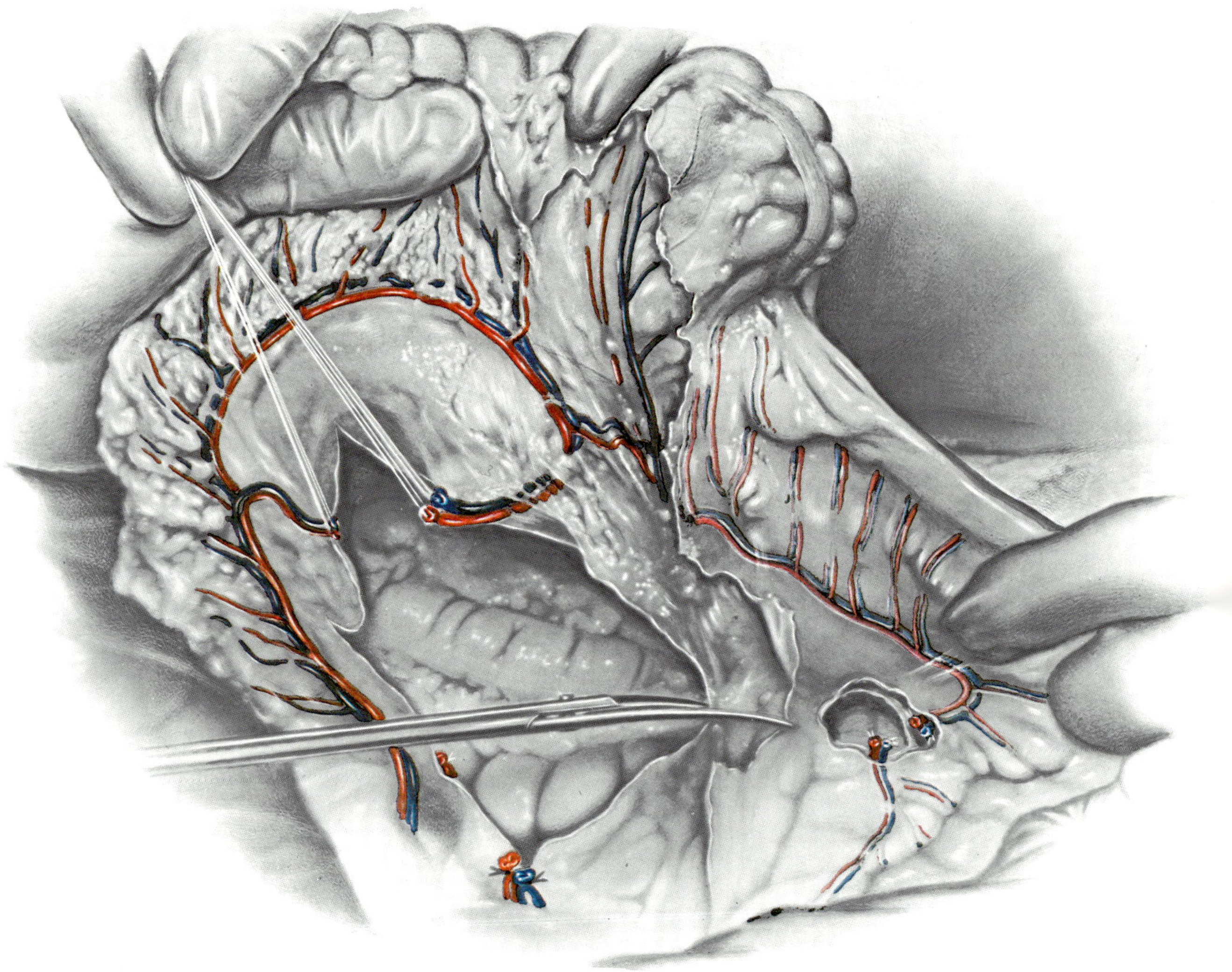

Fig. 638. Mesentery is cut in avascular fields under right half of colon and terminal portion of ileum. Right colic (on left) and ileocolic (in center) arteries and veins and vascular arcade under terminal segment of ileum are ligated and transected.

With the continuity of the intestine restored and the opening in the mesentery between the ileum and the transverse colon sutured, the graft is transposed to the neck through a tunnel formed under the skin or in the anterior mediastinum (Figs. 641 to 643). The free end of the graft is fastened by means of a stitched ligature on a gauze strip at the left mandibular corner (in two-stage esophagoplasty for cicatricial stricture of the esophagus) or 5 to 8 cm above the esophageal stump brought out on the neck or anterior thoracic wall (after Dobromyslov-Torek's operation).

In one-stage esophagoplasty, anastomosis is established between the graft and the cervical esophagus after the abdominal wound has been sutured. An end-to-end

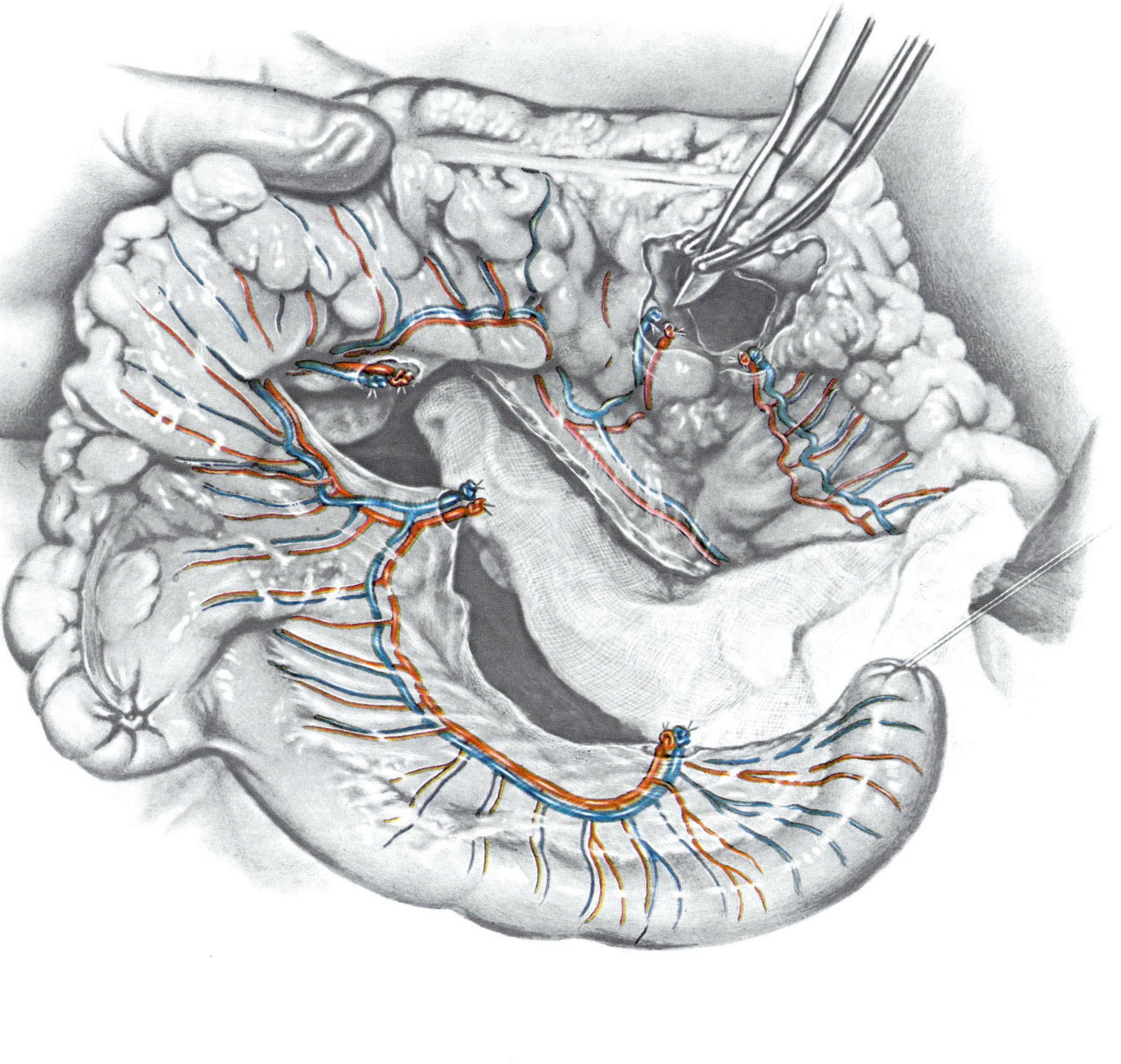

Fig. 639. Riolan's arch to left of middle colic artery is ligated and transected. Ileum is transected and its distal stump closed with sutures. Transverse colon is divided.

anastomosis is created, or the end of the graft is stitched into the side of the cervical esophagus or pharynx depending on the type of the pathological condition of the esophagus and the level of the obstruction.

In cicatricial stenosis of the thoracic esophagus, end-to-end esophagoenterostomy is one of the popular methods. Its technique is as follows. The incision on the neck is made parallel to the medial border of the left sternocleidomastiod muscle. The cervical part of the esophagus is freed from the surrounding tissues by blunt and sharp dissection and held firmly in the wound by a rubber or soft plastic tube. A scalpel is used to make a circular cut in its muscular coat down to the submucous layer nearer to the manubrium of the sternum (Fig. 644).

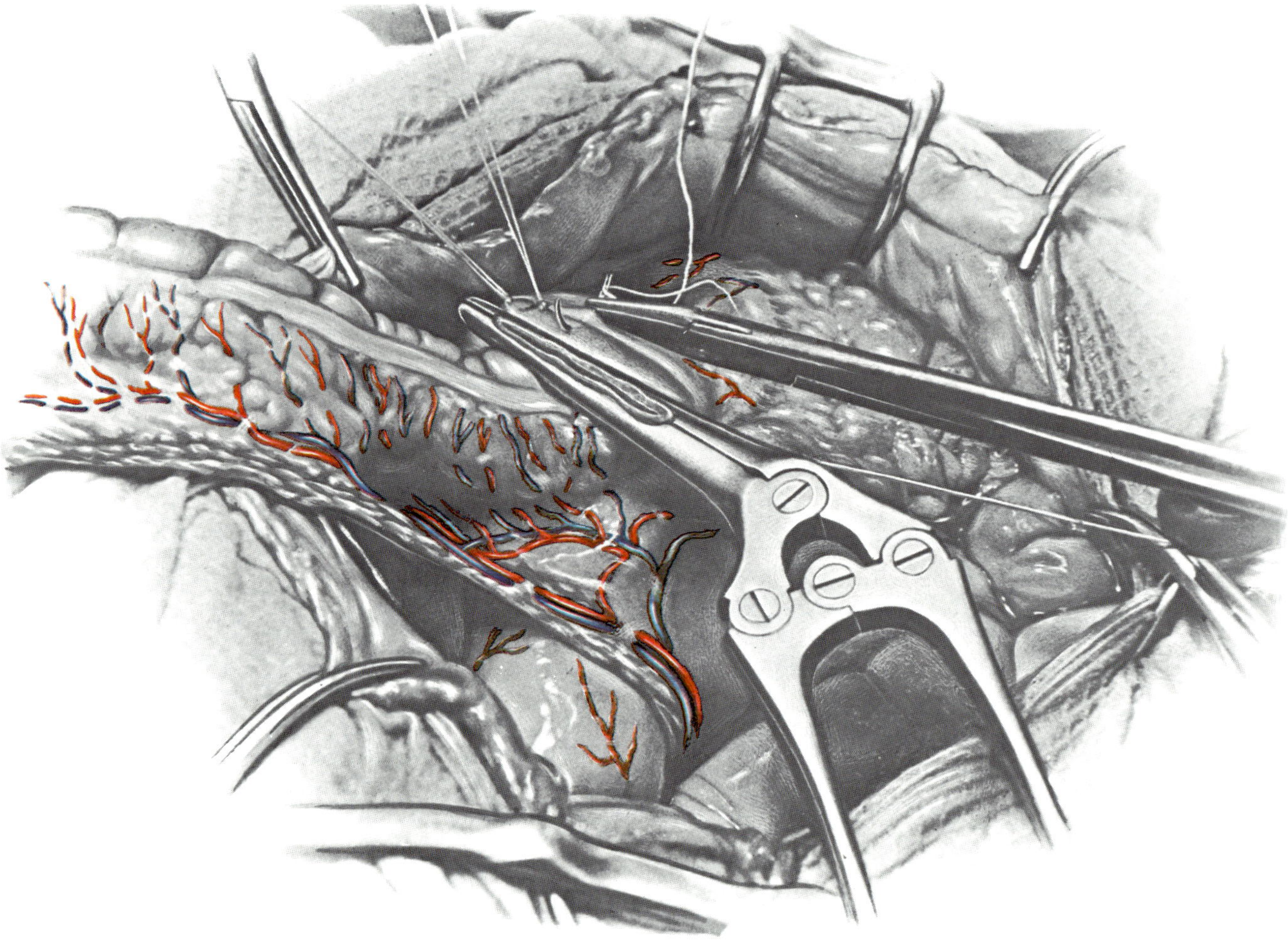

Fig. 640. End-to-side anastomosis between proximal stump of transverse colon graft and stomach.

The edges of the incision are displaced cranially and caudally with a tampon. The submucous and mucous coats are exposed and stitched through with a thread (Fig. 645), with which the nontransected part of the esophagus is ligated.

The esophagus is transected cranially to the stitched ligature (Fig. 646). After treatment with an antiseptic the caudal stump is closed with a single or double row of sutures (Fig. 647) and the cranial stump is anastomosed end to end with the graft by means of double-row interrupted sutures (Fig. 648), the provisional sutures having previously been removed from the ileal stump or its surplus cut away.

Rubber drains are left in the lower corner of the wound. Sutures are placed on the skin.

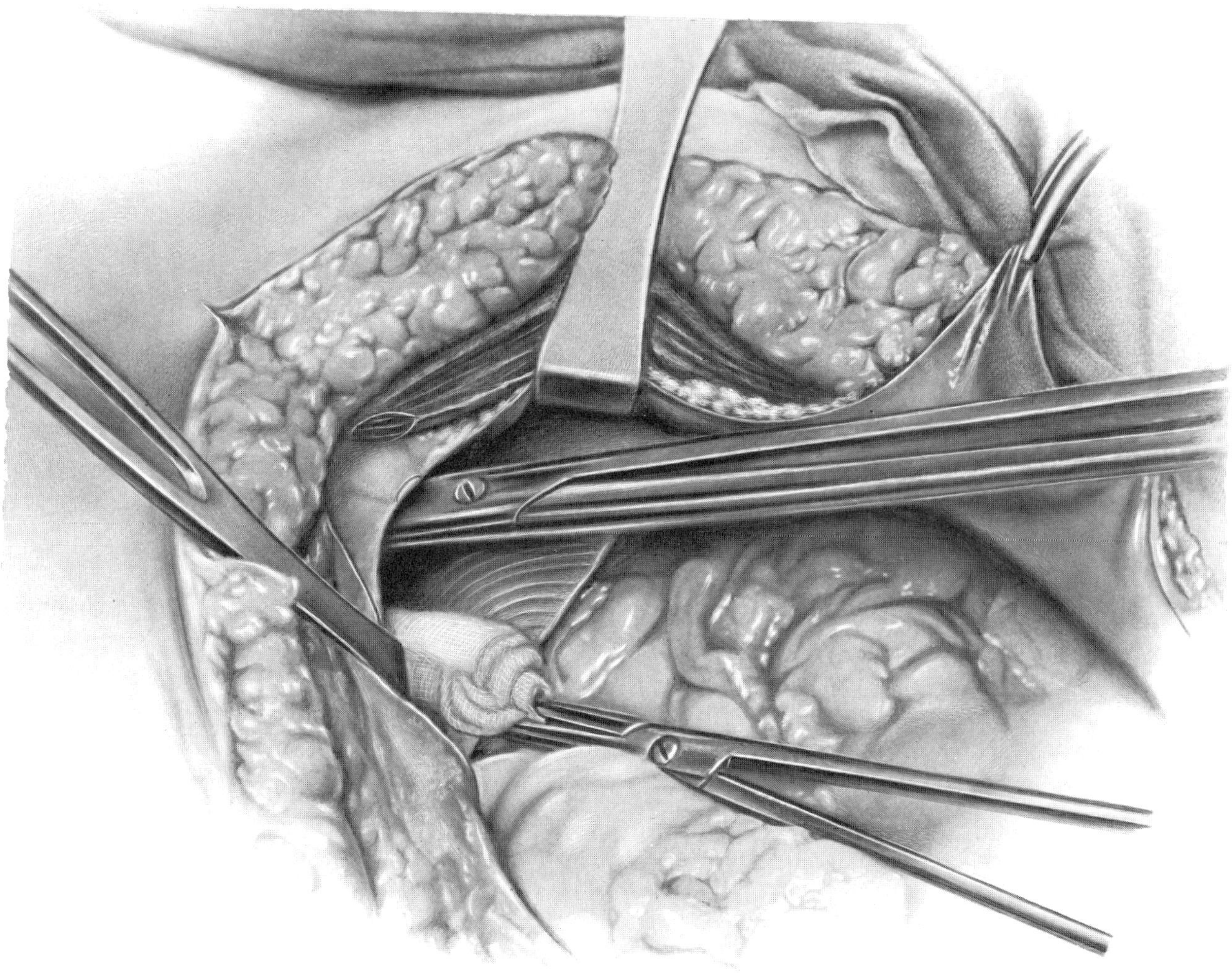

Fig. 641. Diaphragm is cut away for 8 to 10 cm along line of its attachment to anterior thoracic wall below sternal xiphoid process. Tunnel is formed in retrosternal space.

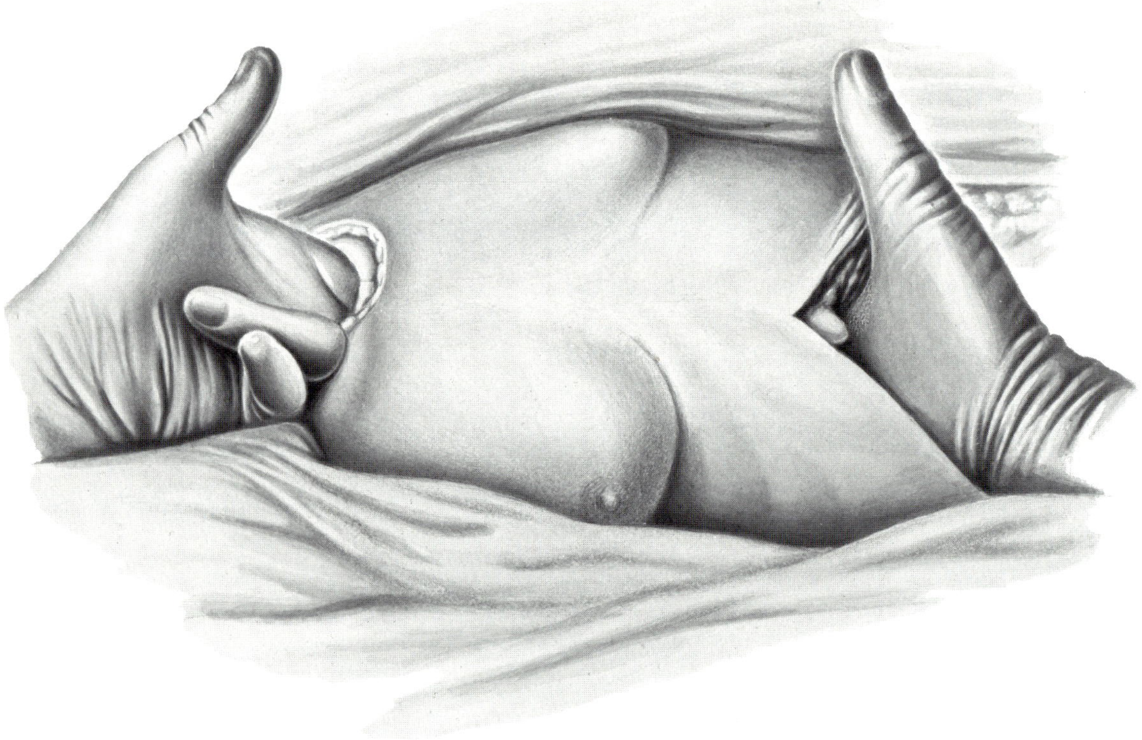

Fig. 642. After incision has been made on neck, retrosternal tunnel is widened with fingers inserted from direction of neck and abdominal cavity, and rare connective tissue strands, which might hinder transpostion of graft to neck through tunnel, are torn.

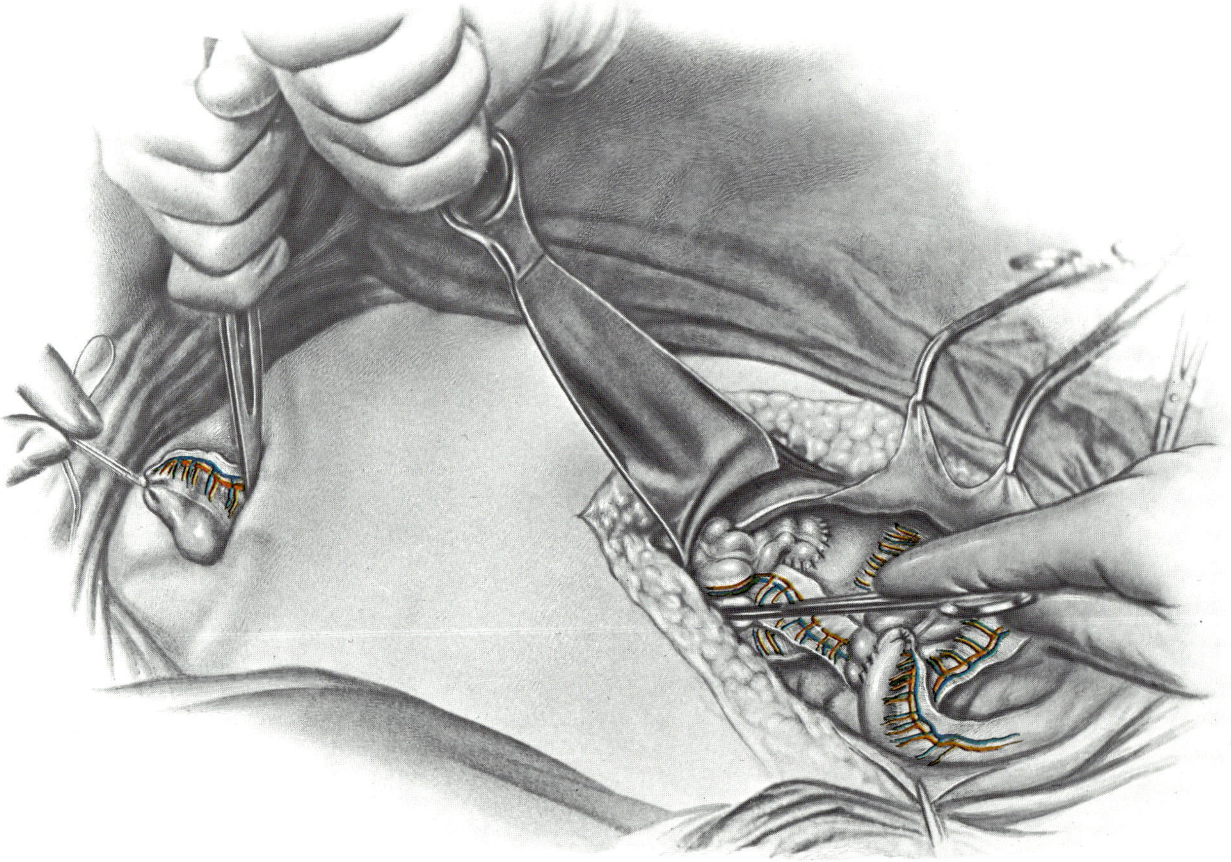

Fig. 643. Hooks have been brought under lower part of sternum and its manubrium. Graft is transposed from abdominal cavity to neck by way of retrosternal tunnel.

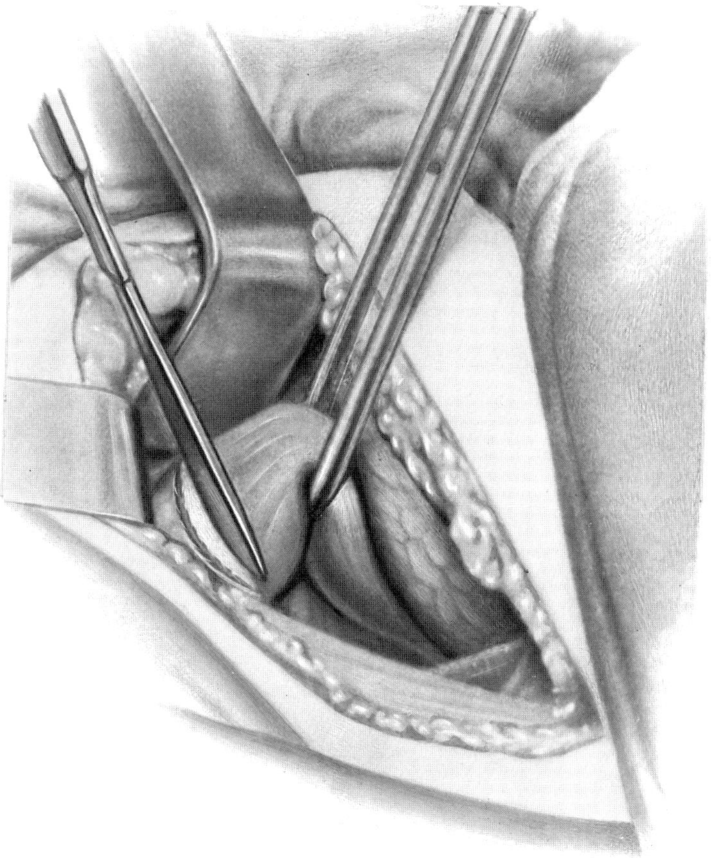

Fig. 644. Circular incision is made in muscular coat of esophagus.

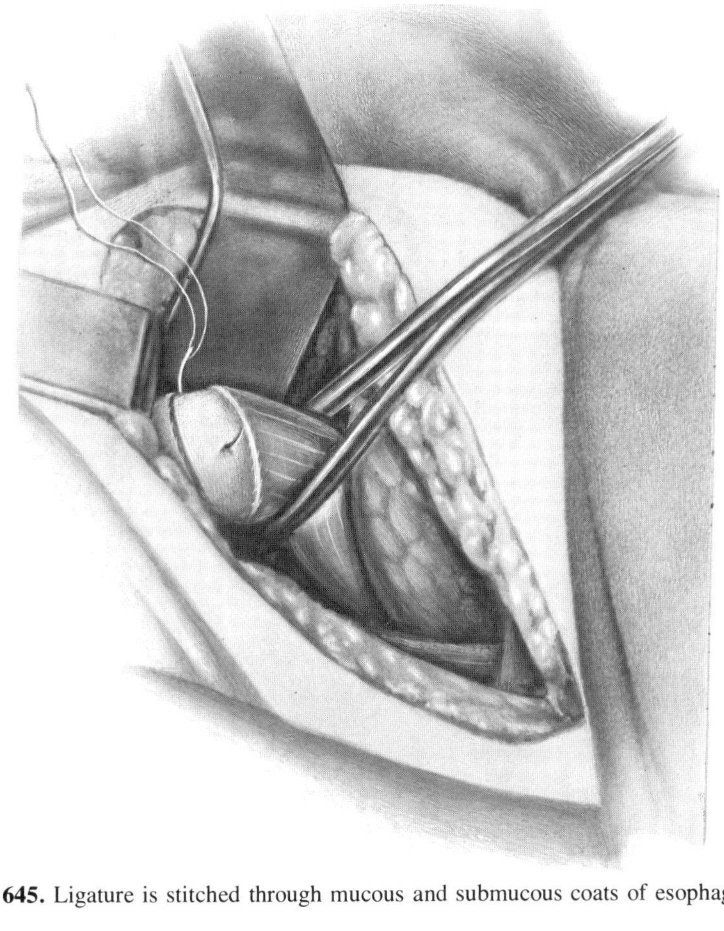

Fig. 645. Ligature is stitched through mucous and submucous coats of esophagus.

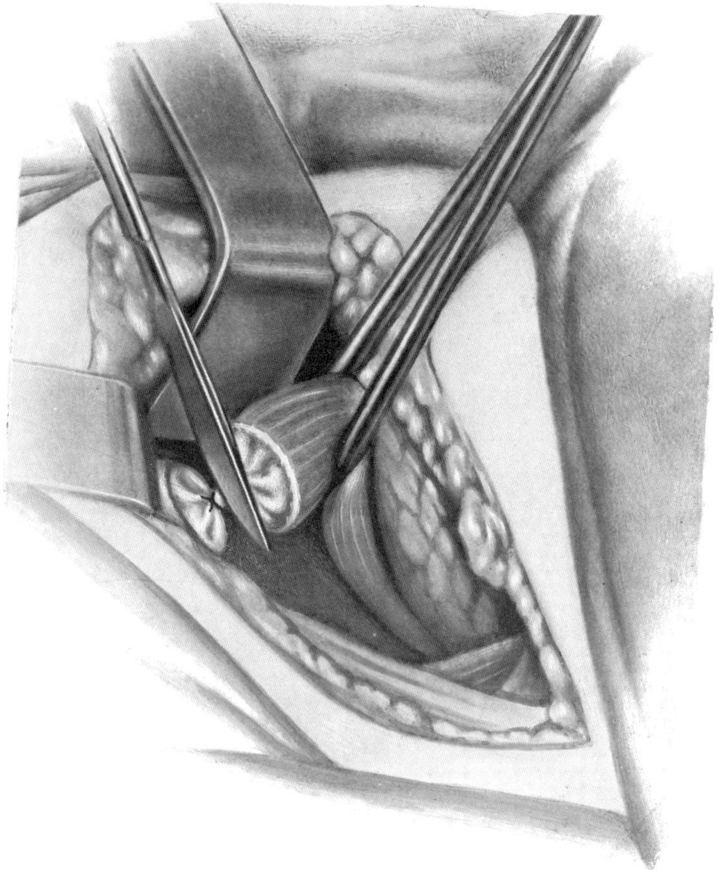

Fig. 646. Cervical esophagus is transected cranially to ligature stitched through it.

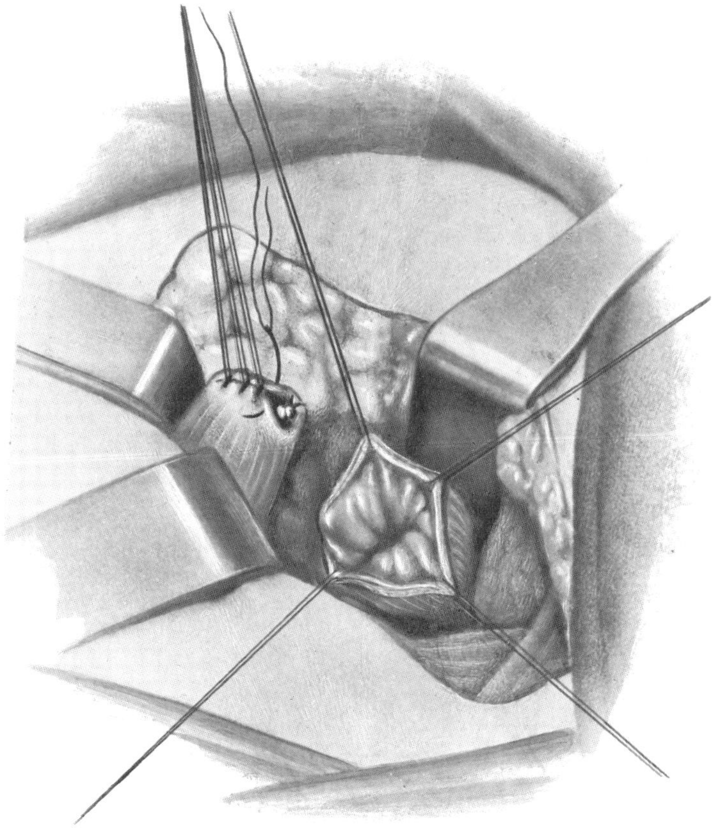

Fig. 647. Caudal esophageal stump is closed with buried musculomuscular sutures. Cranial stump is held fast with ligatures.

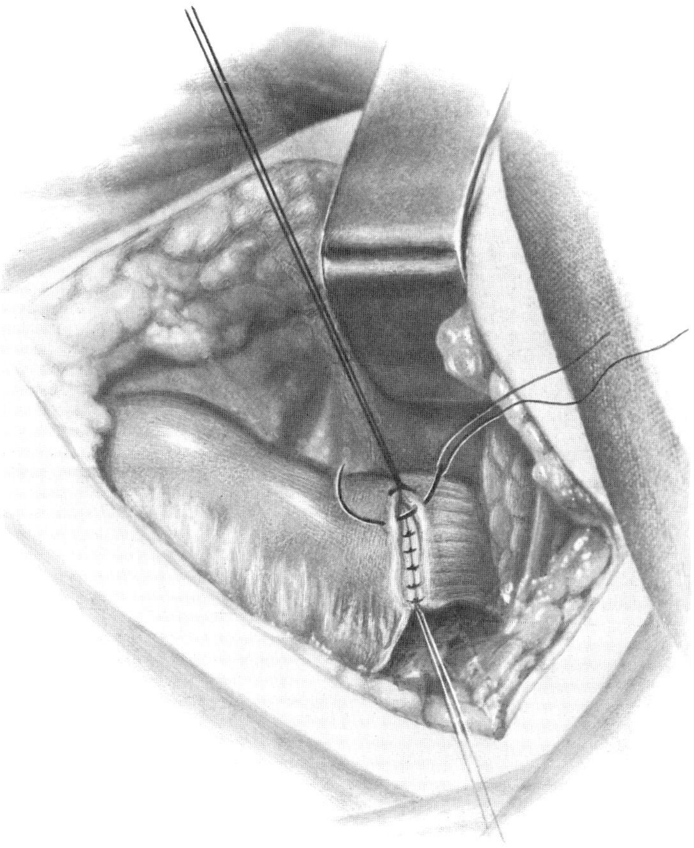

Fig. 648. Second row of sutures is applied to anterior lip of end-to-end esophagoileal anastomosis.

TECHNIQUES FOR MOBILIZING ISOPERISTALTIC GRAFT FROM TRANSVERSE COLON

Median laparotomy is performed with the incision made 3 to 4 cm below the navel.

The greater omentum is separated from the transverse colon in the avascular zone; the left phrenicocolic ligament and the parietal peritoneum in the left lateral canal are transected; and the descending colon and part of the sigmoid are mobilized caudally and medially. The main branches of the middle colic artery and vein are freed from the mesentery of the transverse colon, ligated, and transected. In some cases, to obtain a longer graft, the right colic artery and vein, if present, may be ligated and transected (Fig. 649). The vascular arcade slightly to the right of the middle (or right) colic artery is ligated and transected under the colon, which is then divided at this level. The caudal stump is sutured, while the cranial stump remains clamped until the intestinal anastomosis is established. After the above mentioned vessels are ligated, the transverse colon is supplied

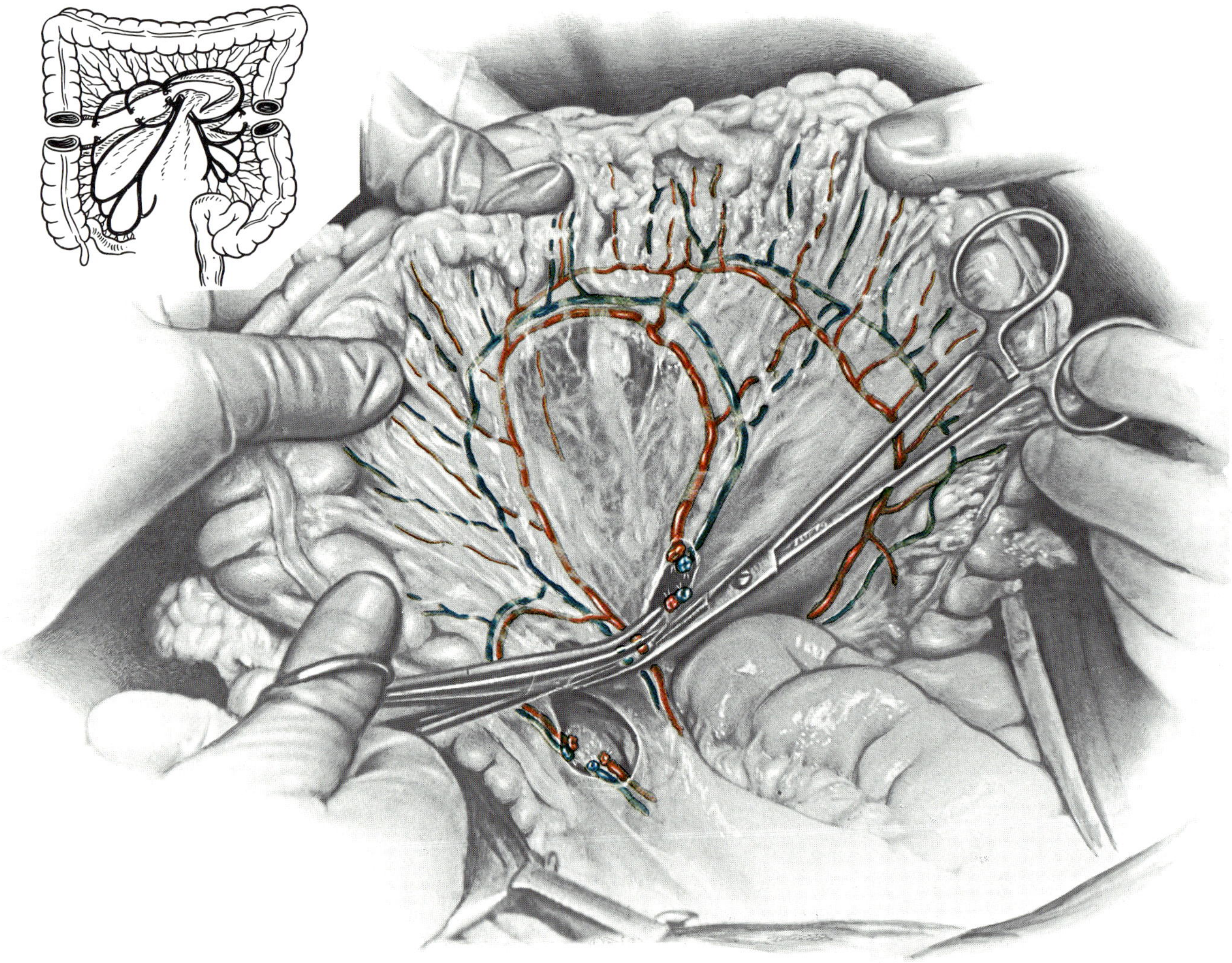

Fig. 649. Middle colic artery and vein and arcade between right colic and ileocolic arteries and veins have been ligated and transected. Right colic artery and vein are transected proximally to their division into branches.

with blood by the left colic artery by way of Riolan's arch and the vascular arcades located between the middle and right colic arteries.

With the vascular arcade between the left colic and sigmoid arteries ligated, the mesentery of the mobilized segment of the transverse colon is divided with scissors (Fig. 650). The colon is transected slightly caudal to the level of the left colic artery.

The stump of the graft formed is anastomosed end to side with the anterior gastric wall (Fig. 651). The continuity of the colon is restored by end-to-end anastomosis between the transverse colon and the sigmoid colon.

If the transverse colon is relatively short while the middle colic artery divides into two branches at a low level, the length of the graft may be increased 4 to 5 cm by transecting the secondary arcade and the mesentery between the main branches of the middle colic artery (Fig. 652). This will make it possible to avoid circulatory disorders when the intestine is transposed to the neck because the slight tightening of the intestine will not be transmitted to its major vessels (Fig. 653).

The subsequent stages of the operation are identical to those described above in esophagoplasty employing the right half of the transverse colon and the ileum.

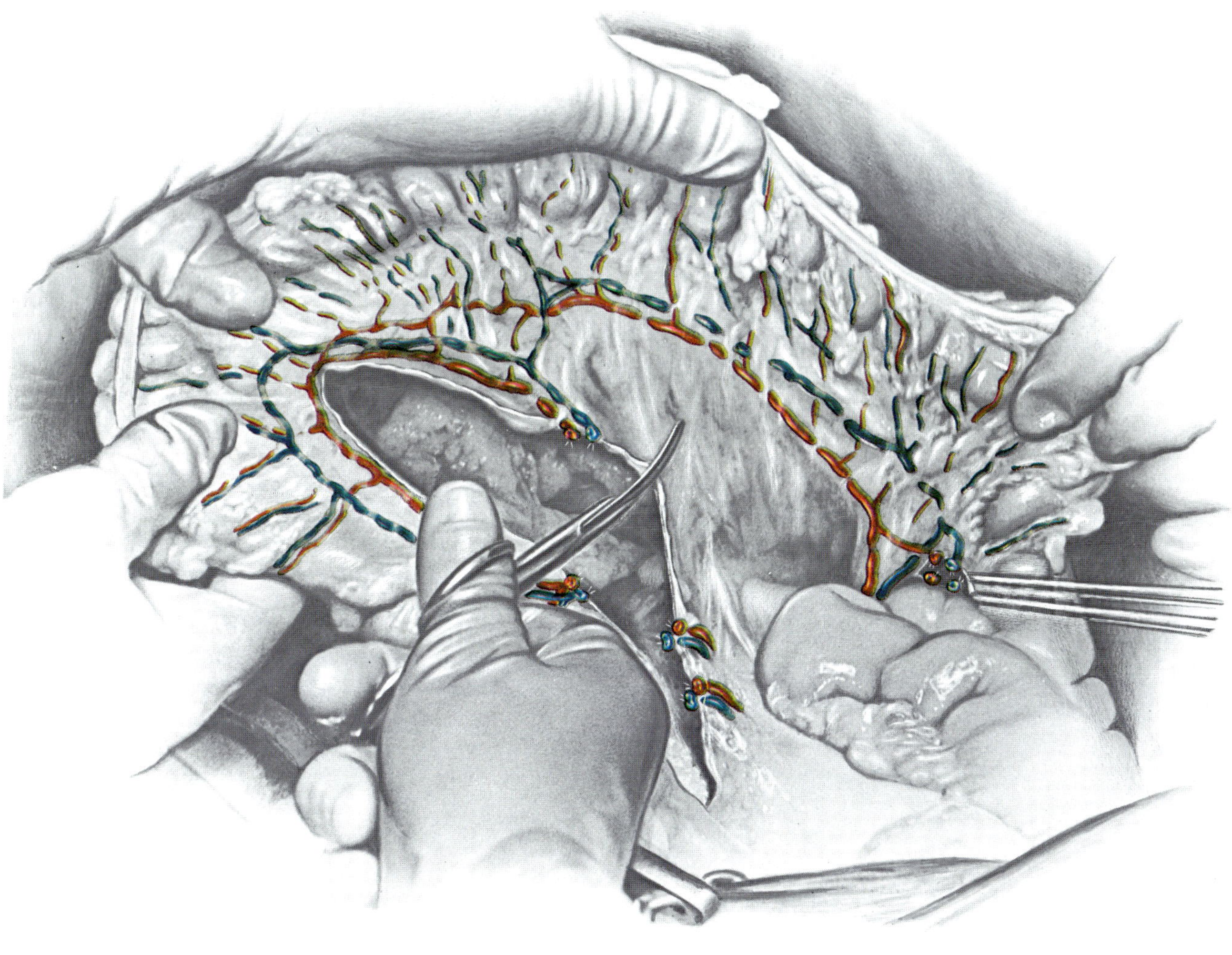

Fig. 650. Mesentery of transverse colon is cut in avascular fields (its incision below Riolan's arch is shown). Vascular arcades between left colic and sigmoid arteries and veins have been ligated and transected.

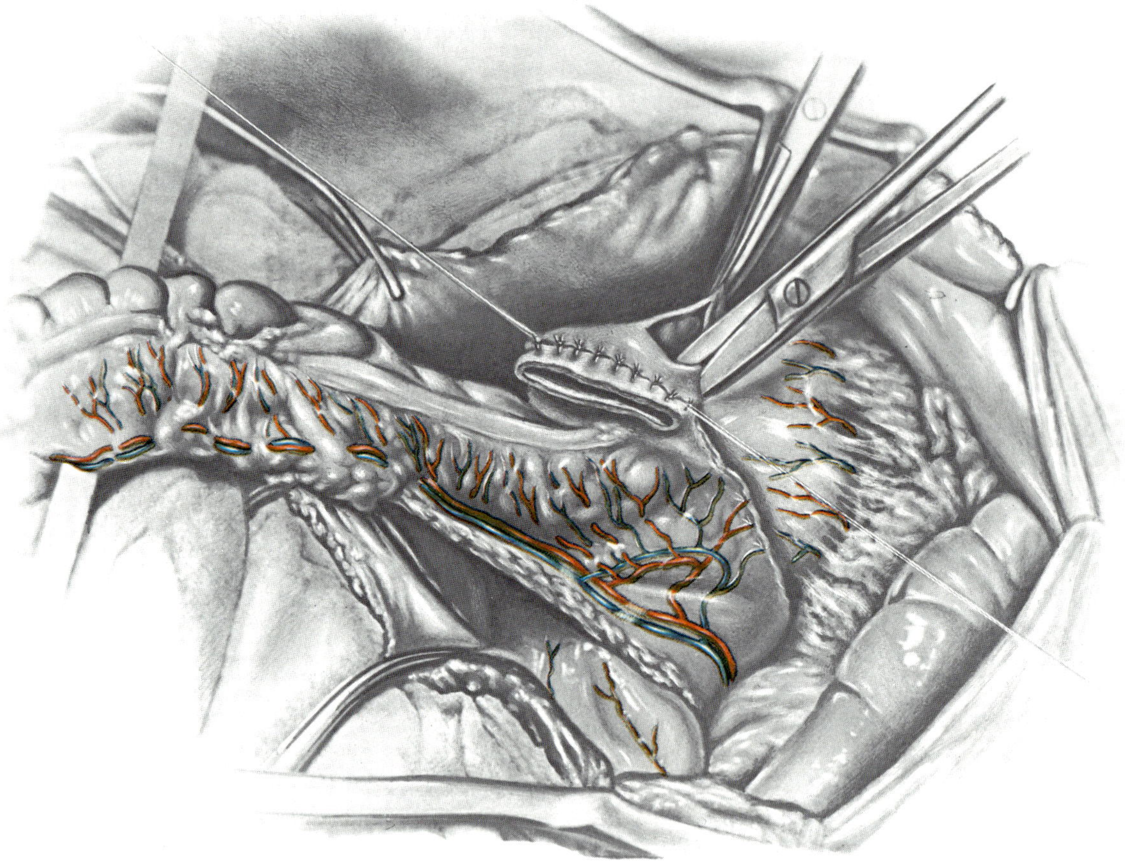

Fig. 651. Creation of end-to-side anastomosis between proximal stump of graft and stomach. Left colic artery and vein extend in base of graft.

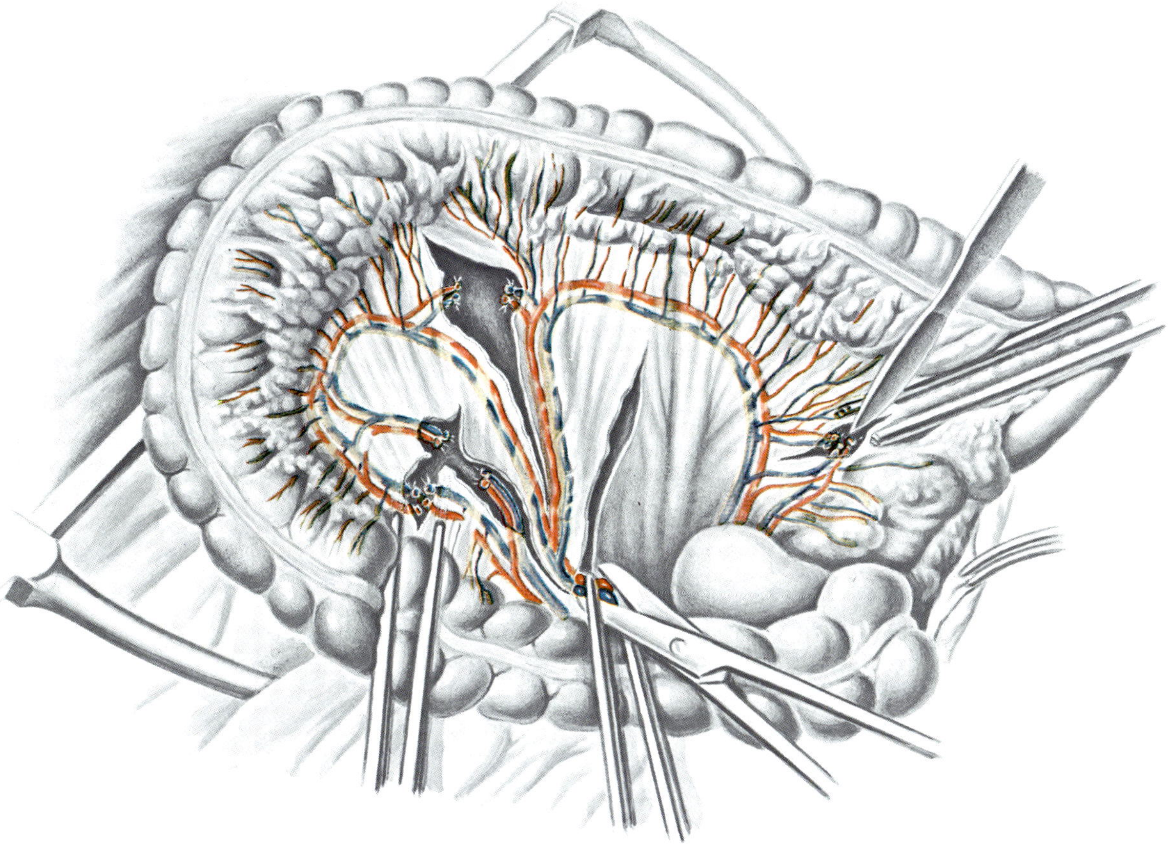

Fig. 652. Sites of transection of colon are bounded by two pairs of clamps. To elongate graft, mesentery is cut in crotch of middle colic artery and vein dividing at a low level. Middle colic artery and vein are transected.

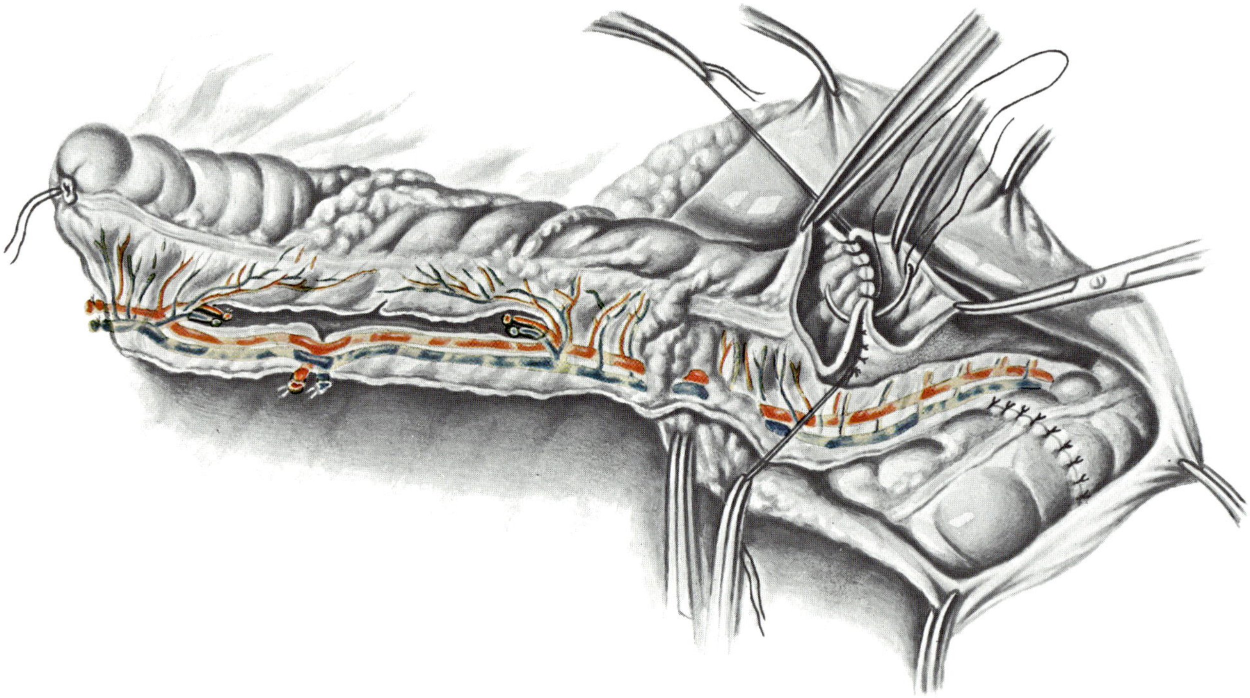

Fig. 653. End-to-end anastomosis between ascending colon and sigmoid colon has been established. Proximal stump of graft is being anastomosed with stomach. After mesentery has been cut below them, both branches of middle colic artery are straightened out almost completely.

PLASTIC SURGERY WITH THE STOMACH

GIANO-HALPERN-GAVRILIU TECHNIQUE OF ANTETHORACIC ESOPHAGOPLASTY WITH SLEEVE GRAFT FORMED FROM GREATER CURVATURE OF STOMACH

The anatomical prerequisites of total esophagoplasty by means of a sleeve graft shaped from the stomach are its sufficiently large greater curvature (from 32 to 60 cm) and well-developed intragastric and extragastric vascular anastomoses.

The abdominal cavity is opened on the midline with an incision made from the xiphoid process of the sternum to a point 3 to 4 cm below the navel. The greater omentum is cut away from the transverse colon in the avascular zone (Fig. 654).

With his left hand the surgeon moves the spleen medially and somewhat caudally, exposing the parietal peritoneum lateral to the spleen. Scissors are used to cut the peritoneum directly at the tail of the pancreas. The

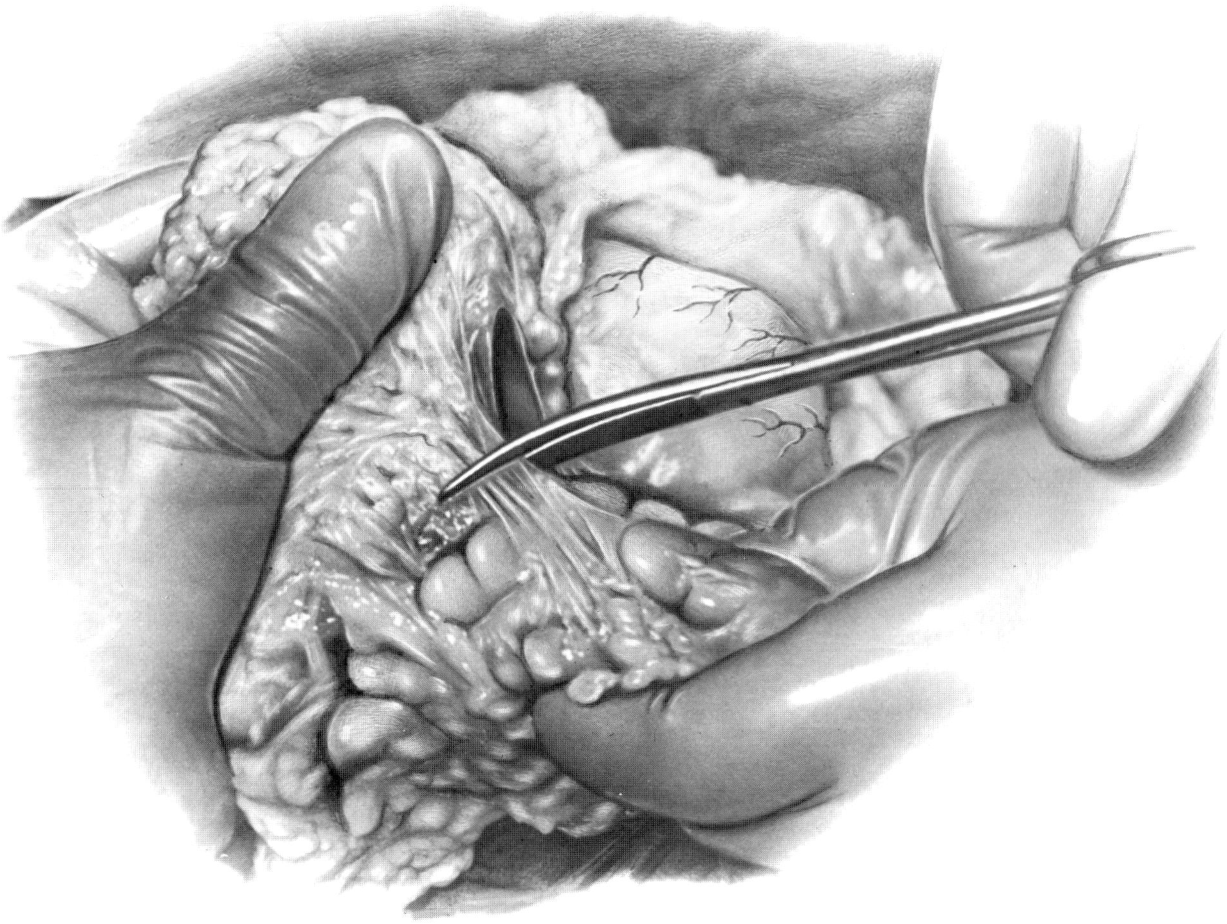

Fig. 654. Greater omentum is cut away from transverse colon in avascular zone.

incision is continued to the phrenicosplenic ligament, which is also transected (Fig. 655).

The tail and body of the pancreas together with the splenic vessels are separated from the posterior abdominal wall to the level of the aorta with the fingers (Fig. 656). The few dense fibrous adhesions found between the pancreas and the posterior abdominal wall are cut with scissors. Great care should be taken during this manipulation not to injure the splenic artery that runs directly along the superior border of the pancreas and gives off numerous branches to it, as well as the splenic vein stretching along the posterior surface of the pancreas below the splenic artery.

In some cases the left adrenal is closely fused with the pancreas, in view of which special caution should be taken with regard to it in mobilizing the tail of the pancreas.

With the head and body of the pancreas separated

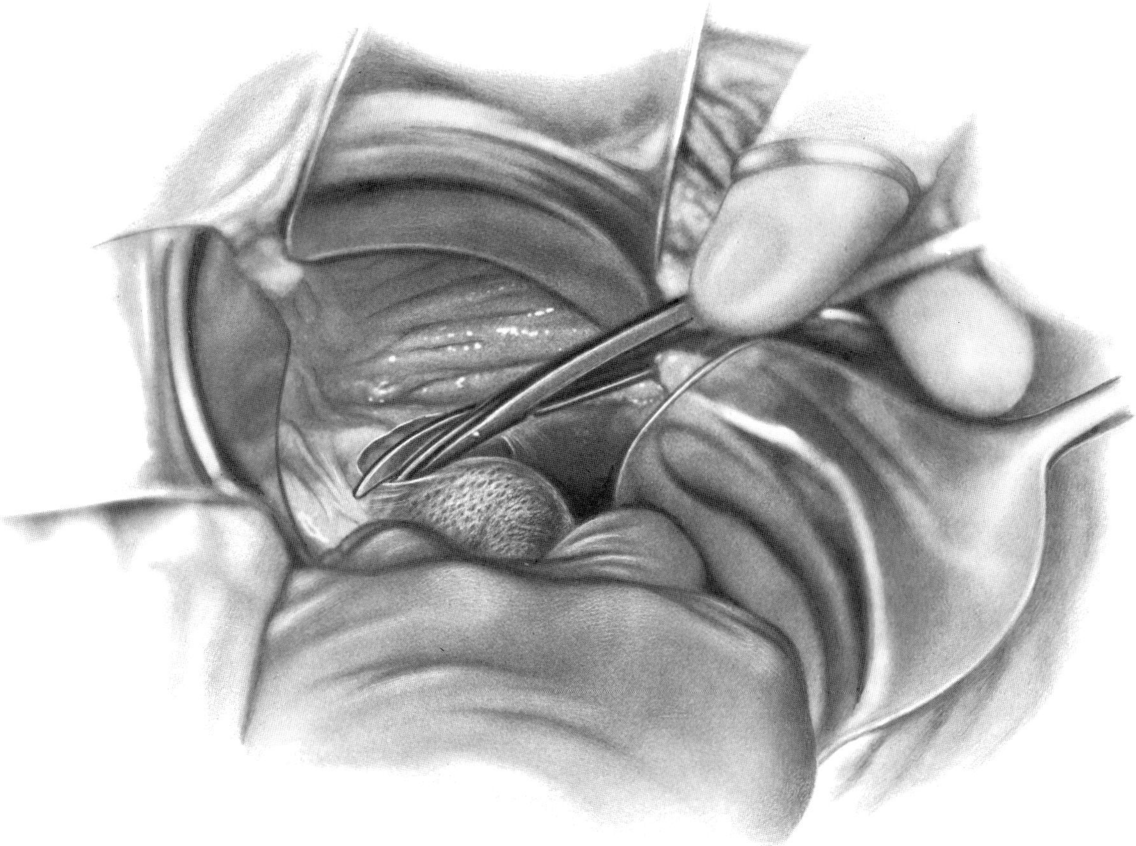

Fig. 655. Phrenicosplenic ligament is transected.

from the posterior abdominal wall, the spleen is dislocated into the wound. Leaving the gastric branches of the splenic arteries intact, the large and small vessels extending to the spleen are successively ligated directly at the hilus of the spleen (and sometimes in its pulp), after which splenectomy is carried out (Fig. 657).

Part of the greater omentum is resected, leaving only a small flap 6 to 12 cm wide connected to the greater curvature of the stomach. The right gastroepiploic artery and vein are ligated and transected close to the pylorus. The future graft is thus provided with blood by the splenic artery through its anastomosis with the left gastroepiploic artery.

The stomach is opened with a 3 to 4 cm long incision made on and perpendicular to the greater curvature about 4 cm to the left of the pylorus (Fig. 658). A rubber tube about 1.5 cm in diameter is introduced into the stomach through this incision and placed along the greater curva-

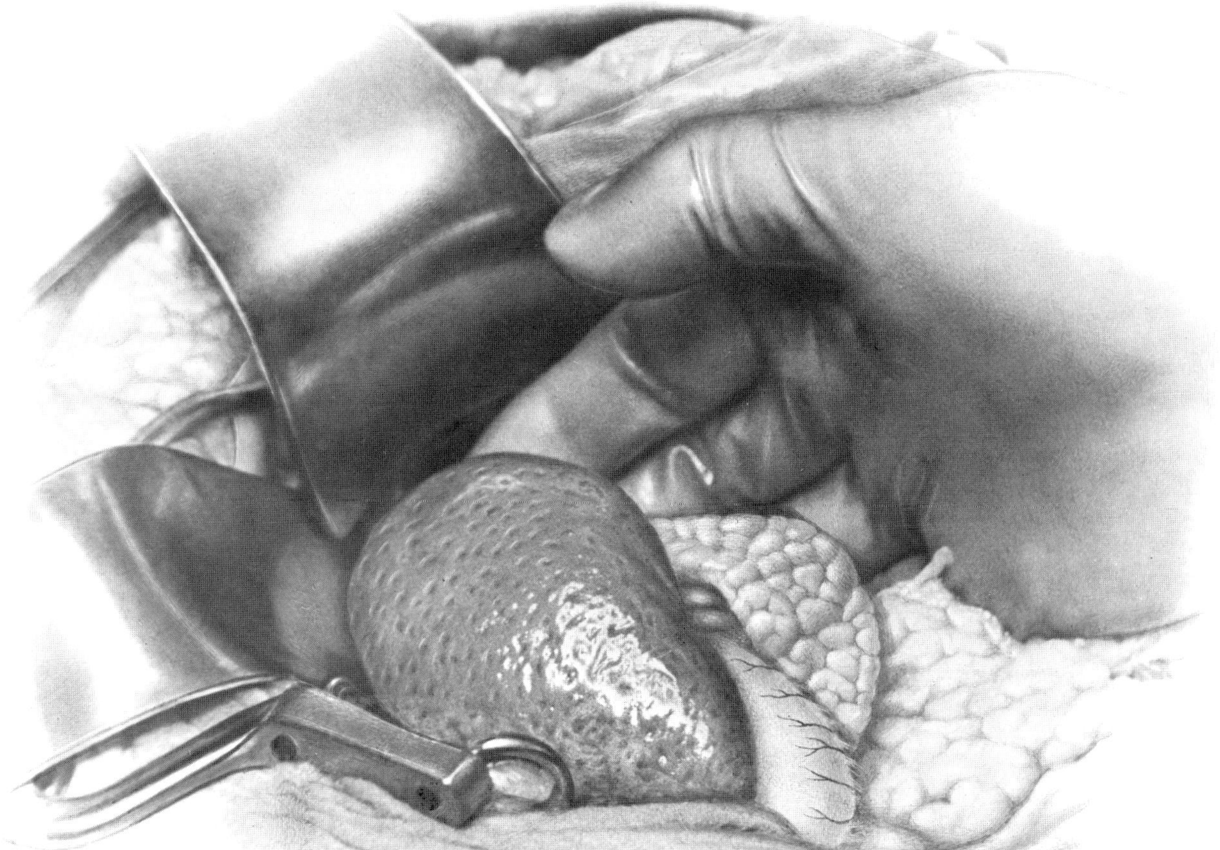

Fig. 656. Tail and body of pancreas are detached from posterior abdominal wall.

ture, slightly stretching the gastric walls over the tube (Fig. 659). The tube is fastened in this position by means of a ligature stitched through the edge of the gastric wound through which the tube is inserted.

It is most convenient to separate the graft from the greater curvature by means of an instrument for creating a gastrointestinal anastomosis (НЖКА). The method of forming the graft here is as follows. One of the detachable parts of the instrument is brought under the posterior wall of the stomach, while the other is placed on the anterior wall along the line of the intended incision, parallel to the tube introduced into the stomach (Fig. 660). Both parts of the instrument are brought together, cutting the anterior and posterior walls of the stomach

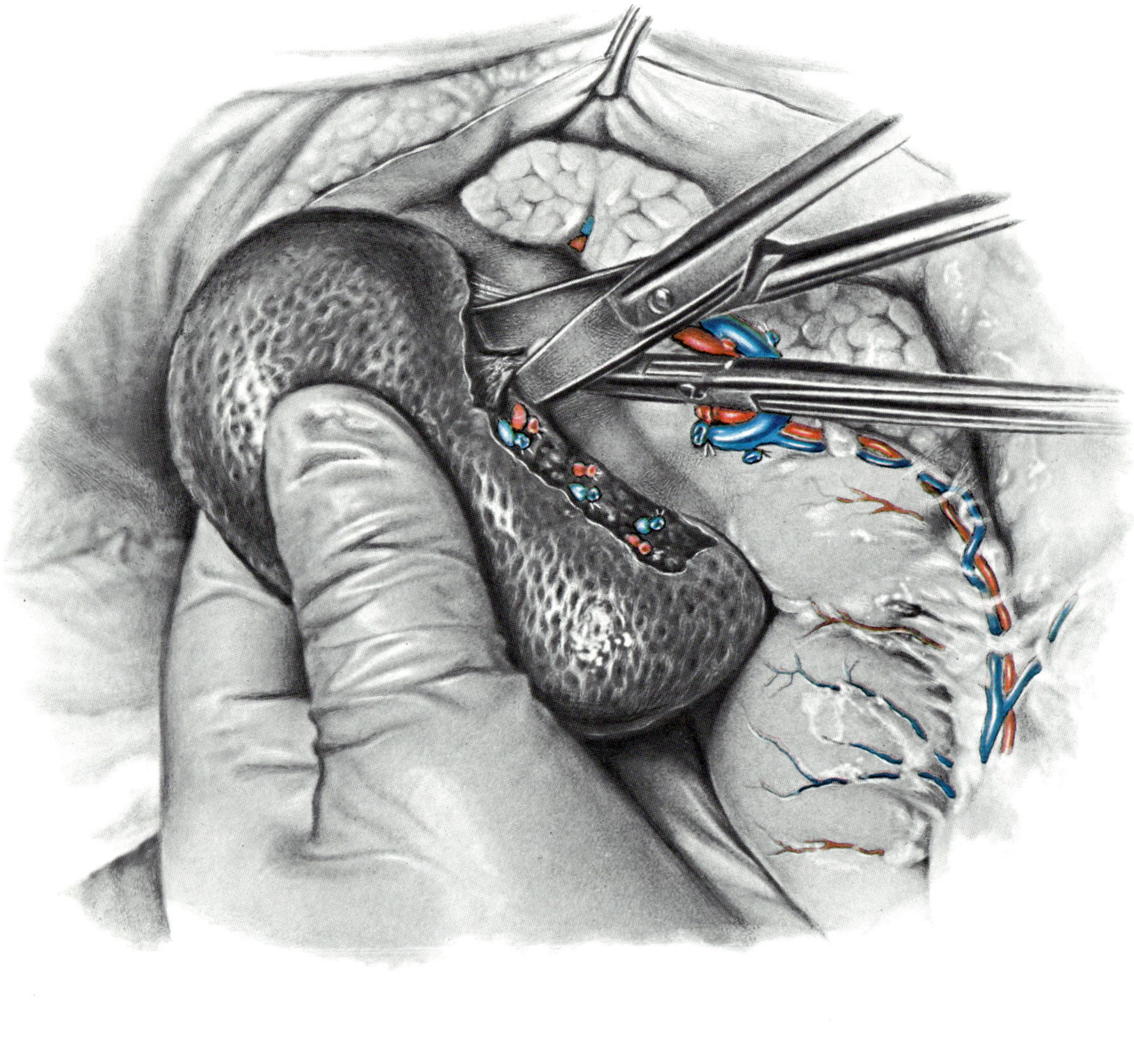

Fig. 657. Splenectomy without disconnecting anastomosis between splenic and left gastroepiploic arteries.

simultaneously for a distance of 7 to 8 cm and stitching them with staples on the side of the future graft and on the remainder of the stomach. After this procedure the edges of the wound prove to be well adapted, and there is no escape of gastric contents. Bleeding from the transected gastric walls is negligible. It is arrested by applying figure-of-eight catgut sutures to the bleeding vessels.

A second row of seroserous interrupted silk or Lavsan sutures is placed on the transected gastric wall (Fig. 661), after which the instrument is again applied and the next portion of the stomach is cut and stitched through (Fig. 662).

To form the necessary graft length, the manipulations are performed in the same order four to six times (Fig.

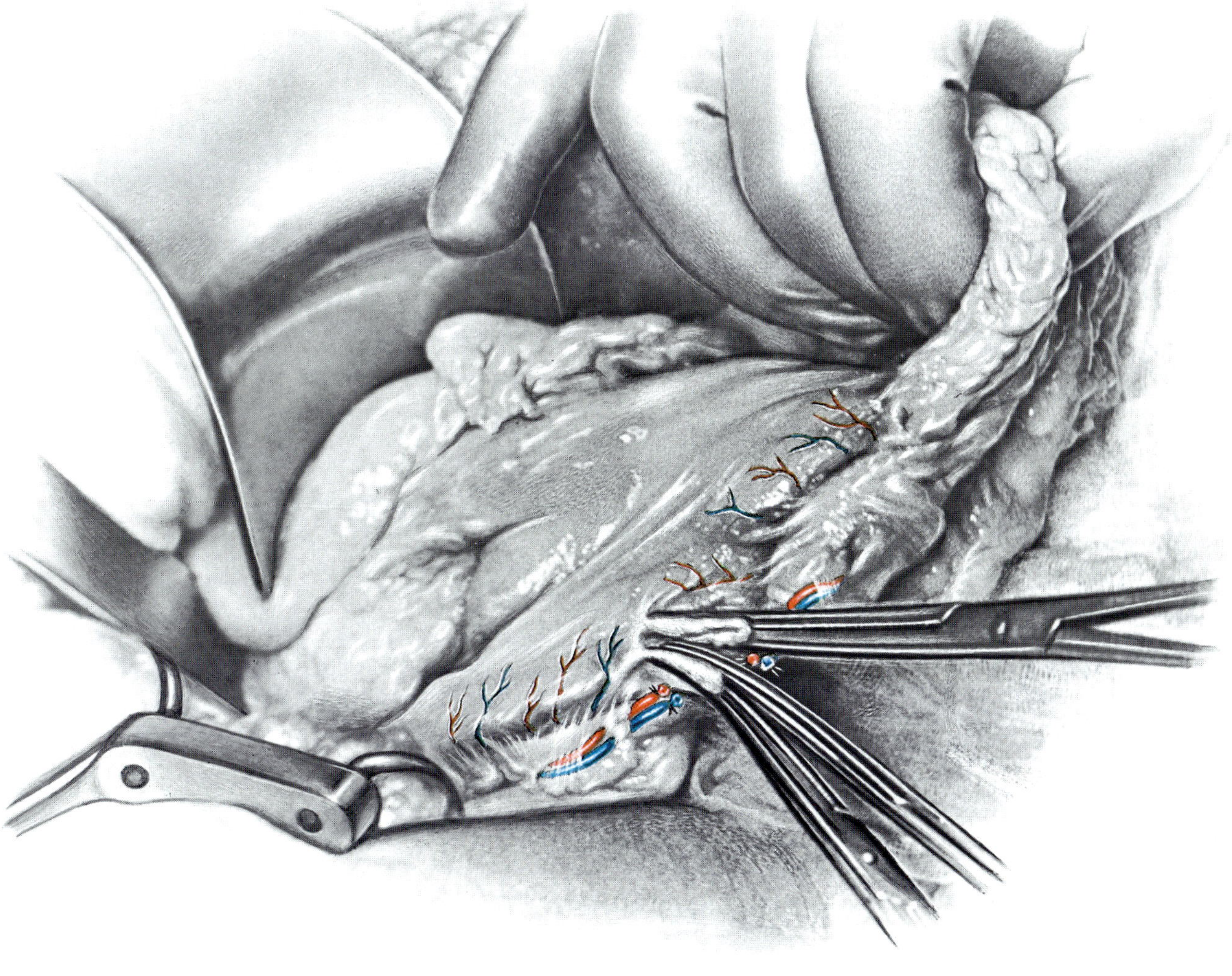

Fig. 658. Right gastroepiploic artery and vein are transected close to pylorus. Gastric wall is cut on greater curvature between two clamps.

663). It is advisable to avoid recharging the same instrument during the operation; four to six instruments should be at hand. The graft may also be formed from the greater curvature of the stomach by means of two apparatuses designed for this purpose by Skobelkin (Figs. 664 to 666 and 668). In some cases an instrument of the УО type (Fig. 667) for stitching small portions of the gastric wall is used. In this case the stomach is cut with a scalpel after the staple suture has been applied.

With the graft separated, a subcutaneous or retro-

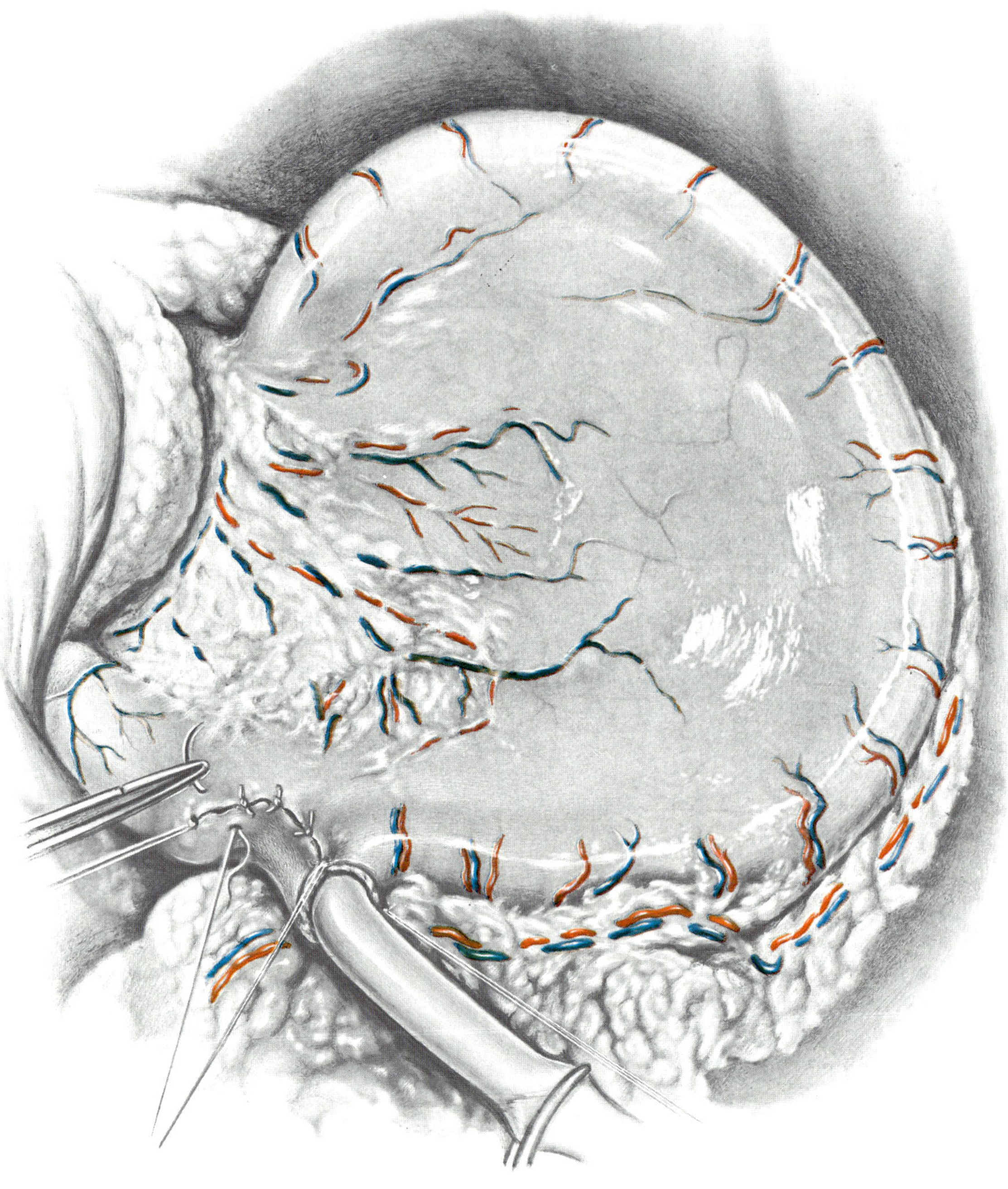

Fig. 659. Thick rubber tube is introduced into stomach through incision.

sternal tunnel is formed (Figs. 669 and 670). The skin overlying the jugular notch of the sternum is cut, and a strong thread or forceps is passed down from the top through the tunnel, and the rubber tube is fastened to it. The tube carrying the graft is then pulled out to the neck through the tunnel (Fig. 671 and 672).

The next stage of the operation comprises the formation of an anastomosis between the graft and the esophagus. Fig. 673 shows the method for anastomosing the graft with the esophageal stump after Dobromyslov-Torek's operation.

The skin is cut around the esophagostoma. The

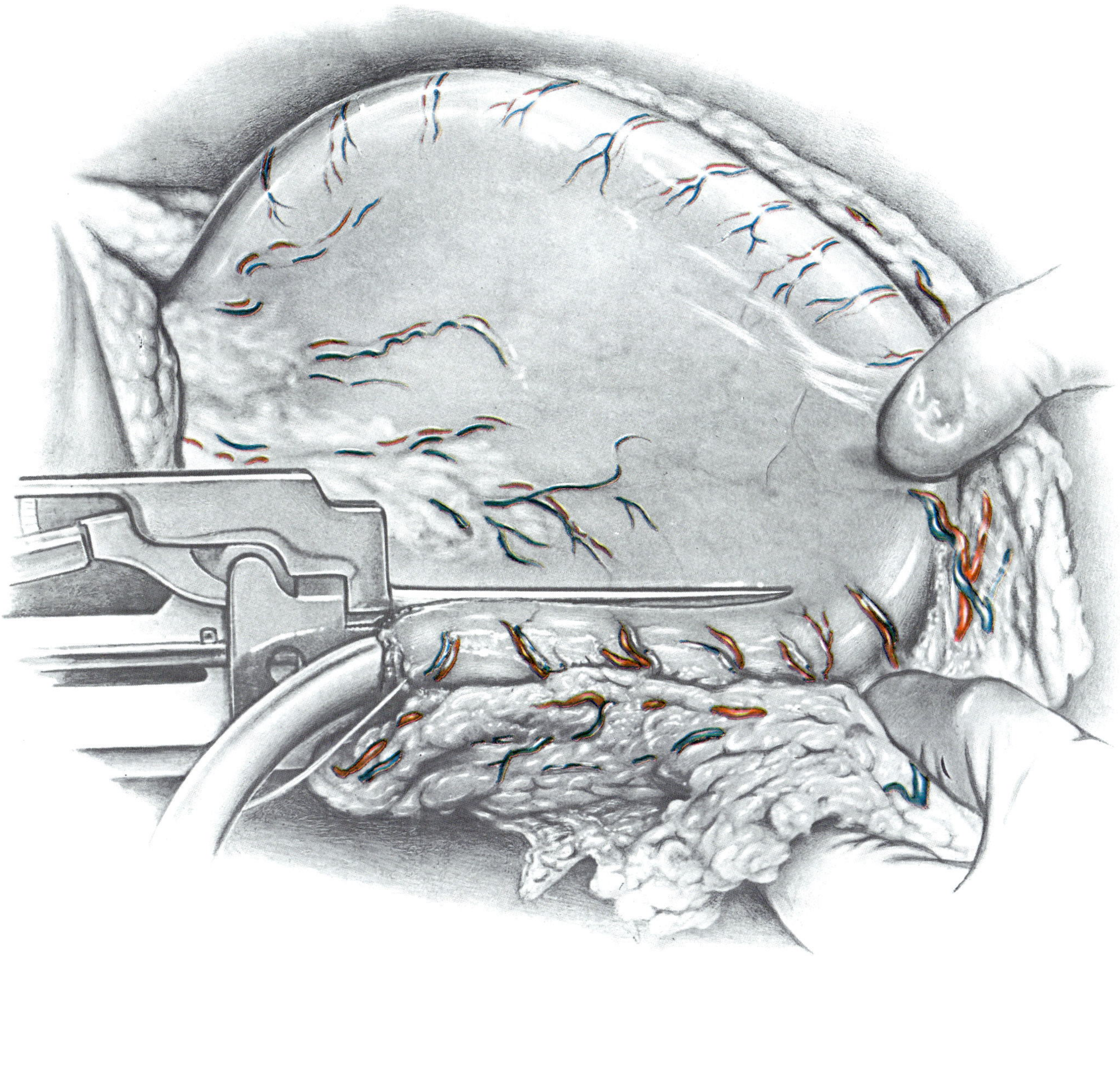

Fig. 660. First portion of stomach is cut parallel to greater curvature with НЖКА instrument.

esophageal stump is closed with interrupted sutures or a stitched ligature, and the posterior external row of sutures is first applied to the graft and the stump. To refresh the edges of the stump, its end is cut away together with the scarred skin. The first row of sutures is applied to the posterior lip of the anastomosis. A rubber tube may be used in forming the anastomosis (Fig. 673), in which case the free end of the tube is passed through the esophageal stump into the mouth. The tube is removed through the mouth after the second row of sutures has been placed on the anterior lip of the anastomosis. The operation is completed by closing the abdominal wound and the skin wound over the esophagogastroanastomosis.

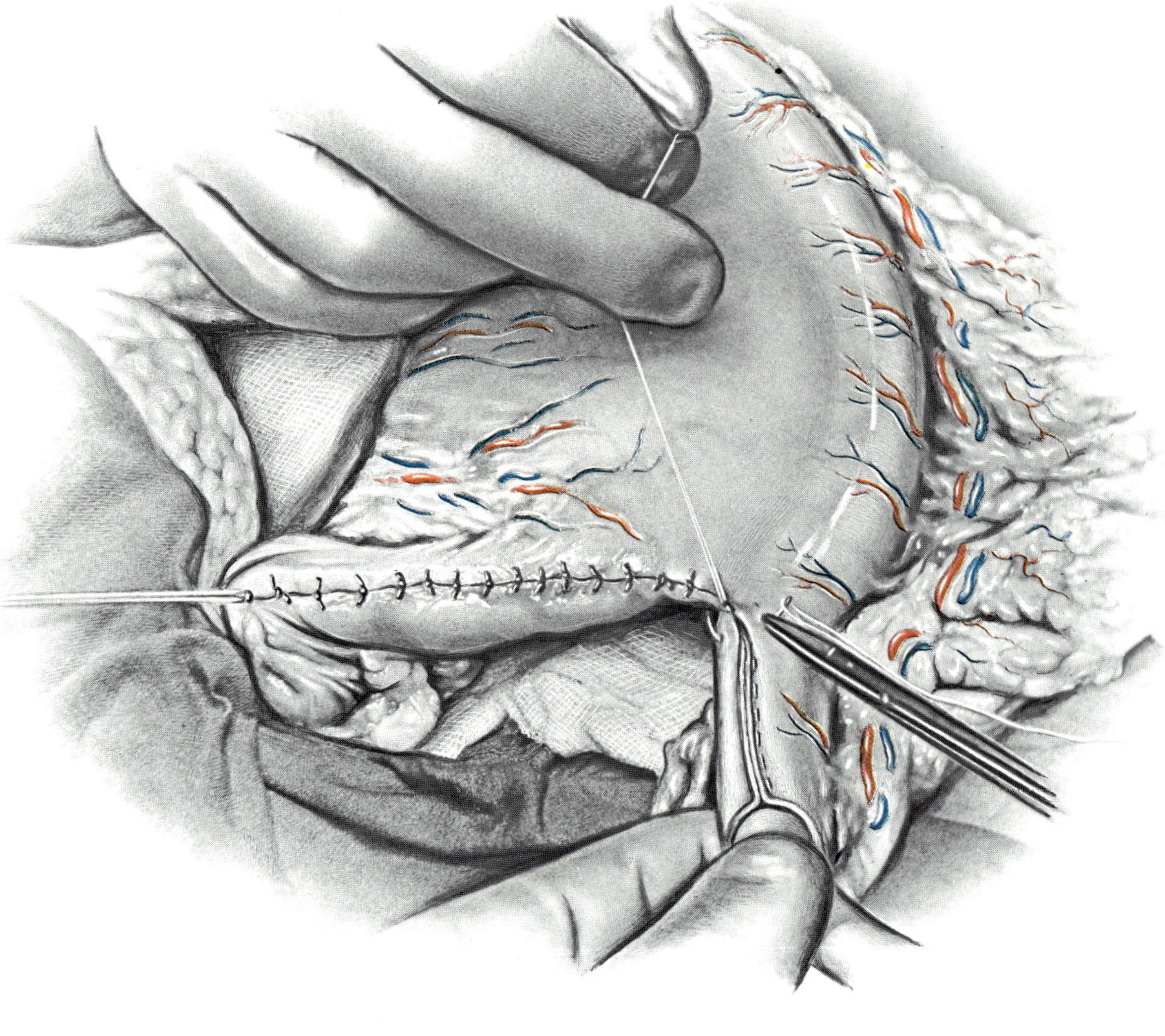

Fig. 661. Second row of sutures is applied to incised walls of stomach over staple suture placed with НЖКА instrument.

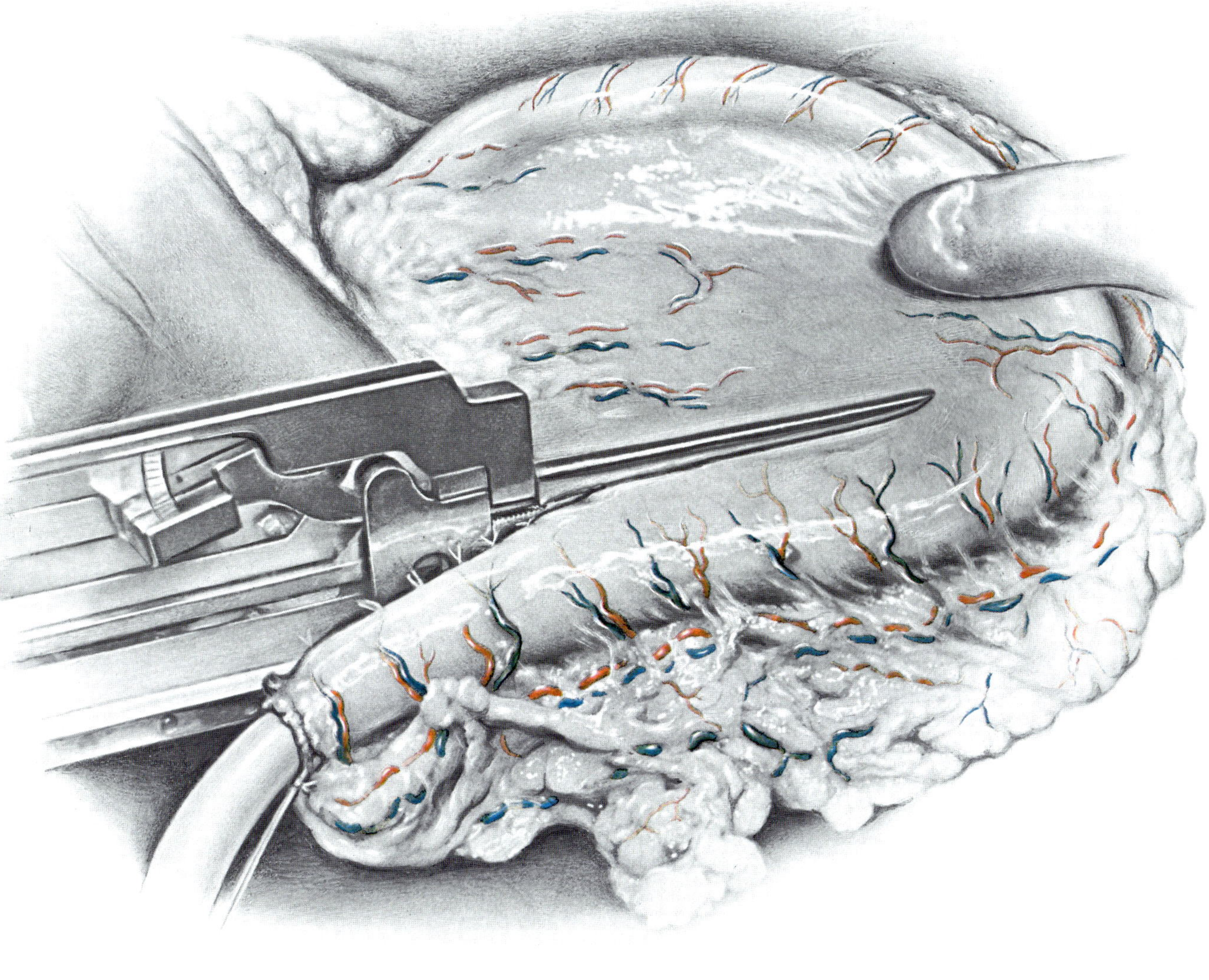

Fig. 662. Second portion of stomach is stitched with НЖКА instrument applied to corner of previously made incision in gastric wall.

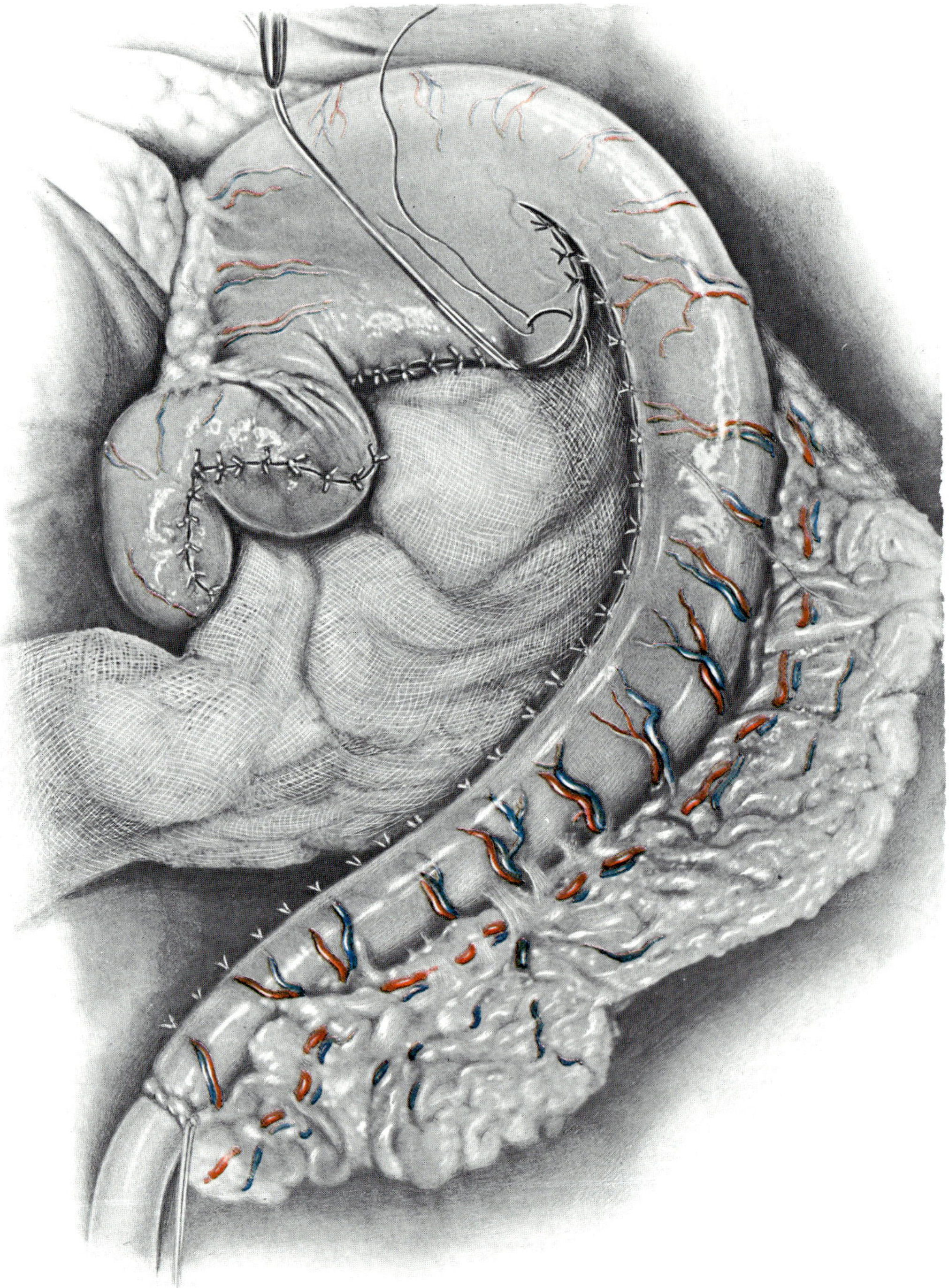

Fig. 663. Sleeve graft has been formed from greater curvature of stomach. Last stitches of second row of sutures are applied to "miniature" stomach.

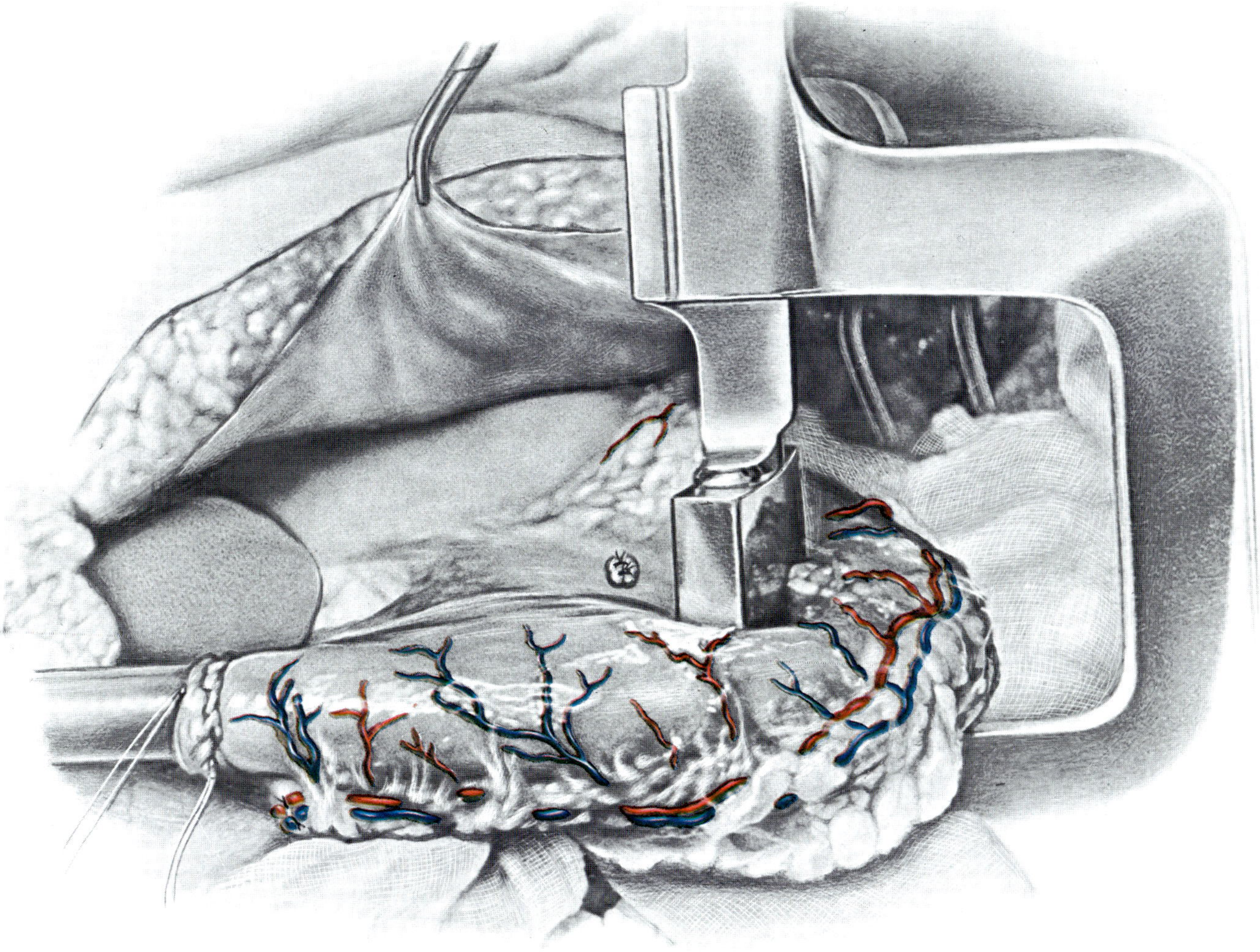

Fig. 664. Gastric wall is cut with first model of Skobelkin's apparatus.

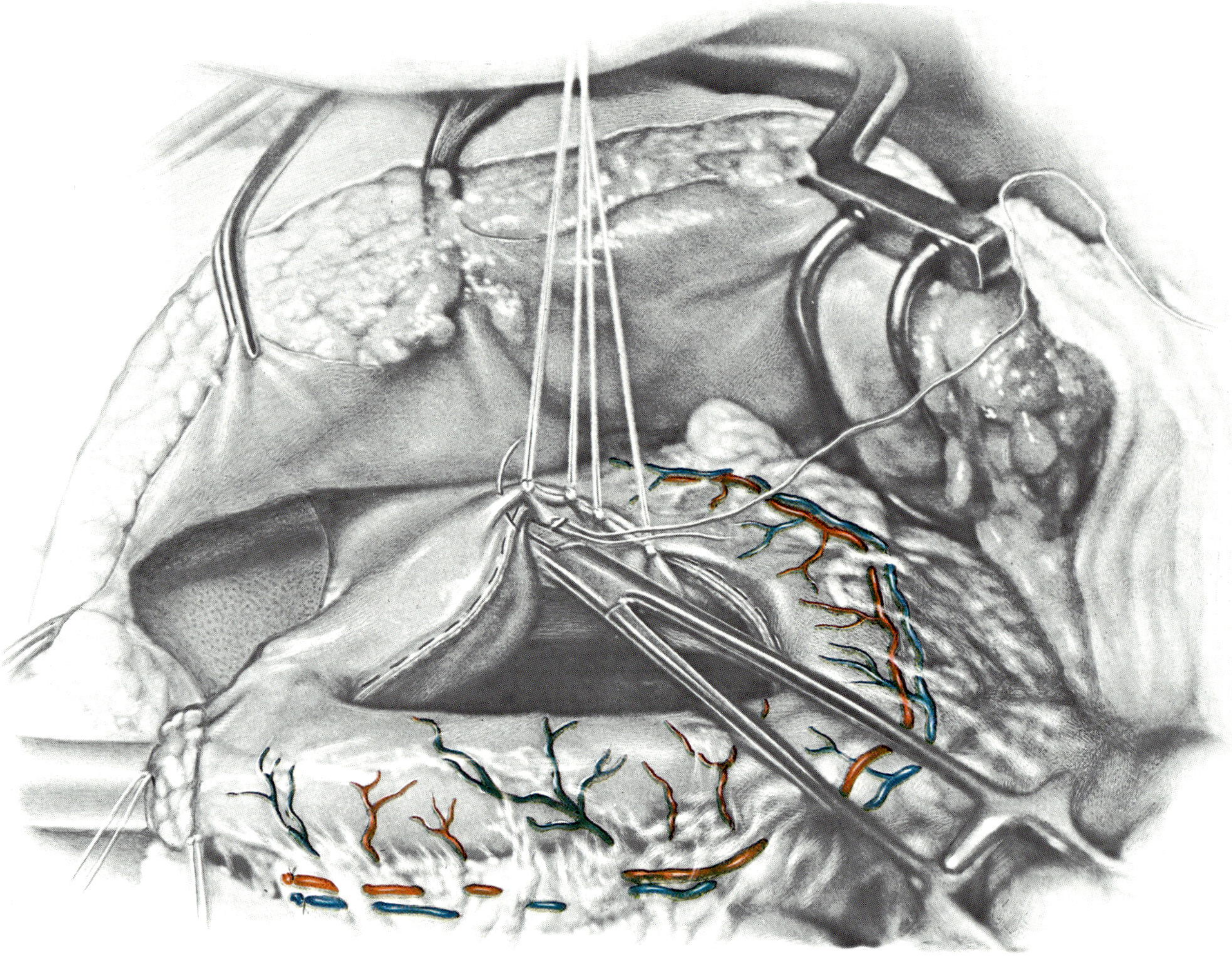

Fig. 665. After stomach has been cut and stitched with metal staples by means of Skobelkin's apparatus, second row of sutures is applied to its wound.

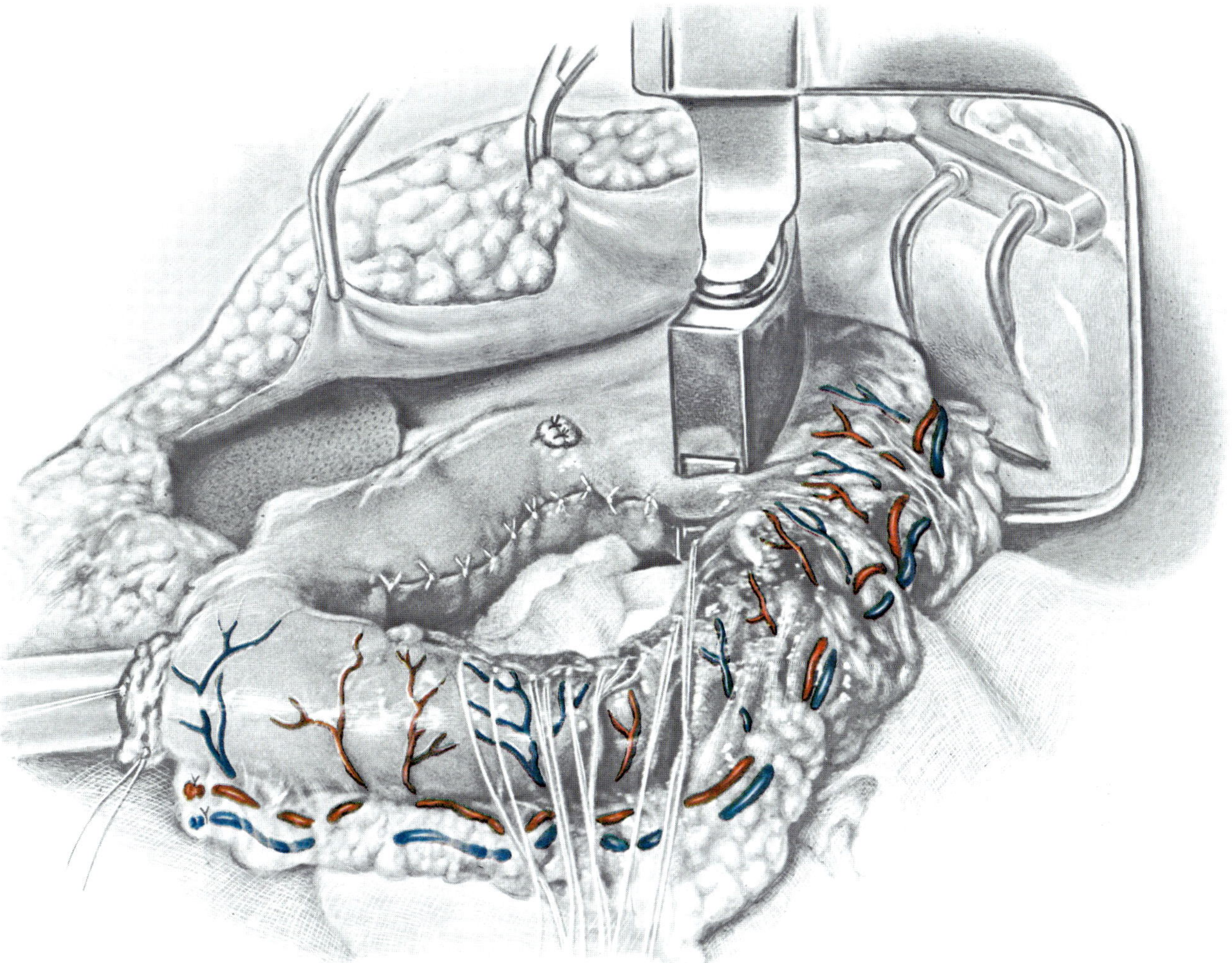

Fig. 666. Second portion of stomach is cut with Skobelkin's apparatus.

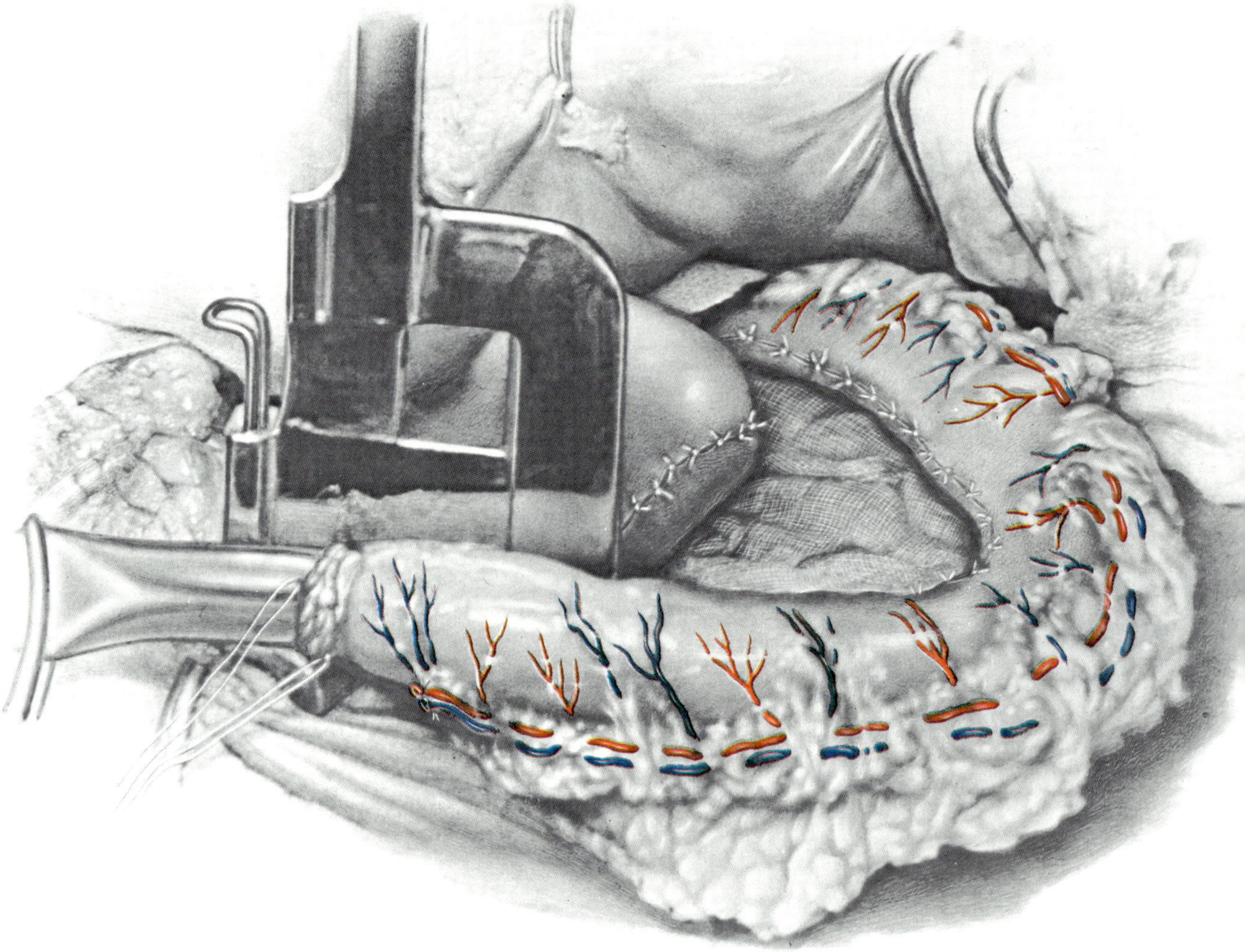

Fig. 667. Gastric wall is stitched close to upper part of graft with the YO instrument.

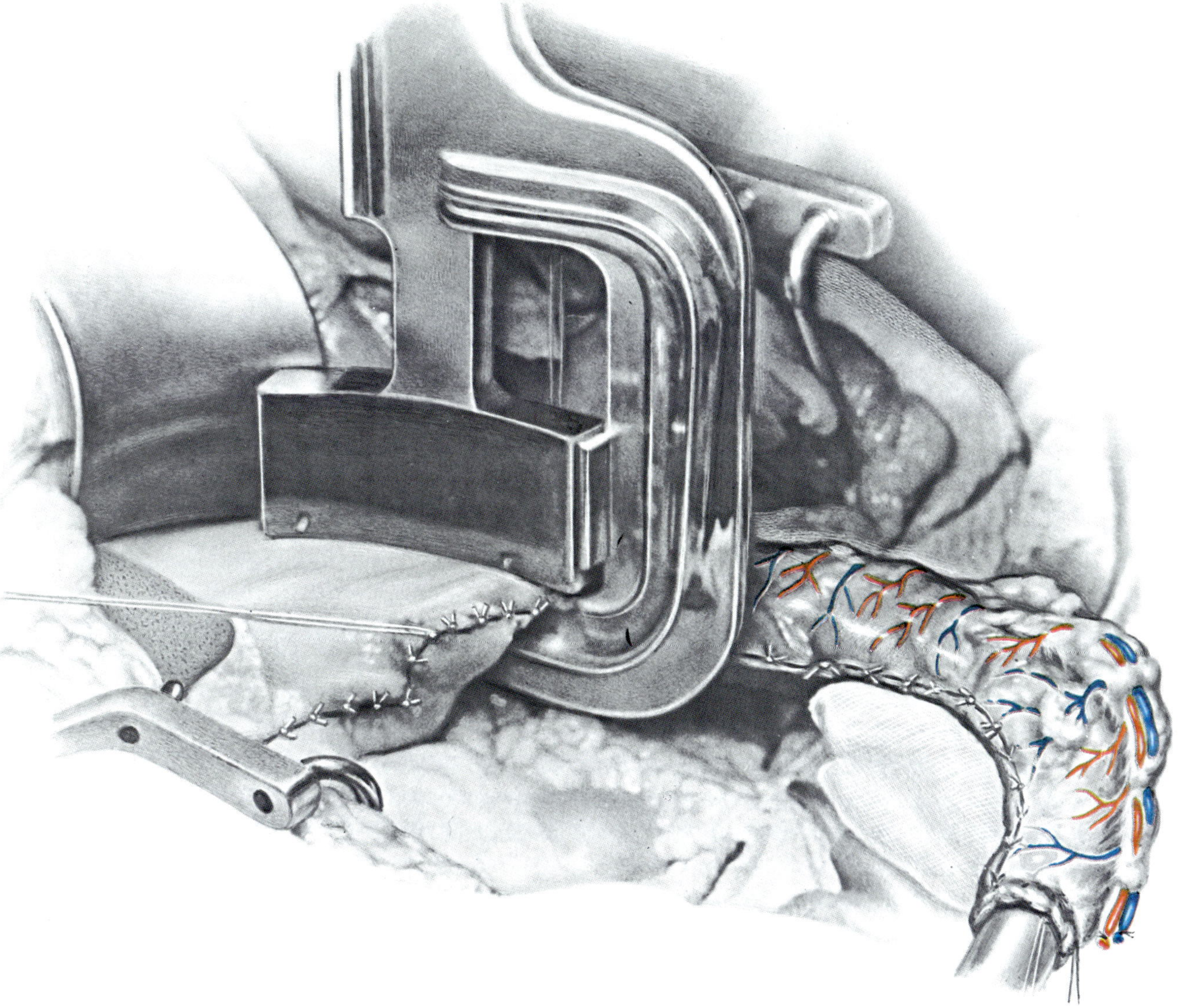

Fig. 668. Gastric wall is cut and stitched close to base of graft by means of second model of Skobelkin's apparatus.

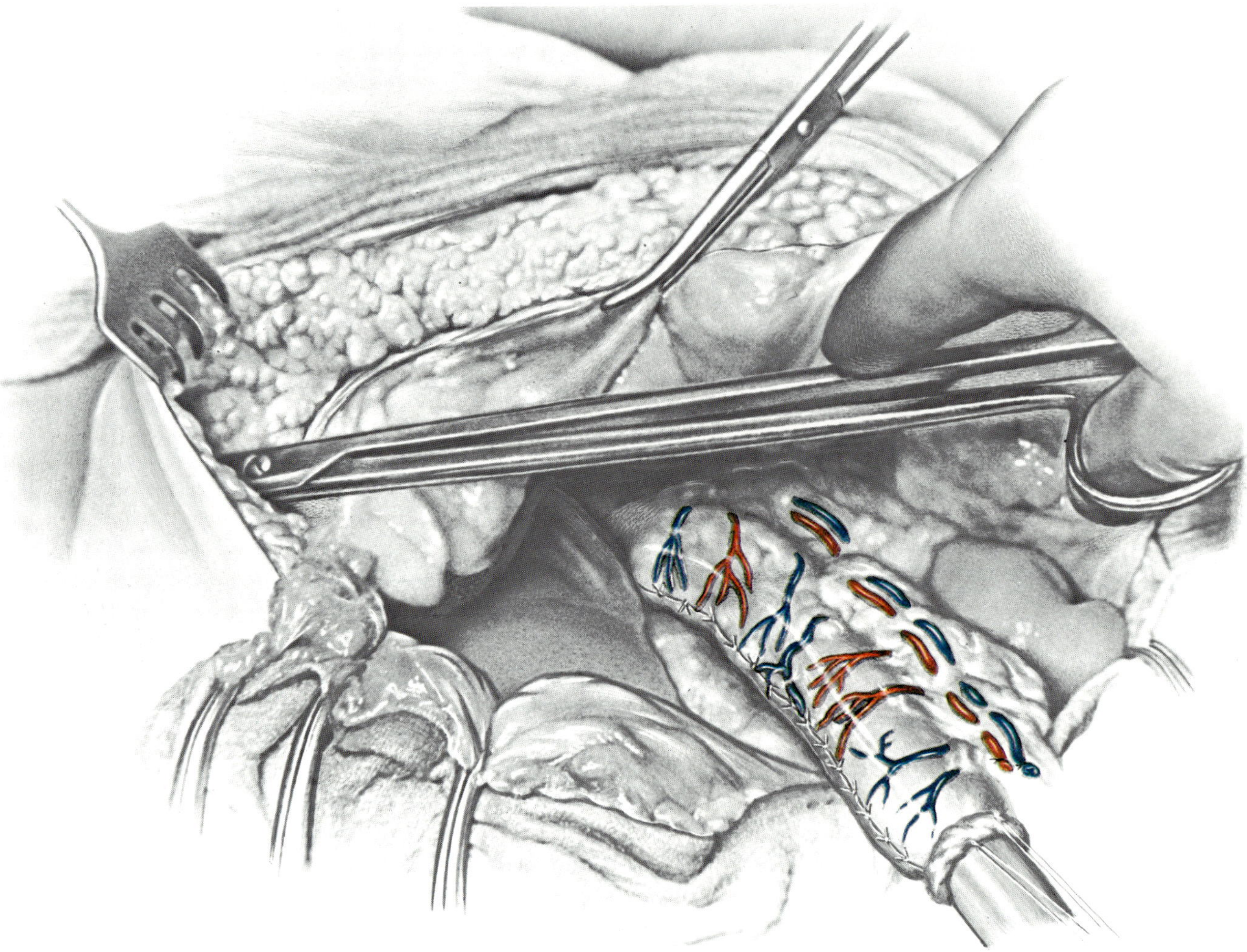

Fig. 669. Subcutaneous tunnel is formed on anterior thoracic wall for transposition of graft to neck. Subcutaneous cellular tissue is separated and cut with long scissors.

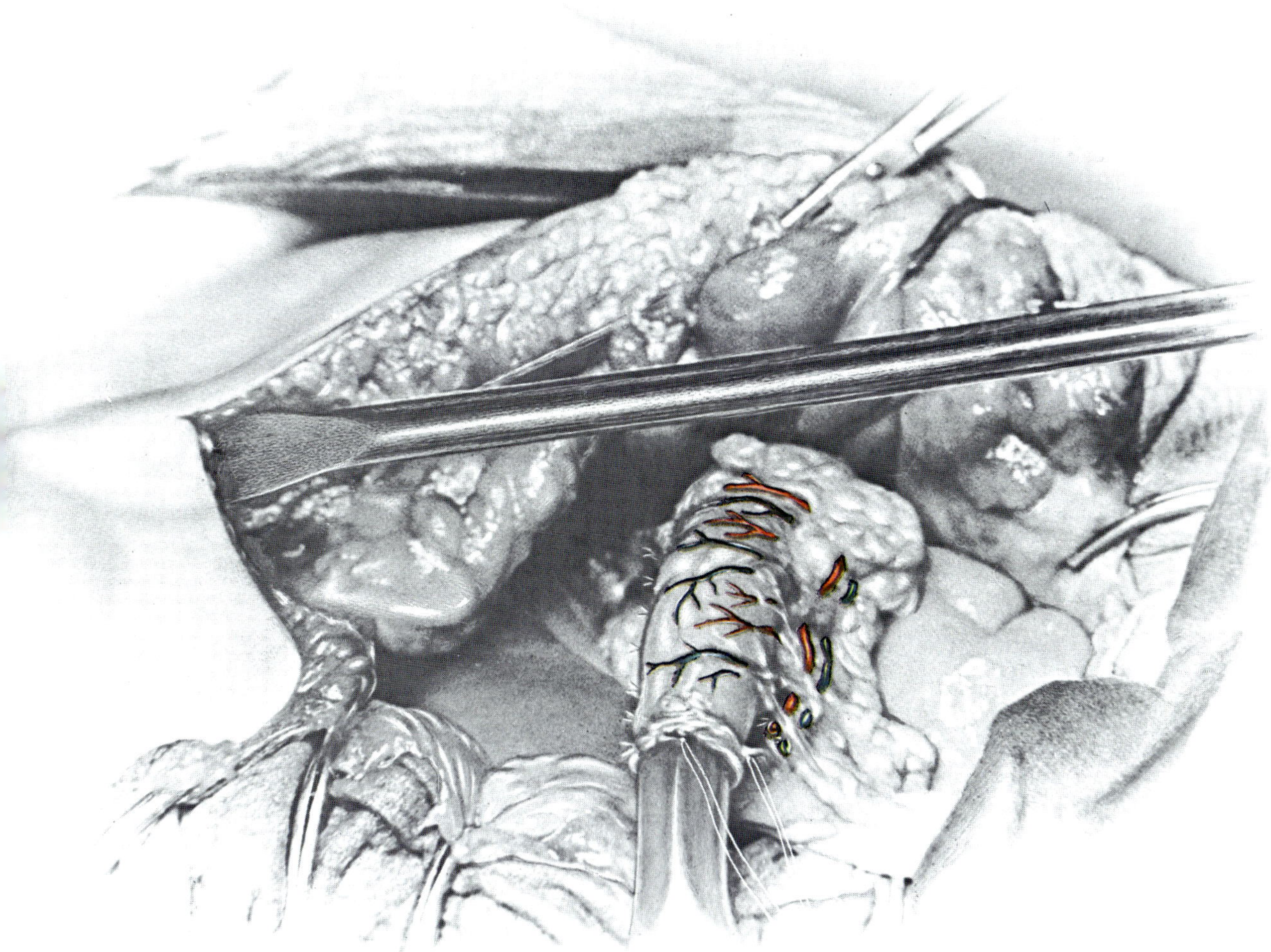

Fig. 670. Subcutaneous tunnel on anterior thoracic wall is made wider with Yudin's lance.

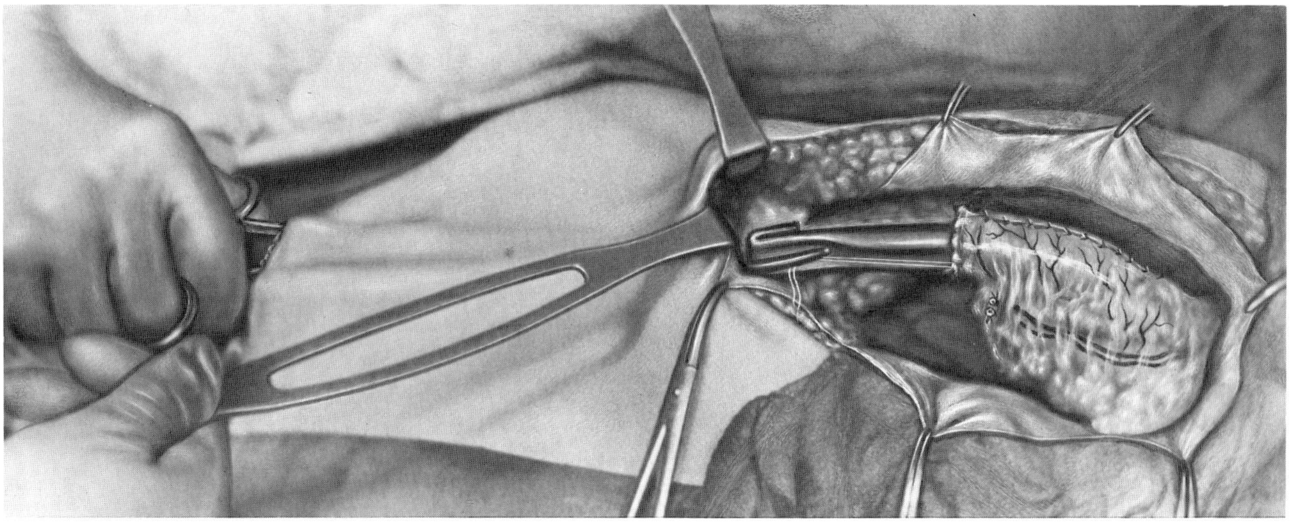

Fig. 671. Dressing forceps are inserted into wound on neck and advanced along subcutaneous tunnel into abdominal cavity; rubber tube and ligature holding graft are grasped with it.

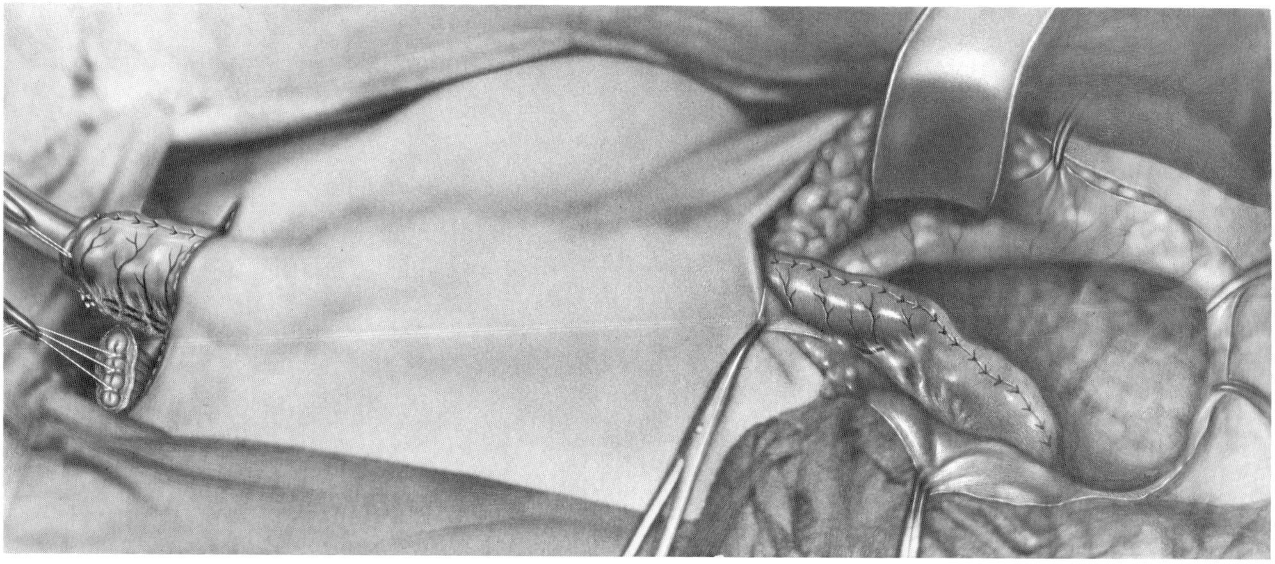

Fig. 672. Graft has been pulled out to neck. Cervical esophagostoma is sutured, and esophageal stump is mobilized for anastomosing with graft.

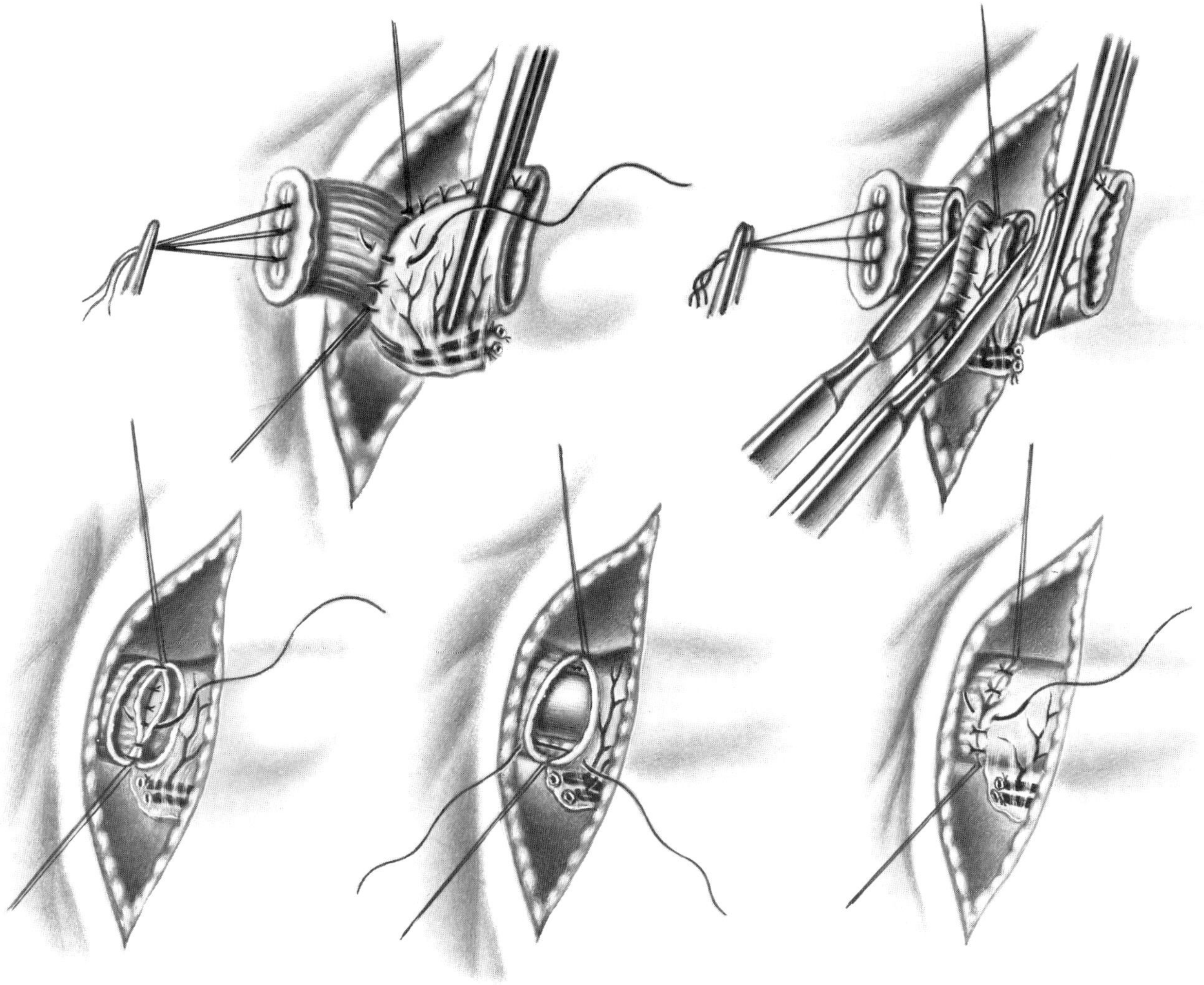

Fig. 673. Stages of establishing anastomosis between proximal esophageal stump formed after Dobromyslov-Torek operation and sleeve graft shaped from greater curvature of stomach.

TECHNIQUES FOR FORMING SLEEVE GRAFT FROM GREATER CURVATURE OF STOMACH AND PROXIMAL DUODENUM AFTER GAVRILIU

The dimensions of the stomach do not always permit tailoring a sleeve graft of the needed length from its greater curvature for transposition to the neck and anastomosing with the cervical esophagus or the pharynx. In such cases the length of the graft may be increased by including the prepyloric part and pylorus of the stomach and the proximal part of the duodenum in it.

The tail and body of the pancreas are mobilized by the above described method, and splenectomy is carried out. The initial portion of the duodenum with the adjoining part of the greater omentum is separated from the surrounding tissues. The pylorus and prepyloric part of the stomach are mobilized along the lesser curvature.

A crushing or soft intestinal clamp is applied to the duodenum, which is then transected 2 to 4 cm caudally to the pylorus (Fig. 674). A rubber tube is introduced

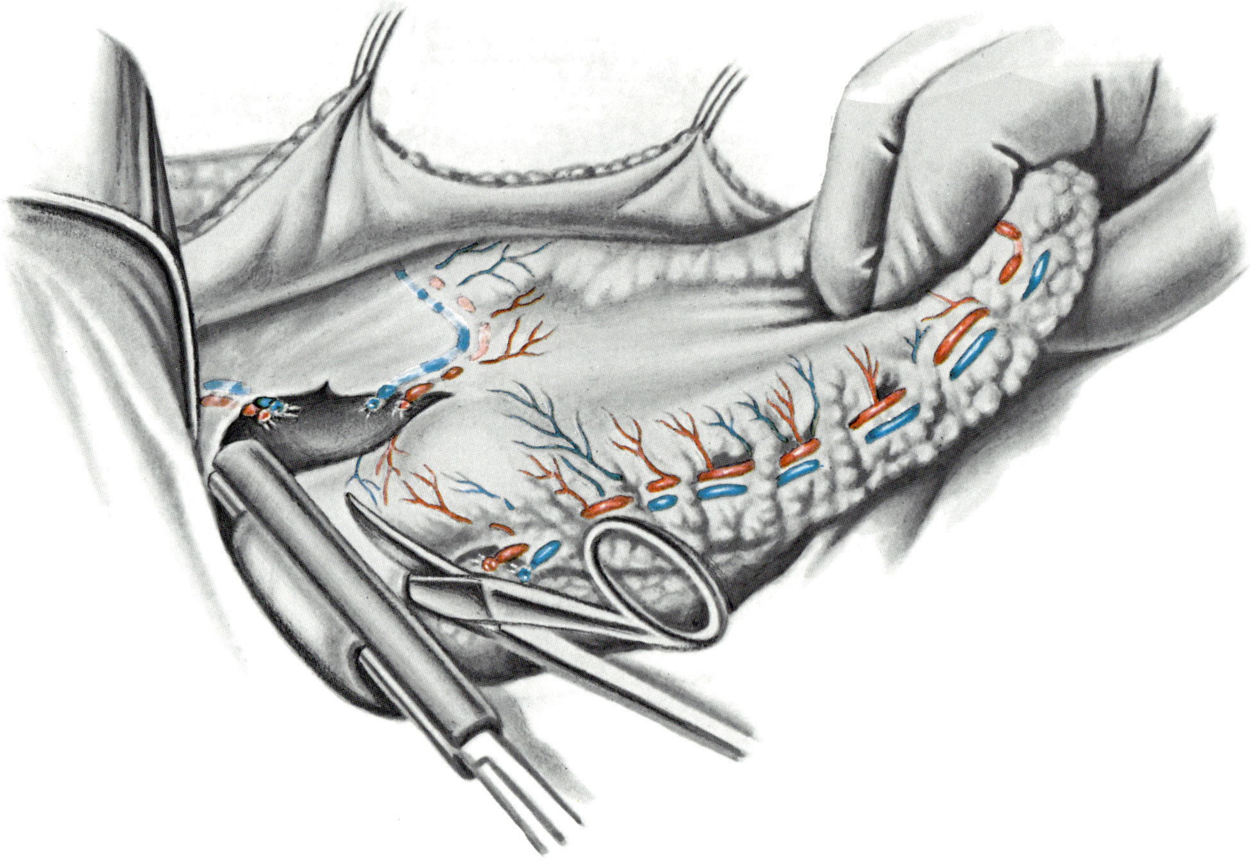

Fig. 674. Duodenum is transected 2 to 4 cm caudally to pylorus.

into the stomach through the pylorus and fastened in the cranial duodenal stump with a ligature (Fig. 675).

An oblique incision is made between two crushing clamps through two thirds of the lumen of the prepyloric part of the stomach. It is passed through the lesser curvature and extended almost to the tube fitted along the greater curvature (Fig. 676).

The right part of the prepyloric incision is closed with double-row sutures, while the left remains clamped until the graft is fully mobilized. All further manipulations in shaping the sleeve graft of the stomach are accomplished with the НЖКА instrument (Fig. 677).

A second row of interrupted seromuscular sutures is applied to the line of the gastric incision (Fig. 678). An end-to-end anastomosis is formed between the distal duodenal stump and the part of the stomach connected with the lesser curvature (Fig. 679). The graft is transposed to the neck through a subcutaneous or retrosternal tunnel and anastomosed with the cervical esophagus or pharynx. Kader's gastrostoma is applied to the "miniature stomach." The abdominal wound is sutured.

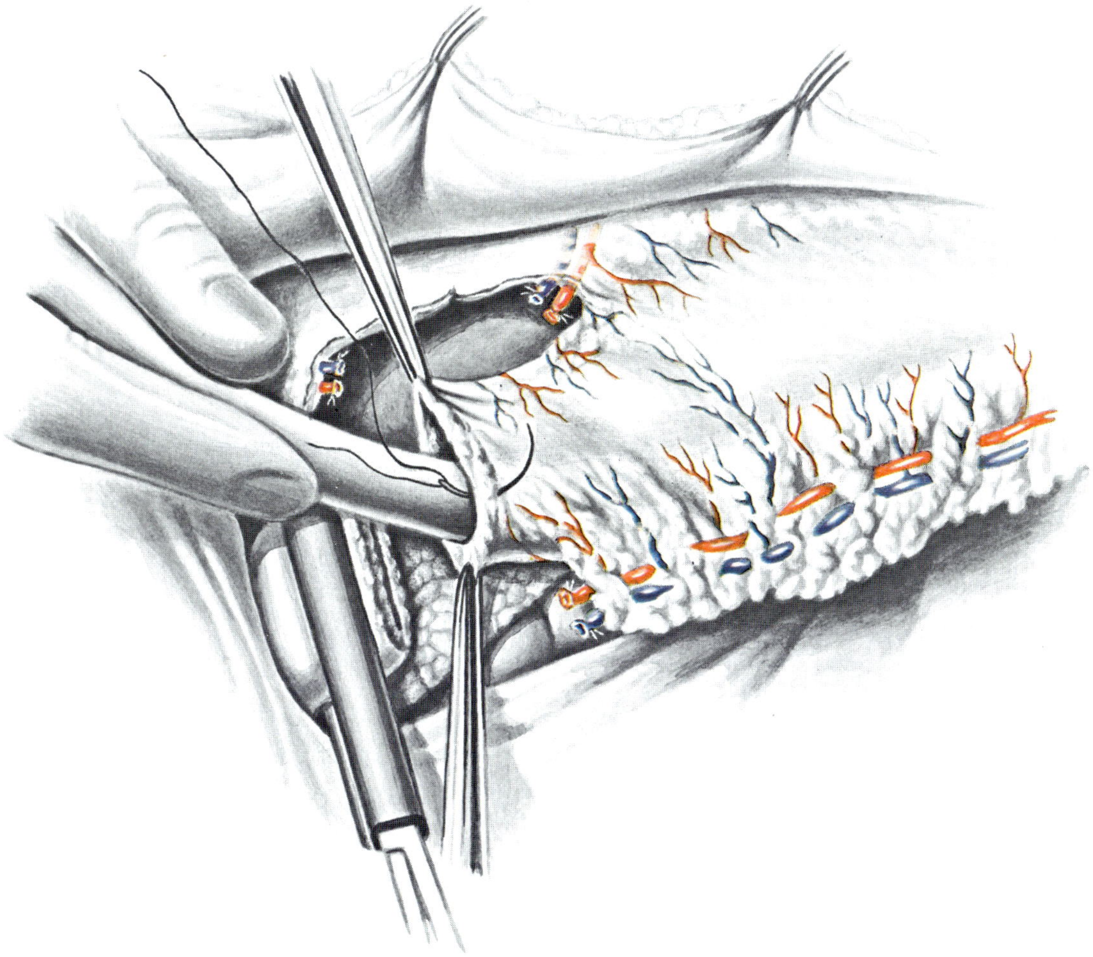

Fig. 675. Rubber tube is passed into stomach through pylorus and placed along greater curvature.

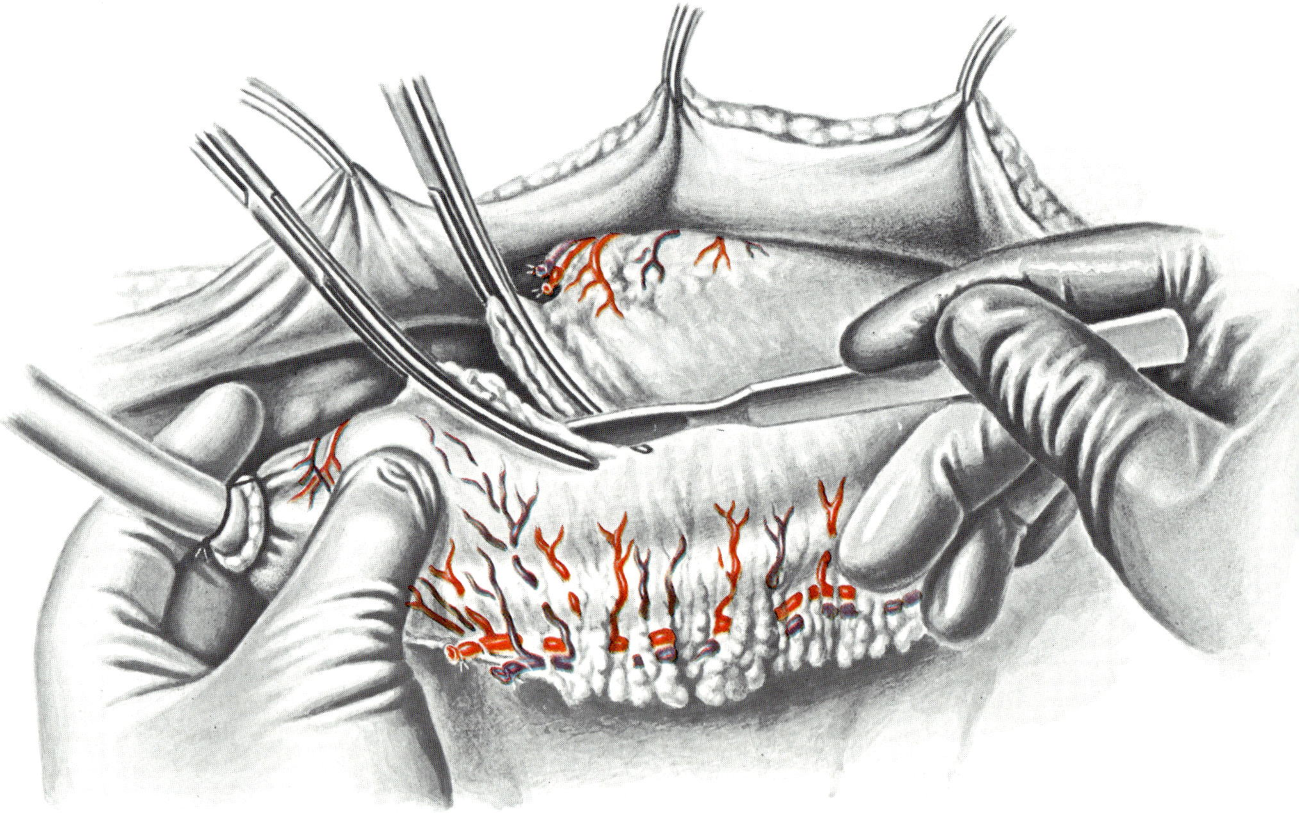

Fig. 676. Prepyloric part of stomach is cut on lesser curvature.

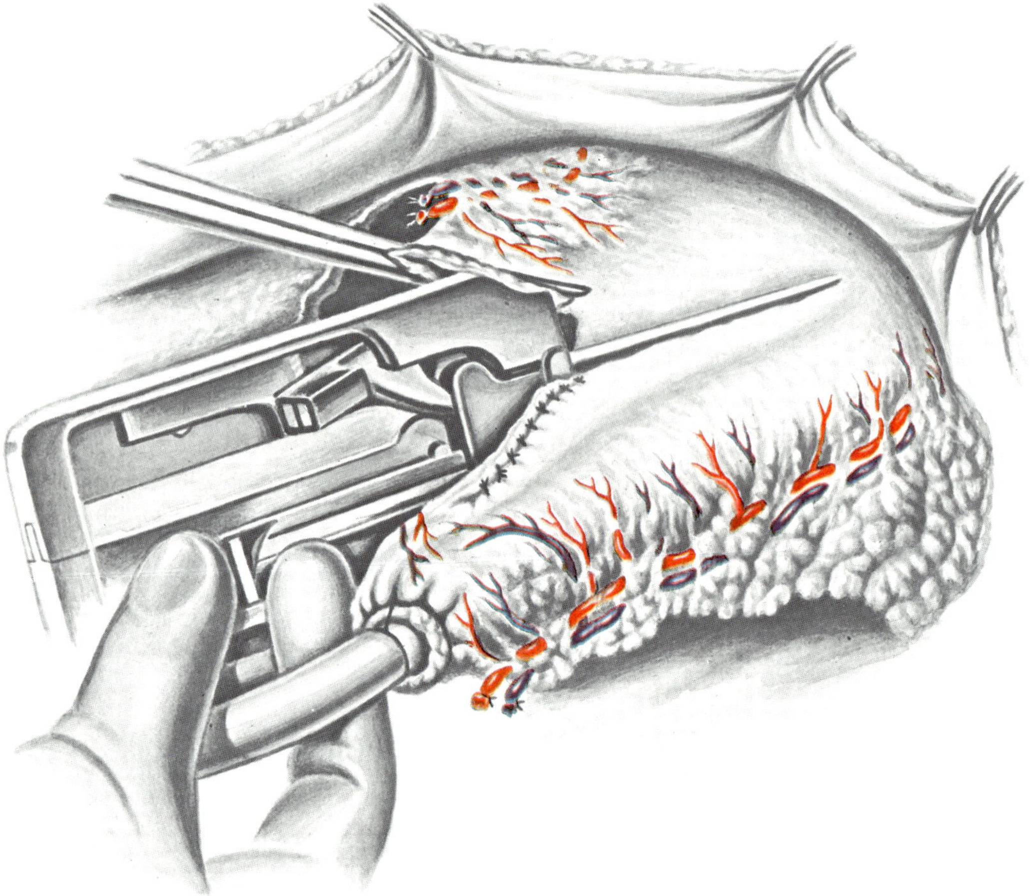

Fig. 677. After closure of prepyloric part of stomach with sutures, sleeve graft is shaped from greater curvature with НЖКА instrument.

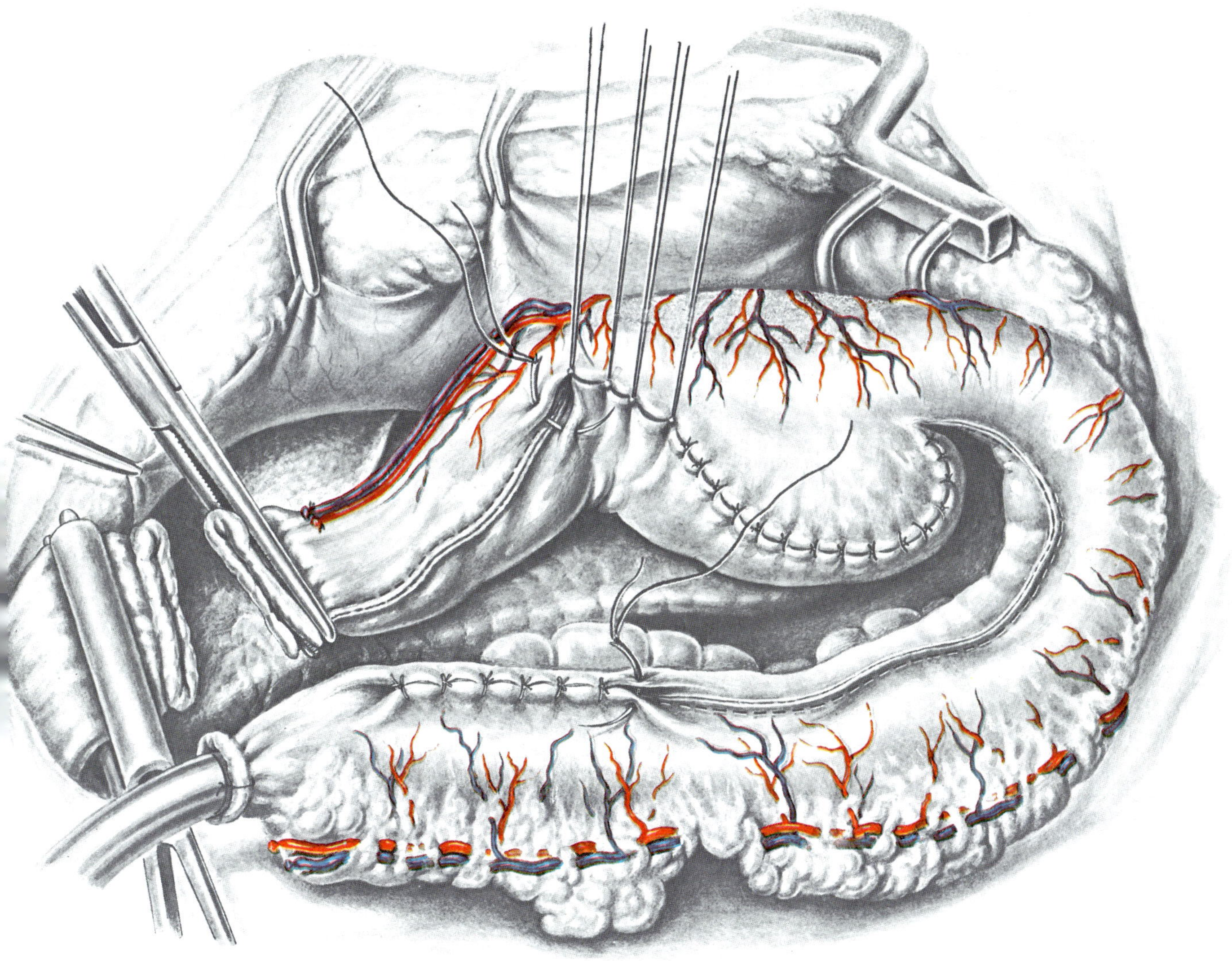

Fig. 678. Staple suture, which had been applied to sleeve graft and remaining part of stomach, is buried by means of interrupted sutures.

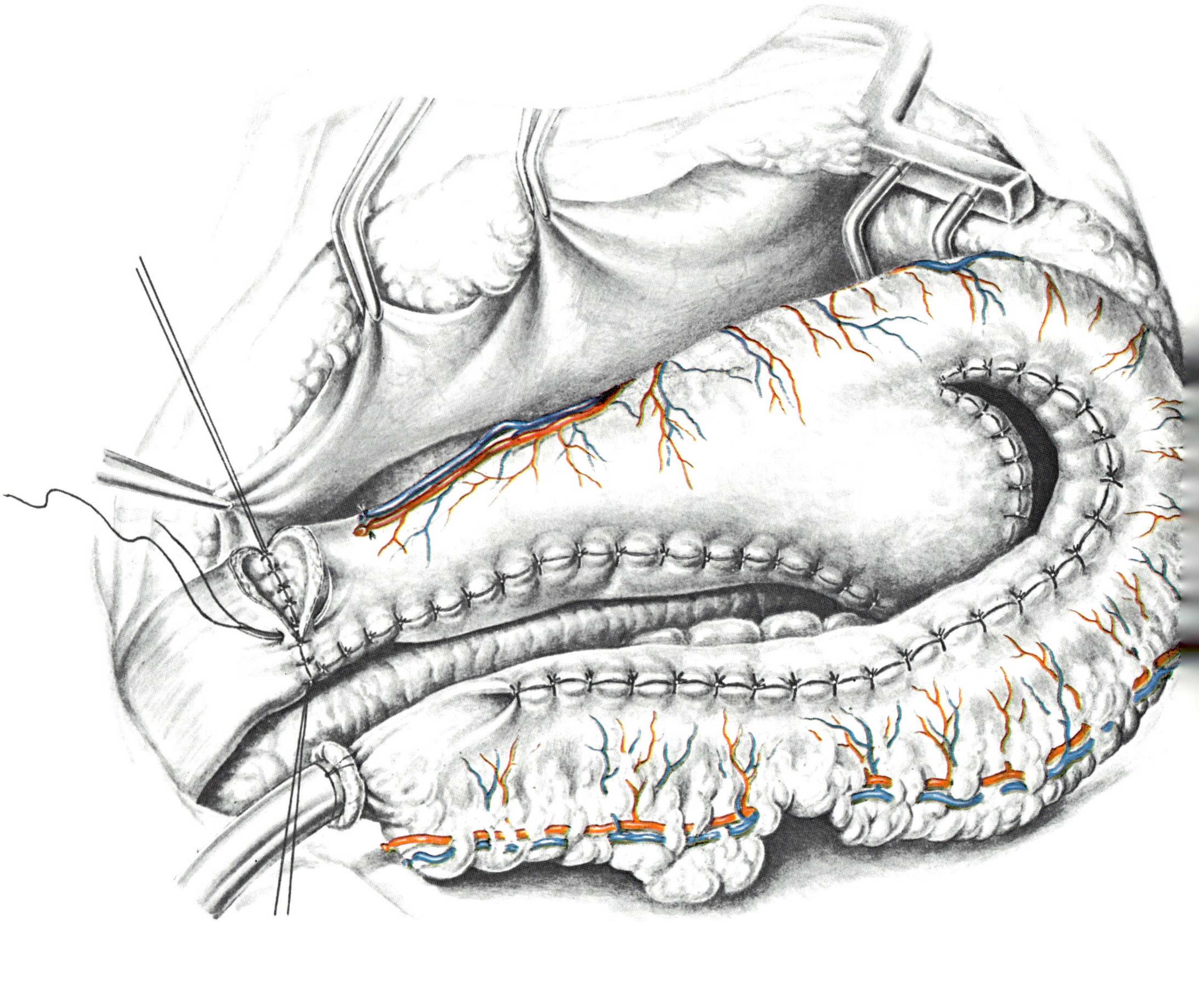

Fig. 679. Creation of end-to-end gastroduodenal anastomosis.

Segmental esophagoplasty

In distinction to total esophagoplasty in which the entire esophagus is replaced by a graft the term *segmental esophagoplasty* stands for operations that restore limited portions (segments) of the esophagus at various levels: in the cervical, in the upper, middle, or lower thoracic, or in the abdominal portion of the esophagus. The operations grouped under the general title "segmental esophagoplasty" comprise esophagoesophagostomy, esophagoenterogastrostomy and esophagoenteroesophagostomy. All these operations envisage the inclusion of intact portions of the esophagus and, in many cases, of the cardia in the performance of the esophagus. In cases with total stricture the precise preoperative diagnosis is only possible with double-contrast study of the esophagus. The examination is conducted with the patient in a horizontal position, and the contrast medium is introduced simultaneously into the esophagus through the mouth and in the retrograde direction through the gastrostoma along a tube inserted through an esophagoscope (Fig. 680).

Segmental plastic surgery of the esophagus is conducted predominantly on patients with malignant diseases of the esophagus, such as cicatricial stenosis consequent upon chemical burns, peptic strictures, and congenital atresia.

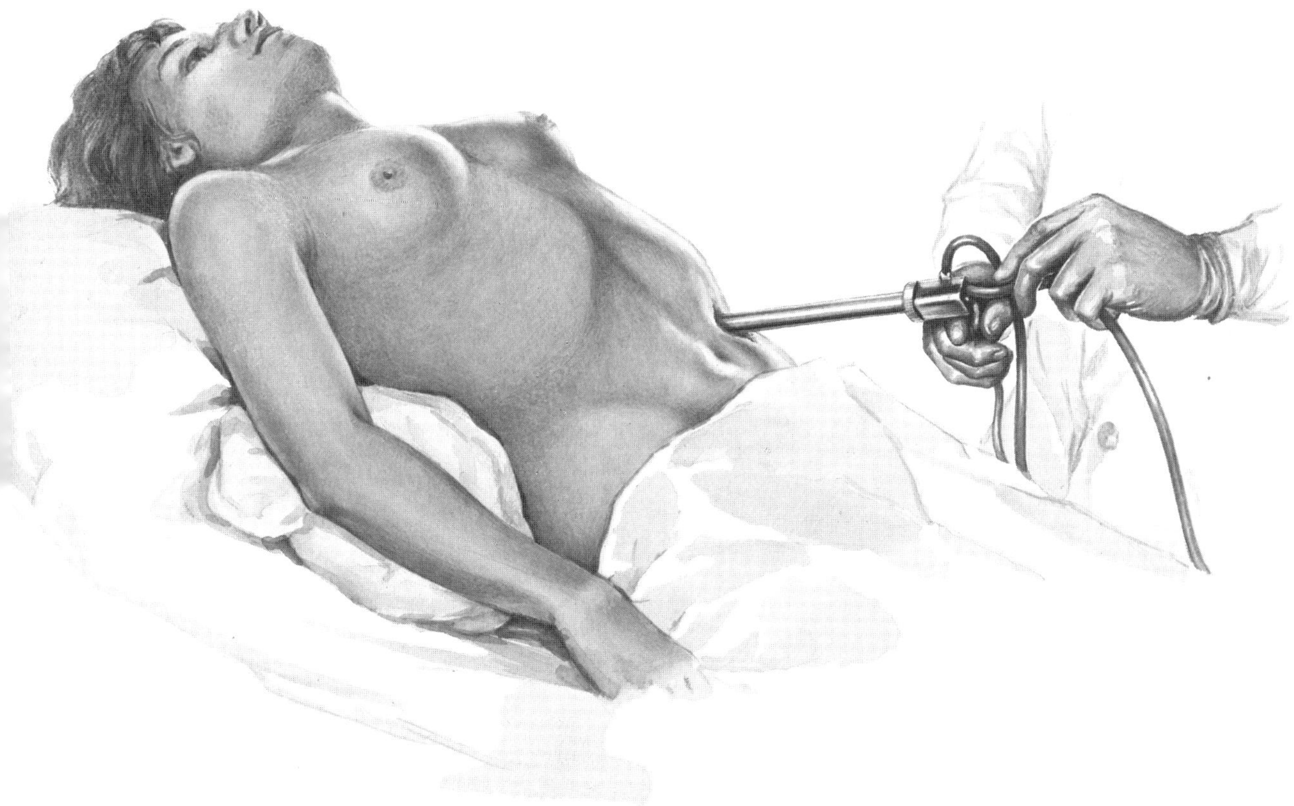

Fig. 680. Introduction of esophageal tube through endoscope for retrograde roentgenoesophagoscopy.

ESOPHAGOESOPHAGOSTOMY

"THREE-FOURTHS" ESOPHAGOESOPHAGOSTOMY

"Three fourths" esophagoesophagostomy is an operation commonly performed in cicatricial stricutre of no longer than 3 cm.

The approach to the esophagus is determined by the level of the cicatricial stenosis in the thoracic or cervical portion. In separating the esophagus from the surrounding tissues, a gastric tube introduced into it may help to determine the upper boundary of the narrowing. Mediastinotomy is performed, the level of the stricture is determined, and the esophagus is held with a rubber tube or a gauze strip and separated from the mediastinal tissues for 5 to 7 cm (Fig. 681). It is essential to leave the main branches of the vagus nerves intact. The anterior wall of the esophagus is cut with a scalpel directly above and along the entire length of the stricture (Fig. 682). The edges of the incision are drawn apart with traction sutures. The first row of interrupted sutures or a continuous suture is applied transversely through all the esophageal coats (Fig. 683). The second row of interrupted sutures is applied through the submucous and muscular coats (Fig. 684). The mediastinal pleura is either left unsutured or closed with widely spaced stitches. The mediastinum and pleural cavity are drained by means of a tube in a transthoracic approach or by means of rubber bands in a cervical approach. The thoracic wound is closed. The wound in the neck is sutured to the level of the rubber drains.

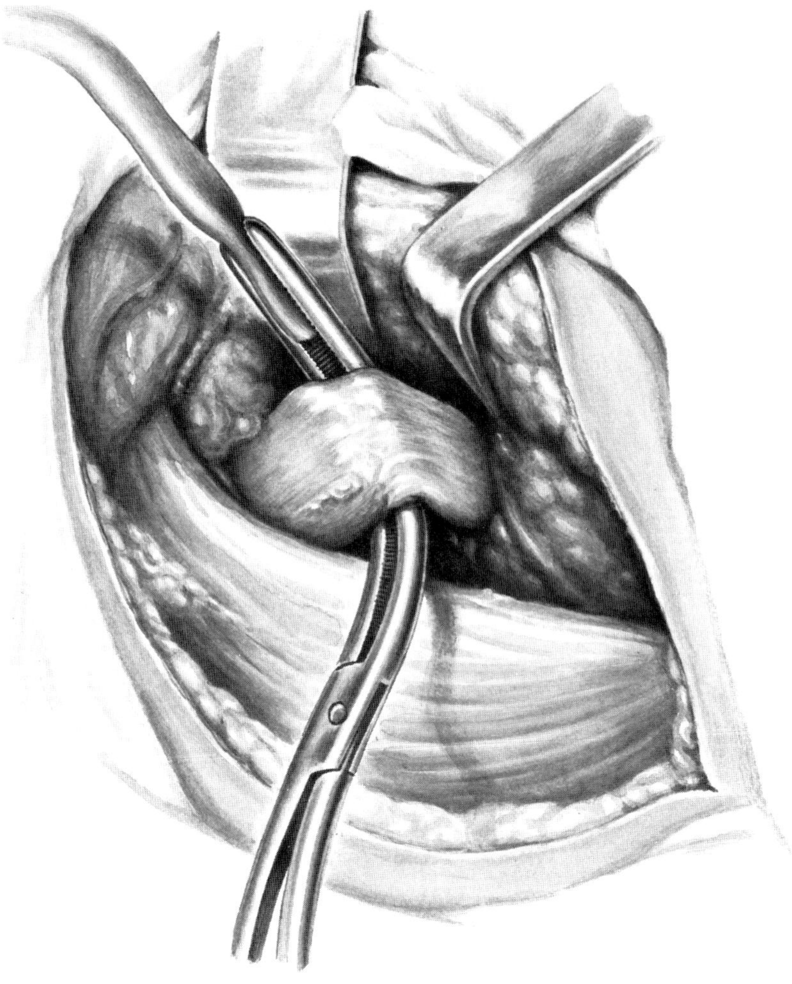

Fig. 681. Fixation of esophagus in region of stricture on rubber tube.

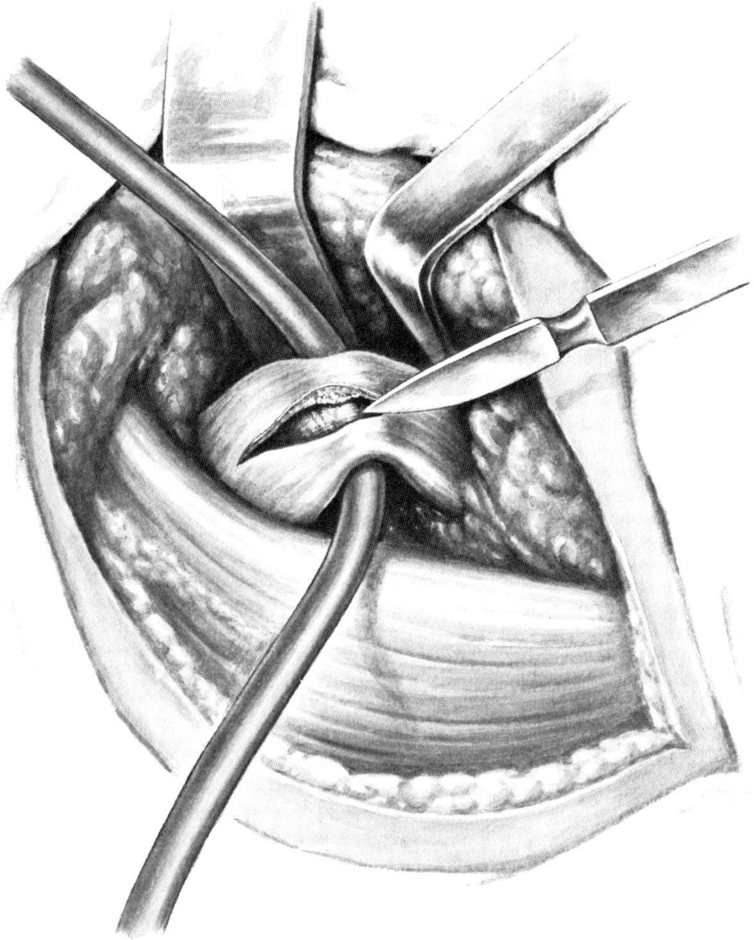

Fig. 682. Esophageal wall is cut lengthwise through stricture.

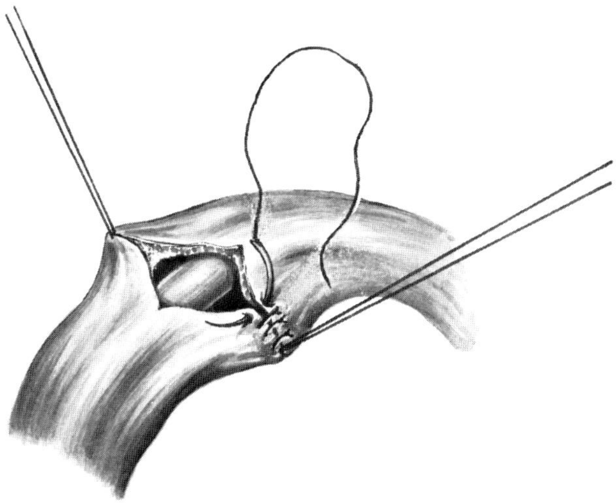

Fig. 683. Transverse inner sutures stitched through all coats of esophageal wall.

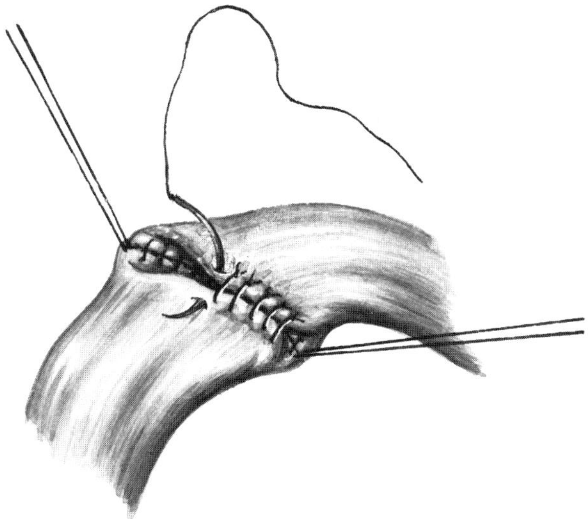

Fig. 684. Application of inner row of buried sutures to muscular coat of esophagus.

SIDE-TO-SIDE ESOPHAGOESOPHAGOSTOMY

In severe suprastenotic dilatation of the esophagus another type, the side-to-side anastomosis, may be created. It is possible in any part of the esophagus, the cervical included, if the stricture is no longer than 2 to 3 cm.

The esophagus is separated from the tissues of the mediastinum and held by two loops; its anterior wall is cut transversely above and below the stricture (Fig. 685).

If the distance between the two incisions is no longer than 1.5 cm, interrupted sutures are applied to the edges of the incisions through all the esophageal coats (Fig. 686). When the distance between the incisions is greater, it is necessary to approximate their inner margins first by means of musculomuscular sutures. Interrupted sutures are then applied through all coats of the anterior lip of the anastomósis (Fig. 687). The line of the anastomosis is covered with interrupted musculomuscular sutures.

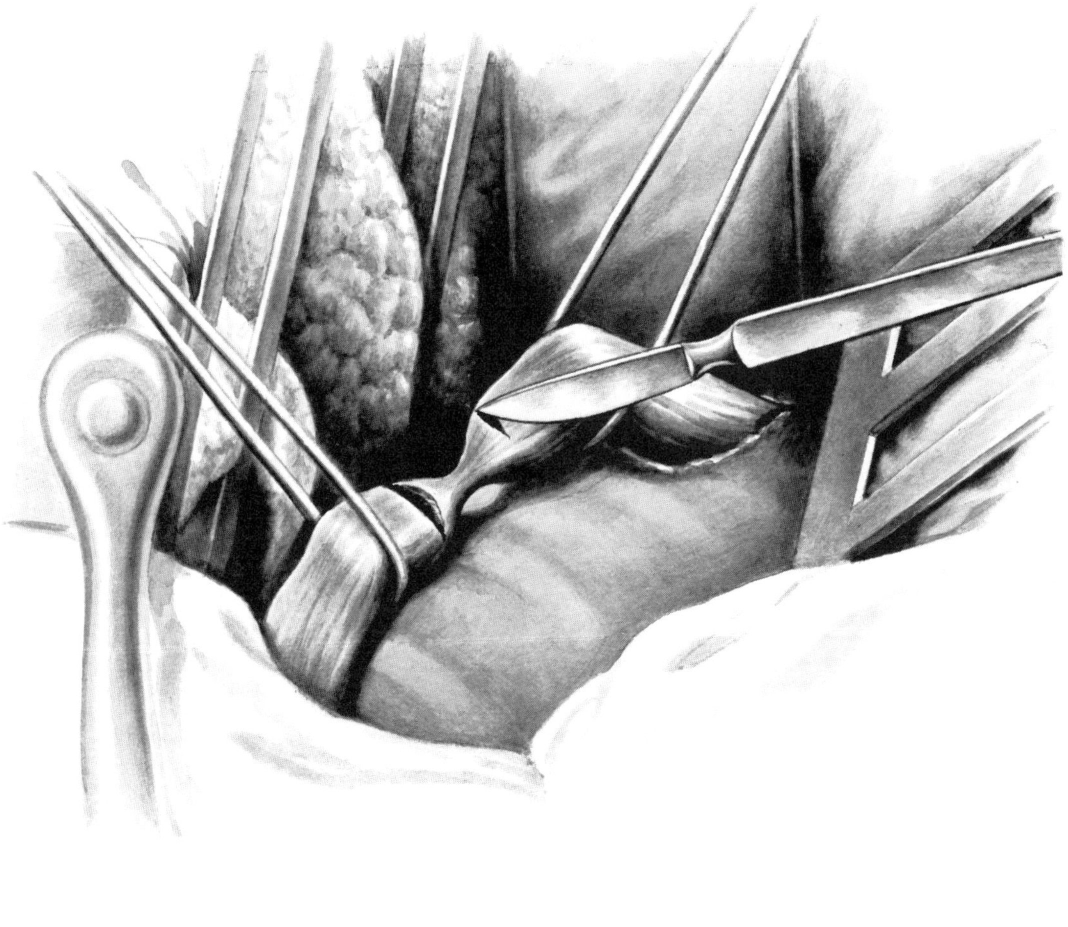

Fig. 685. Transverse incisions along half of esophageal circumference above and below stricture.

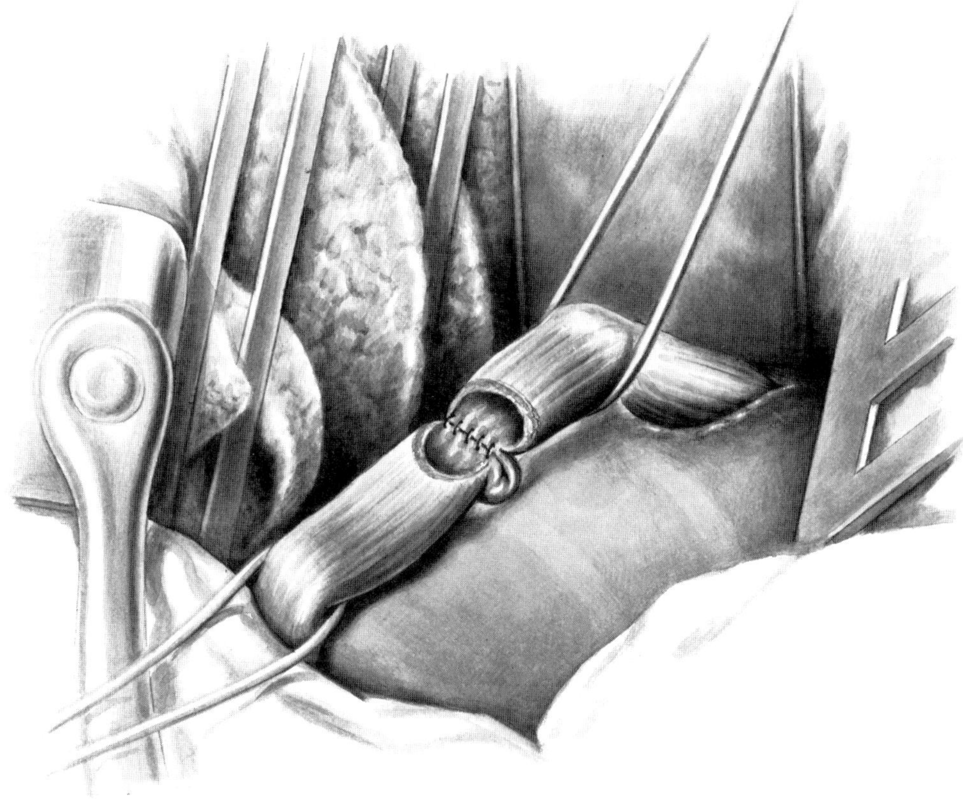

Fig. 686. Sutures applied to posterior lip of esophagoenteric anastomosis.

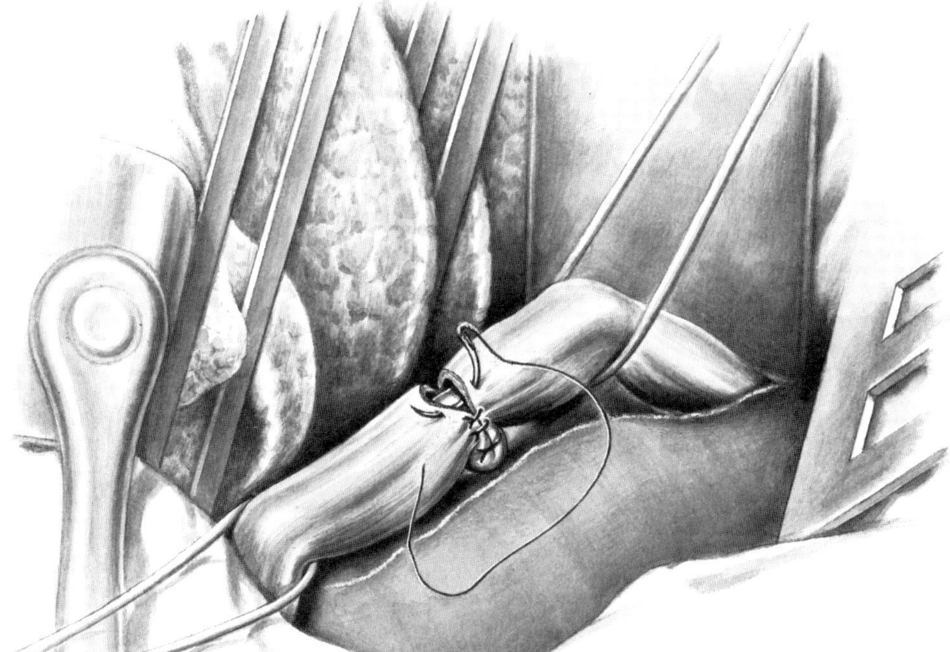

Fig. 687. Application of inner sutures to anterior lip of anastomosis.

DIRECT ANASTOMOSIS IN ATRESIA OF ESOPHAGUS

The most commonly employed operations in atresia of the esophagus are direct intrathoracic esophageal anastomosis or transposition of the upper esophageal segment to the neck with the formation of a cervical esophagostoma and gastrostoma after Kader. Transposition of the esophagus is performed when the diastasis between the esophageal segments is more than 1.5 cm, in cases with high atresia (at the level of the sixth and seventh cervical vertebrae), and in the absence or considerable underdevelopment of the lower esophageal segment. If there is a tracheoesophageal fistula, it should be corrected irrespective of the type of operation to be undertaken.

Direct end-to-side anastomosis is usually carried out when the upper and lower segments of the esophagus touch each other, overlap, or when the diastasis between them does not exceed 1 to 1.5 cm and also when there exists a considerable discrepancy between their diameters.

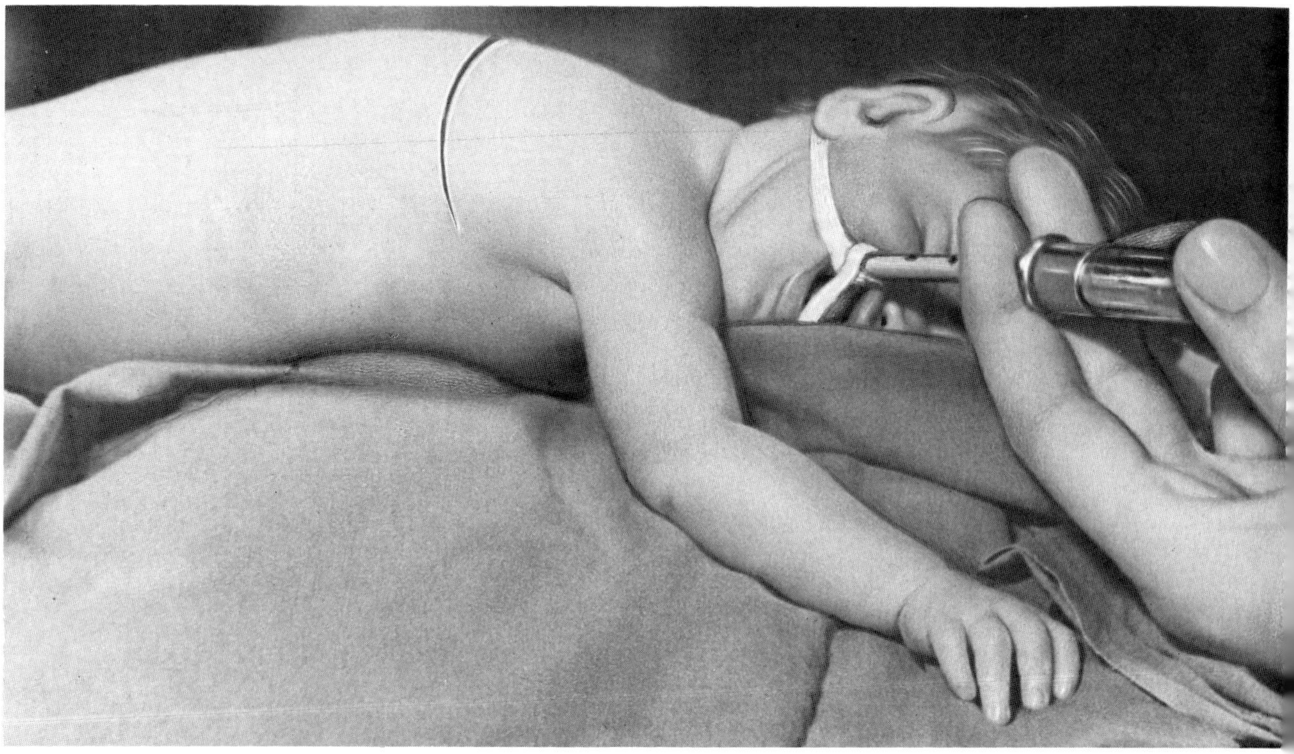

Fig. 688. Position of patient and operative approach (posterolateral thoracotomy in fifth intercostal space).

Right lateral or posterolateral thoracotomy through the fifth intercostal space or the seat of the fifth rib (Fig. 688) and mediastinotomy are performed. The arch of the azygos vein is tied with two ligatures and transected between them (Fig. 689). The caudal segment of the esophagus is separated from the surrounding tissues, and the orifice of the tracheoesophageal fistula is closed by tying the esophagus close to the tracheal wall with two ligatures (Fig. 690) and transecting it in between (Fig. 691).

Dissection of the cranial esophageal segment becomes easier if a rubber or a soft plastic tube is introduced into it through the nose.

The ends of the esophagus are approximated by applying interrupted musculoadventitial sutures with an atraumatic needle transversely to the posterior wall of the cranial esophageal segment and obliquely or lengthwise to the posterior wall of the caudal segment (Fig. 692). Incisions are then made in the anterior walls of both esophageal segments 2 to 3 mm above and below and

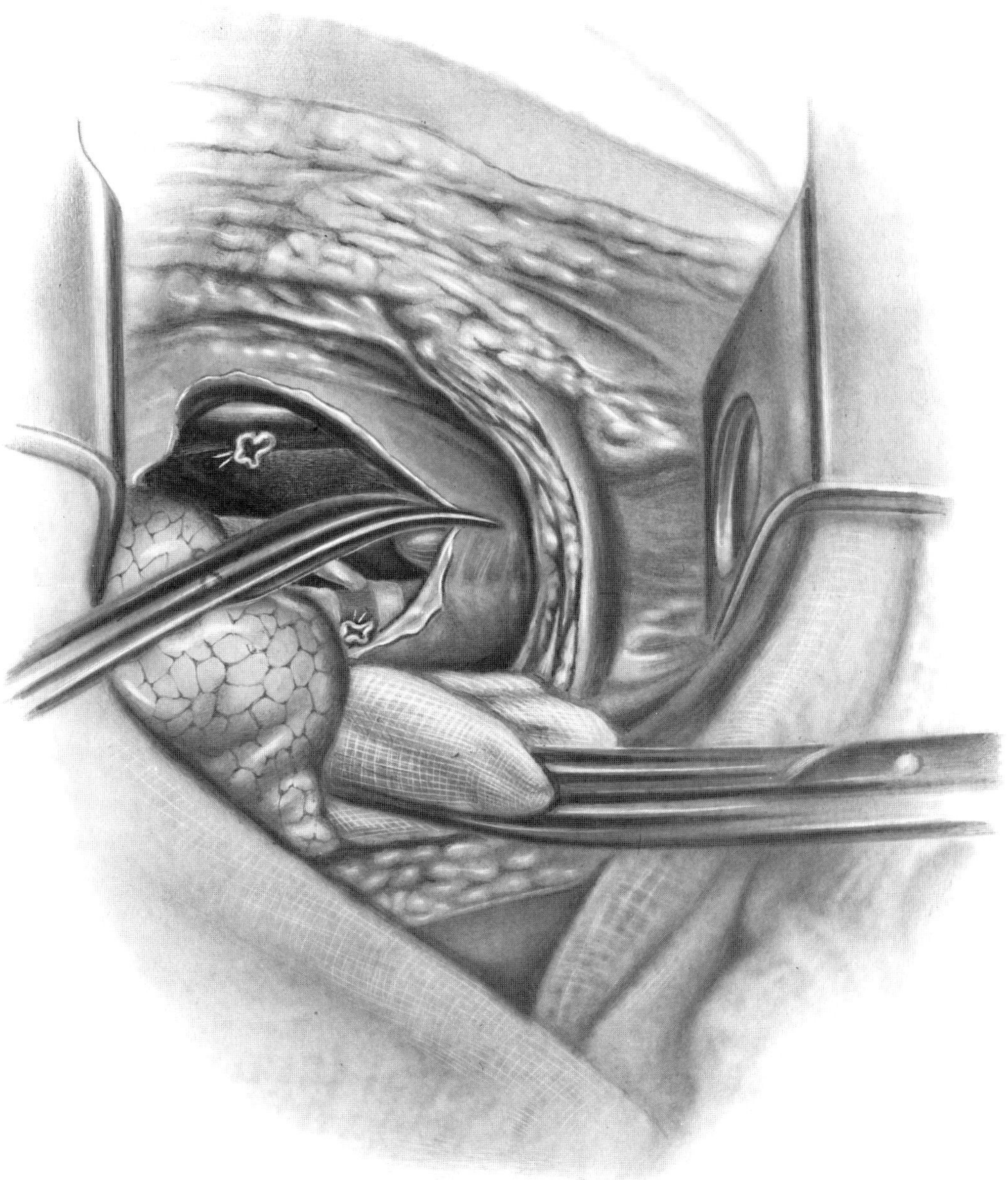

Fig. 689. Mediastinotomy at level of esophageal atresia. Azygos vein has been ligated and transected.

parallel to the suture (Fig. 693). Interrupted sutures are passed through all the coats of the posterior lip of the anastomosis (Fig. 694). The tube is passed from the upper esophageal segment into the lower and then into the stomach (Fig. 695), and interrupted sutures are placed through all the coats of the anterior lip of the anastomosis on it (Fig. 696). The creation of the anastomosis is completed by placing interrupted sutures on the muscular or adventitial layer of the anterior walls of the esophageal segment (Fig. 697).

In some cases a different technique may be used for establishing end-to-end anastomosis. Two or three stitches are made through the muscular and submucous coats of each of the opposing esophageal ends about

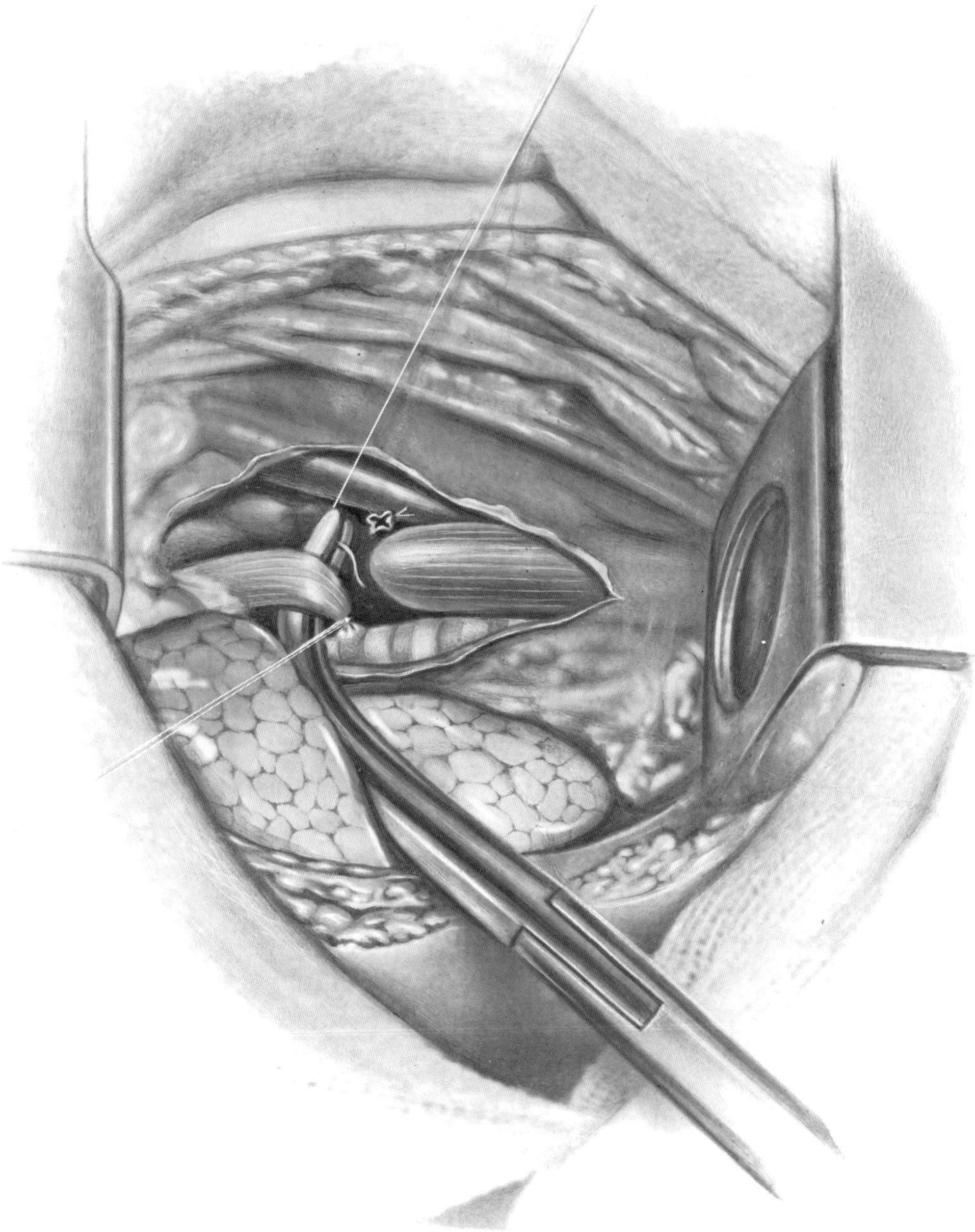

Fig. 690. Esophagus is tied with two ligatures close to tracheoesophageal fistula.

1 to 1.5 cm from their edges. The last stitch is made 1.5 to 2 mm from the margin of the incision of the muscular coat. When each pair of opposite threads is tied, the edges of the cut esophagus are brought together and inverted into its lumen. In this case a second row of sutures is not applied. In mild tension of the esophageal segments each is attached to the paravertebral fascia with two or three interrupted sutures. The line of the sutures is covered with the remnants of the mediastinal pleura. The pleural cavity is completely closed.

A tube is inserted into the stomach through the nose and left there for two or three days for feeding the child in the postoperative period, or Kader's gastrostoma is formed.

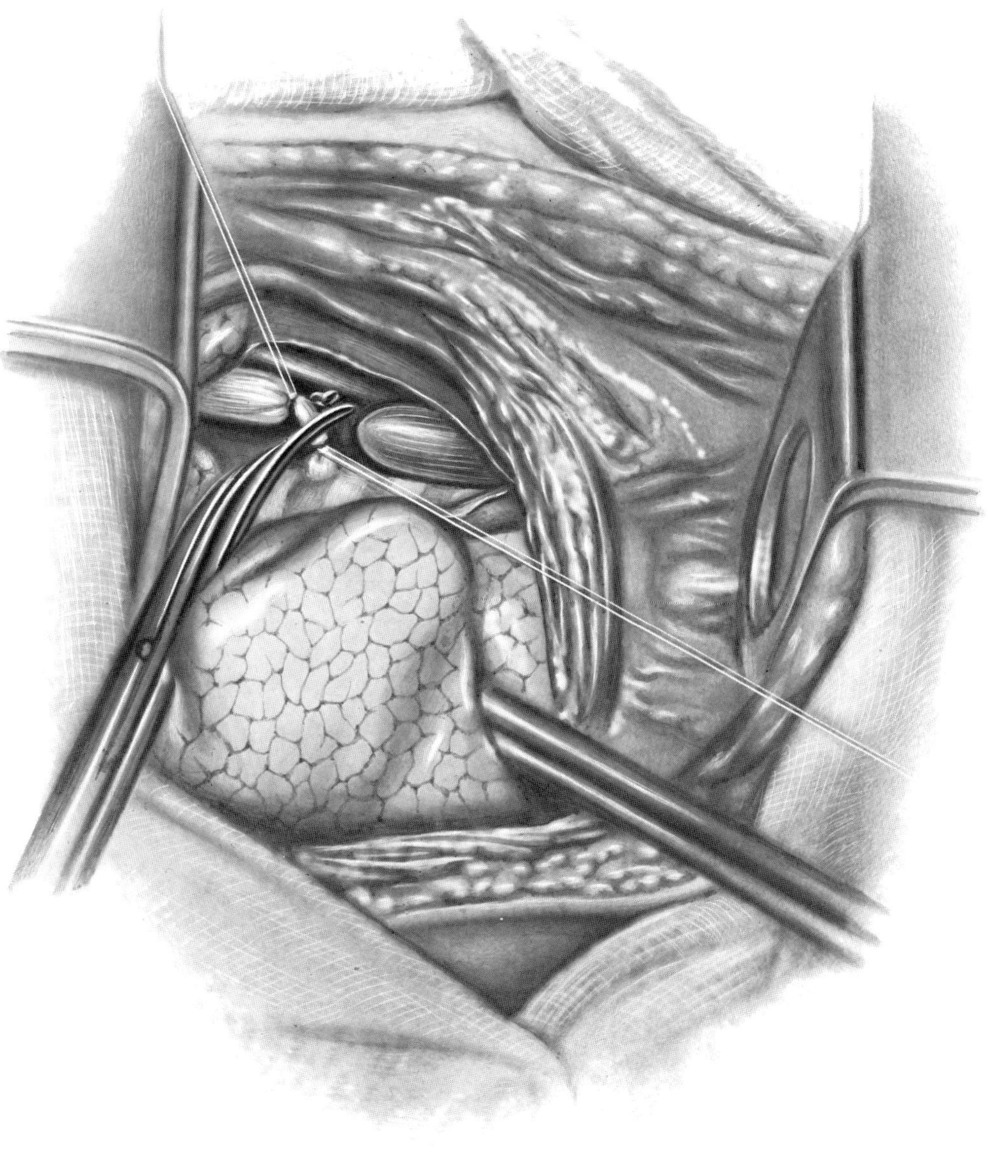

Fig. 691. Transection of esophagus between two ligatures.

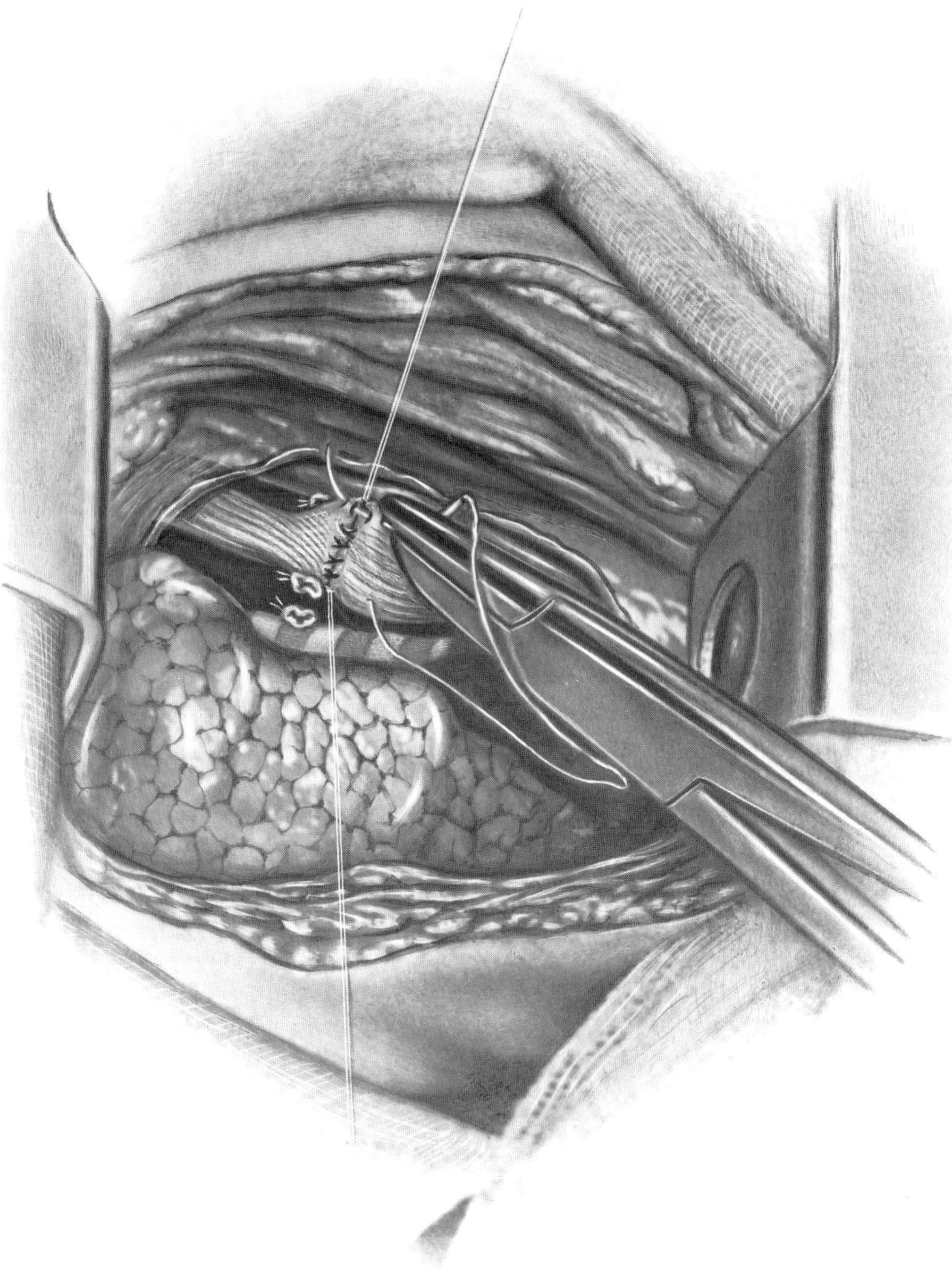

Fig. 692. Application of posterior row of sutures through muscular coats of esophagoesophageal anastomosis.

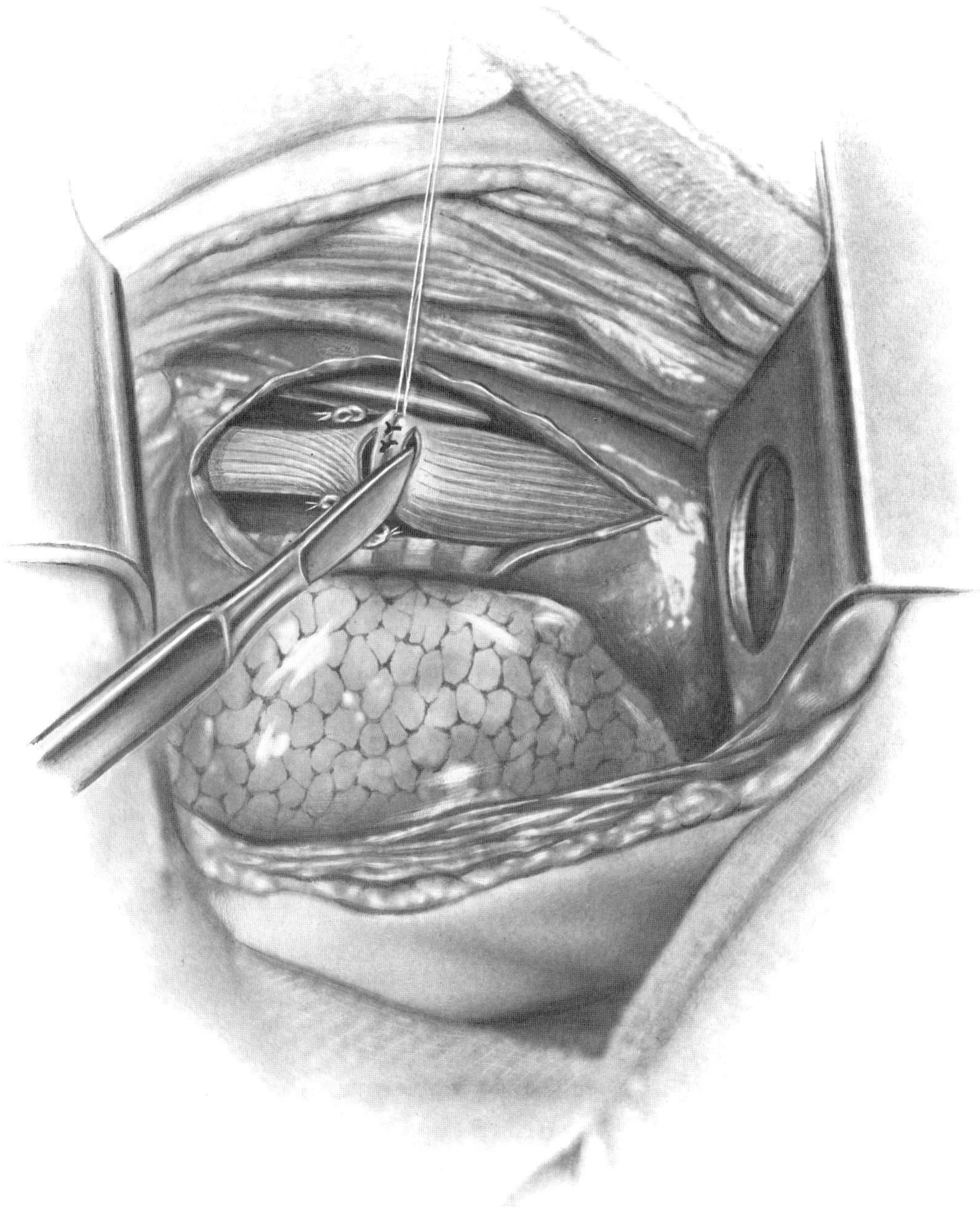

Fig. 693. Transverse incisions made in anterior walls of upper and lower esophageal stumps parallel to line of posterior musculoadventitial sutures.

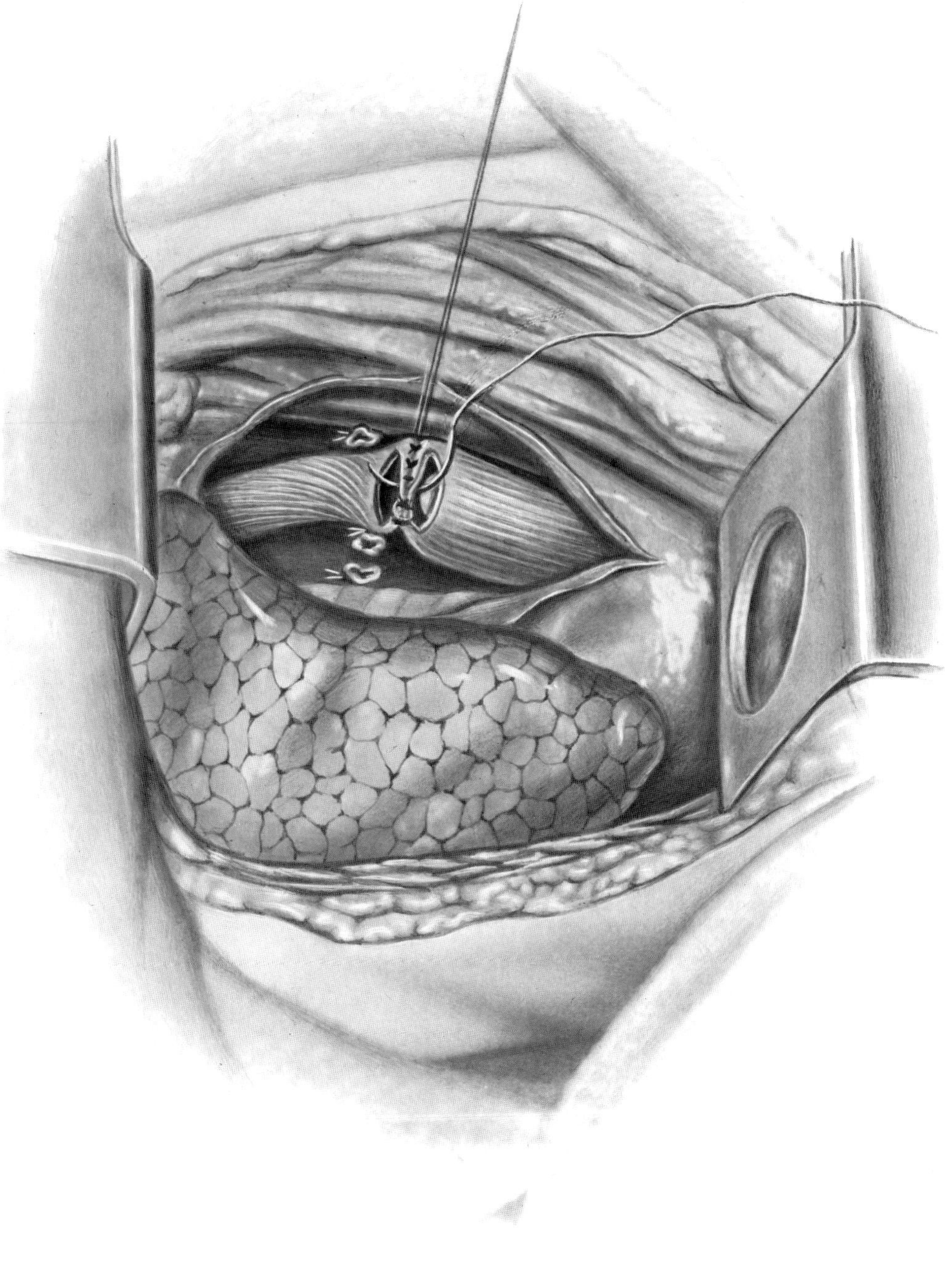

Fig. 694. Interrupted sutures are placed through all coats of posterior lip of esophageal anastomosis.

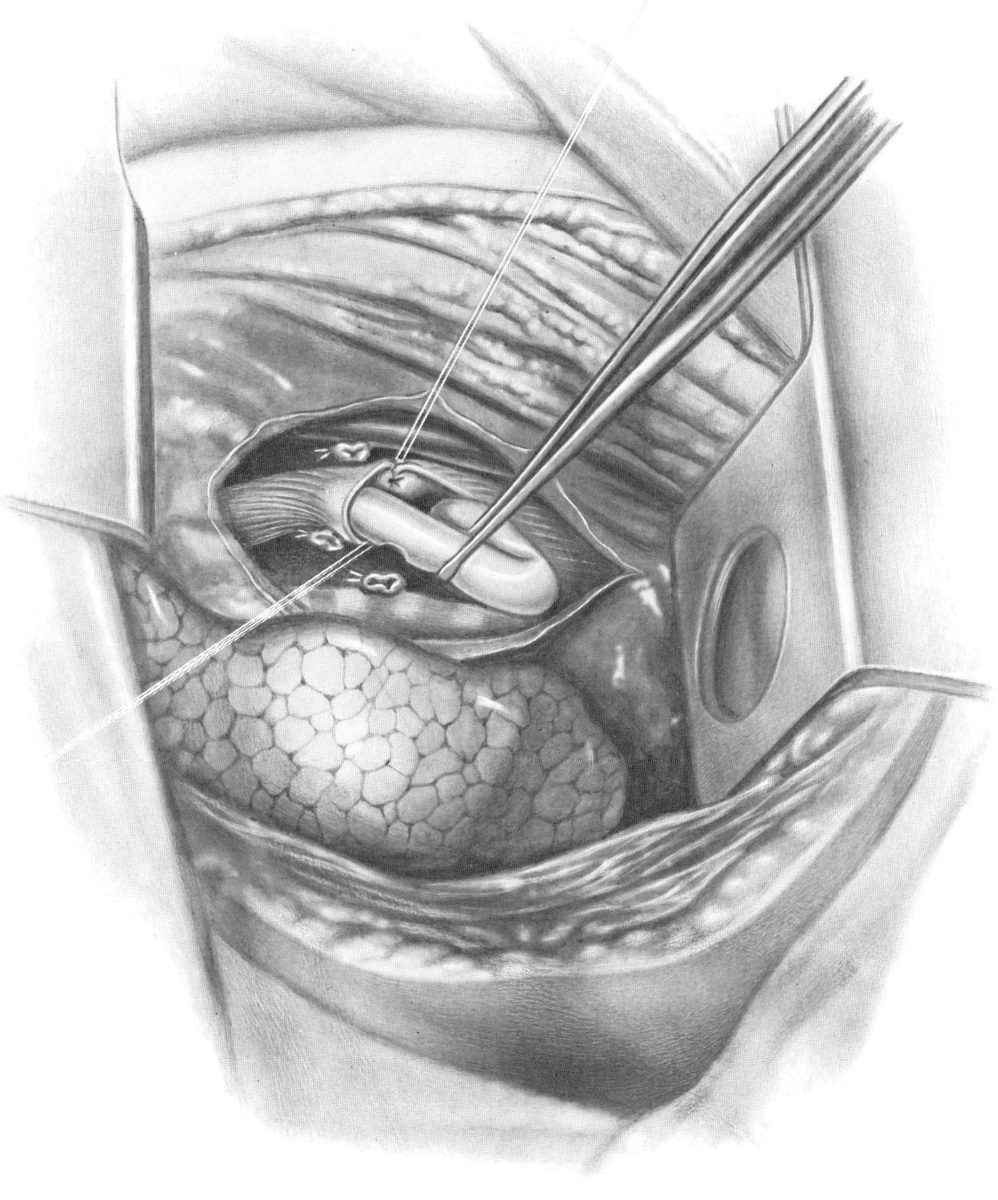

Fig. 695. Rubber tube is passed through mouth into upper and then into lower stumps of esophagus.

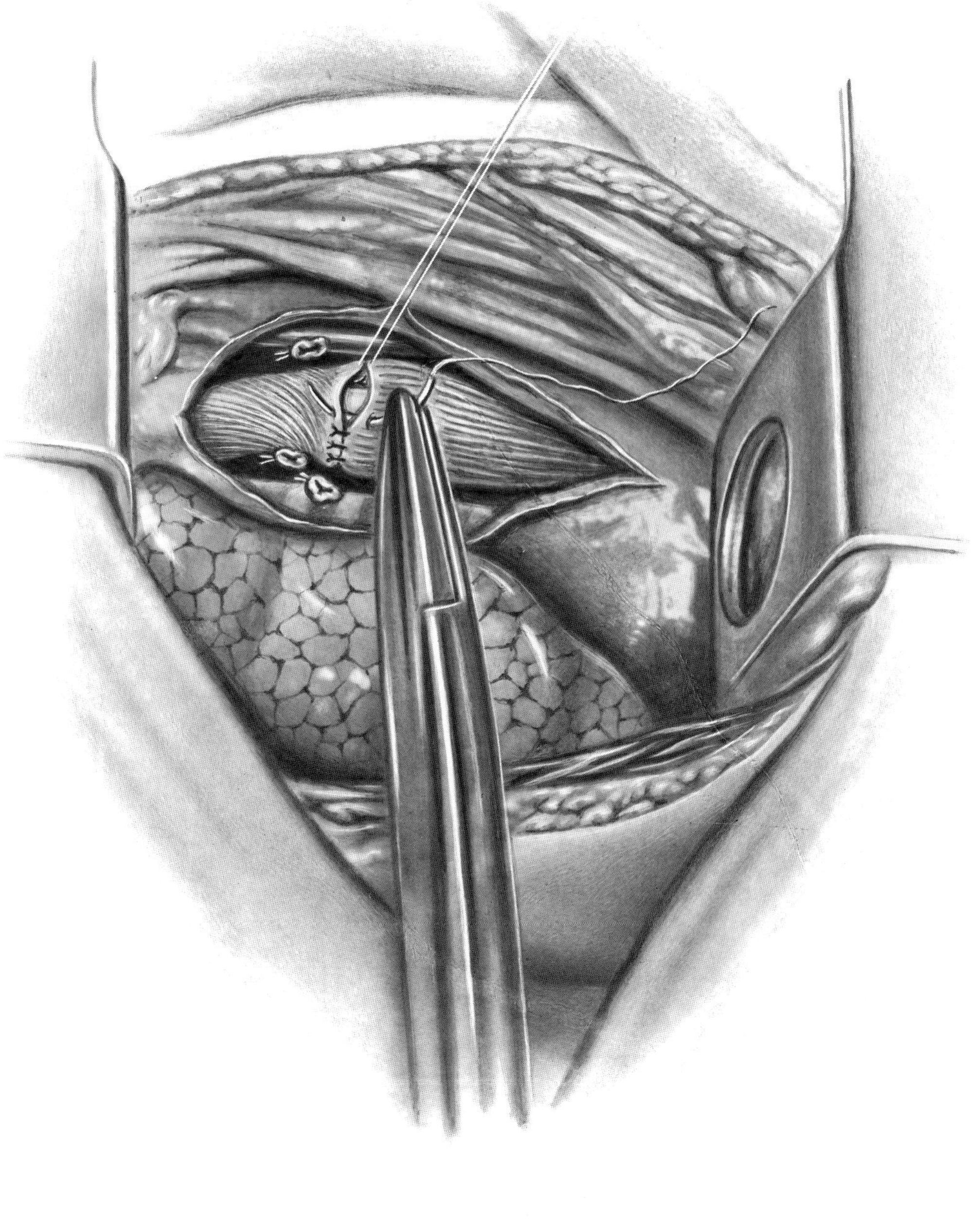

Fig. 696. Interrupted sutures are placed through all coats of anterior lip of anastomosis.

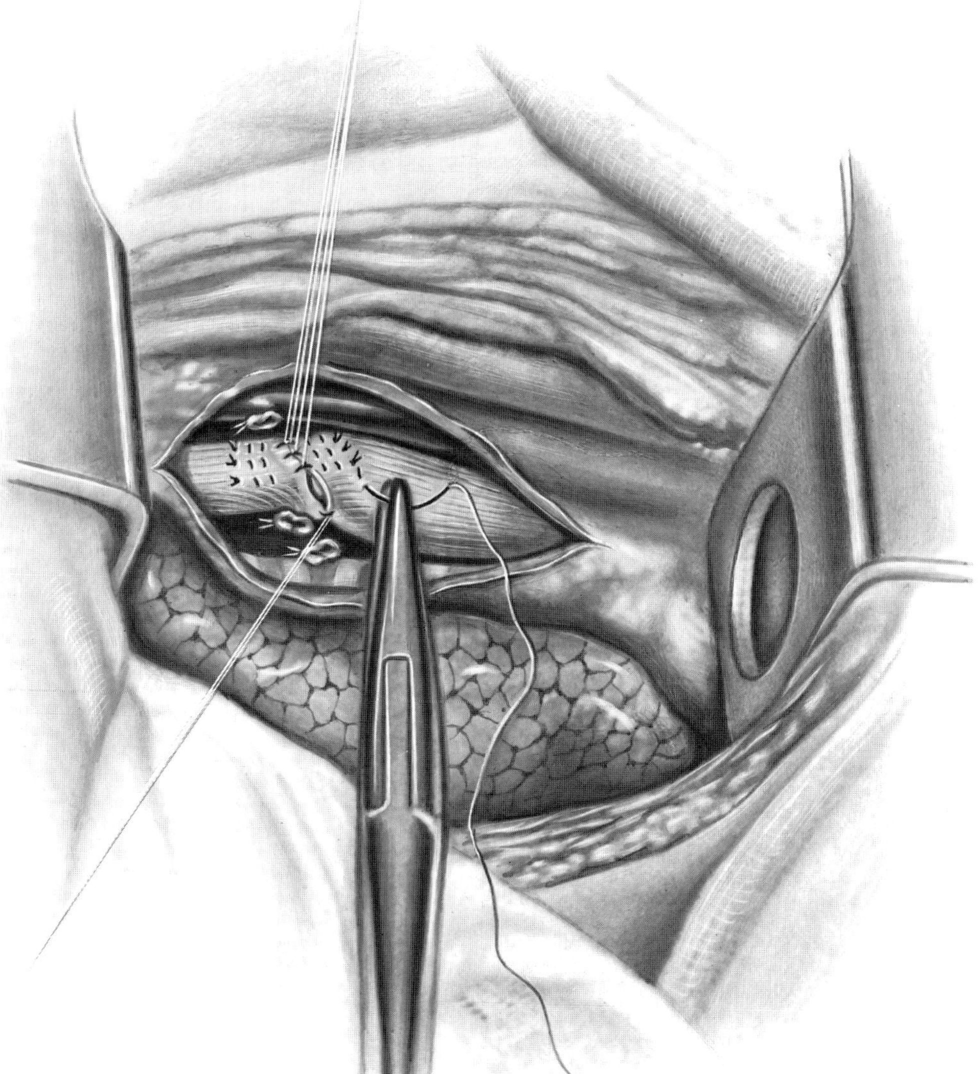

Fig. 697. Single-row three-stitch inverting suture formed with "threads stitched in opposite directions."

INTRAPLEURAL PLASTIC SURGERY WITH THE INTESTINE

PLASTIC SURGERY WITH ANTIPERISTALTIC LOOP OF LEFT HALF OF TRANSVERSE COLON

This type of esophagoplasty is conducted in cicatricial stricture of the lower and middle parts of the thoracic esophagus.

The operation begins with superior median laparotomy and mobilization of the graft. The omentum is cut away from the transverse colon in the avascular zone, the left phrenicocolic ligament is transected, and the left parts of the large intestine are mobilized. The vascular arcade between the left colic and sigmoid arteries and then the left colic artery and vein are ligated and transected (Fig. 698). The mesentery of the transverse colon is cut below Riolan's arch in the avascular area to the middle colic artery (Fig. 699).

The descending colon is transected between two

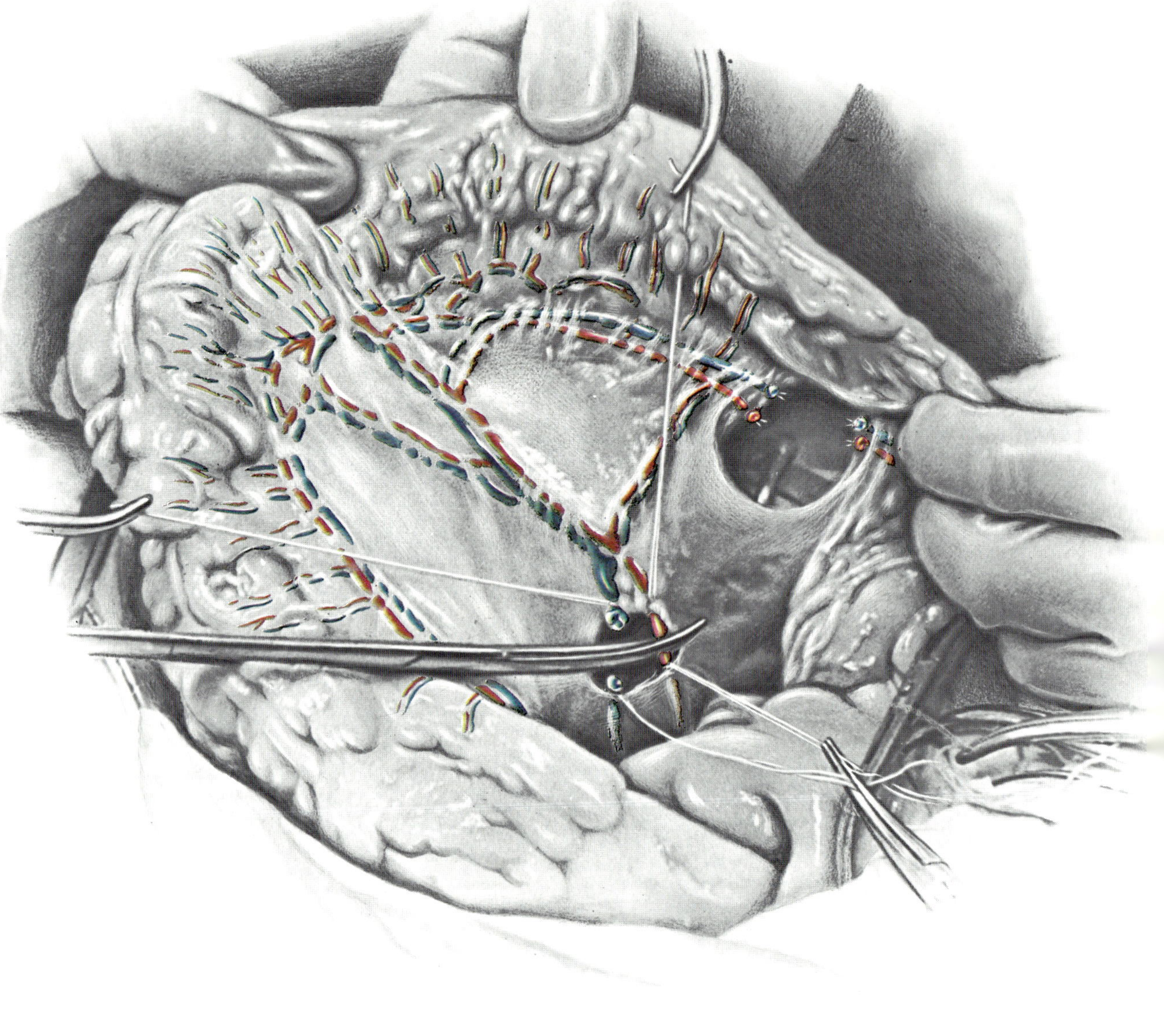

Fig. 698. Transection of left colic artery.

clamps at the level of the divided vascular arcade (Fig. 700). The central end of the colon is first closed with a continuous catgut suture (Fig. 701), which is then buried with interrupted silk sutures or in a purse-string suture. The intestine and the vascular arcade below are again transected slightly to the right of the main trunk of the middle colic artery. End-to-end anastomosis is formed between the remaining right part of the transverse colon and the sigmoid colon with three rows of interrupted silk sutures (Fig. 702).

With the anastomosis between the ends of the colon established, end-to-side anastomosis is created between the lower (right) stump of the graft formed and the anterior wall of the stomach (Fig. 703). It is formed by means of a double row catgut or silk suture closer to the smaller curvature of the subcardiac part of the stomach (Fig. 704).

The graft is placed under the left or the right half of the diaphragm (depending on the side thoracotomy is performed), and a gastrostoma is formed by Kader's

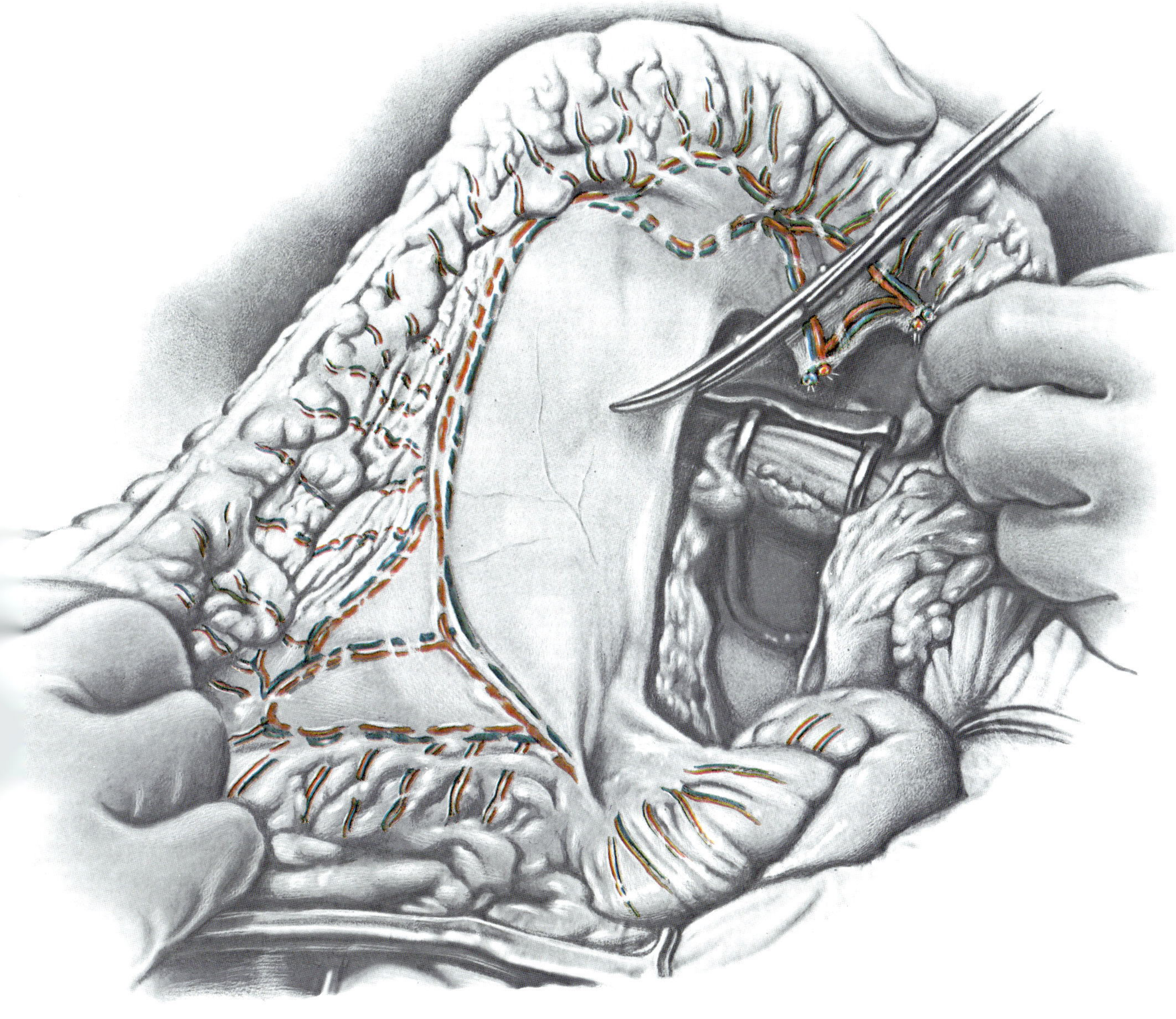

Fig. 699. Mesentery of colon is cut in avascular field below Riolan's arch.

(Figs. 705 and 706) or Witzel's technique. The gastrostomy tube is brought out through a separate stab wound in the abdominal wall slightly to the left of the median wound, which is then closed completely, layer by layer. Right or left thoracotomy is conducted corresponding to the level of the esophageal stricture. The mediastinal pleura is cut. The level of the stricture is determined by palpating the end of a tube inserted through the mouth and esophagus until it abuts the stricture. The anterolateral wall of the esophagus is mobilized at this level for 5 to 6 cm.

The diaphragm is cut in its ventromedial part. The free end of the colon graft is passed into the pleural cavity through the opening in the diaphragm and anasto-

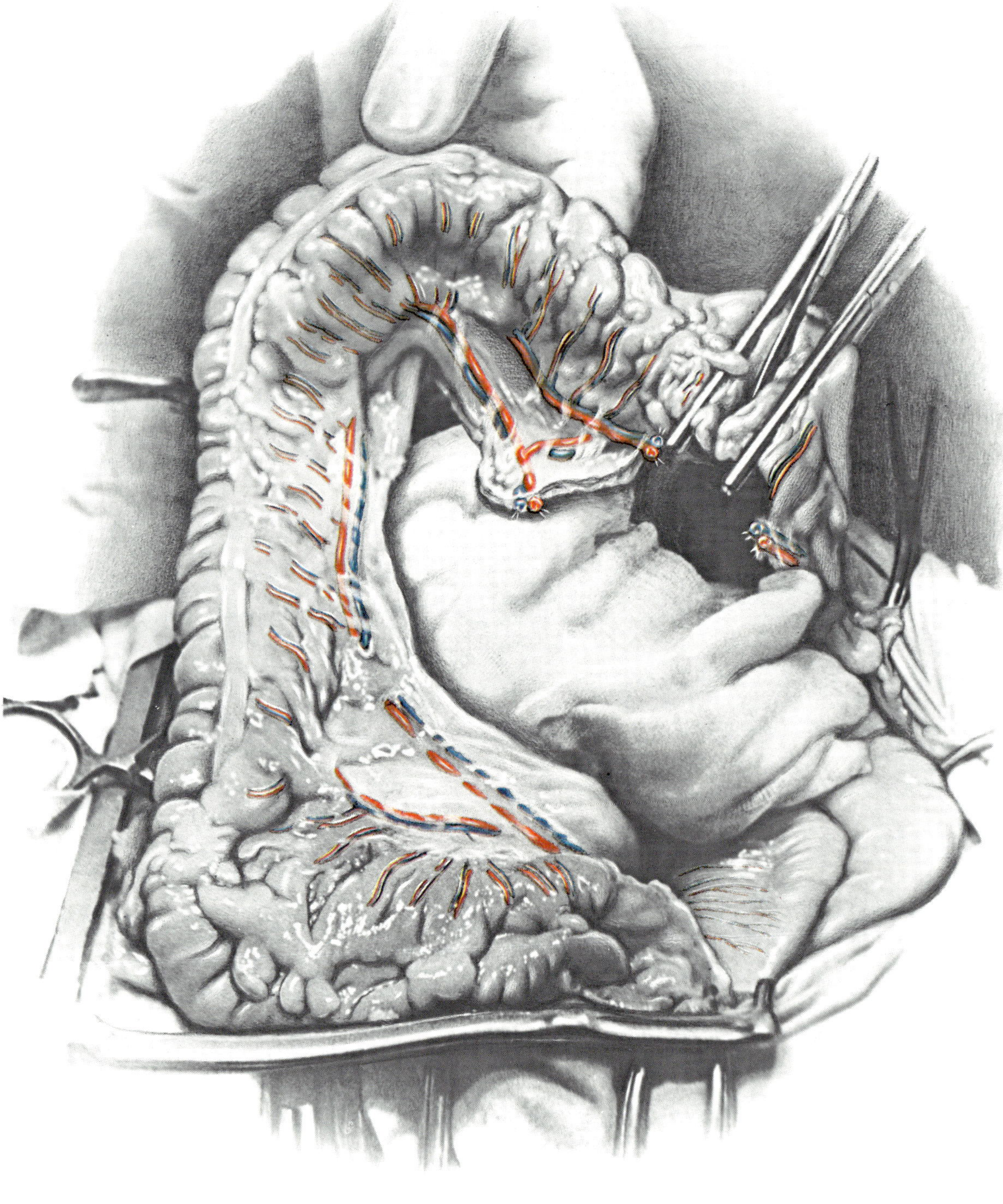

Fig. 700. Transection of descending colon.

mosed side to side (Figs. 707 and 708) or end to side (less frequently) with the esophagus by means of a double row of interrupted silk sutures. In rare cases the stricture is resected or the esophagus is transected above it, and end-to-end invagination anastomosis is established between the cranial end of the esophagus and the graft. The caudal end of the esophagus is closed with sutures. The opening in the diaphragm is closed before the graft. The edges of the diaphragmatic incision are attached to the graft with interrupted, widely spaced sutures.

The mediastinal pleura is not sutured to avoid the formation of purulent abscesses if the anastomosis fails. The wound in the thoracic wall is completely sutured layer by layer.

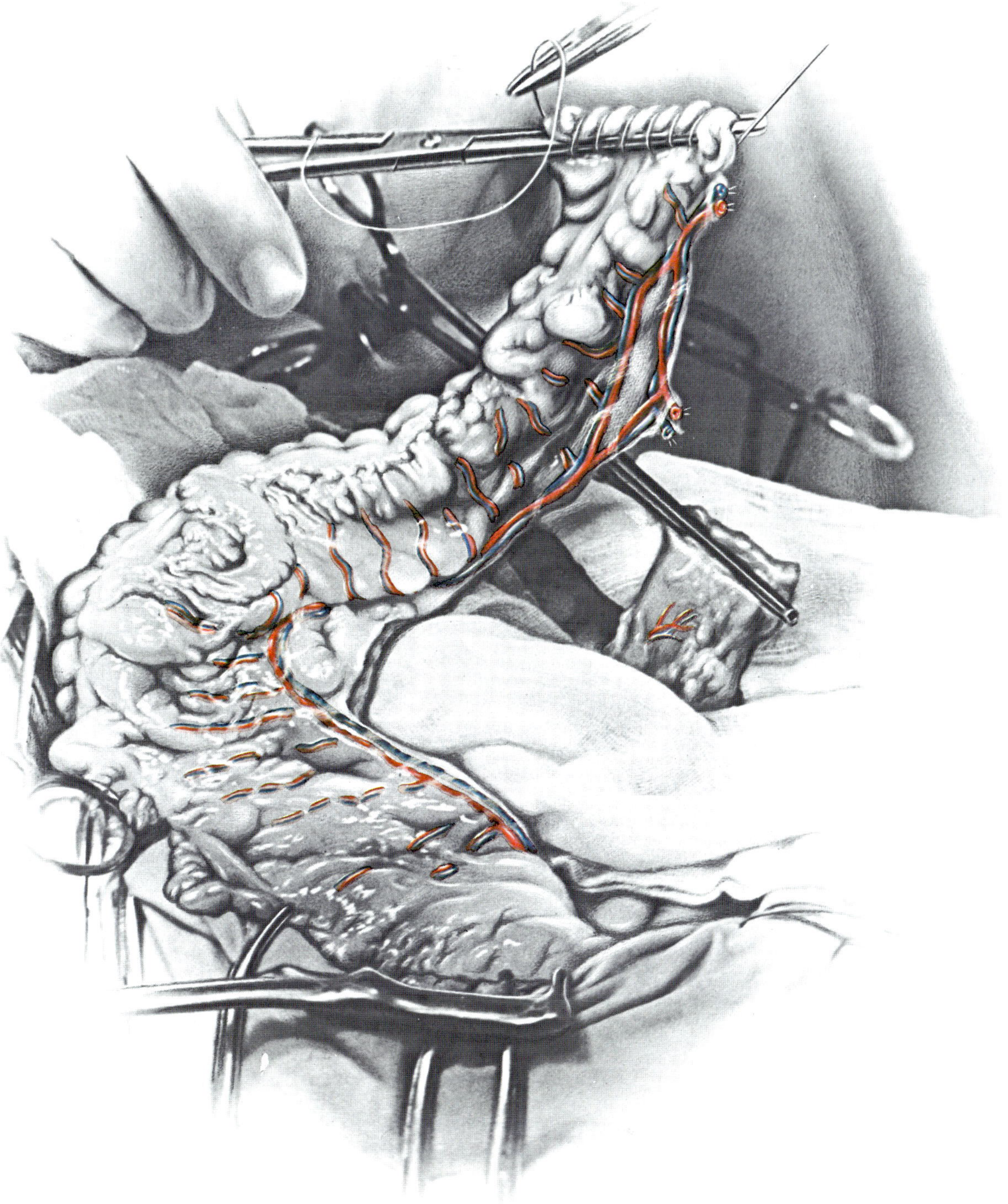

Fig. 701. Central end of graft is closed with continuous catgut suture.

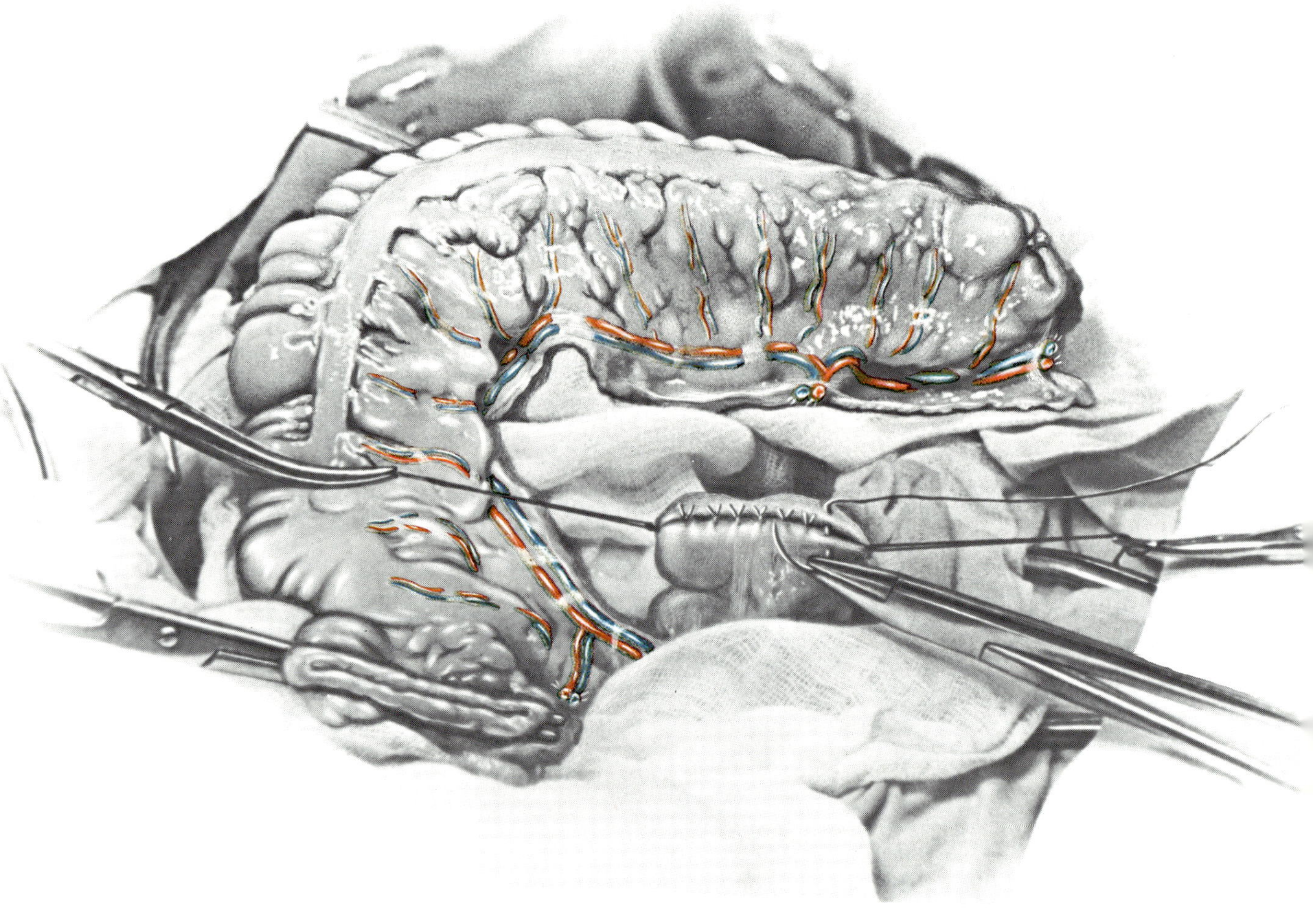

Fig. 702. Colon is transected a second time to right of middle colic artery. End-to-end anastomosis is formed between stomach and graft.

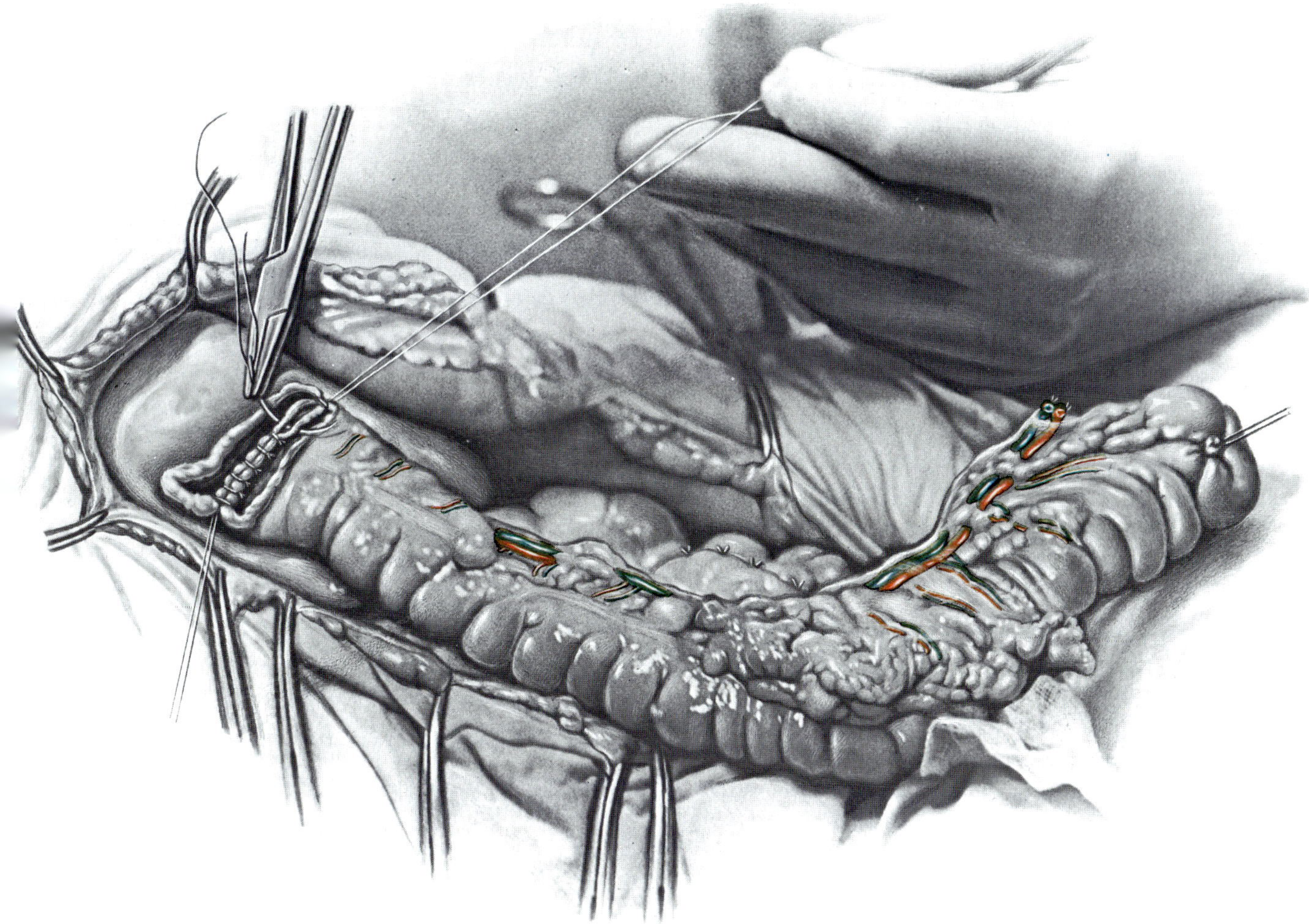

Fig. 703. Sutures are applied to posterior lip of anastomosis between stomach and graft.

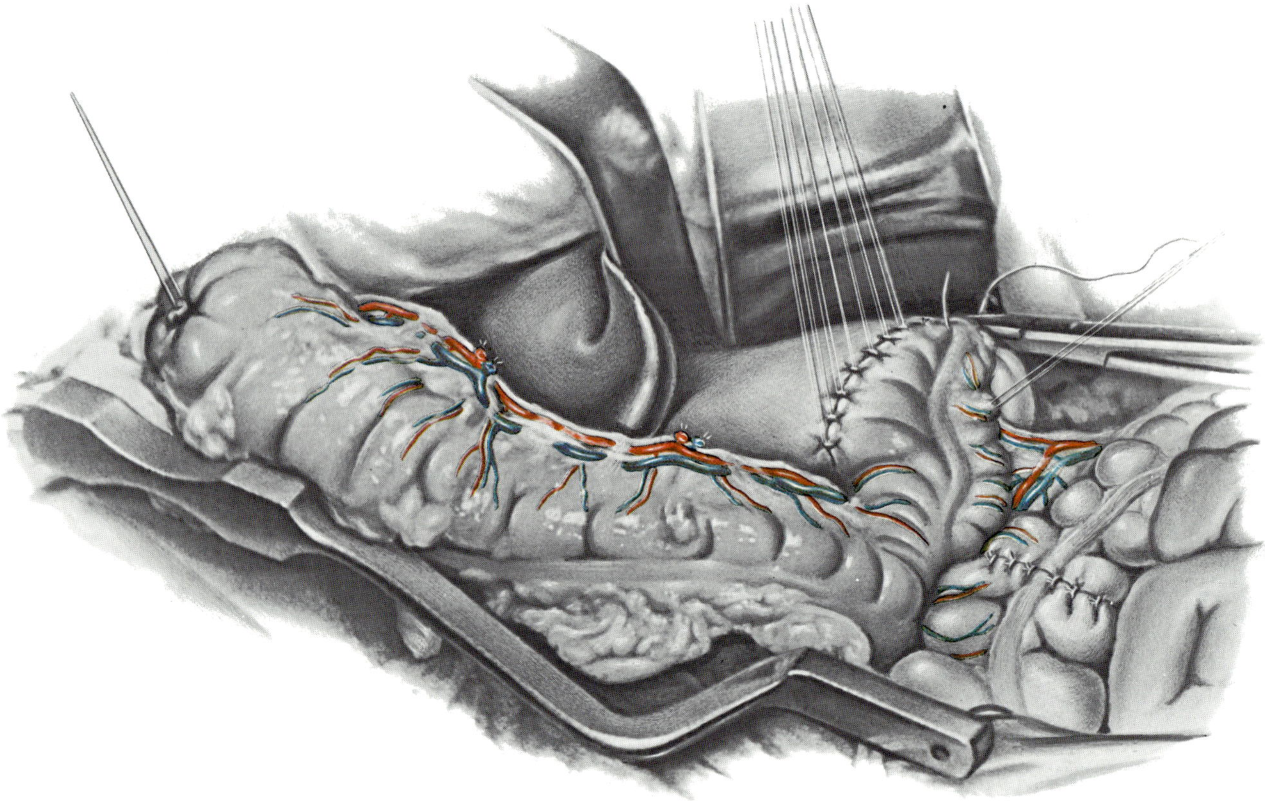

Fig. 704. Anastomosis between stomach and graft is completed with second row of sutures. Anastomosed transverse colon and sigmoid colon are shown on right.

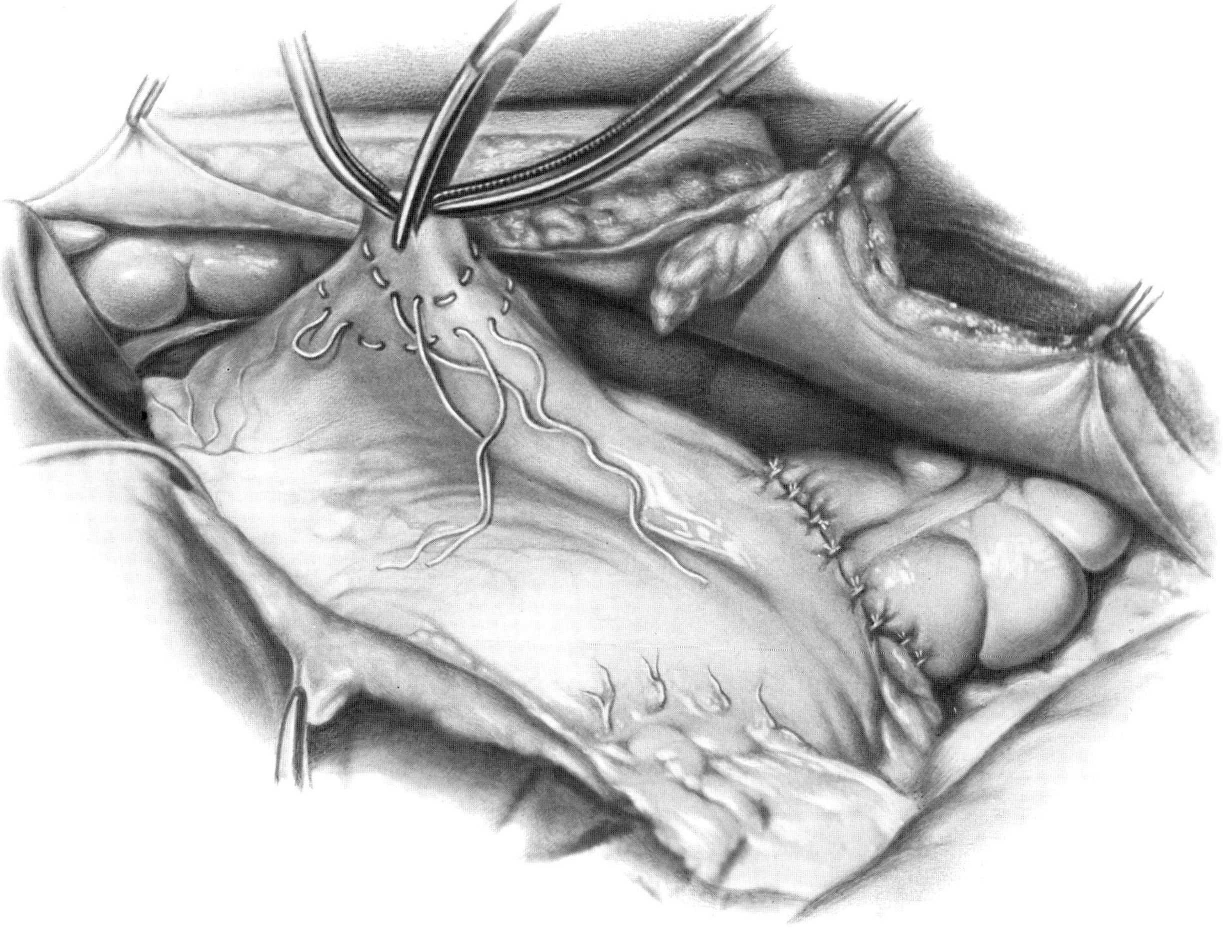

Fig. 705. Stage in formation of Kader's gastrostoma. Graft is placed into subdiaphragmatic space of abdominal cavity. Stomach is opened.

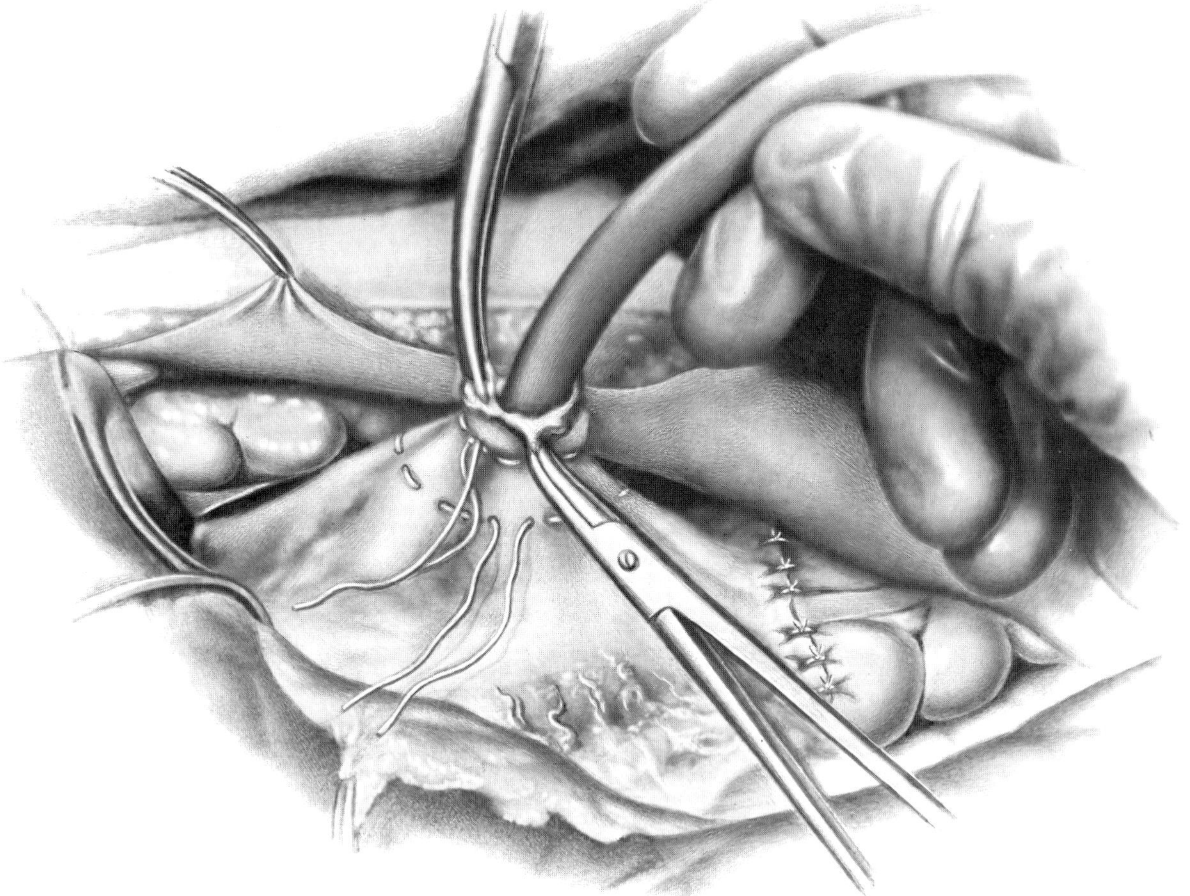

Fig. 706. Rubber tube is inserted into stomach.

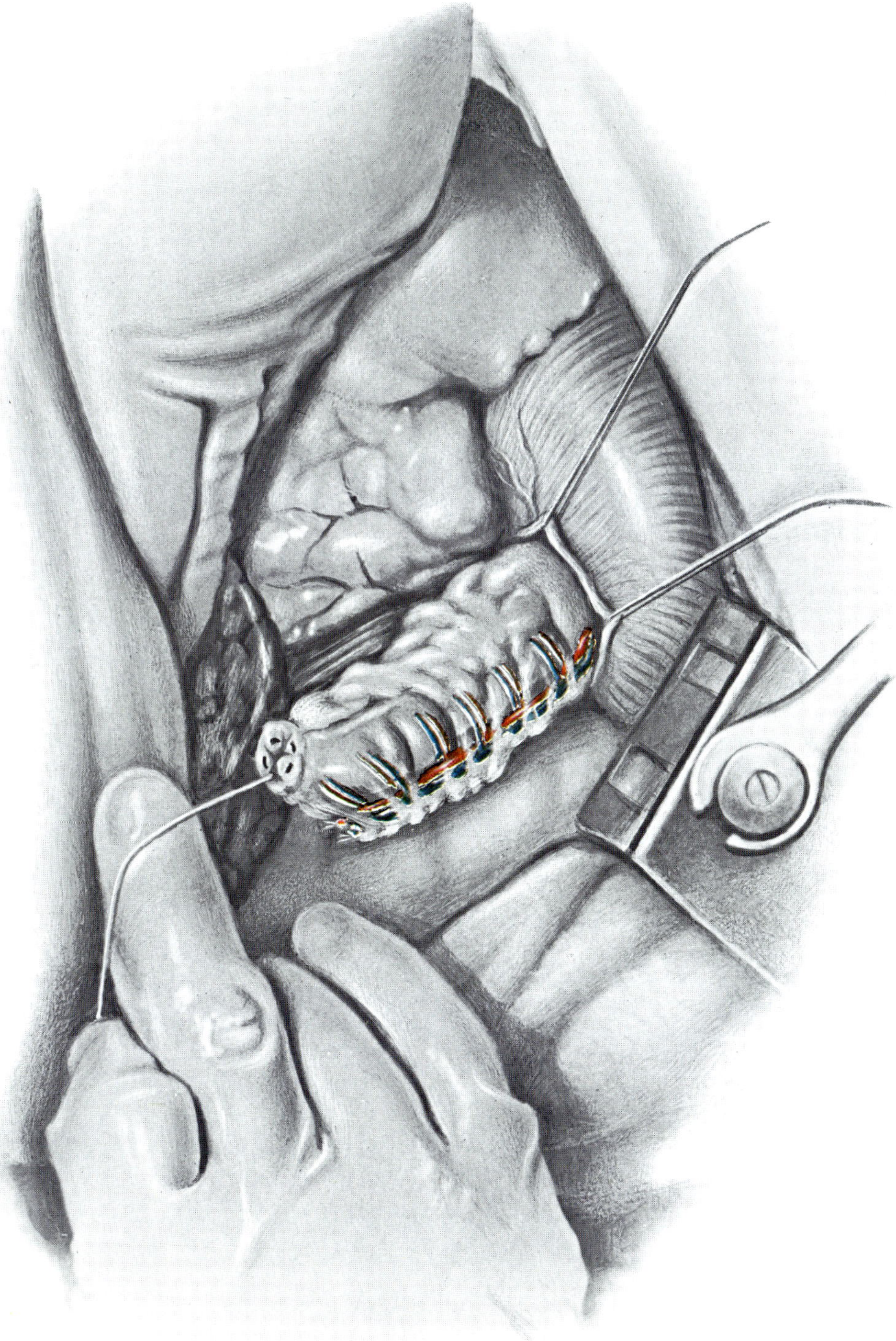

Fig. 707. Intestinal graft is transposed into right pleural cavity through cut in diaphragm.

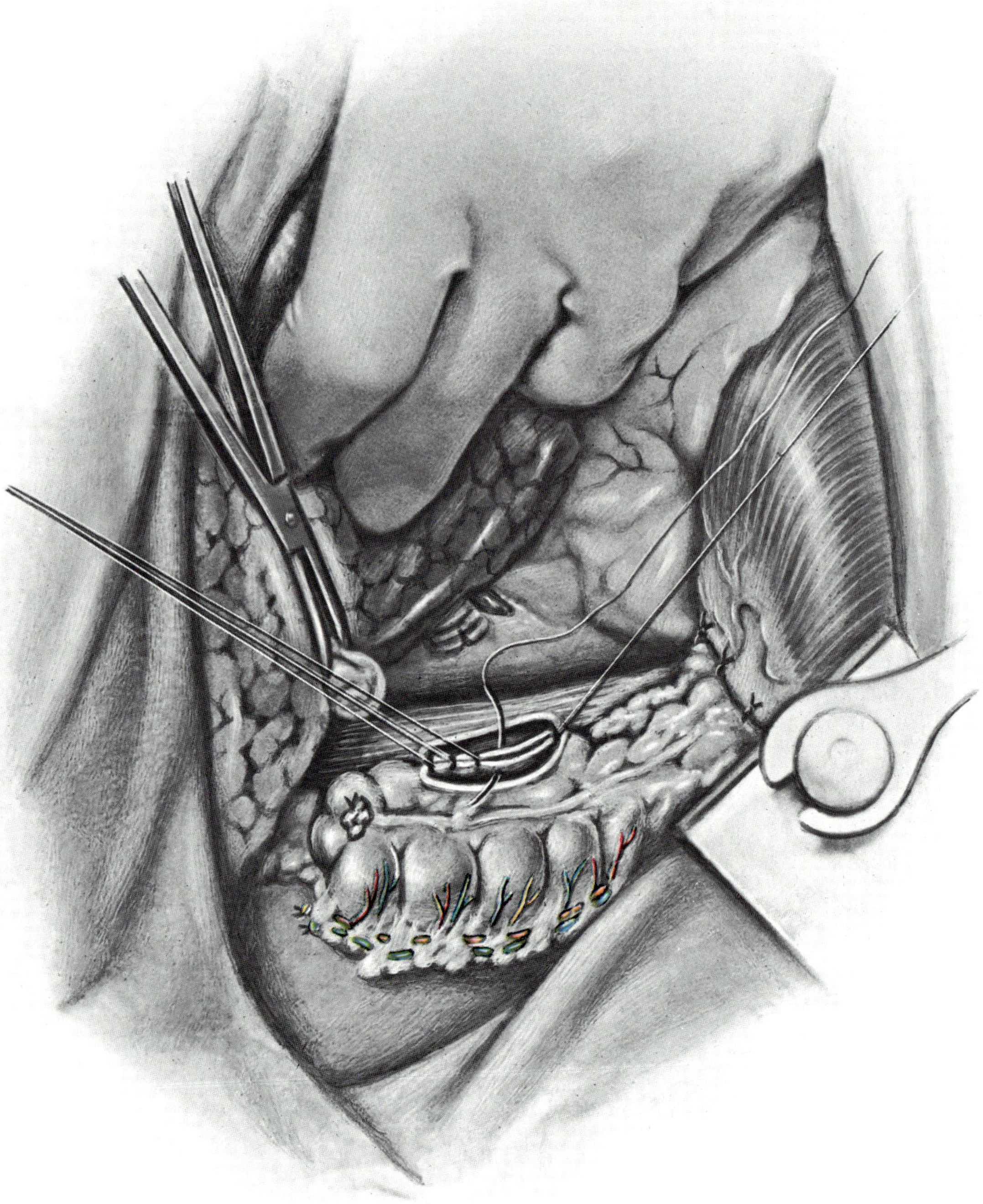

Fig. 708. Application of sutures to posterior lip of esophagoentericanastomosis.

PLASTIC SURGERY OF CERVICAL ESOPHAGUS WITH INTESTINAL GRAFTS

PLASTIC SURGERY WITH SHORT GRAFT OF SMALL INTESTINE ON LONG VASCULAR PEDICLE

The operation begins with superior median laparotomy. The initial part of the small intestine is brought out into the wound, and the mesenteric vessels are examined. If the anatomical situation is favorable, mobilization of the graft is begun.

The first traction ligature is stitched through the mesentery at the level of the cranial end of the future intestinal graft 12 to 15 cm from Treitz's ligament, or a thin rubber tube is brought under the intestine through a stab wound of the mesentery. A second traction ligature is also applied 10 to 15 cm caudal to the first. Both ligatures limit the loop of the small intestine to the

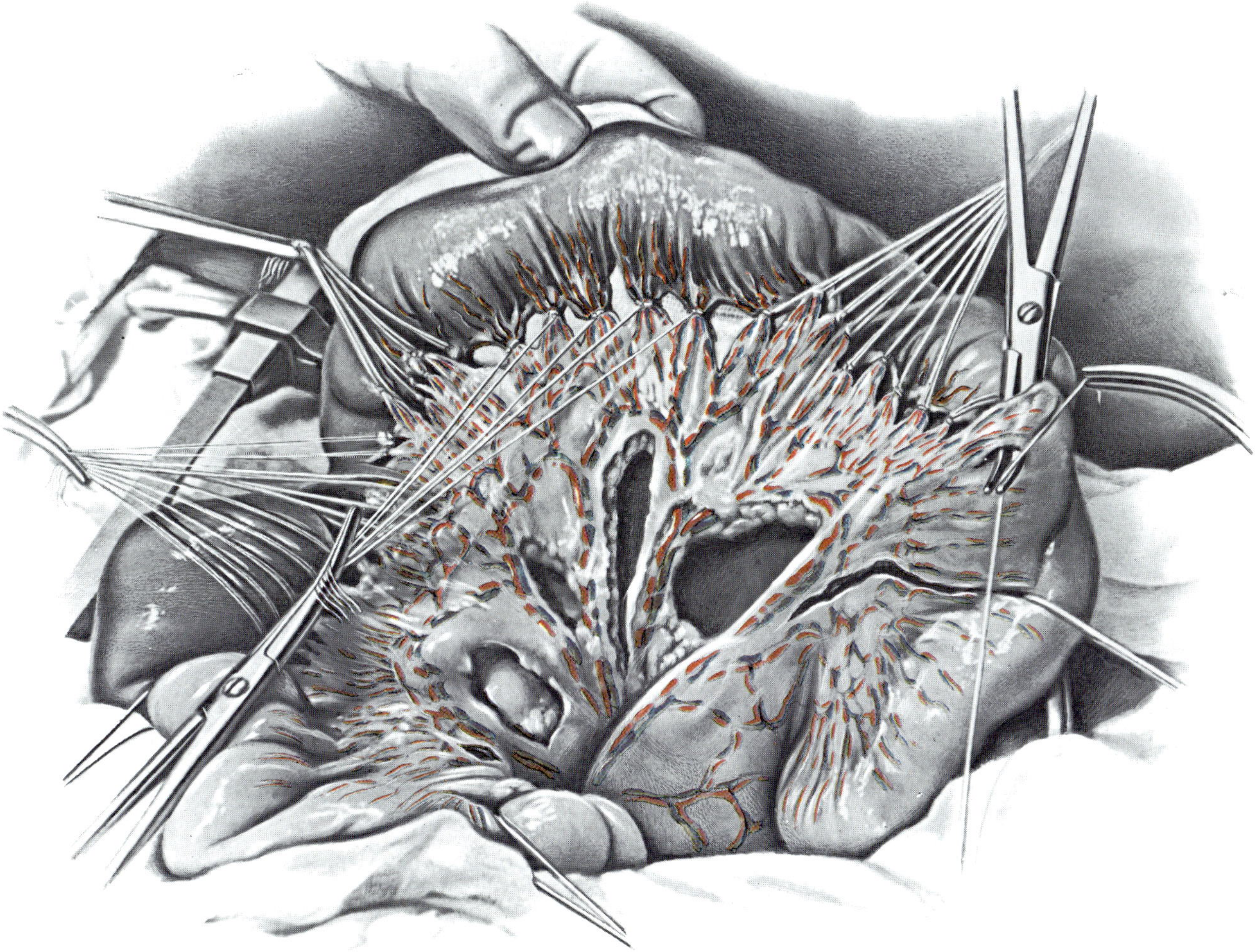

Fig. 709. Radial vessels are prepared for ligation and transection. Ligation of straight vessels below part of small intestine to be resected.

length necessary for replacing the esophageal segment.

A third traction ligature is applied in a similar manner 25 to 30 cm caudal to the second. This third ligature is 2 to 3 cm caudal to the radial artery, which is to be left in the base of the vascular pedicle of the future graft. Beginning with the second limiting traction ligature, all straight vessels are ligated immediately under the intestine in the caudal direction to the level of the third traction ligature (Fig. 709). At the place where the last ligature is applied, the intestine is cut transversely between two crushing clamps (Fig. 710).

The loop of the small intestine deprived of its blood supply because of the ligation of the vessels is cut away from the mesentery (Fig. 711). The small intestine is transected once again at the level of the second traction ligature.

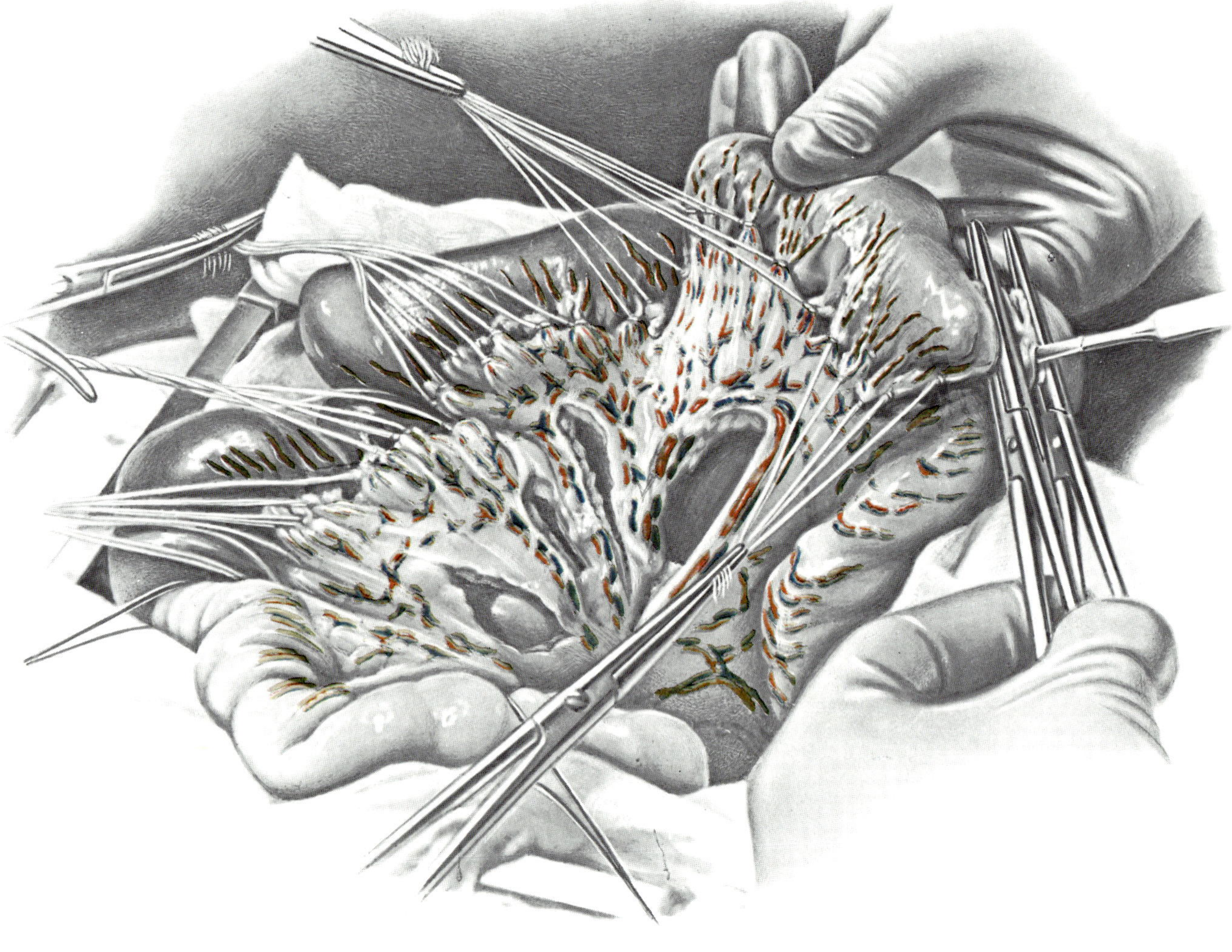

Fig. 710. Small intestine is transected at level of base of vascular pedicle of future graft.

Three, rarely four, radial mesentery vessels are consecutively tied and transected beginning at the level of the first traction ligature. The radial artery and vein located at the level of the third traction ligature are left intact to supply the graft with blood (Fig. 712).

The small intestine is again transected between two crushing clamps at the level of the first traction ligature limiting the cranial end of the graft (Fig. 713). The ligatures are cut away from the straight vessels, and the stumps of the graft are closed with purse-string sutures to avoid contamination of the subcutaneous or retrosternal tunnel through which the graft will be transposed to the neck. The continuity of the small intestine is restored by end-to-end anastomosis of its cranial and caudal stumps left after the resection of the graft (Figs. 714 and 715). To avoid tightening the vessels of the

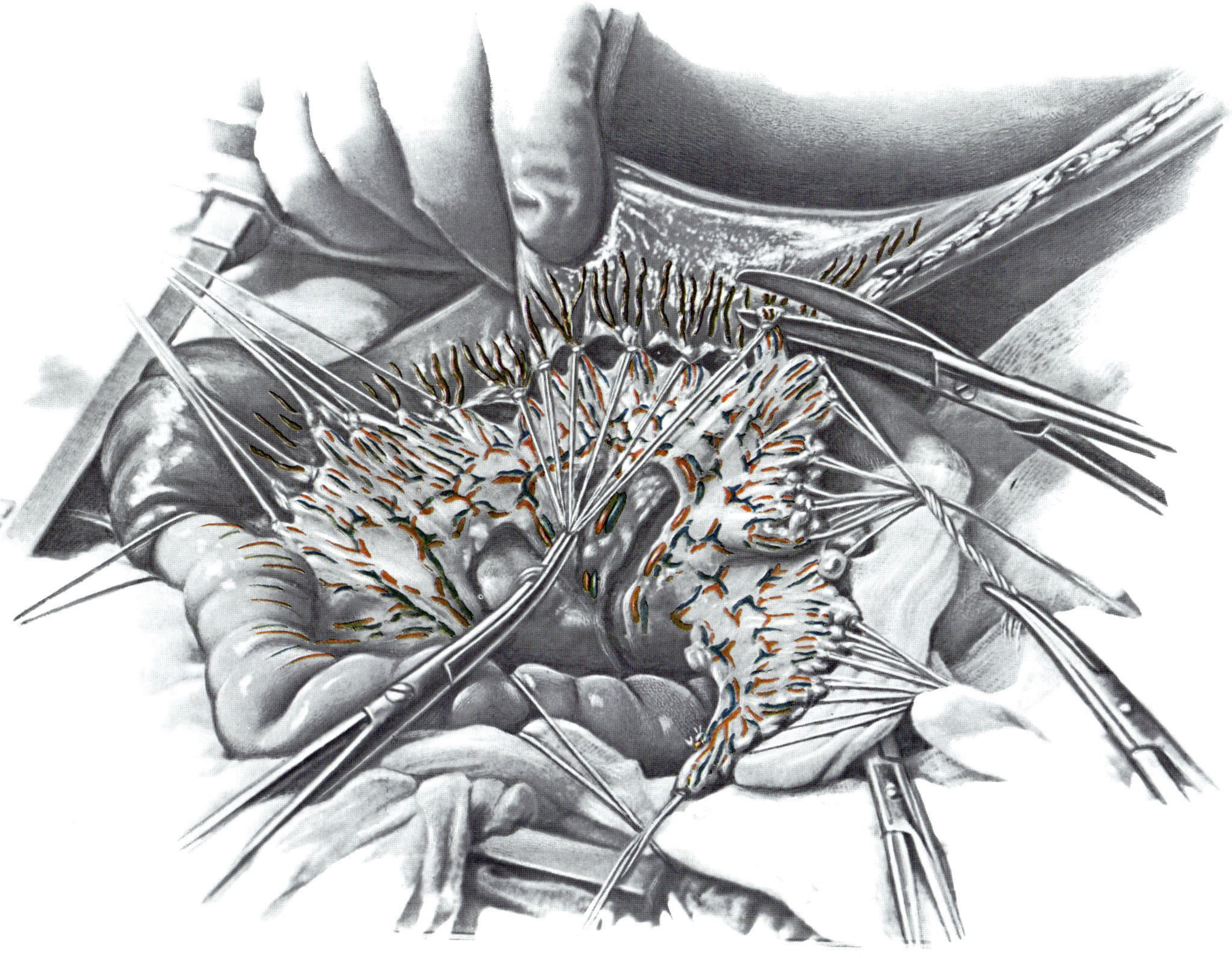

Fig. 711. Segment of small intestine deprived of blood supply is cut away from mesentery above vascular arcades.

graft, the root of the mesentery of the small intestine is stitched to the upper corner of the wound in the abdominal wall (Fig. 716).

A tunnel is formed under the skin or in the anterior mediastinum through which the graft is transposed to the neck. With the cervical esophagus freed from the surrounding tissues, end-to-side anastomosis is first created between the lower end of the graft and the esophagus (below the esophageal stricture) (Figs. 717 and 718), and then the cranial end of the graft is anastomosed with the side of the pharynx above the stricture (Fig. 719). The wounds of the abdominal cavity and neck are sutured layer by layer. Until the enteroesophageal anastomosis heals, the patient is fed through the gastrostoma created prior to or at the same time as esophagoplasty. In some cases with severe chemical burns of the pharynx, not only swallowing but normal respiration is impaired

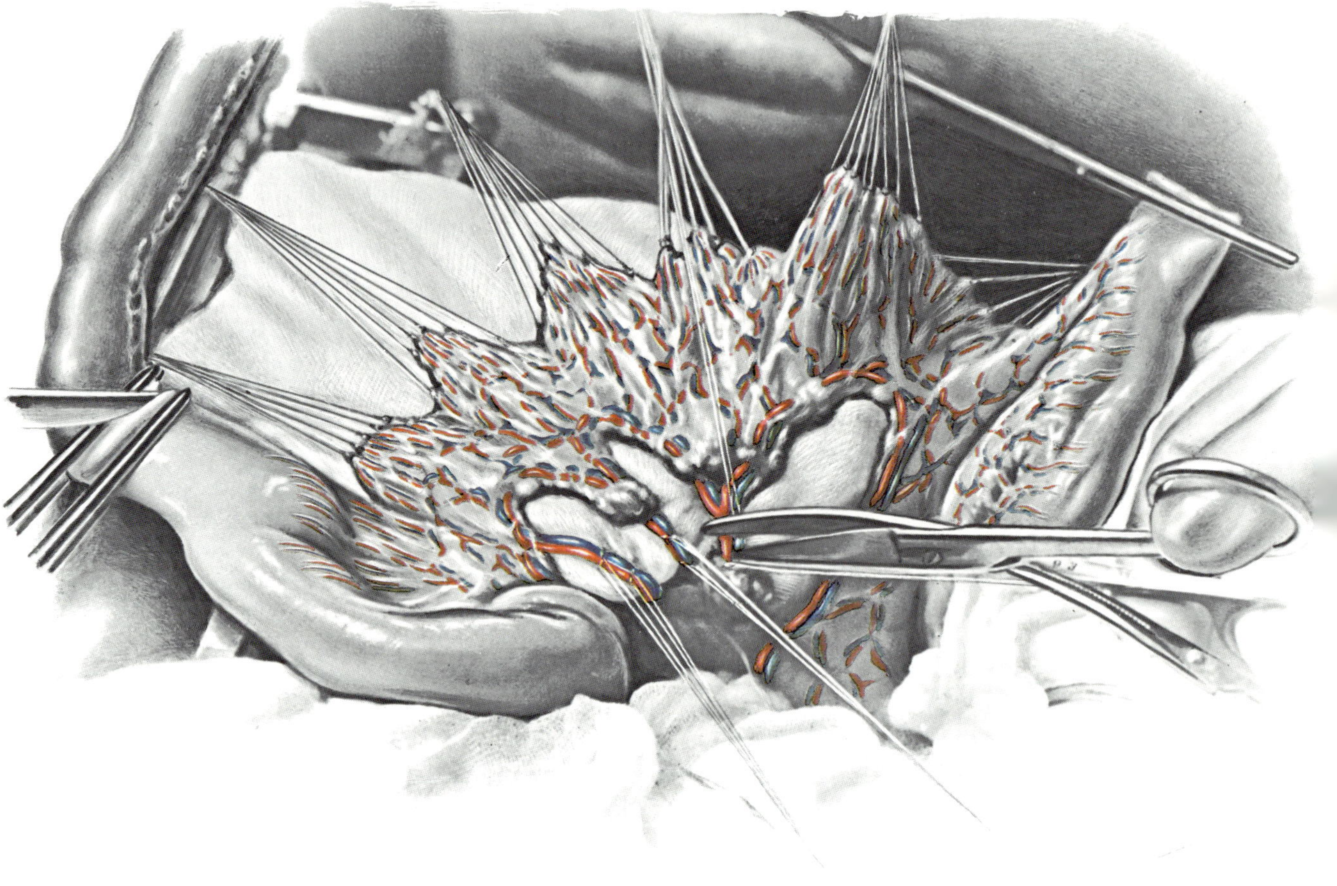

Fig. 712. Intestinal segment deprived of blood supply us cut away from graft. Three pairs of radial vessels below vascular pedicle of graft are transected between two ligatures.

due to scars at the entrance into the larynx and adhesions of the lateral walls and apex of the epiglottis with the posterior pharyngeal wall. The following operation is commonly performed in such cases.

Anterior suprahyoid pharyngotomy is performed (Fig. 720) without or (less frequently) with resection of the left horn of the hyoid bone. The epiglottis embedded in the cicatricial adhesions is stitched through with one, two, or three ligatures in its free portion and gradually separated from the cicatrices with scissors, keeping to its margin all the time. Single catgut sutures are applied to the wound along the margin of its mucous coat, and only after this the formation of anastomosis of the intestinal graft with the posterolateral wall of the pharynx may be begun. The operation is completed by closing the wound on the neck, leaving one or two drains in it for 24 hours.

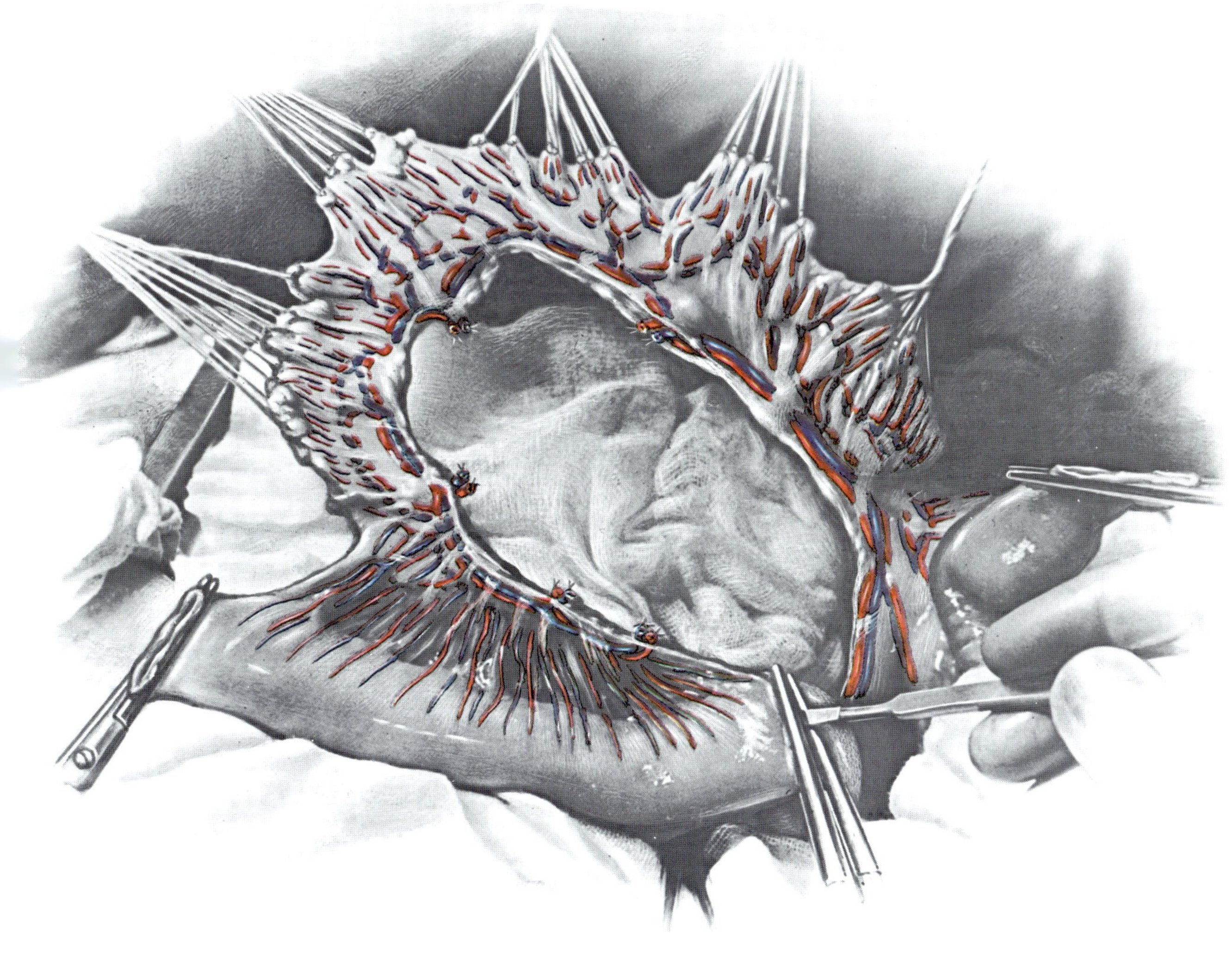

Fig. 713. Upper portion of graft is resected from afferent loop of small intestine.

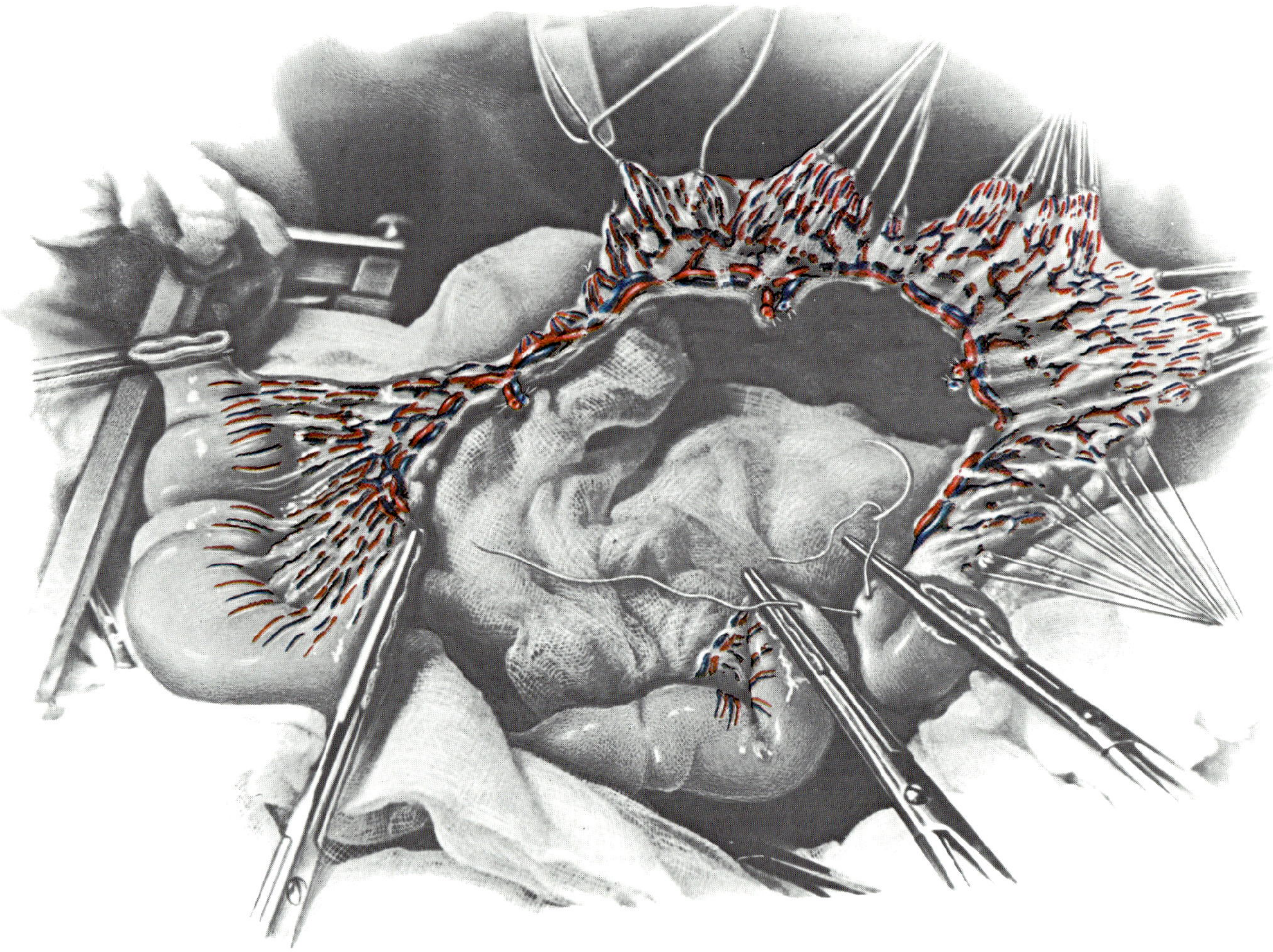

Fig. 714. Ligatures are cut away from straight vessels. Stumps of afferent and efferent portions of small intestine are brought together. First suture is applied to enteroentericanastomosis.

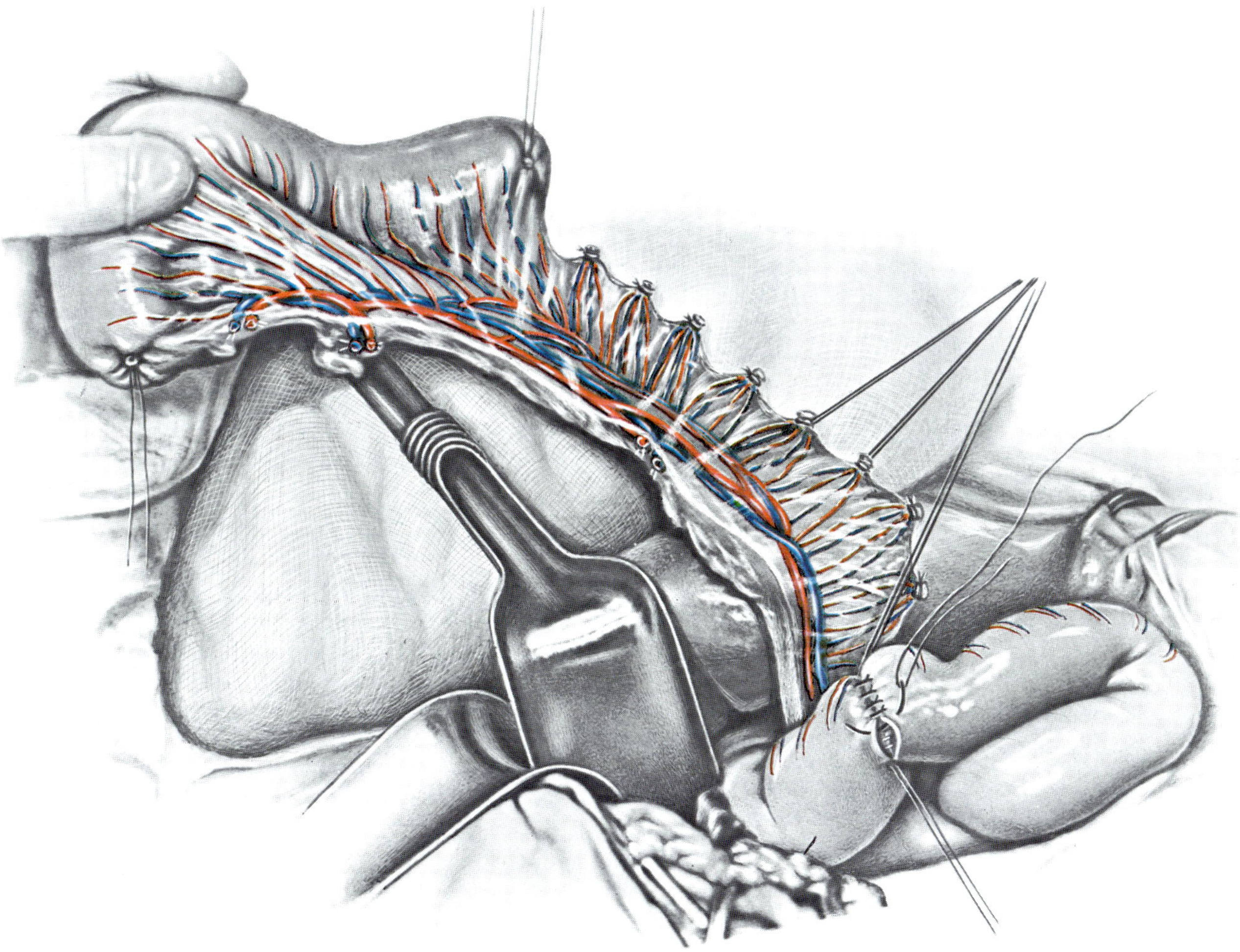

Fig. 715. Continuity of small intestine is restored by end-to-end anastomosis. Stumps of graft are closed with purse-string suture.

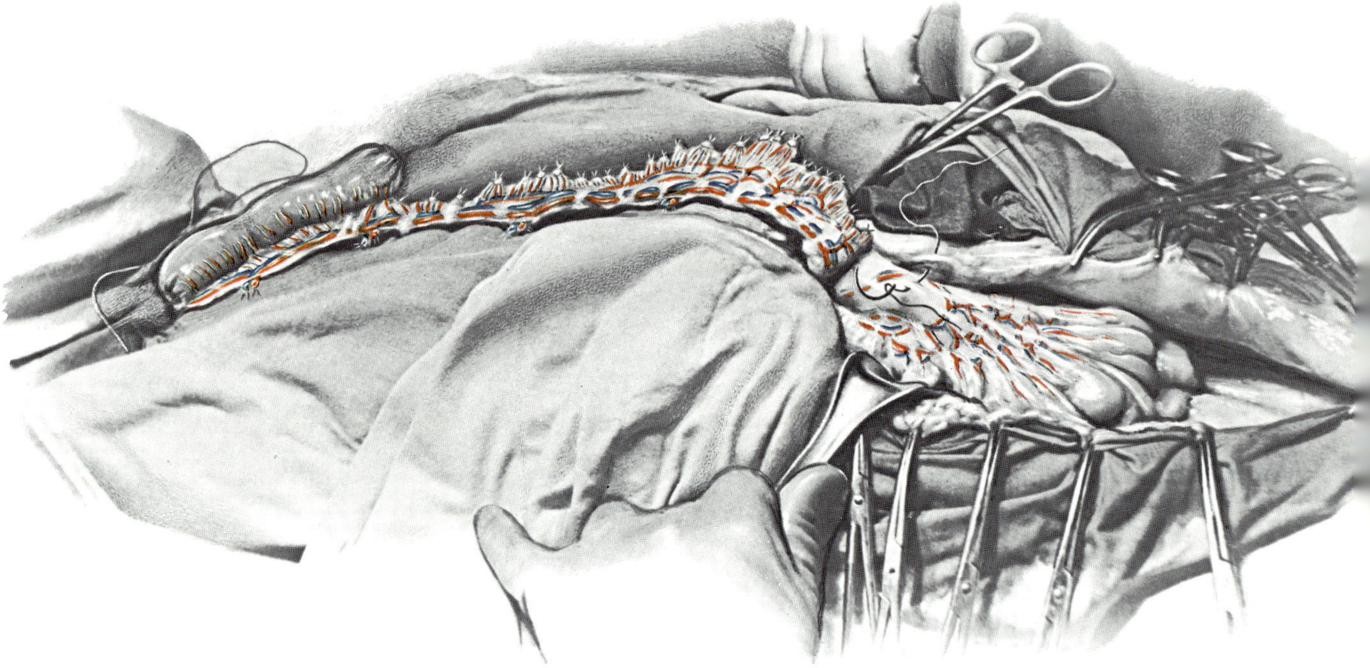

Fig. 716. Graft is transposed to neck with certain tightening of vascular pedicle. To correct this, root of mesentery is mobilized by Petrov-Khundadze method and attached with interrupted sutures to aponeurosis in upper corner of abdominal wound.

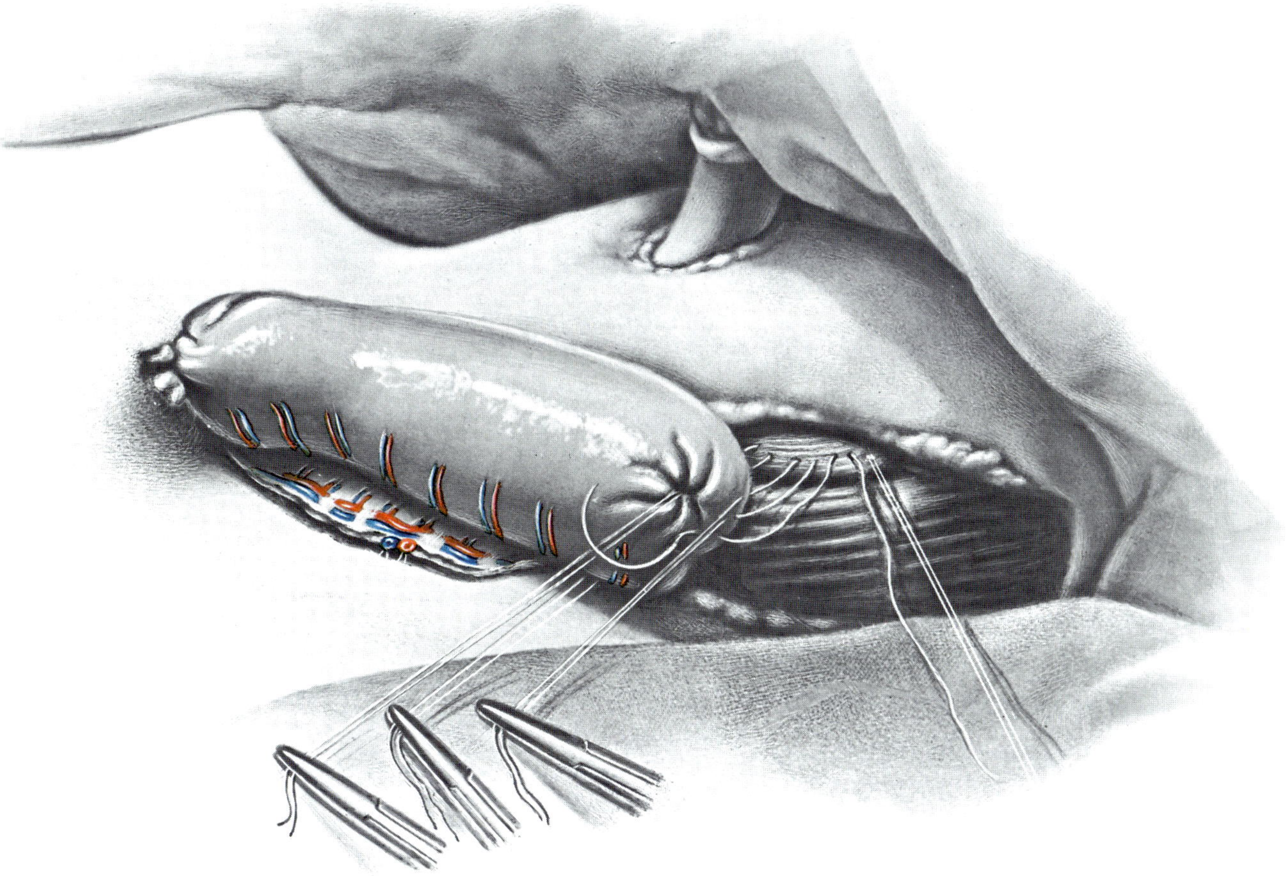

Fig. 717. Graft is transposed to neck through subcutaneous tunnel. Application of outer sutures to posterior lip of anastomosis between peripheral end of graft and esophagus below stricture.

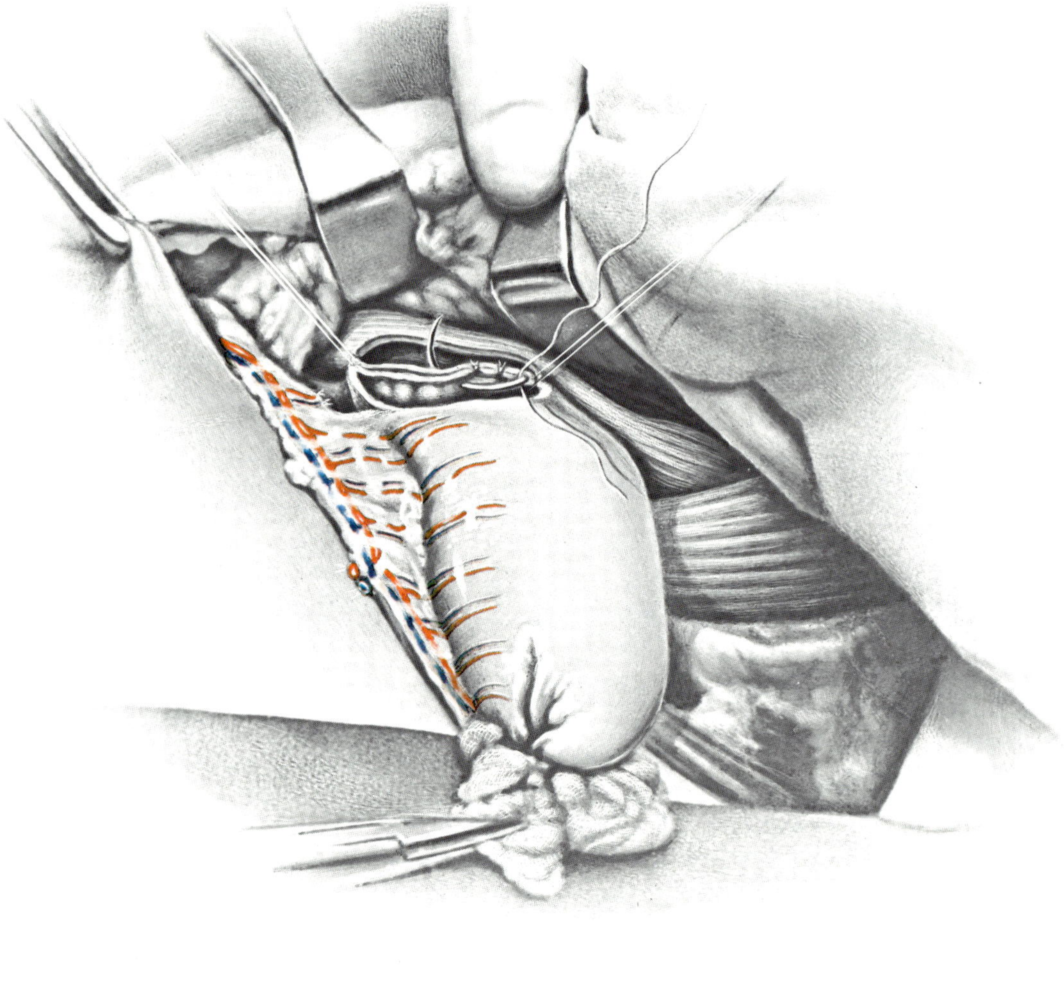

Fig. 718. Application of inner sutures to posterior lip of end-to-side anastomosis between lower end of graft and esophagus. Upper part of graft's vascular pedicle is seen protruding from subcutaneous tunnel.

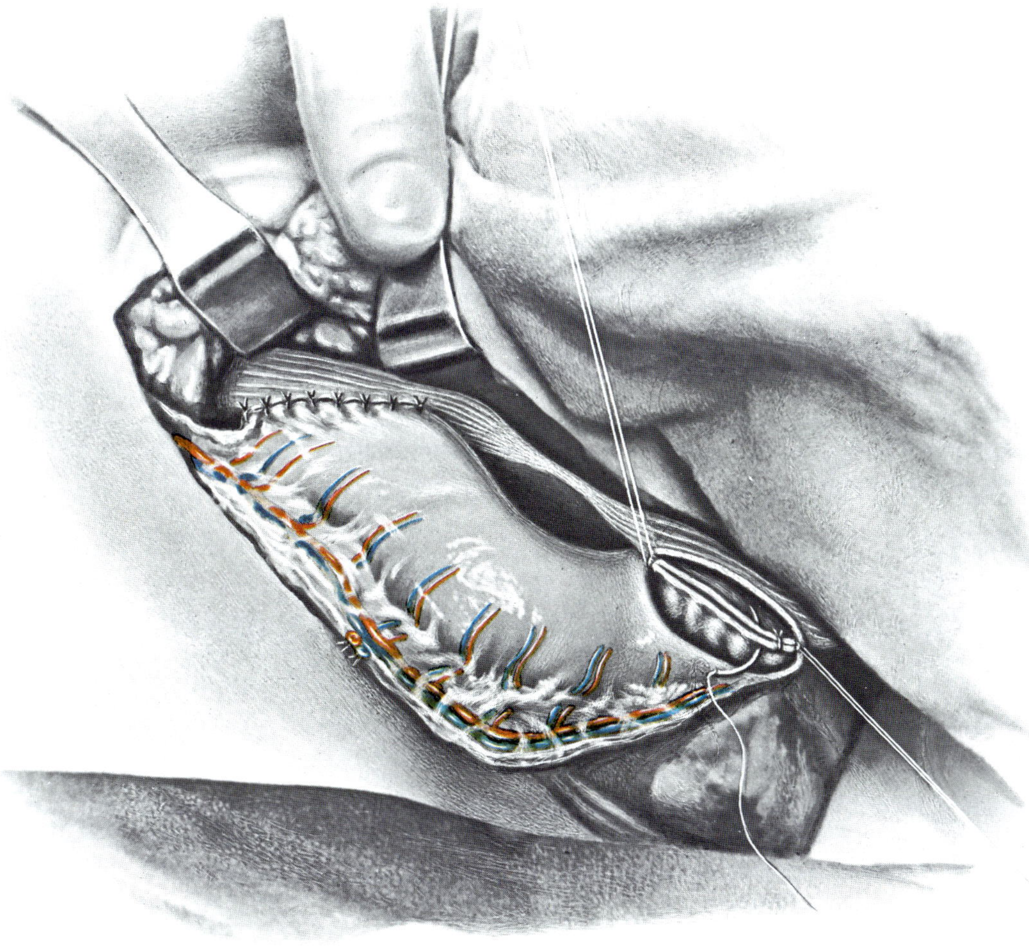

Fig. 719. Creation of anastomosis between upper end of graft and lateral wall of pharynx above stricture.

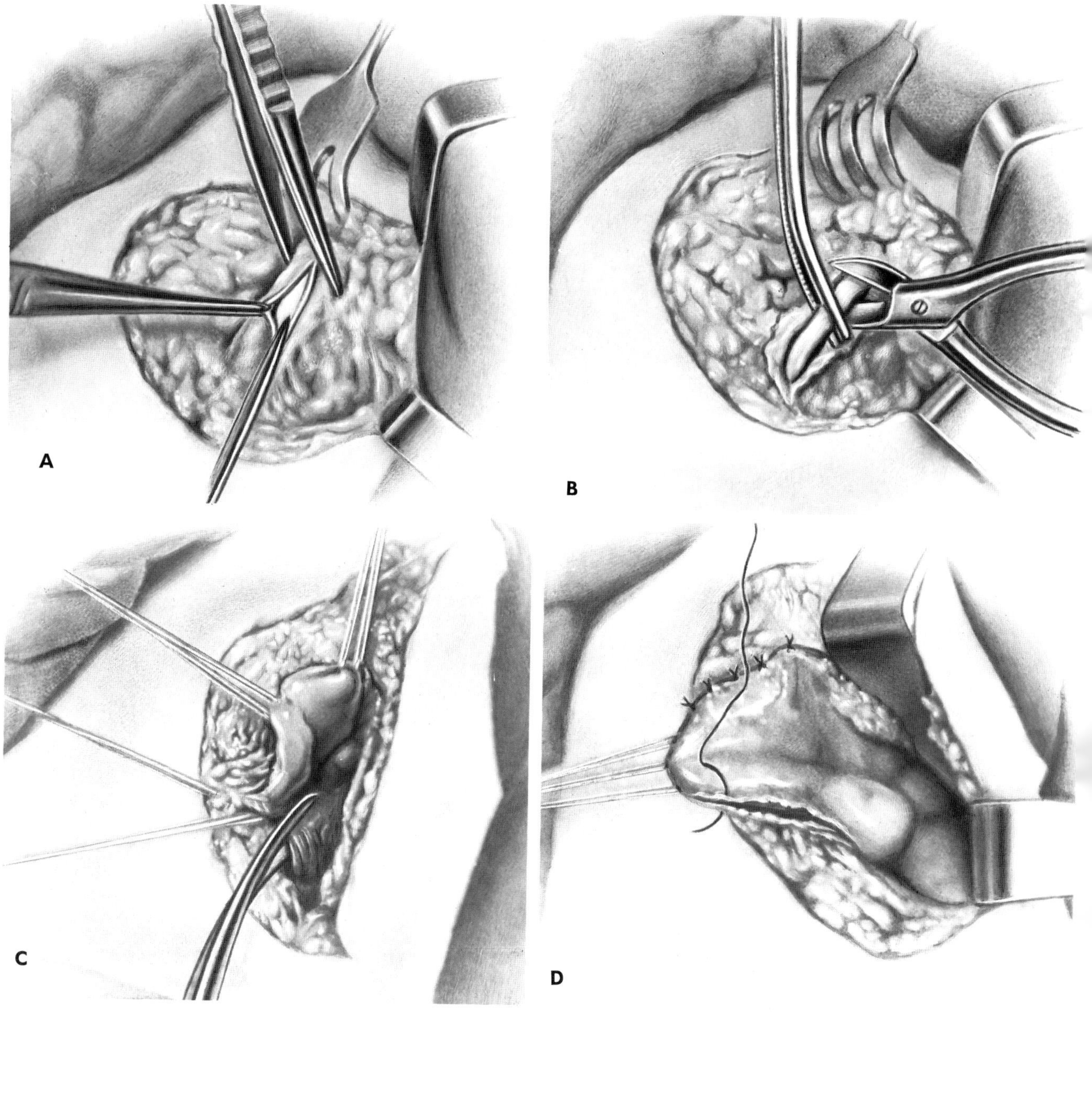

Fig. 720. Separation of epiglottis from scars. **A,** Periosteum of left horn of hyoid bone is cut. **B,** Left horn of hyoid bone is resected. **C,** Epiglottis is freed from adhesions. **D,** Edges of epiglottic mucosa are sutured.

TECHNIQUES FOR FORMING SHORT COLON GRAFT ON LONG VASCULAR PEDICLE

This type of esophagoplasty is employed in short cicatricial strictures of the pharynx and cervical esophagus, for completing retrosternal or antethoracic total esophagoplasty when the graft of the small intestine or stomach is of insufficient length, and in segmental plastic surgery of the superior and middle portions of the esophagus.

Superior median laparotomy is carried out. The greater omentum is separated from the transverse colon. The segment of the descending or sigmoid colon of the required length for repairing the defect in the esophagus is marked off by two threads stitched through the mesentery or by two thin rubber tubes.

Beginning from the cranial thread, all the straight vessels are tied consecutively with separate ligatures directly under the descending colon and the left half of the transverse colon above Riolan's arch to the level of the right branch of the middle colic artery (Fig. 721).

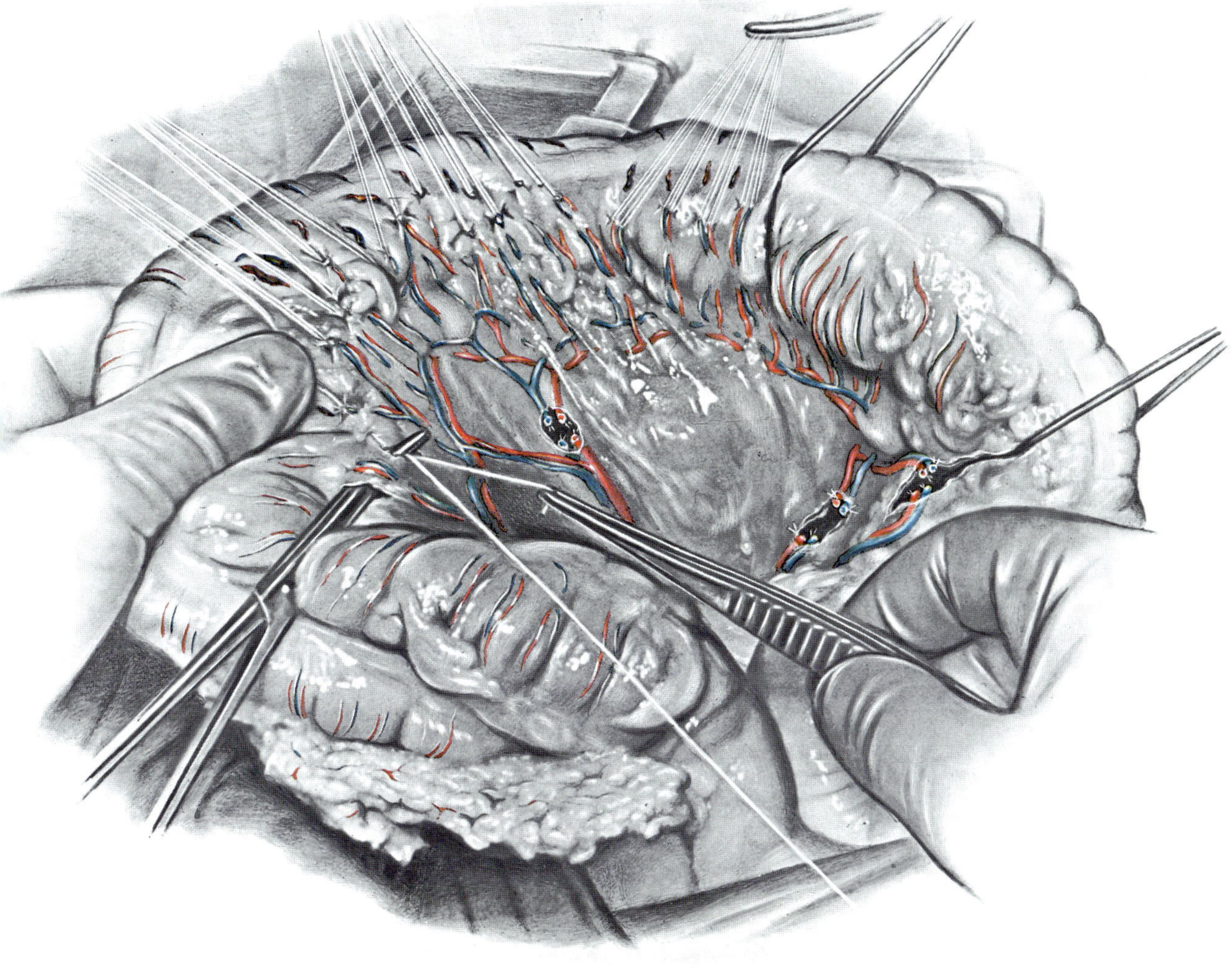

Fig. 721. Segment of colon to be transposed to neck for repairing esophageal defect is delimited with rubber loops. Straight vessels are ligated above Riolan's arch.

After that the left colic artery and vein and the vascular arch below the ligature delimiting the cranial end of the future graft are tied and transected. If there is a well-developed vascular arch between the right and left branches of the middle colic artery and between the branches of the corresponding vein, then the left branches of this artery and vein may also be tied and transected to elongate the vascular pedicle of the graft. This should not be done in the absence of a good anastomosis.

The segment of the colon deprived of blood supply is first transected between one of the pairs of crushing clamps (Fig. 722). The mesentery is held by ligatures remaining from the time the straight vessels had been tied. This part of the colon is now separated from the mesentery with scissors up to the next pair of crushing clamps, between which it is again transected, and the ischemic segment is removed (Fig. 723).

The mesentery is cut away with scissors from the posterior abdominal wall under the graft and Riolan's

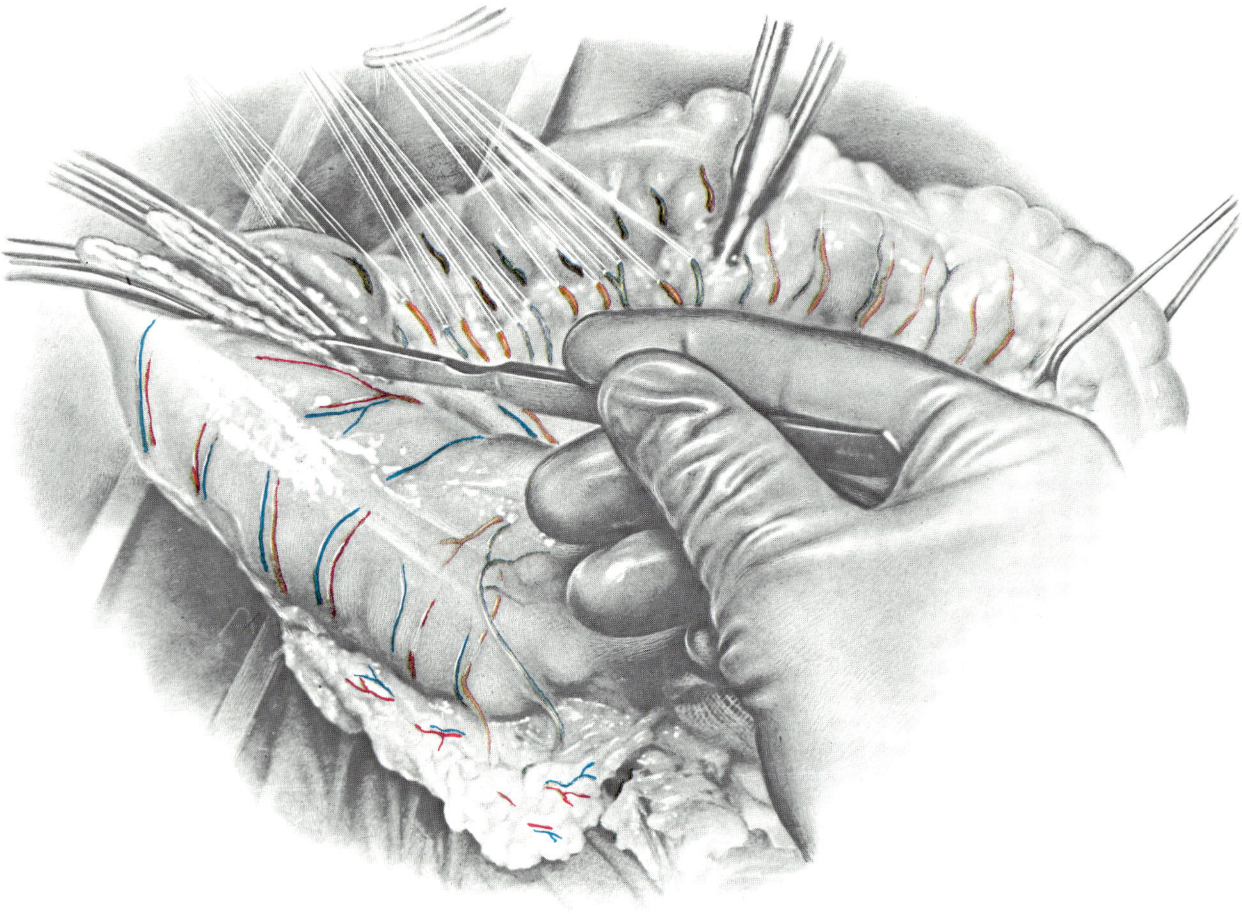

Fig. 722. Colon is transected at level of last right ligature applied to straight vessels of mesentery.

arch and parallel to them in the avascular fields up to the middle colic artery. The sigmoid colon is then transected between two crushing clamps above the tied vascular arcade where the cranial end of the future graft had been delimited by the ligature (Fig. 724). The ligatures are cut off from the vascular pedicle of the graft (Fig. 725), and both stumps of the graft are closed with a purse-string suture to prevent contamination of the tunnel with the intestinal contents during transposition of the graft. The continuity of the intestine is restored by end-to-end anastomosis of the right half of the transverse colon and the sigmoid colon. After transposition of the graft to the neck, the abdominal wound is sutured. The purse-string suture is cut away from the stump of the graft, and first the lower and then the upper anastomoses are formed between the graft and the esophagus with the ends of the graft sutured into its side, bypassing the stricture (Fig. 726).

In using a short segment of the colon, total esophagoplasty is accomplished by anastomosing its lower stump with the upper stump of the graft employed earlier.

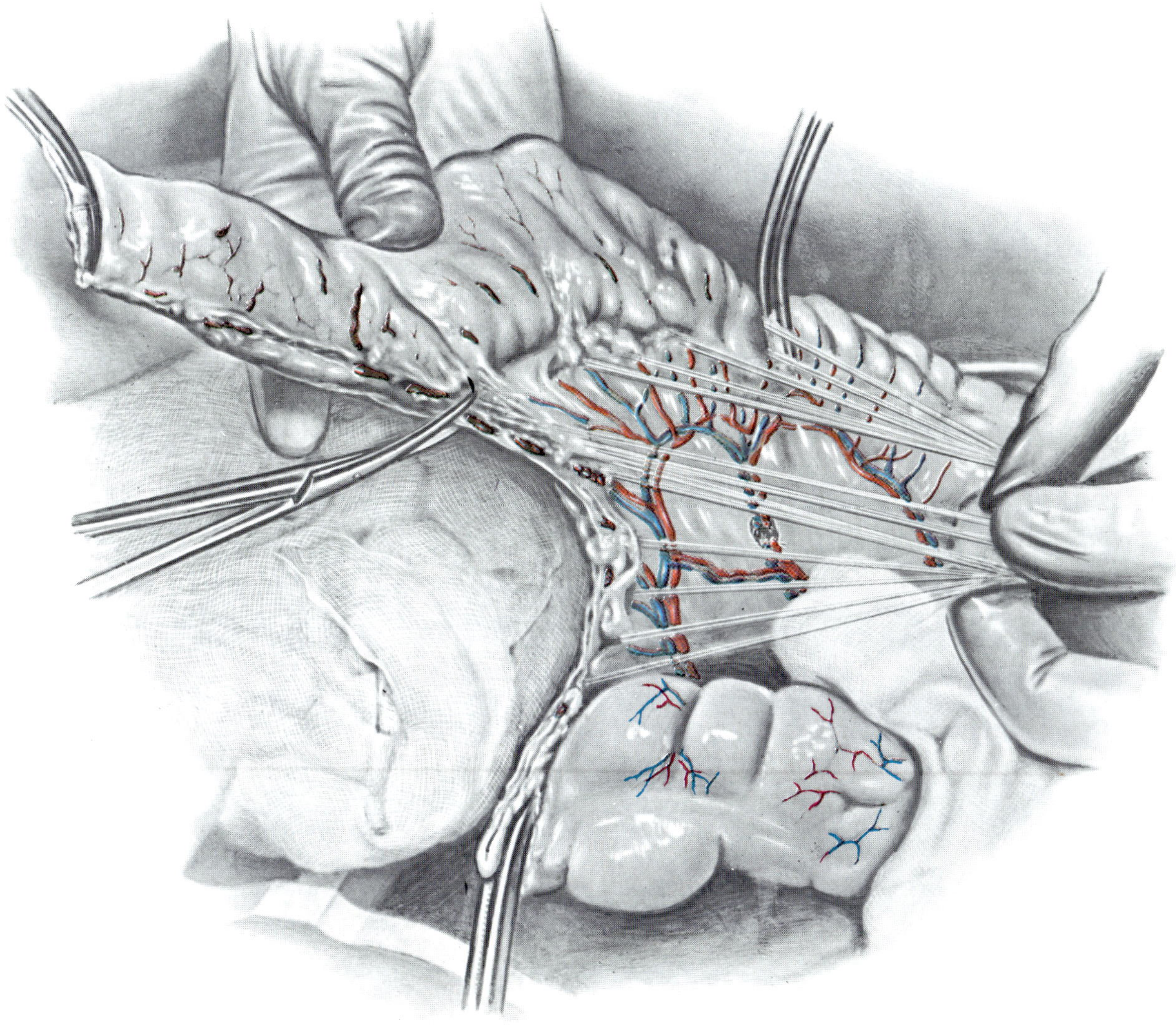

Fig. 723. Segment of colon deprived of blood supply is resected above Riolan's arch.

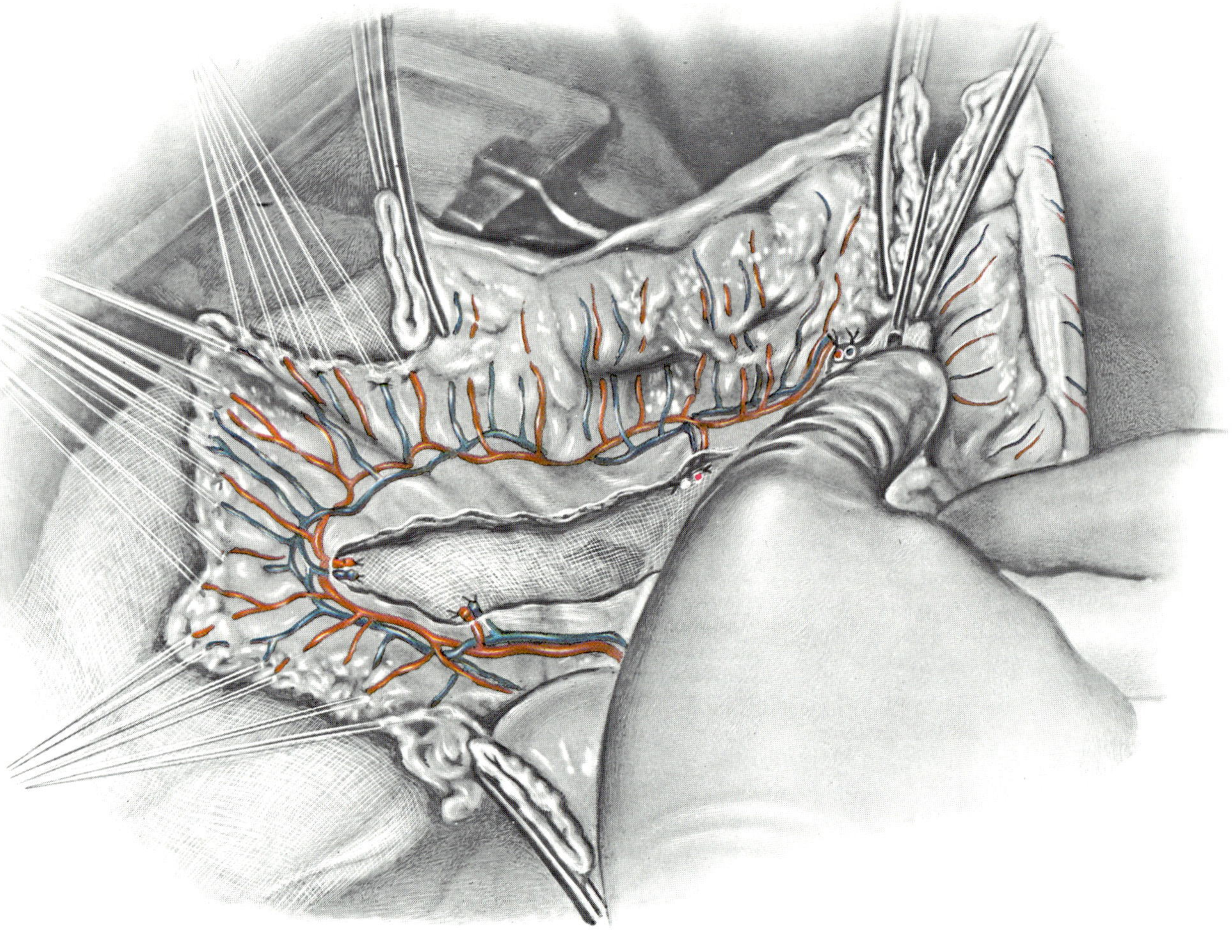

Fig. 724. Transection of colon at upper boundary of graft.

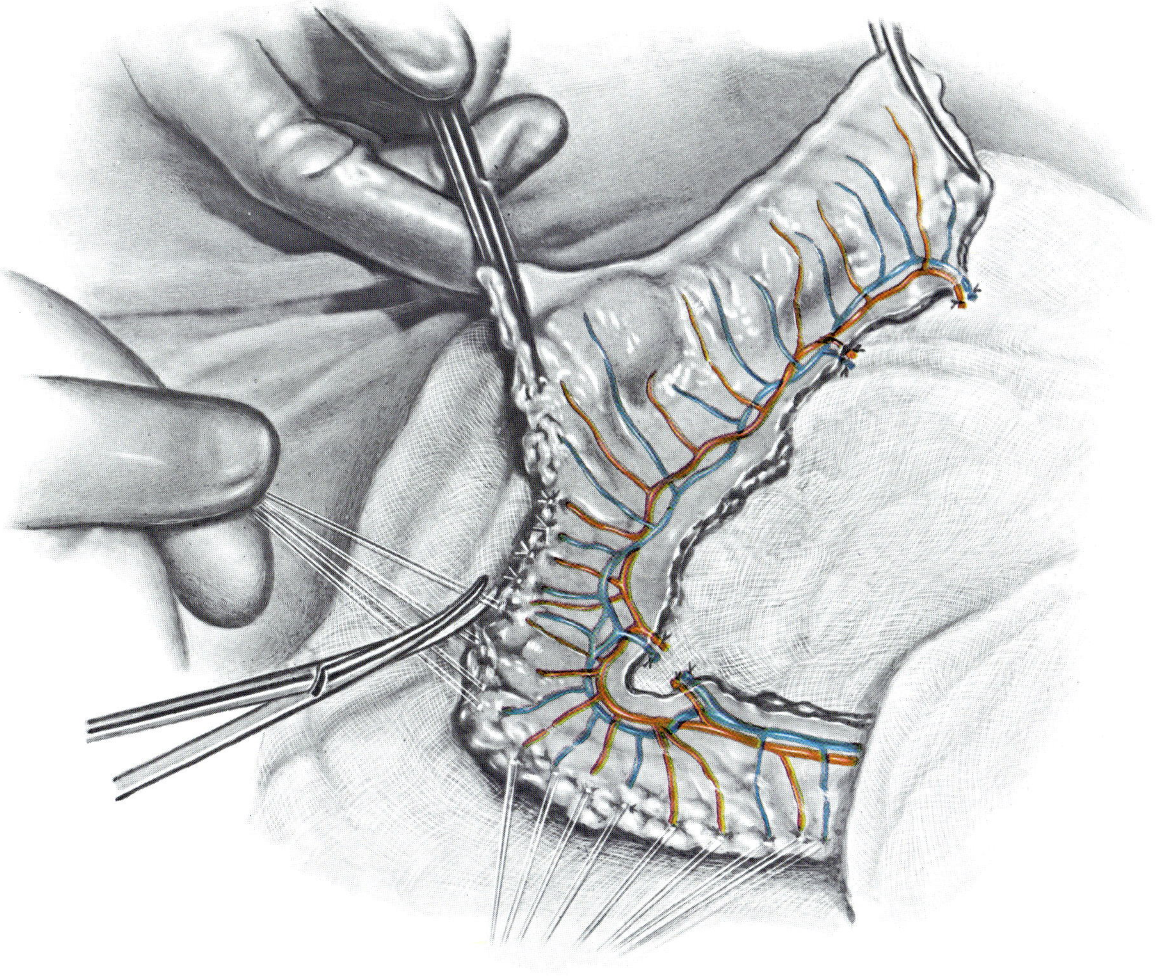

Fig. 725. Ligatures are cut off from ligated straight vessels of graft's pedicle.

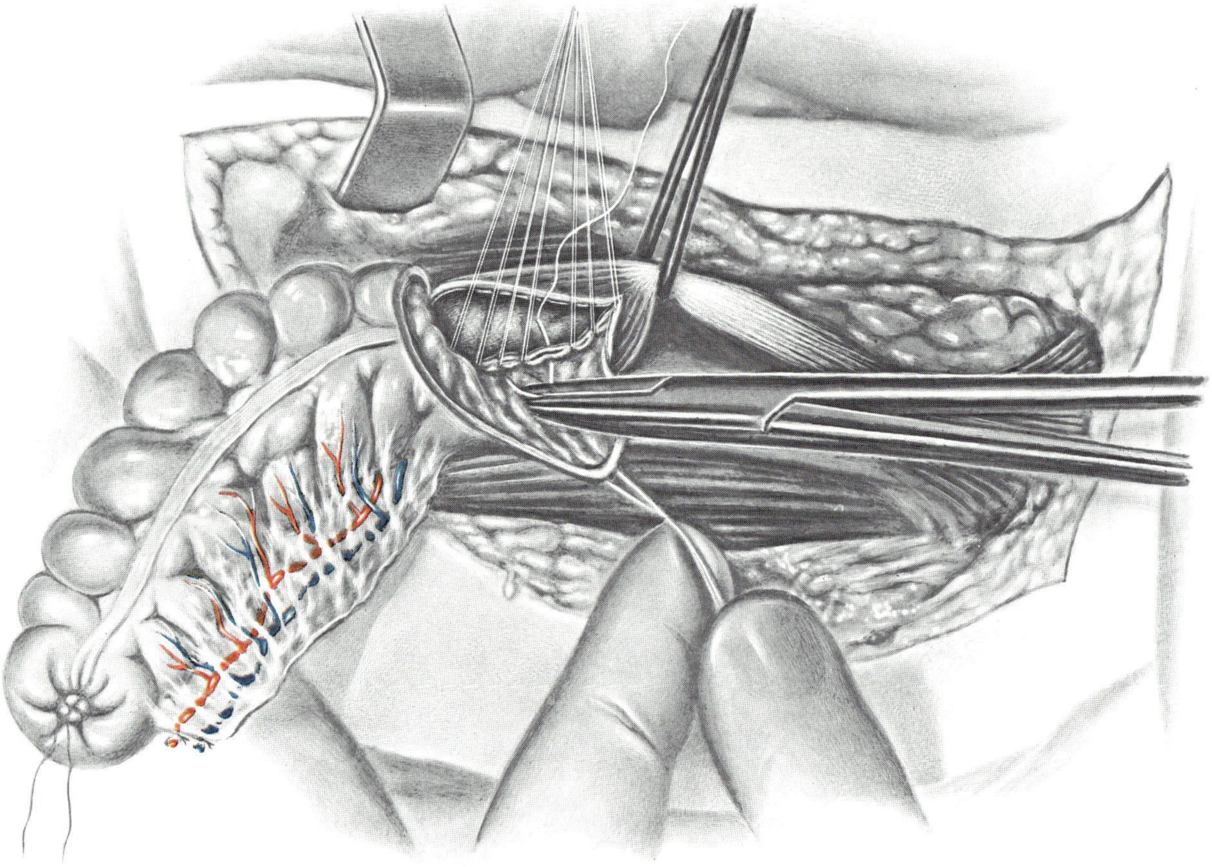

Fig. 726. Formation of anastomosis between lower stump of graft and esophagus.

OPERATIONS IN CARDIOSPASM

CARDIOPLASTY WITH DIAPHRAGMATIC GRAFT AFTER PETROVSKY

Transpleural approach in the seventh intercostal space is employed.

The pleural cavity is opened; the pulmonodiaphragmatic ligament is transected; and the inferior lobe of the lung is moved cranially. The defect formed in the lower part of the mediastinal pleura after transection of the ligament is slightly widened with scissors to expose the left wall of the lower part of the esophagus.

The middle part of the diaphragm is held with two clamps, and a Π-shaped flap with its base facing the esophageal hiatus, but short of it by 2 to 3 cm, is shaped from its anterolateral area (Fig. 727). The flap is cut in such a way as to preserve the large veins and arteries in it. The left anterior portion of the phrenicoesophageal ligament is destroyed by the blunt and sharp techniques; the lower part of the esophagus is freed from the medi-

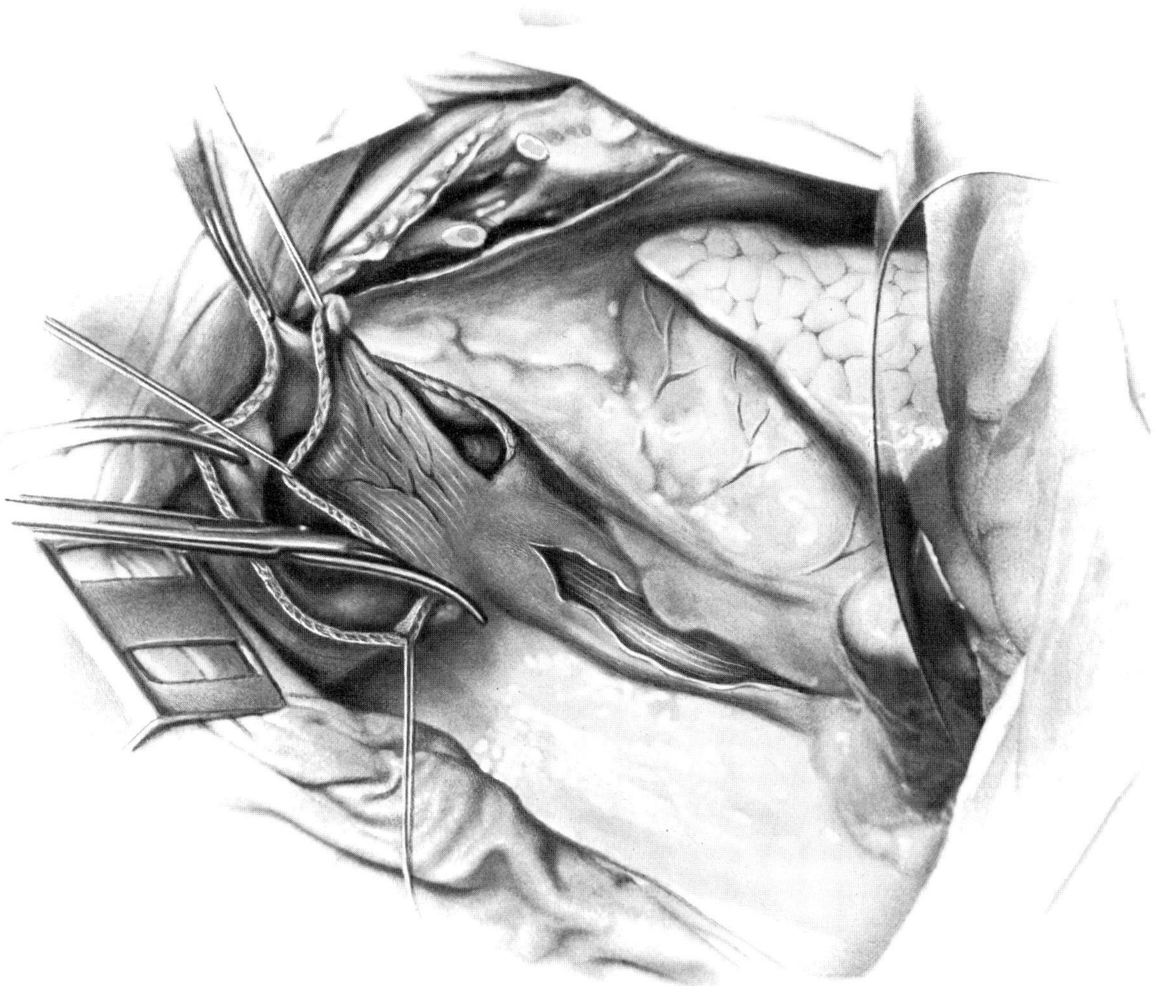

Fig. 727. A Π-shaped muscular flap is tailored from diaphragm.

astinum and held with a thin rubber tube or gauze strip. By pulling the tube or strip the abdominal portion of the esophagus and cardia are drawn out into the pleural cavity through the esophageal hiatus. The muscular coat, 4 to 6 cm above the cardia, is cut transversely with a scalpel down to the submucous coat along approximately one third of the esophageal circumference (Fig. 728). A second incision is then made in the muscular coat, in the longitudinal direction this time, from the middle of the transverse incision to the cardia and below it 0.5 to 1.0 cm (Fig. 729). The edges of this T-shaped incision in the muscular coat of the lower esophagus and cardia are drawn slightly apart, exposing the submucous coat of the esophagus. The few transverse muscular fibers remaining on it are transected with a scalpel without injuring the submucous and mucous coats of the esophagus. The anterior wall of the subcardiac part of the stomach is invaginated into the esophageal cavity with one or

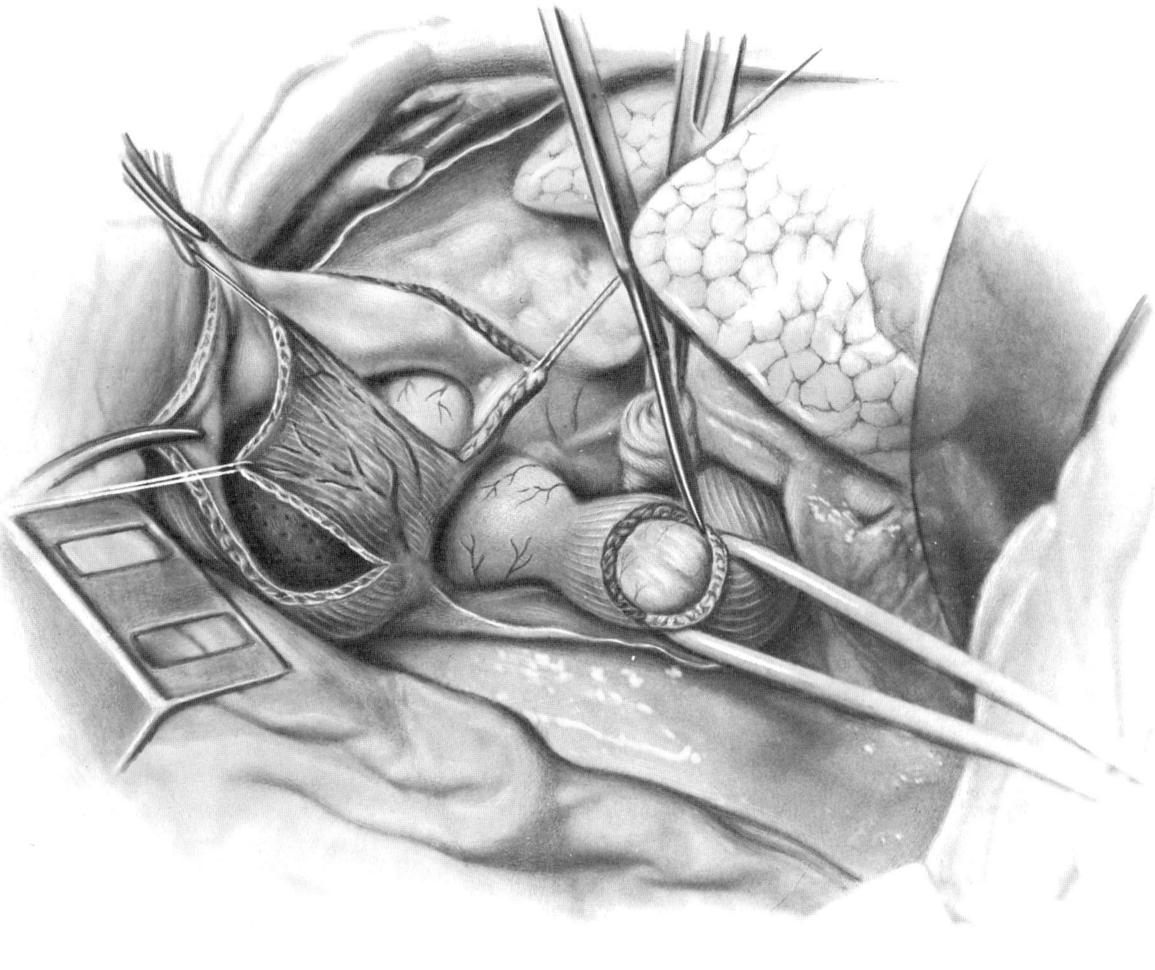

Fig. 728. Anterior left part of esophageal muscular coat above constriction is cut transversely.

two fingers inserted into the abdominal cavity through the incision in the diaphragm, achieving a certain distension of the cardia in this way (Fig. 730).

Fine interrupted sutures of Lavsan or silk are applied with atraumatic needles between the base of the Π-shaped diaphragmatic flap and the seromuscular coat of the cardia (Fig. 731). The edges of the diaphragmatic flap are then stitched to the edges of the incision in the esophageal muscular coat along the entire perimeter (Fig. 732).

The bared area of the submucous coat is thus fully wrapped in the Π-shaped diaphragmatic flap.

The defect formed in the diaphragm after tailoring the flap is repaired with interrupted sutures (Fig. 733). Widely spaced sutures are applied to the mediastinal pleura. A drain is left in the pleural cavity. The wound in the thoracic cage is completely closed.

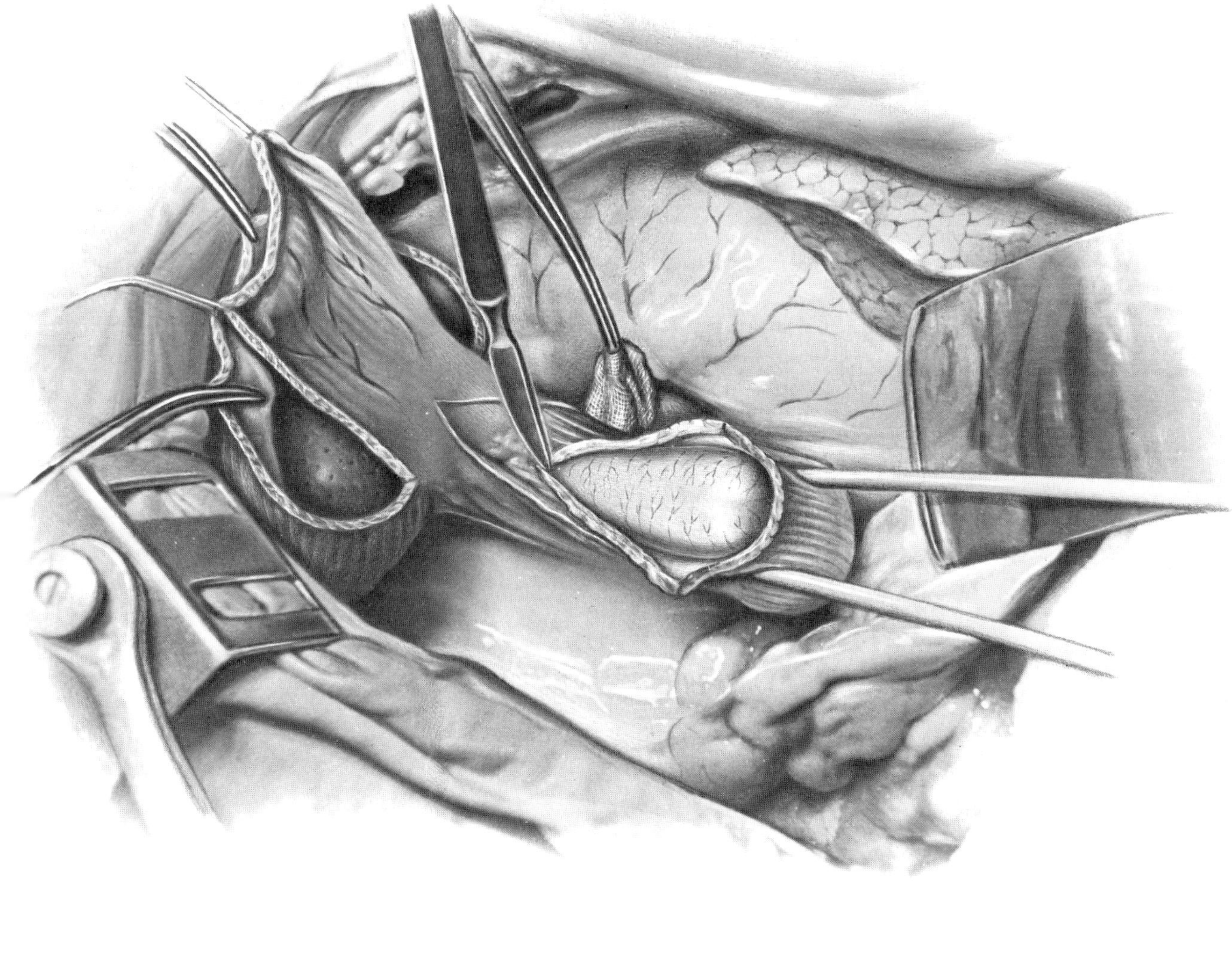

Fig. 729. Muscular coat of esophagus and cardia is cut lengthwise through constricted part down to subcardiac part of stomach.

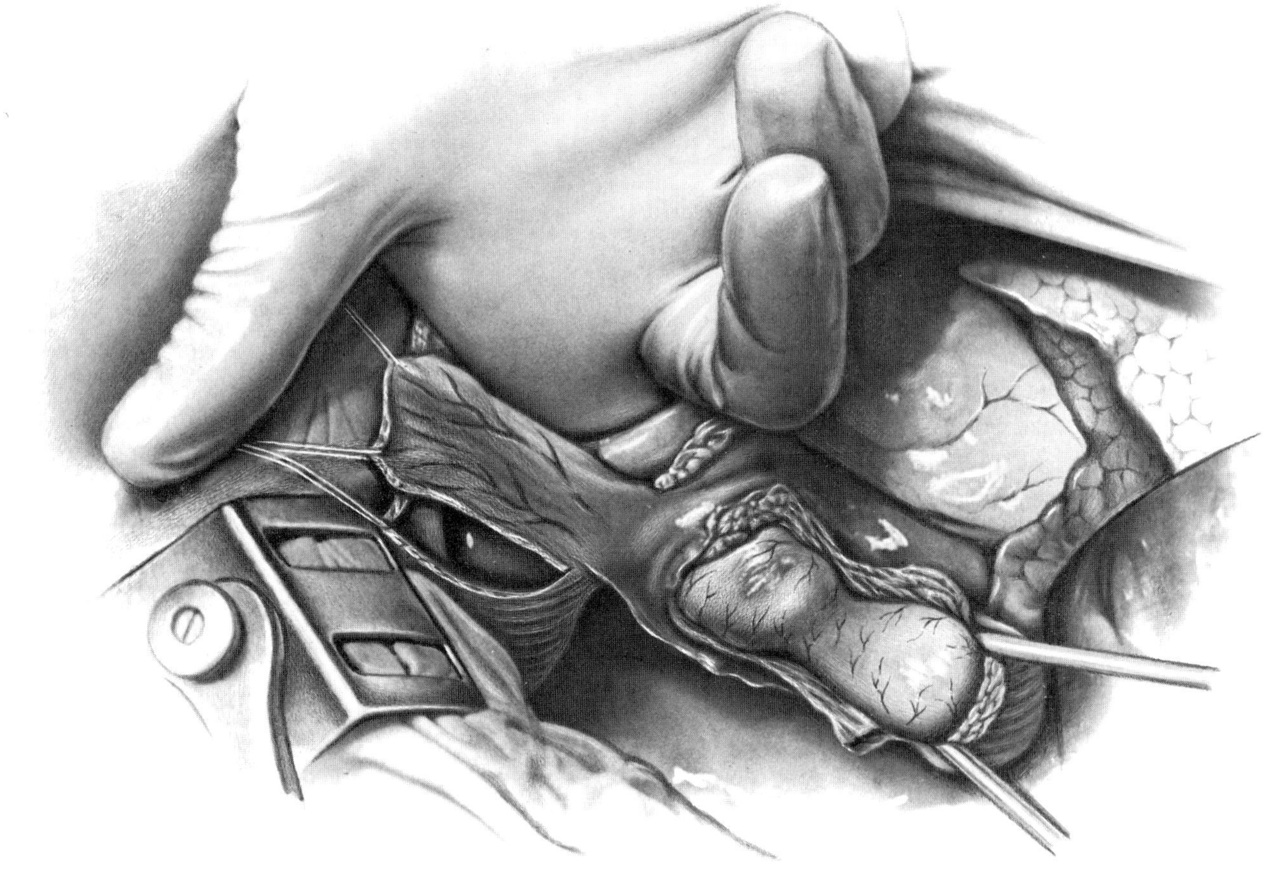

Fig. 730. Constricted segment of lower esophagus and cardia is distended with finger invaginating anterior wall of stomach into esophageal lumen.

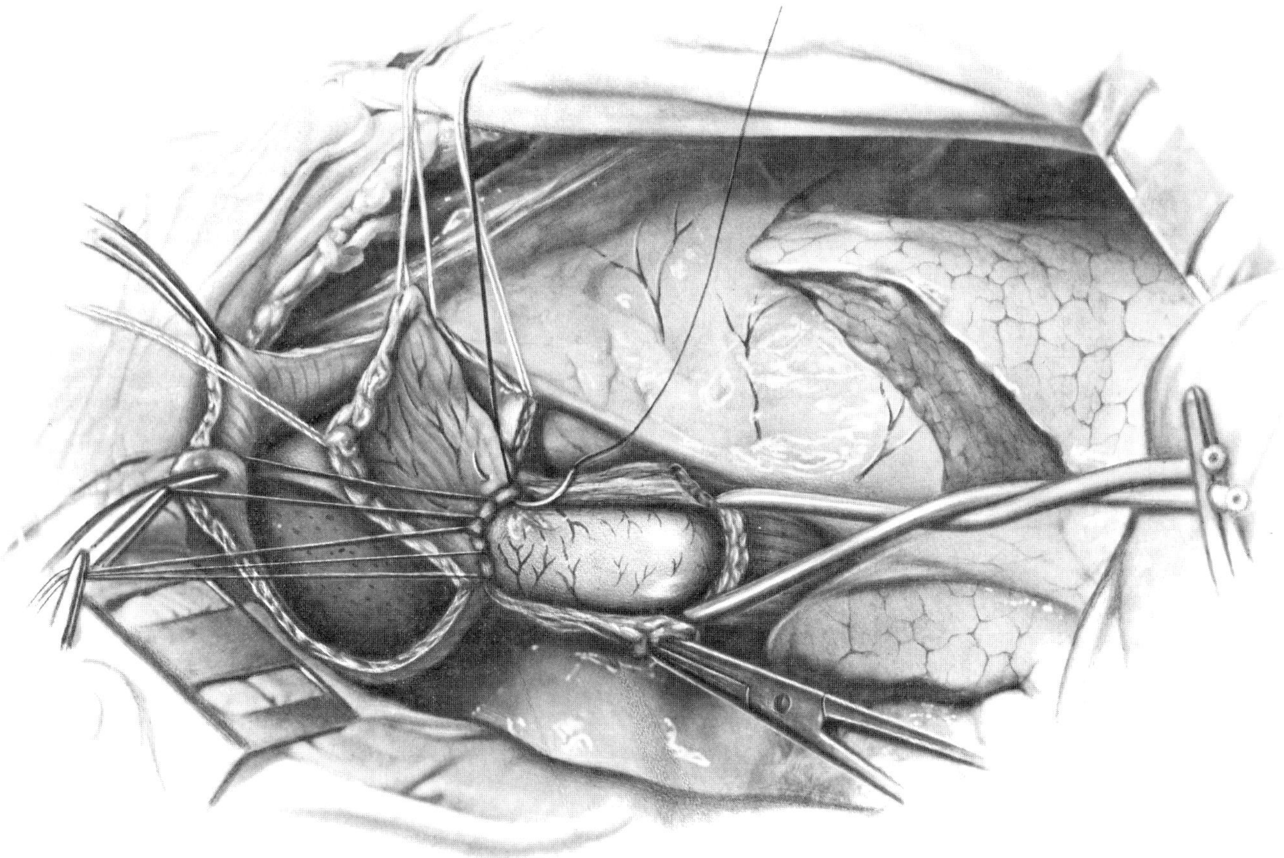

Fig. 731. Base of Π-shaped diaphragmatic flap is stitched to edge of incised seromuscular coat of cardiac portion of stomach.

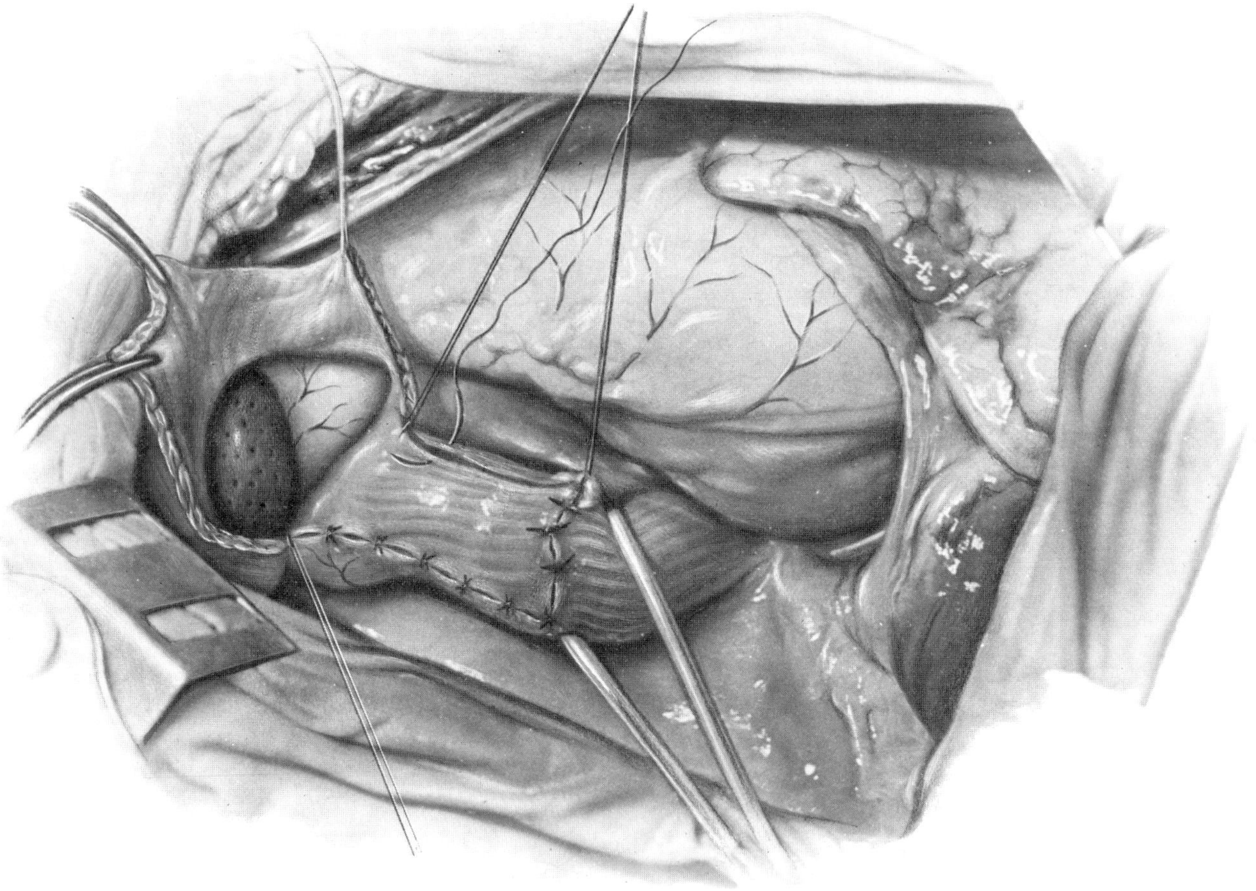

Fig. 732. Diaphragmatic flap is stitched to edges of incised esophageal muscular coat.

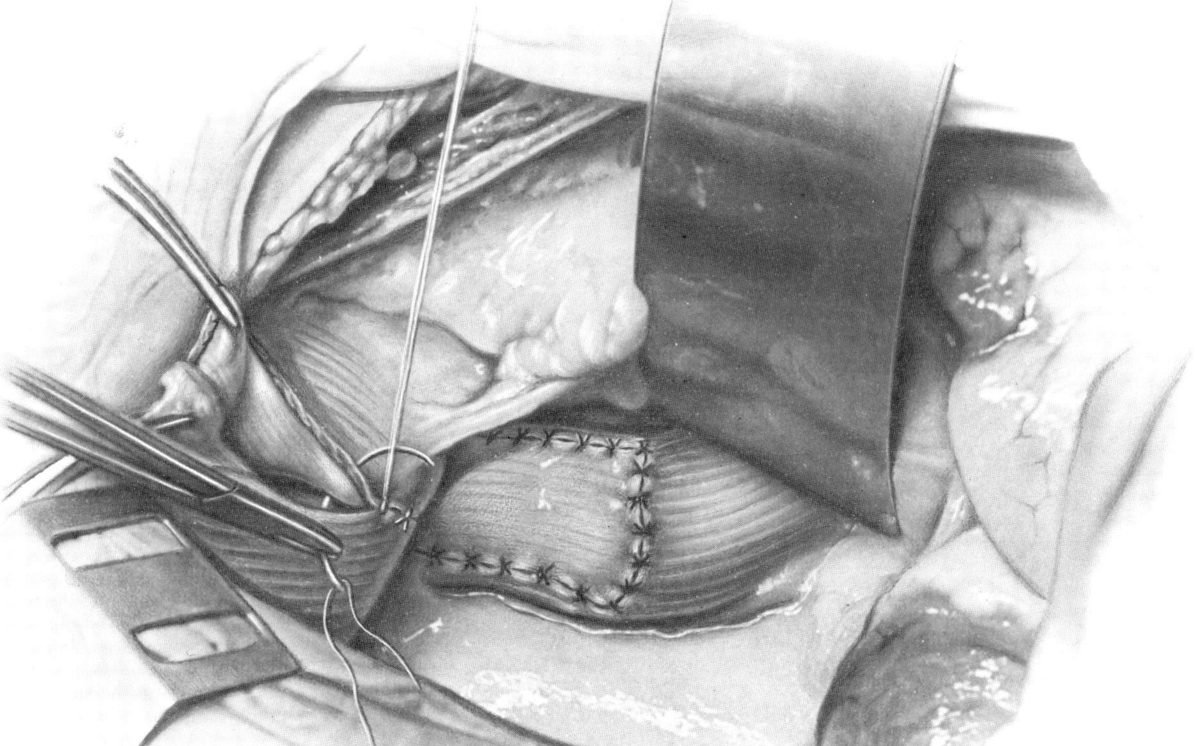

Fig. 733. Defect in muscular coat of lower esophageal segment and cardia has been repaired. Defect in diaphragm is sutured.

EXTRAMUCOUS CARDIOMYOTOMY (HELLER'S OPERATION)

The operation is performed through superior median laparotomy or left thoracotomy in the seventh intercostal space.

After the constricted segment of the esophagus has been mobilized from the mediastinal tissue, a 6 to 8 cm longitudinal incision is made in the muscular coat from the distended part of the esophagus and down to the cardia and stomach. The edges of the cut muscular coat are drawn apart, exposing the intact mucous membrane of the esophagus and cardia, which prolapses easily into the wound (Fig. 734). The operation is thus terminated. The wound in the thoracic (or abdominal cavity) is fully closed.

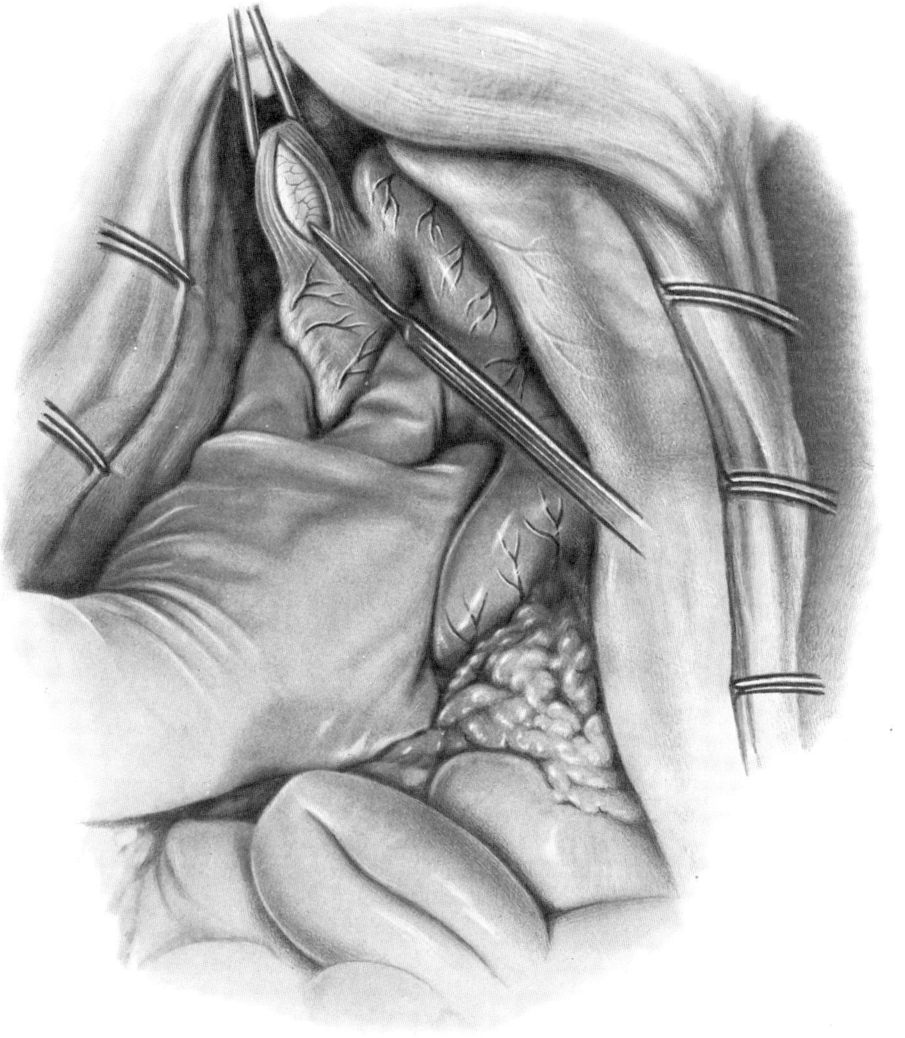

Fig. 734. Extramucous cardiotomy through abdominal approach.

OPERATIONS IN DIVERTICULA

The surgical approach to an esophageal diverticulum is determined by its location. In a pharyngoesophageal (Zenker's) diverticulum, usually localized on the left posterior wall of the pharyngoesophageal junction, most surgeons prefer to use an incision along the anterior border of the left sternocleidomastoid muscle. Right anterolateral thoracotomy in the fifth or sixth intercostal space is convenient for the management of bifurcation diverticula located on a level with the third to fifth thoracic vertebrae, usually on the right anterior wall of the esophagus. The patient is placed on the left side with a small bolster under the middle part of the thoracic cage. In an epiphrenic diverticulum it is expedient to approach the esophagus through the seventh intercostal space on the left or right depending on the location of the pouch.

Two operations are commonly used, namely, diverticulectomy (excision of the diverticulum) or invagination of the diverticulum after Girard.

DIVERTICULECTOMY

After the esophagus is freed from the mediastinum, the diverticulum is held with fenestrated forceps and separated from its adhesions with the surrounding tissues by blunt and sharp techniques (Fig. 735). Introduction of air into the esophageal lumen through a tube helps to detect the pouch. If the neck of the diverticulum is thin (5 mm at most), a circular ligature may be applied to it at the esophageal wall, and the diverticulum may

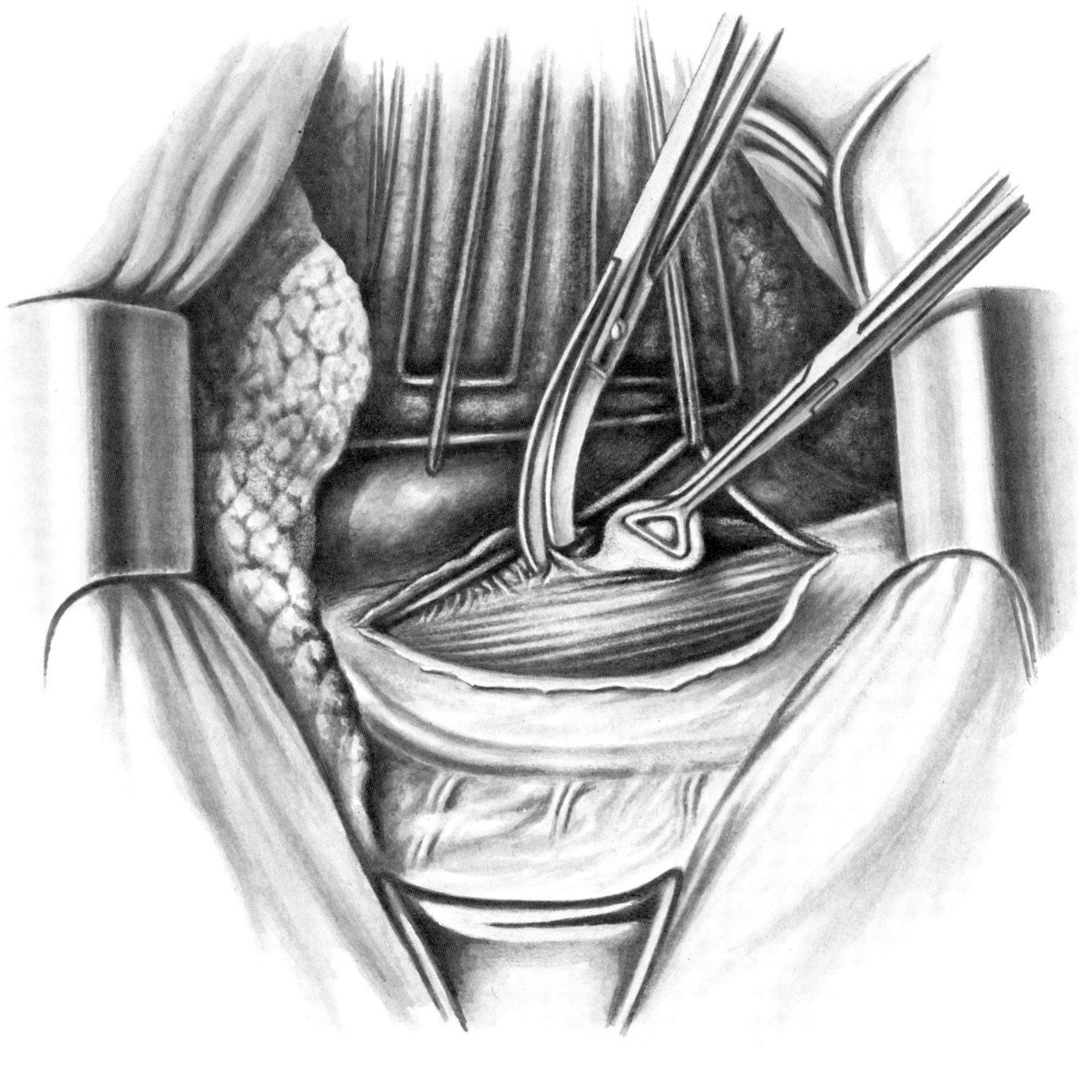

Fig. 735. Esophageal diverticulum is held with fenestrated forceps, and adhesions between it and mediastinal tissues are cut.

be cut away and buried muscular sutures applied to the muscular coat. A wide neck of the diverticulum is clamped with a Satinsky-type clamp directly at the esophageal wall, under which the neck is stitched through with a continuous mattress catgut suture (Fig. 736). After the diverticulum has been cut away and the clamp has been removed, the same thread is used to apply a lock-stitch suture through all the coats. The third row of interrupted silk or Lavsan sutures is applied to the muscular coat of the esophagus (Fig. 737).

When diverticulectomy is carried out on the thoracic esophagus, the line of the suture is covered with the mediastinal pleura (Fig. 738) or with a muscular flap of the diaphragm as in Petrovsky's cardioplasty. The pleura below the esophageal wound is not sutured so as to provide for the drainage of the mediastinum through the pleural cavity.

After diverticulectomy on the thoracic esophagus, rubber drains are left in the neck wound for one or two days.

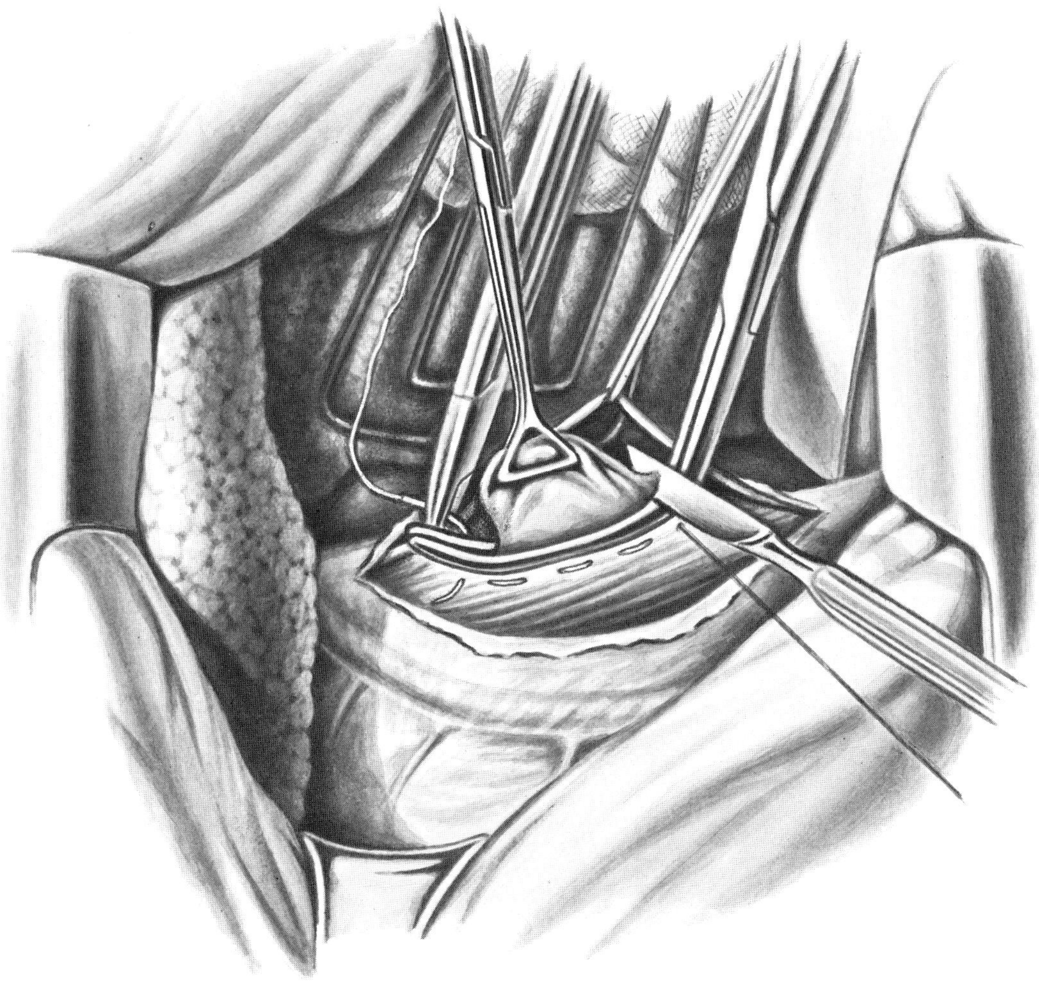

Fig. 736. Neck of diverticulum is stitched through with continuous mattress catgut suture under Satinsky's clamp and then cut off.

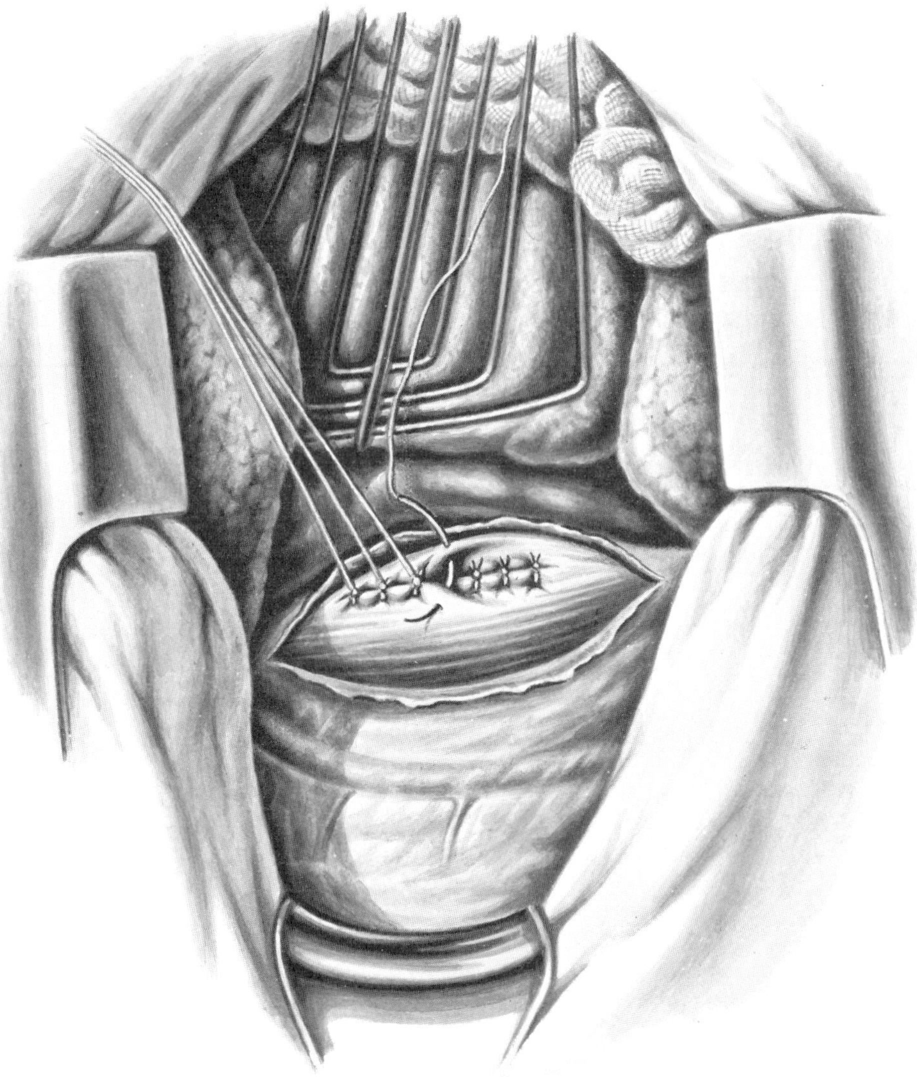

Fig. 737. Application of third row of interrupted buried sutures to muscular coat of esophagus.

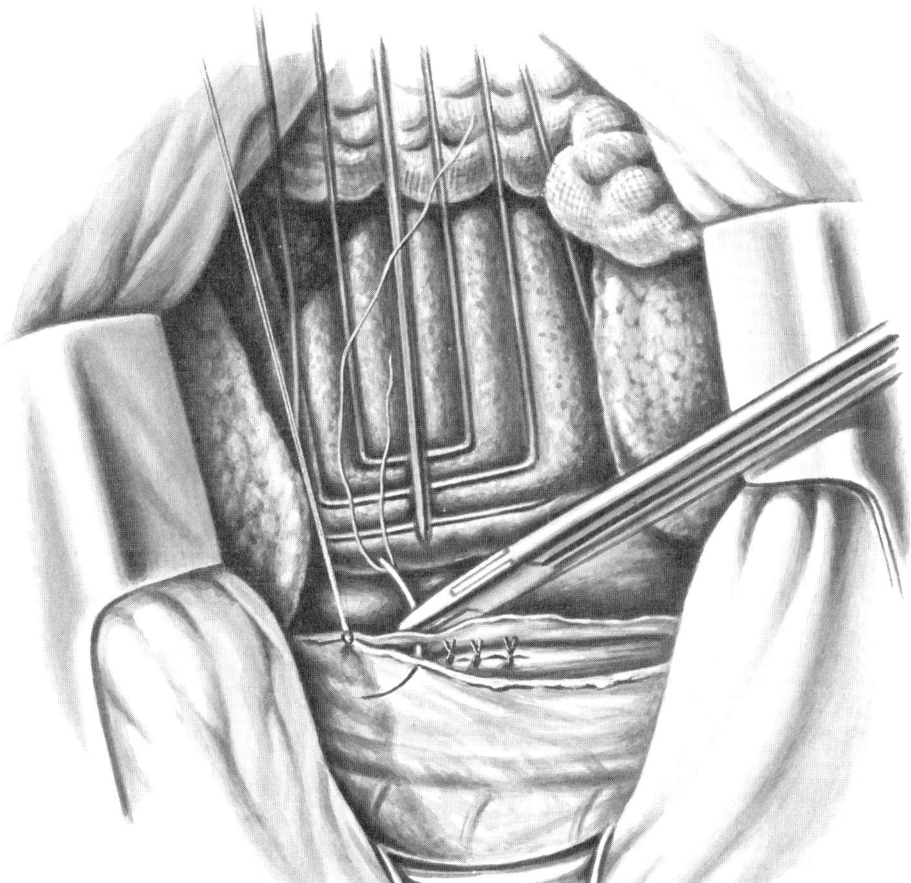

Fig. 738. Mediastinal pleura is sutured.

DIVERTICULUM INVAGINATION

The mobilization of the diverticulum in this operation is identical with that described above.

After it is freed from adhesions by means of a tampon or spade, the diverticulum is invaginated into the esophageal lumen. A few interrupted silk sutures or (when the diverticulum has a thin neck) a purse-string or Z-shaped suture is applied to the site of invagination with the thread passed through the muscular and submucous coats of the esophagus (Fig. 739). All the subsequent stages of the operation are carried out as described for diverticulectomy.

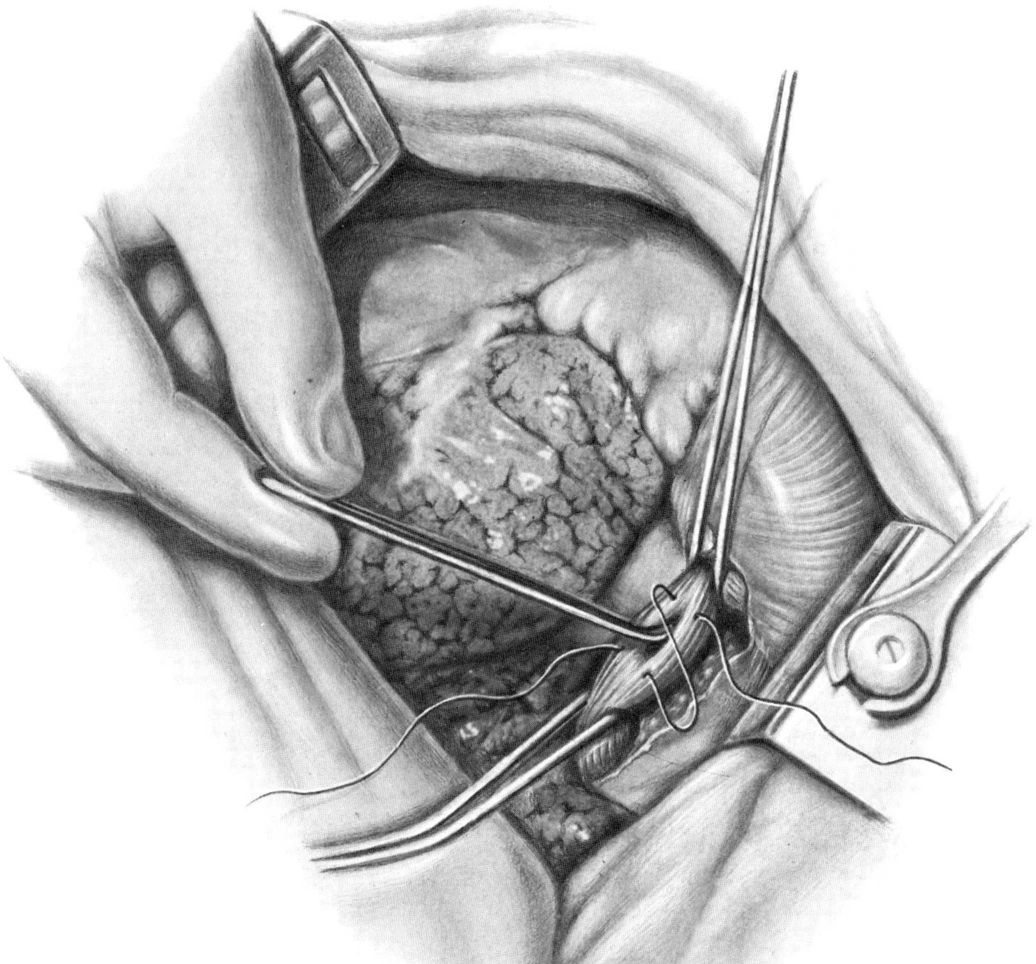

Fig. 739. Z-shaped suture is applied to muscular coat of esophagus over neck of invaginated diverticulum.

CLOSURE OF ESOPHAGEAL RUPTURES

In the first two or three hours following injury to the esophageal walls with foreign bodies, instruments, etc., it is permissible to suture the wound using local tissues (a muscular flap, the lung, a flap of the diaphragm or the gastric wall).

The approach to the esophagus is determined by the level at which the defect in its wall is located, whether it is the right or left wall that is injured and which surrounding tissues or cavities (right or left pleural, or the abdominal cavity) are involved in the pathological

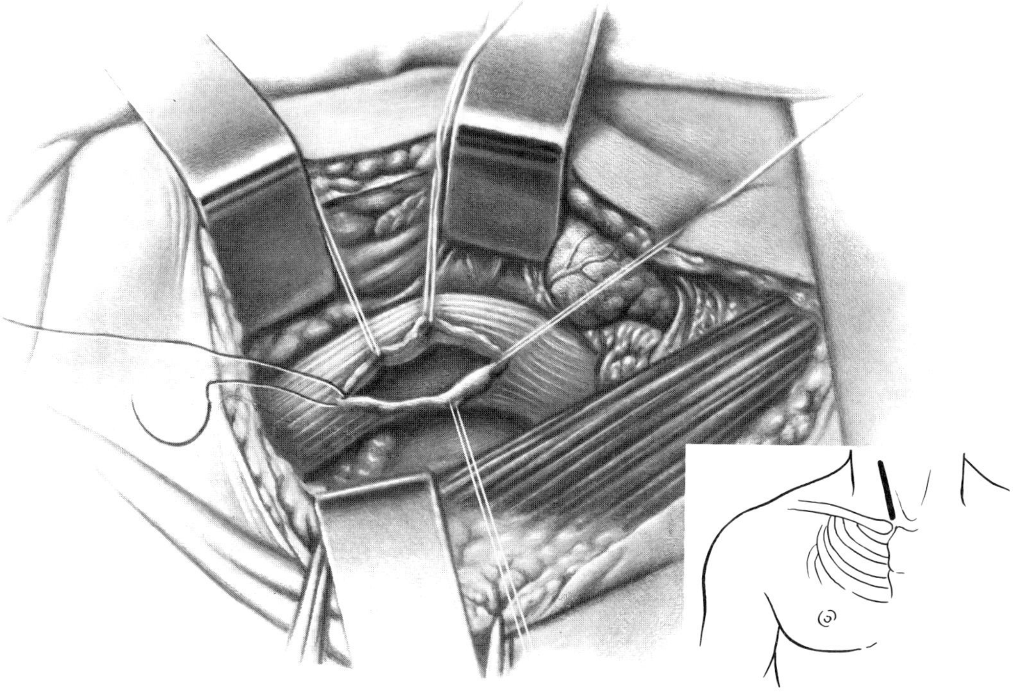

Fig. 740. Edges of esophageal wound are held with catgut traction sutures.

processes caused by the injury. The technique for closing an instrumental rupture of the right wall of the cervical esophagus is shown in Figs. 740 to 743.

A right approach along the medial border of the sternocleidomastoid muscle is used.

An incision is made through the skin, platysma, and anterior and posterior walls of the sheath of the sternocleidomastoid muscle close to its medial border, and the muscle is moved laterally. The omohyoid and sternothyroid muscles are transected. The superior (and, whenever necessary, the inferior also) thyroid artery is ligated with two ligatures and transected between them. The neurovascular bundle is drawn laterally with blunt hooks while the thyroid gland and trachea are drawn medially. The lateral wall of the larynx and the posterior surface of the spine serve as guidepoints in locating the esophagus.

When its posterior wall is injured, it is expedient to mobilize the esophagus along its entire circumference and hold it with rubber loops. This should not be done if the lateral wall is injured.

With the lateral and partly the anterior and posterior walls of the esophagus freed, chromicized catgut traction sutures are applied to the edges of the wound through all the coats (Fig. 740). The rupture is sutured on a tube to avoid narrowing the esophageal lumen. If the wound is small, a rubber tube is introduced into the esophagus through the mouth. In cases with a large rupture, the tube may be introduced into the esophagus through the wound (Fig. 741). The esophageal wound is closed lengthwise. The first row of interrupted chromicized catgut or silk sutures is stitched through all the coats (Fig. 742); the second row is applied only to the muscular coat.

To prevent the escape of the esophageal contents into

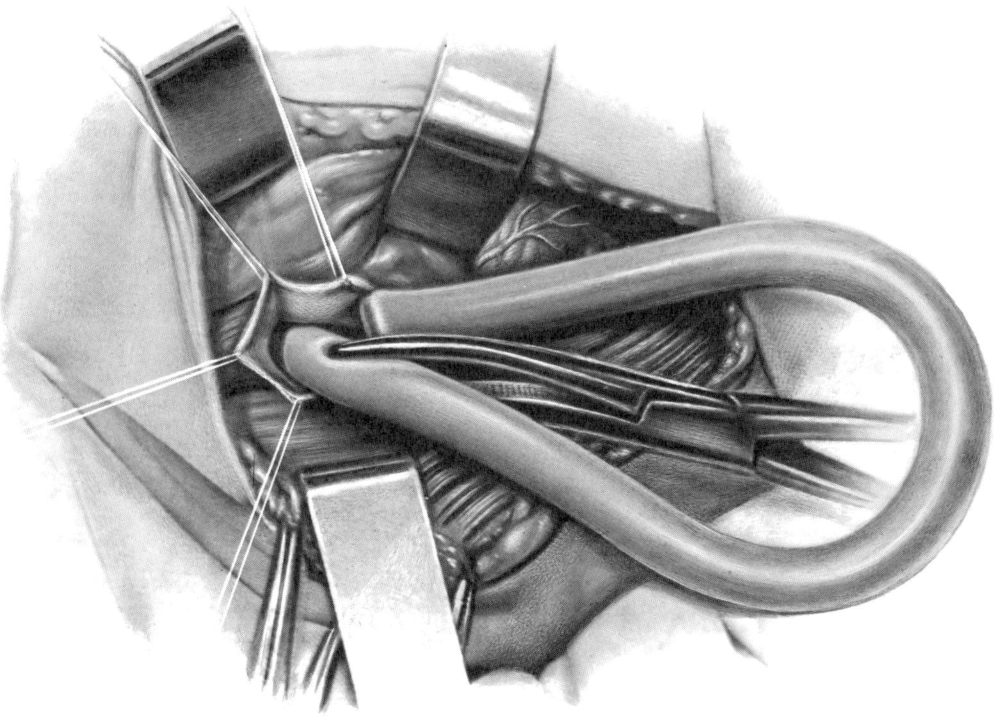

Fig. 741. Introduction of tube into esophagus through wound in its cervical part.

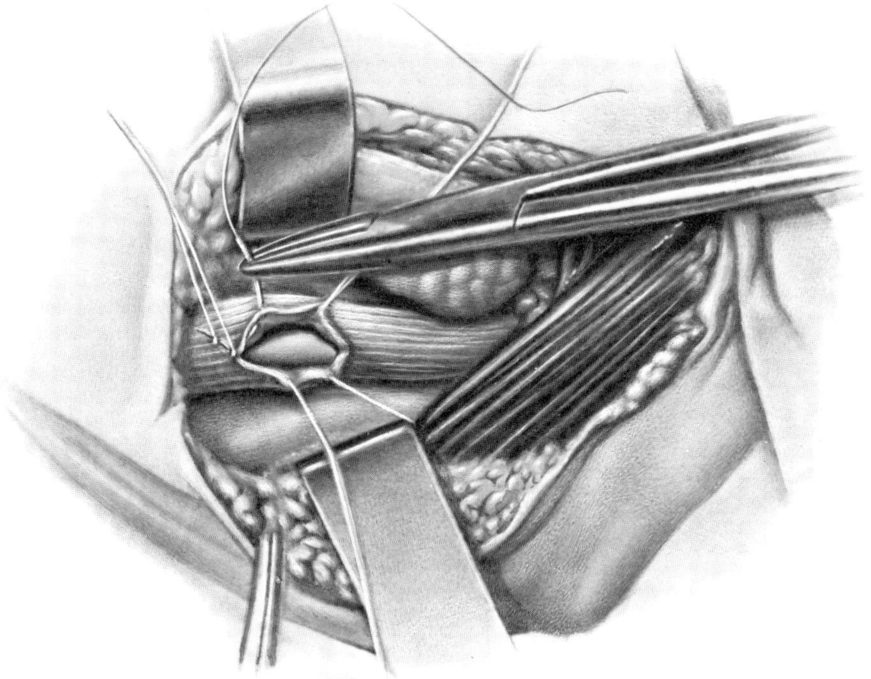

Fig. 742. First row of interrupted sutures is applied through all coats of esophagus.

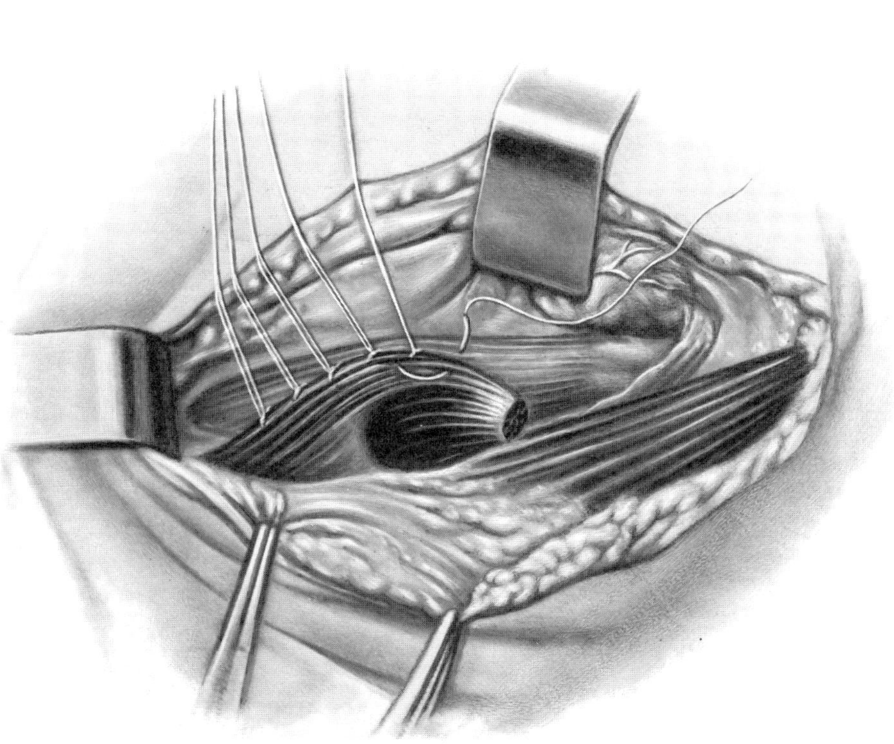

Fig. 743. Flap of sternocleidomastoid muscle is stitched to esophagus over sutured wound.

the wound on the neck, the line of the suture is covered with a flap formed from the medial part of the sternocleidomastoid muscle. The medial head of this muscle is cut in its tendinous part close to its origin from the manubrium sterni. The cut portion of the muscle is detached in the cranial direction. The pedicle muscular graft formed is stitched to the esophagus with two rows of sutures, one of which is dorsal and the other ventral to the line of the closed esophageal wound (Fig. 743). Antibiotics are introduced into the neck wound, which is then sutured to the level of the rubber drains brought up to the posterolateral wall of the esophagus.

In injury to the thoracic esophagus a right or left transpleural approach is employed. Wide mediastinotomy is performed and the esophagus separated from the mediastinal cellular tissue. Rubber loops are brought under the esophagus, and the rupture is sutured by the method described. The tissue of the lung may be used to make the line of the suture more airtight. It is wrapped around the esophagus in the region of the wound and fastened to it with sutures (Fig. 744).

The line of the sutures on the lower thoracic and abdominal portions of the esophagus is made airtight by means of a П -shaped diaphragmatic flap of a fundoplication cuff.

After the wound in the thoracic esophagus is closed, the mediastinal pleura is ot sutured, or very widely spaced sutures are applied to it. Drains are left in the mediastinum and pleural cavity. The wound on the thoracic wall is sutured.

Extirpation of the esophagus (an operation of the Dobromyslov-Torek type) is indicated in cases with extensive injury to the thoracic esophagus and when a long period has elapsed after the trauma occurred.

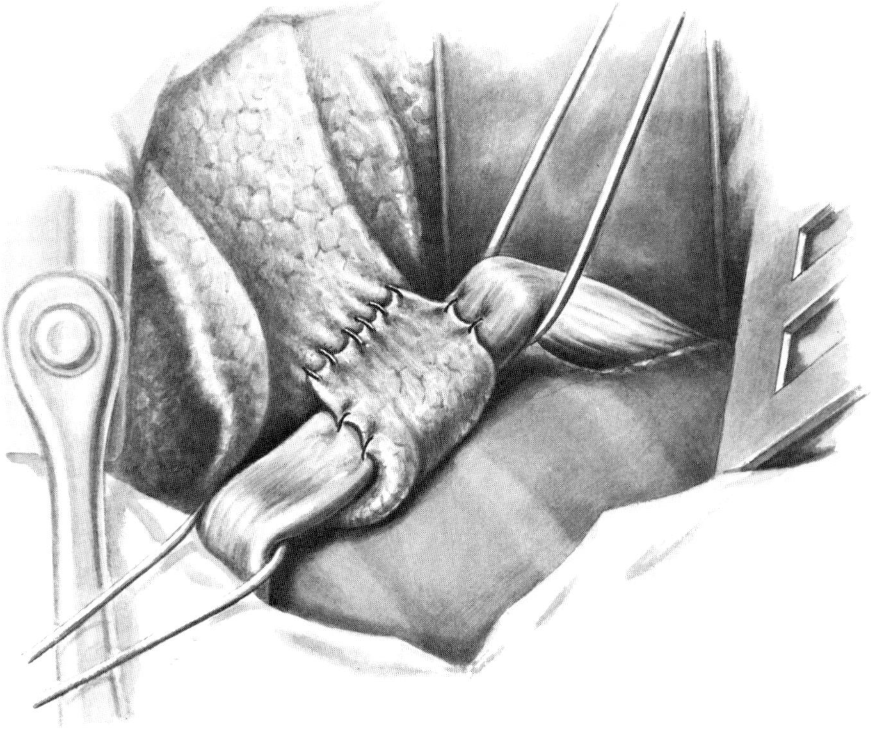

Fig. 744. Line of suture on esophagus is covered with border of lung.

OPERATIONS IN BLEEDING FROM VARICOSE VEINS OF THE ESOPHAGUS AND CARDIA

STITCHING THE VARICES

Approach by means of superior median laparotomy is used. The coronary ligament of the liver is transected. The left hepatic lobe is drawn aside to the right. This can be done only if the cirrhotic liver is relatively small. A drastically enlarged and firm liver that cannot be moved is shifted caudally after the hepatodiaphragmatic ligament has been divided, and the assistant keeps it in this position throughout the subsequent stages of the operation.

The serous and muscular coats of the stomach are cut transversely 3 to 4 cm below the cardia (Fig. 745), and the edges of the wound are slightly drawn apart with a tampon. Each exposed arterial and venous vessel of the gastric submucous coat is stitched through with two silk

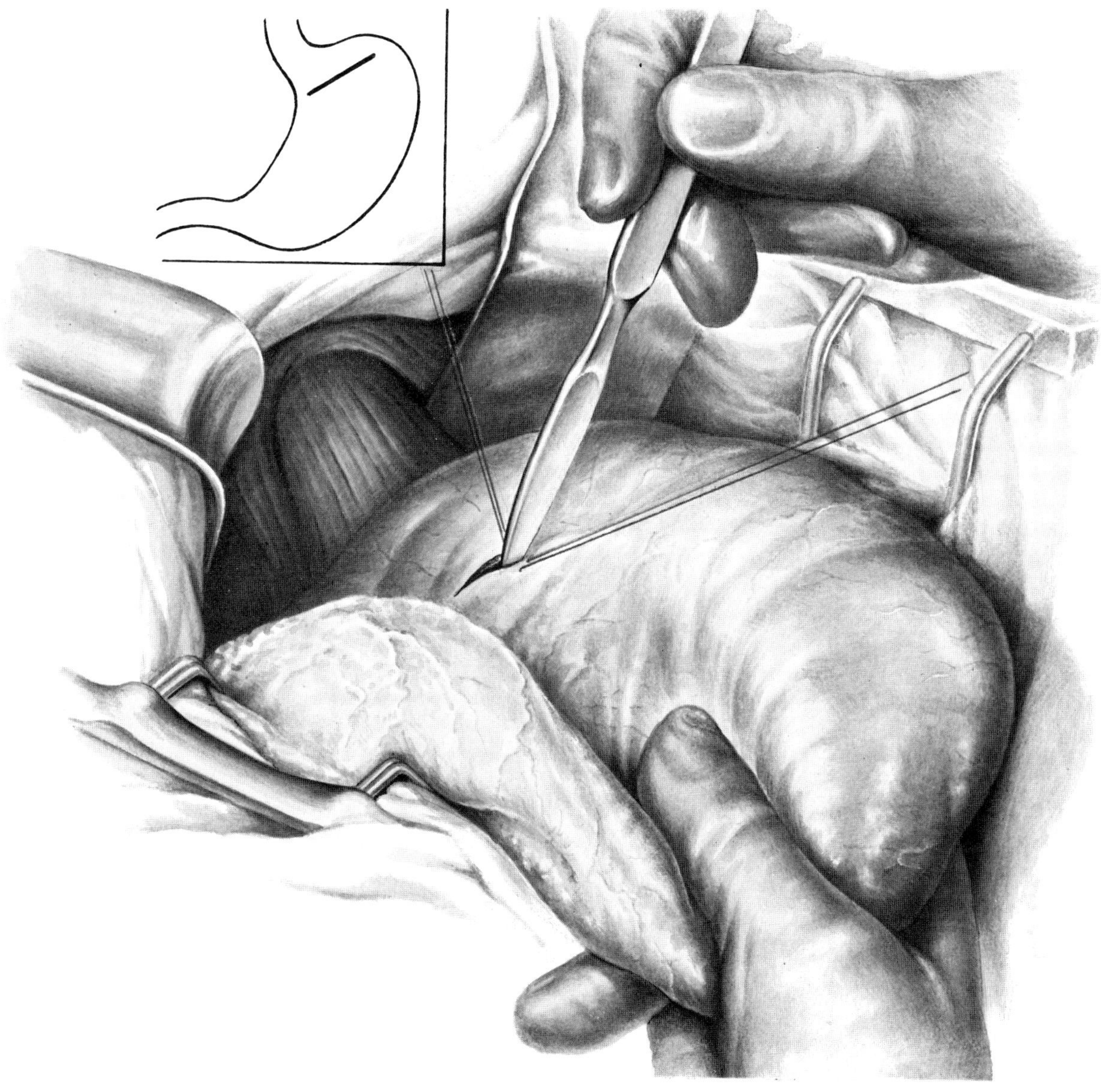

Fig. 745. Incision is made through serous and muscular coats of subcardiac part of stomach.

ligatures and transected between them. The opened cavity of the stomach is emptied by means of an aspirator. Ligatures are stitched through for the additional arrest of bleeding from the edges of the gastric wound. The gastric wound is opened with blunt hooks. Each swollen vein in the region of the cardia and inferior esophagus is stitched through with several separate ligatures passed through the mucous and submucous coats (Fig. 746). On completion of this stage of the operation the gastric wound is closed, first with a continuous catgut blanket hemostatic suture, and then with interrupted seroserous sutures. The abdominal wound is completely sutured layer by layer.

Varicose esophageal veins may also be sutured through a left transthoracic approach in the seventh or eighth intercostal space. In such instances the esophagus is mobilized for a distance of 8 to 10 cm above the diaphragm. The esophagus is opened with a 5 to 6 cm longitudinal incision. The edges of the incision are held by traction sutures, and each trunk of the varicose veins of the esophagus and cardia is stitched through several times at intervals of 1 to 1.5 cm consecutively. The esophageal wound is then closed with a double-row suture. A drain is left in the thoracic cavity, and the wound in the thoracic wall is sutured.

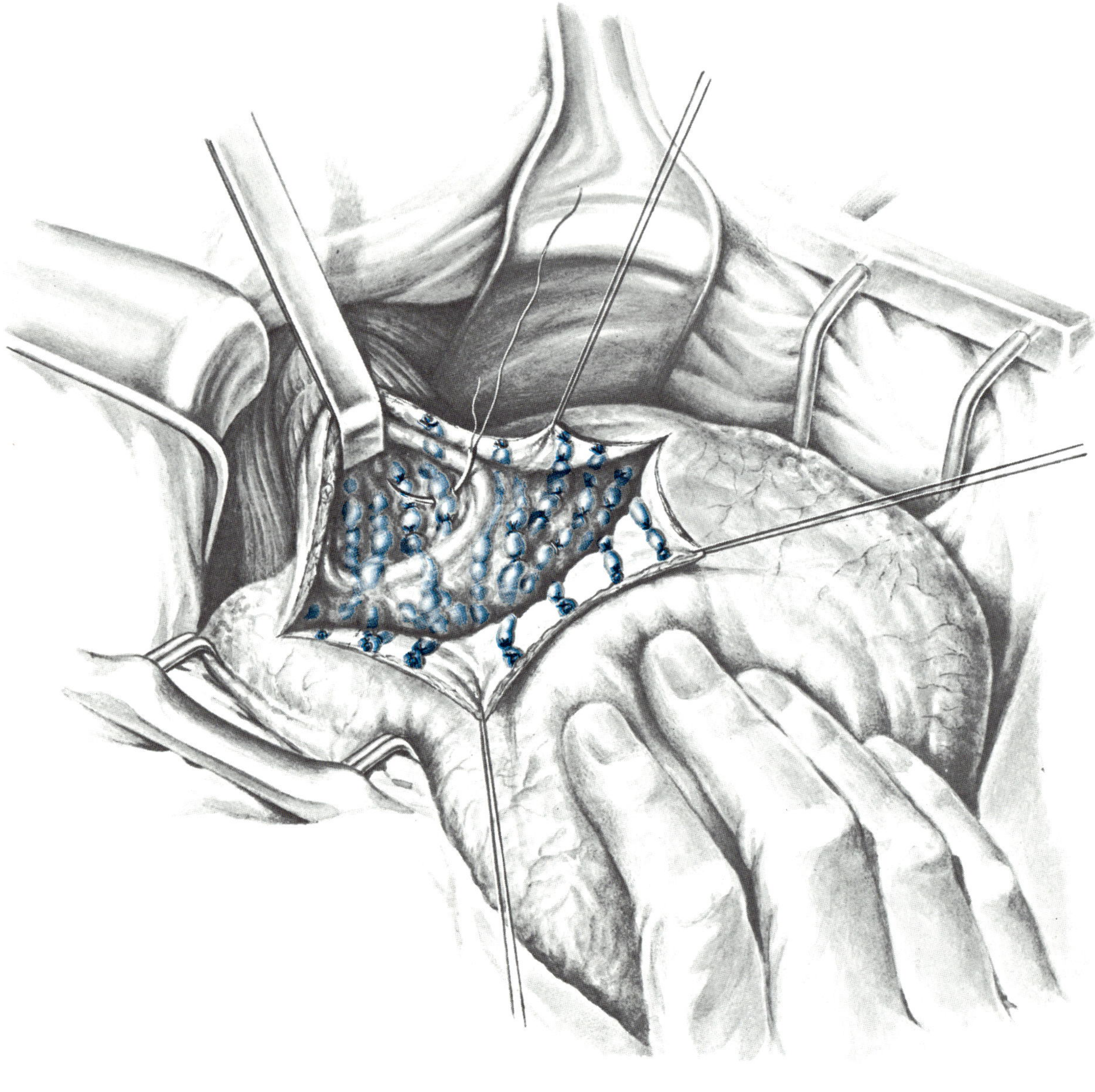

Fig. 746. Varices in proximal portion of stomach and abdominal esophagus are stitched through.

OPERATIONS ON THE DIAPHRAGM

Four approaches are used in surgical interventions on the diaphragm: (1) transabdominal, of which median laparotomy (extended, whenever necessary, below the navel) and paramedian and oblique subcostal incisions are currently most popular; these approaches ensure good access to the anterolateral, posterolateral, and central portions of the diaphragm; (2) transthoracic, among which wide intercostal incisions are employed most commonly; an incision in the seventh or eighth intercostal space (particularly with transection of the costal arch) provides sufficient freedom for operating on all the parts of the corresponding half of the diaphragm; with the pathological process localized in the lateral part of the dome, however, incision in the ninth intercostal space is most convenient; (3) thoracoabdominal approaches of the type of thoracophrenolaparotomy have no substantial advantage over a wide intercostal approach with division of the costal arch and are now hardly used due to their marked traumatic character; (4) combined approaches; if it is found that the entire operation cannot be performed through the laparotomy applied, the wound in the abdominal wall is sutured after completion of interabdominal manipulations and thoracotomy is undertaken.

In various transphrenic interventions, as in operations on the diaphragm, it is desirable to take into account the routes followed by the branches of the phrenic nerve. Fig. 747 schematically represents the rational (with due consideration for the peculiarities of innervation) incisions of the diaphragm recommended by Merendino and coauthors (1956).

Before the diaphragm is cut, it is held with two clamps, between which a small incision is made with scissors and then extended in the required direction. All bleeding vessels are clamped with hemostatic forceps and sutured.

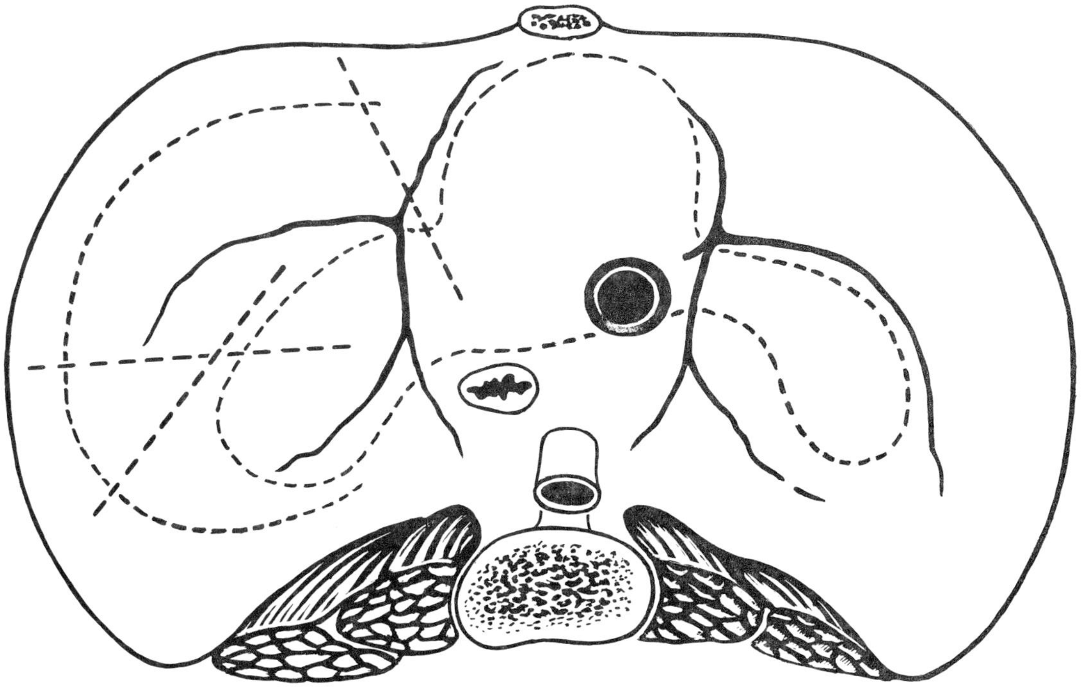

Fig. 747. Schema of incisions of diaphragm. (After Merendino et al., 1956.)

CLOSURE OF DIAPHRAGMATIC WOUNDS

Isolated injuries to the diaphragm are rare; that is why the operative approach is determined by the concomitant damage to the thoracic or abdominal organs. Laparotomy is undertaken when there are clinical signs of injury to the abdominal organs. In predominance of symptoms of damage to the thoracic organs an incision in the seventh or eighth intercostal space is made.

Stab or incised wounds in the diaphragm are closed with interrupted sutures placed 0.5 to 1.0 cm from each other. In extensive wounds and crushing of the diaphragm, nonviable tissues are excised. If a large defect of the diaphragm results, several traction sutures are applied to its edges for drawing them together, thus making its repair easier (Fig. 748).

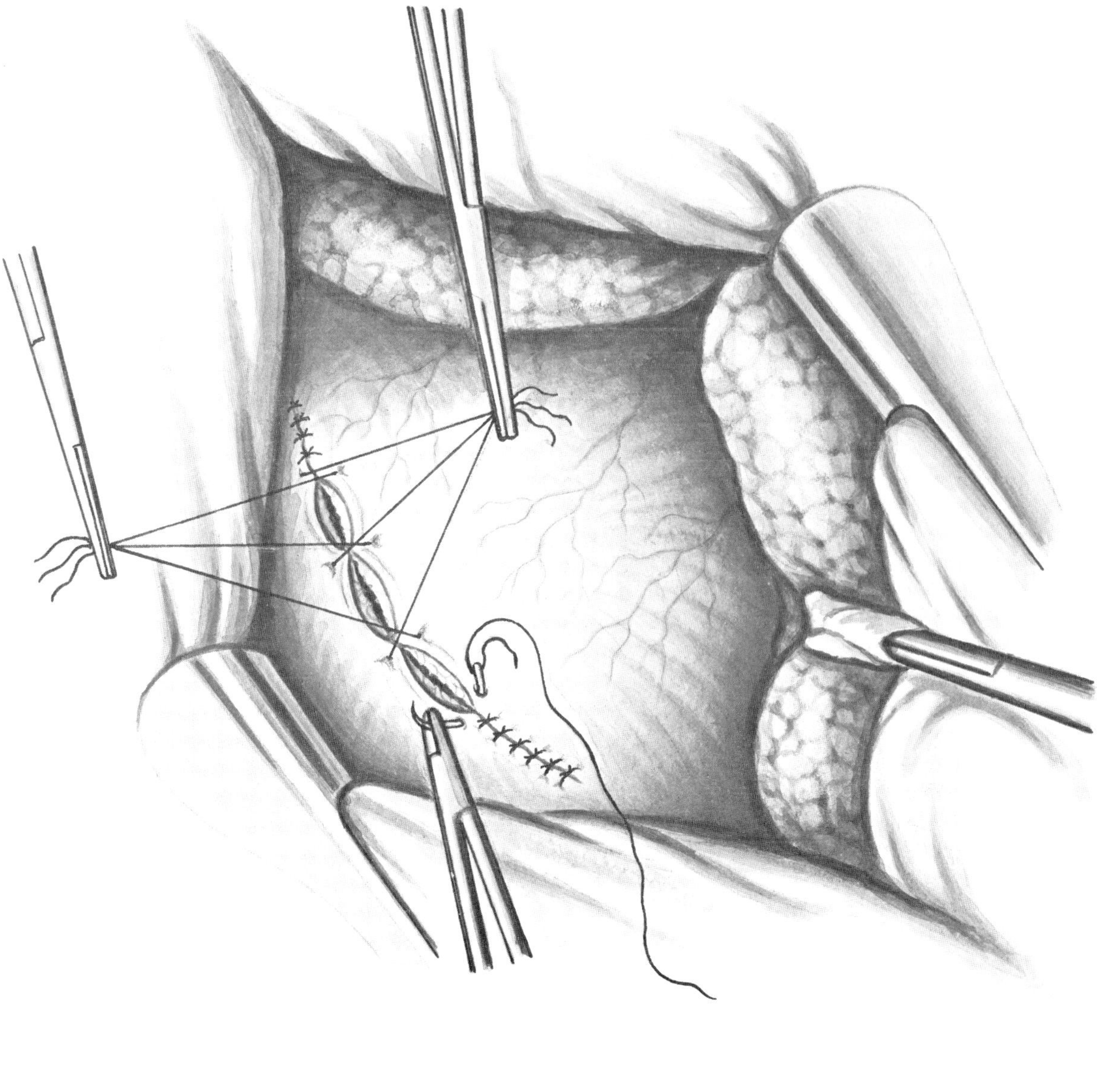

Fig. 748. Diaphragmatic wound is closed with sutures while its edges are brought together by means of traction sutures.

REMOVAL OF TUMORS AND CYSTS OF THE DIAPHRAGM

Primary isolated tumors and cysts of the diaphragm are rare occurrences. Involvement of the diaphragm is usually of secondary character, with the tumors or cysts spreading to it from neighboring organs. Benign tumors and cysts of the diaphragm are resected through a transthoracic intercostal approach by enucleation or economical excision with small areas of diaphragmatic tissue left on the removed structures (Fig. 749). The wound is closed with interrupted sutures (Fig. 750). In malignant lesions the diaphragm is extensively resected with removal of healthy tissues. In such cases the wound may be closed by the above described manipulation with the application of traction sutures. In large lesions of the diaphragm, alloplastic closure of the defect may be necessary (see below).

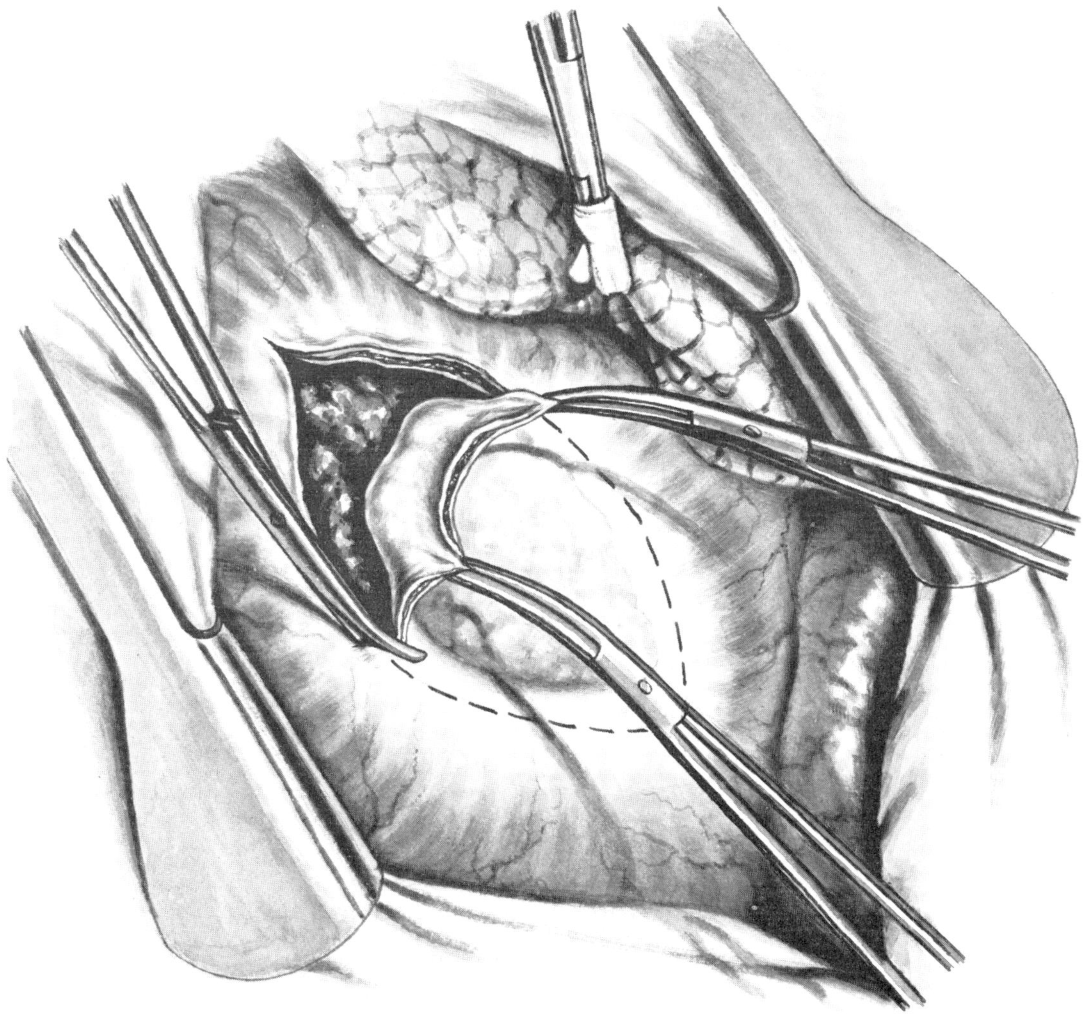

Fig. 749. Resection of new growth of diaphragm.

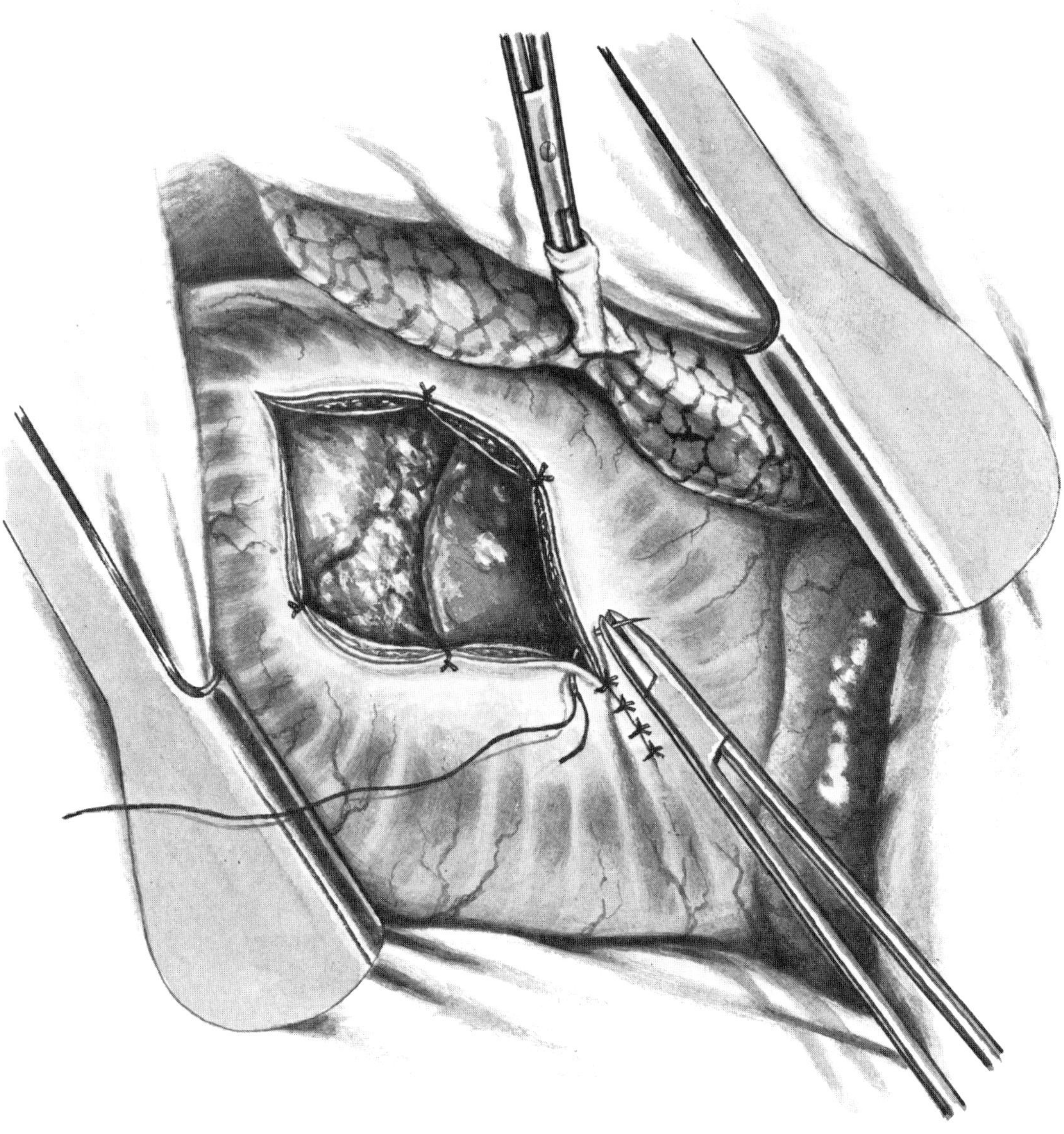

Fig. 750. Defect formed in diaphragm after resection of new growth is sutured.

PLASTIC SURGERY IN TRAUMATIC DIAPHRAGMATIC HERNIAS

In traumatic diaphragmatic hernias the defect may be localized in any part of the diaphgram. An operative approach through the seventh or eighth intercostal space is applied, with transection of the costal arch whenever necessary. Traumatic hernias are usually attended with more or less severe adhesions between the abdominal organs and the diaphragm, the inner surface of the thoracic wall, and the pericardium and lungs; these adhesions are separated by the sharp and blunt techniques. Then the margins of the hernial aperture are freed by cutting the adhesions that had prolapsed with the organs (Fig. 751). After reduction of the abdominal

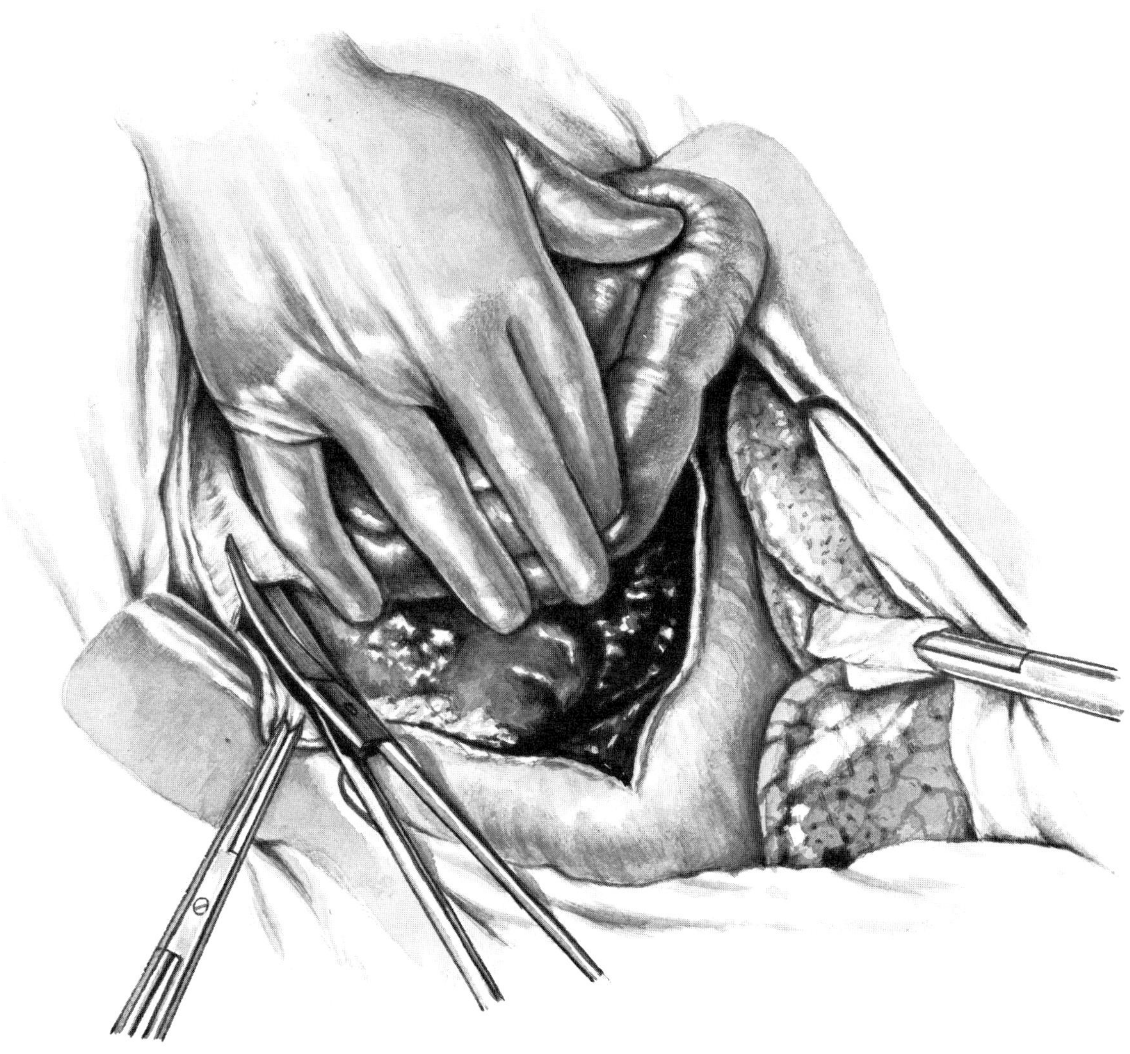

Fig. 751. Separation of adhesions in region of hernial aperture.

organs, interrupted Halsted sutures are applied to the edges of the diaphragmatic defect (Fig. 752) so that they will be duplicated when the threads are tied, for which purpose a second row of interrupted sutures is placed (Fig. 753).

In some cases with total rupture of the diaphragm, its edges become fused to the thoracic wall and the pericardium. This makes it seem that there is no diaphragmatic dome at all. In such instances the tissue of the diaphragm may be drastically thin. The following manipulation may be performed then: a plate of alloplastic material is stitched with interrupted sutures to healthy portions of the diaphragm at a considerable distance from the margins of the defect. After that, sutures are applied to the edges of the defect, passing the threads through the alloplastic prosthesis too (Figs. 754 and 755).

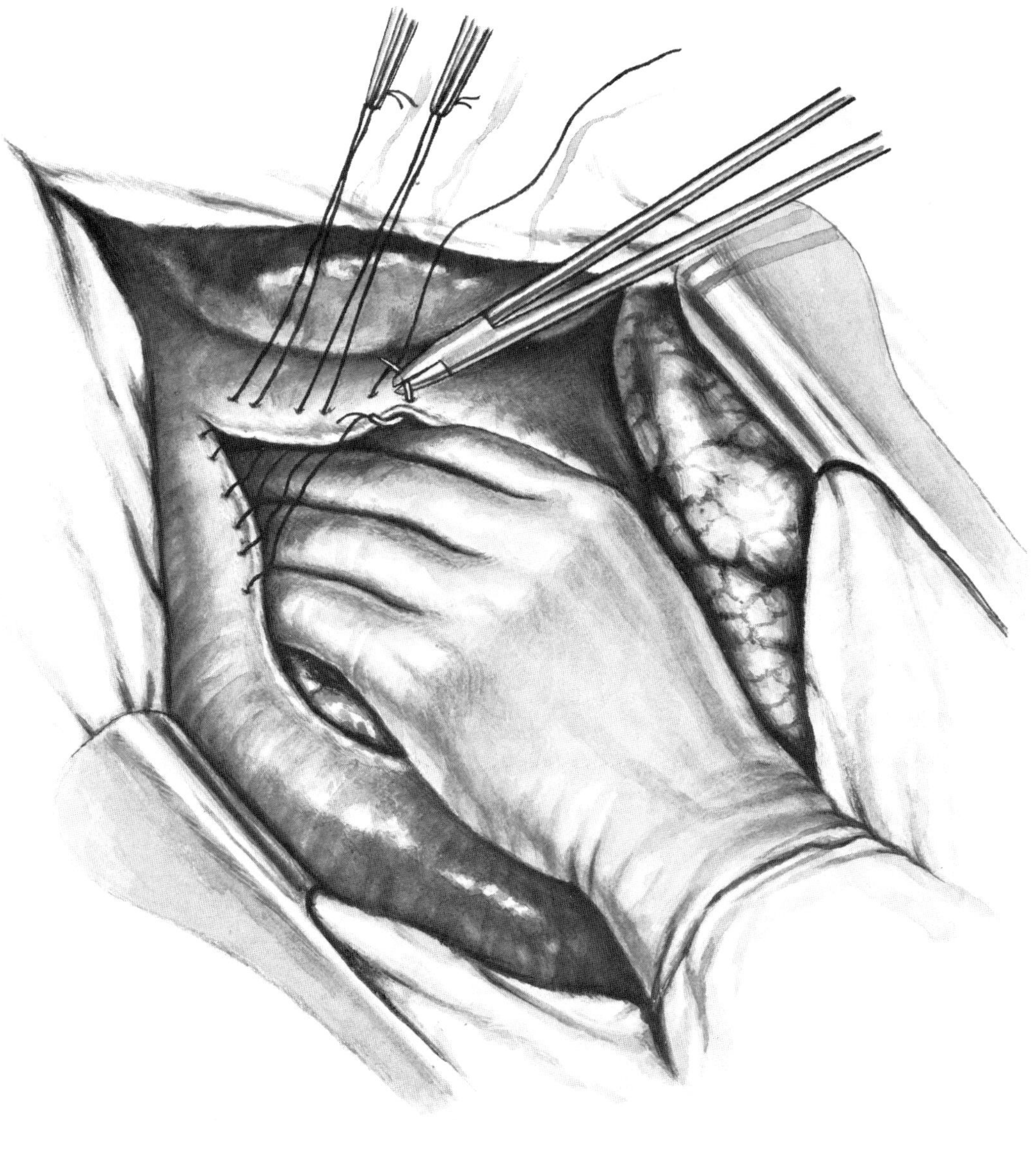

Fig. 752. Closure of hernial aperture with Halsted sutures.

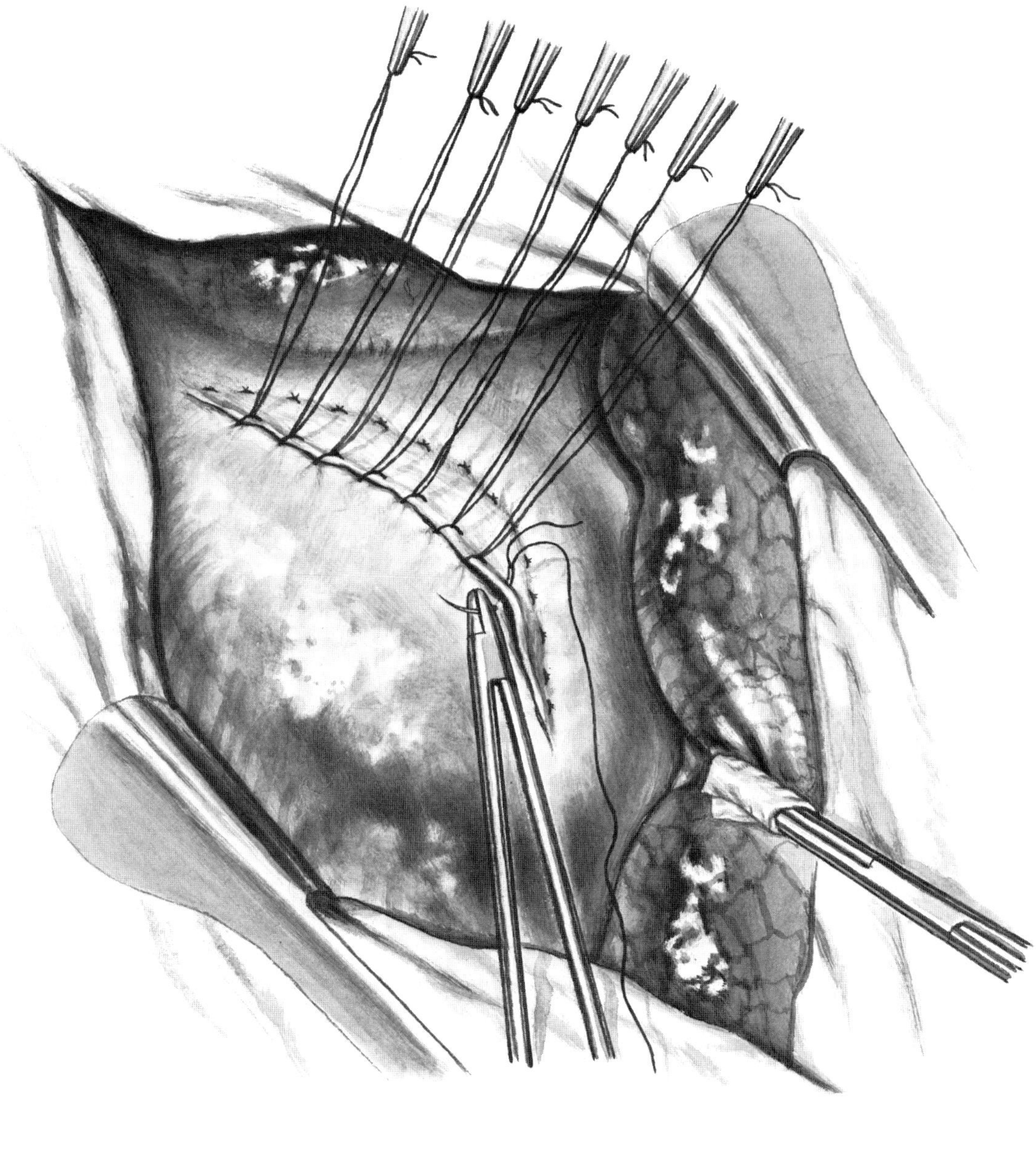

Fig. 753. Duplication of diaphragmatic edges.

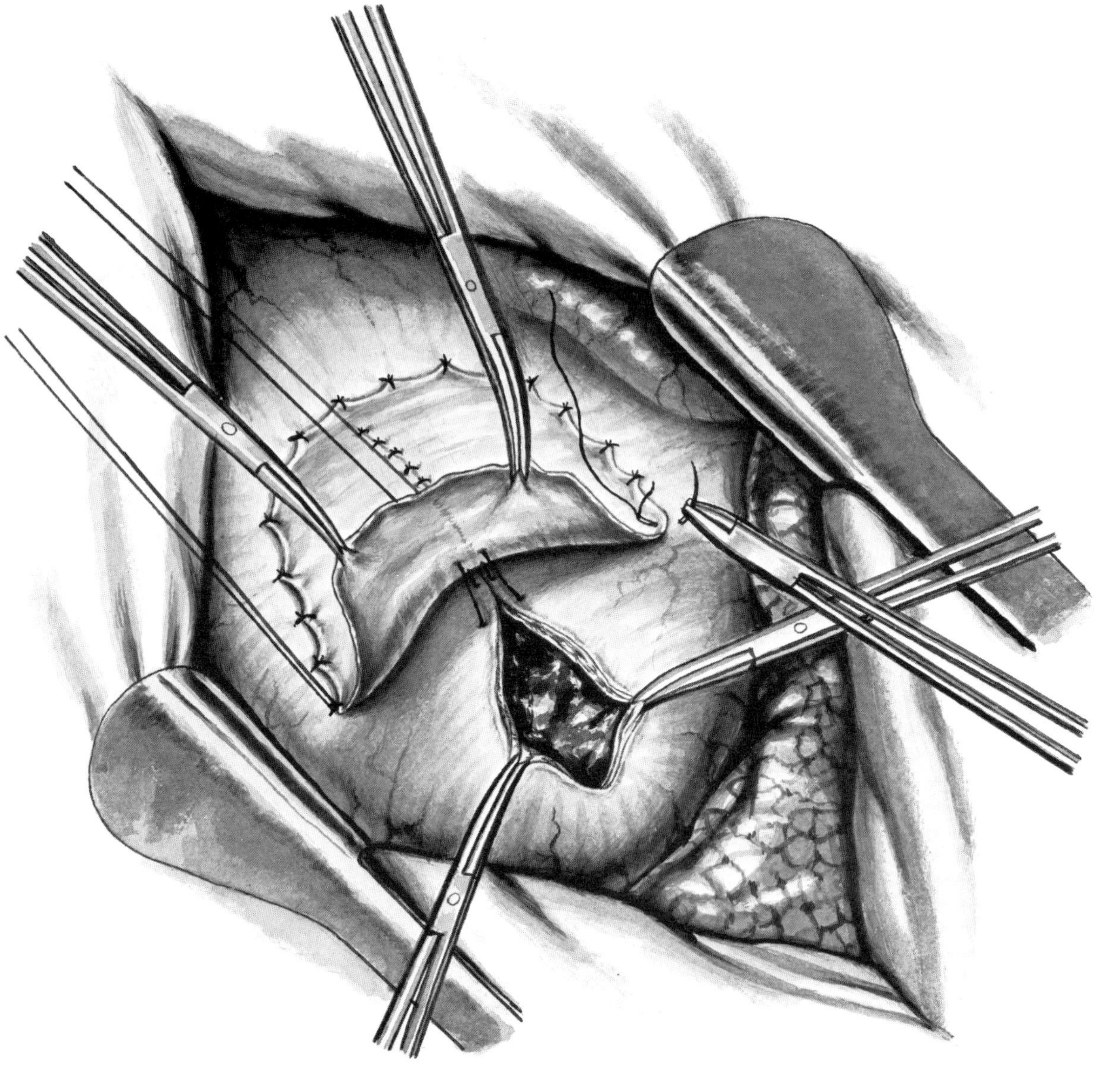

Fig. 754. Sutires applied to diaphragm are reinforced with alloplastic prosthesis.

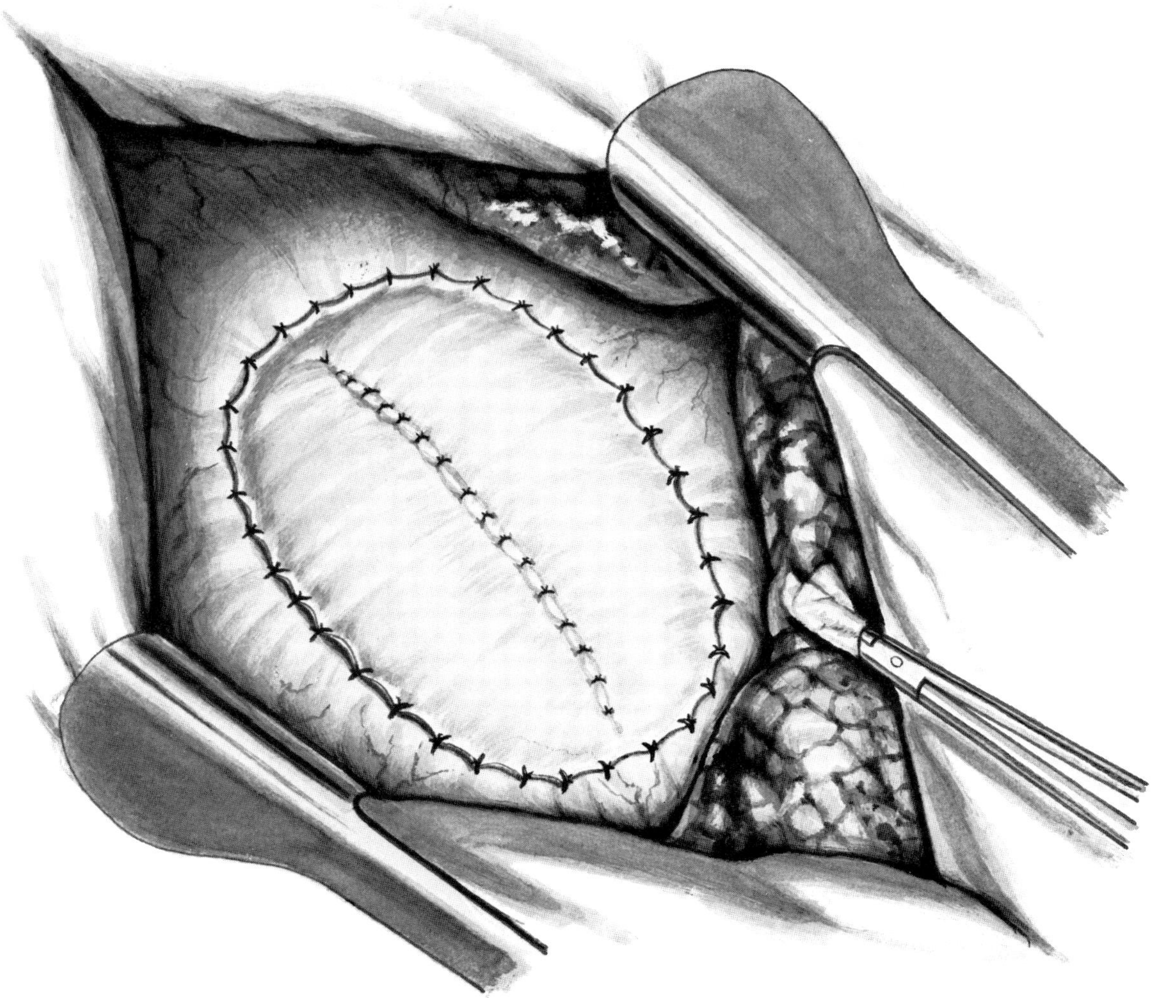

Fig. 755. Plastic surgery of diaphragm with alloplastic prosthesis is completed.

PLASTIC SURGERY IN CONGENITAL FALSE DIAPHRAGMATIC HERNIAS (DEFECTS)

Congential diaphragmatic pseudohernias, lacking a hernial sac, are subdivided into aplasia and partial defects in the diaphragm (Fig. 756). The choice of the operative approach is determined by the location and size of the defect. On newborn infants and infants under 12 months the operation is usually performed through superior median laparotomy or an oblique subcostal incision. These approaches are also used in adults in posterolateral cleft defects. The transpleural approach is employed in defects on the right side and in the absence of the whole dome when alloplastic material has to be used for reconstructing the diaphragm.

Adhesions between the prolapsed organs and the hernial aperture often have to be separated in adults

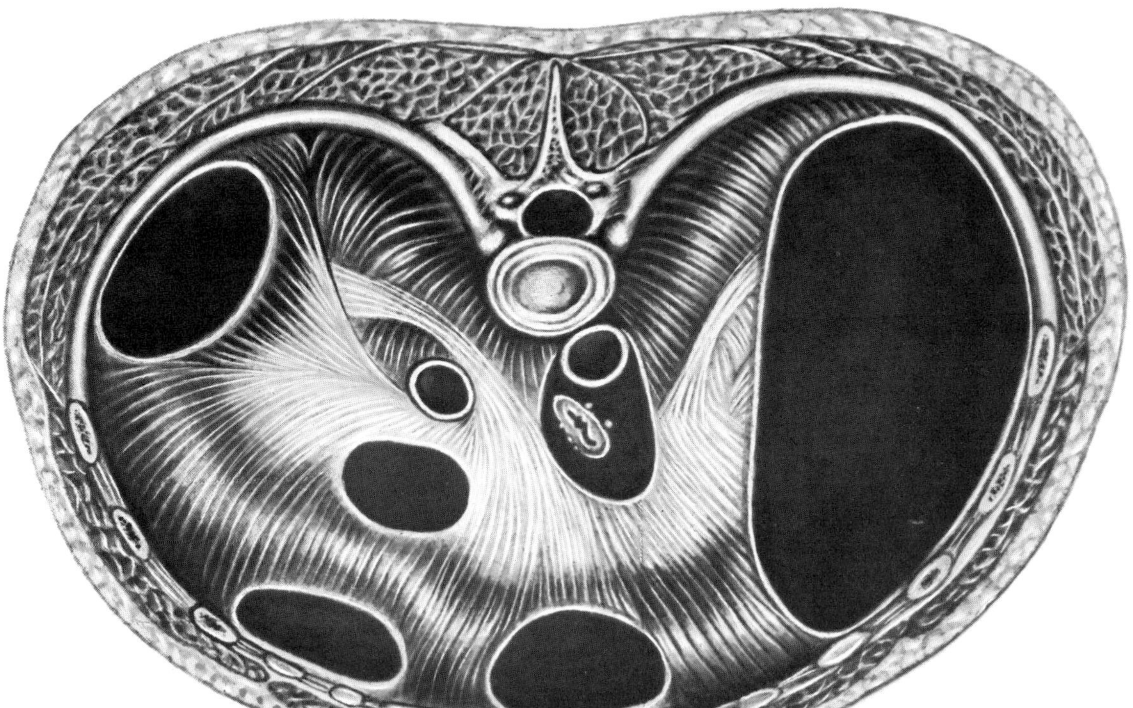

Fig. 756. Congenital defects in diaphragm.

(Fig. 757). If it is difficult to reduce the herniated abdominal organs through a narrow defect, the diaphragm is partly cut and the wound widened with hooks. With the organs brought back into the abdominal cavity, the defect is sutured with duplication of the edges (Fig. 758). A catheter is left between the layers of the diaphragm for continued aspiration (Fig. 759).

In a large anterolateral or posterolateral diaphragmatic defect, which is difficult to suture from the abdomen, a transthoracic approach is used. When alloplasty is necessary, the material is sutured to the diaphragm with interrupted sutures placed at some distance from the edge of the defect (Fig. 760). When the use of alloplastic materials may be avoided, the defect should be repaired only with the patient's own tissues.

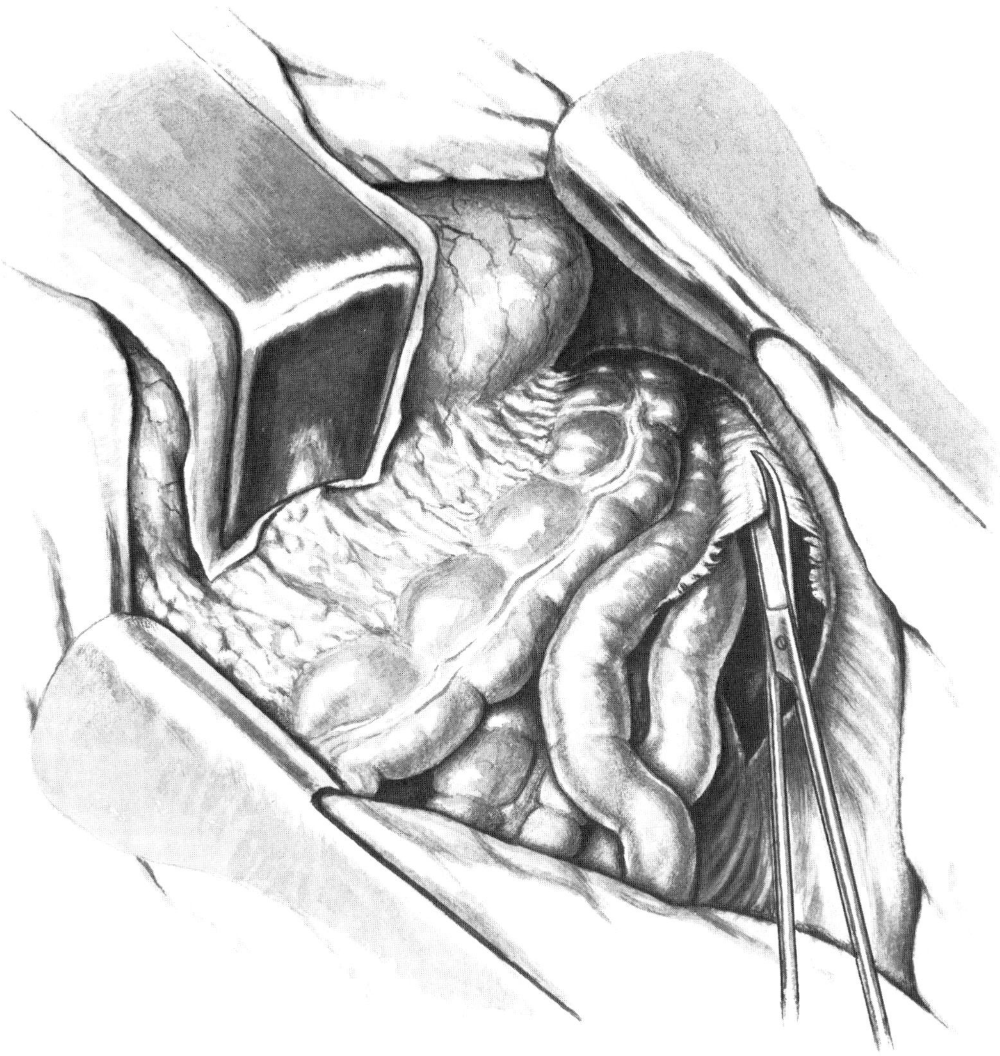

Fig. 757. Separation of adhesions between abdominal organs and hernial aperture.

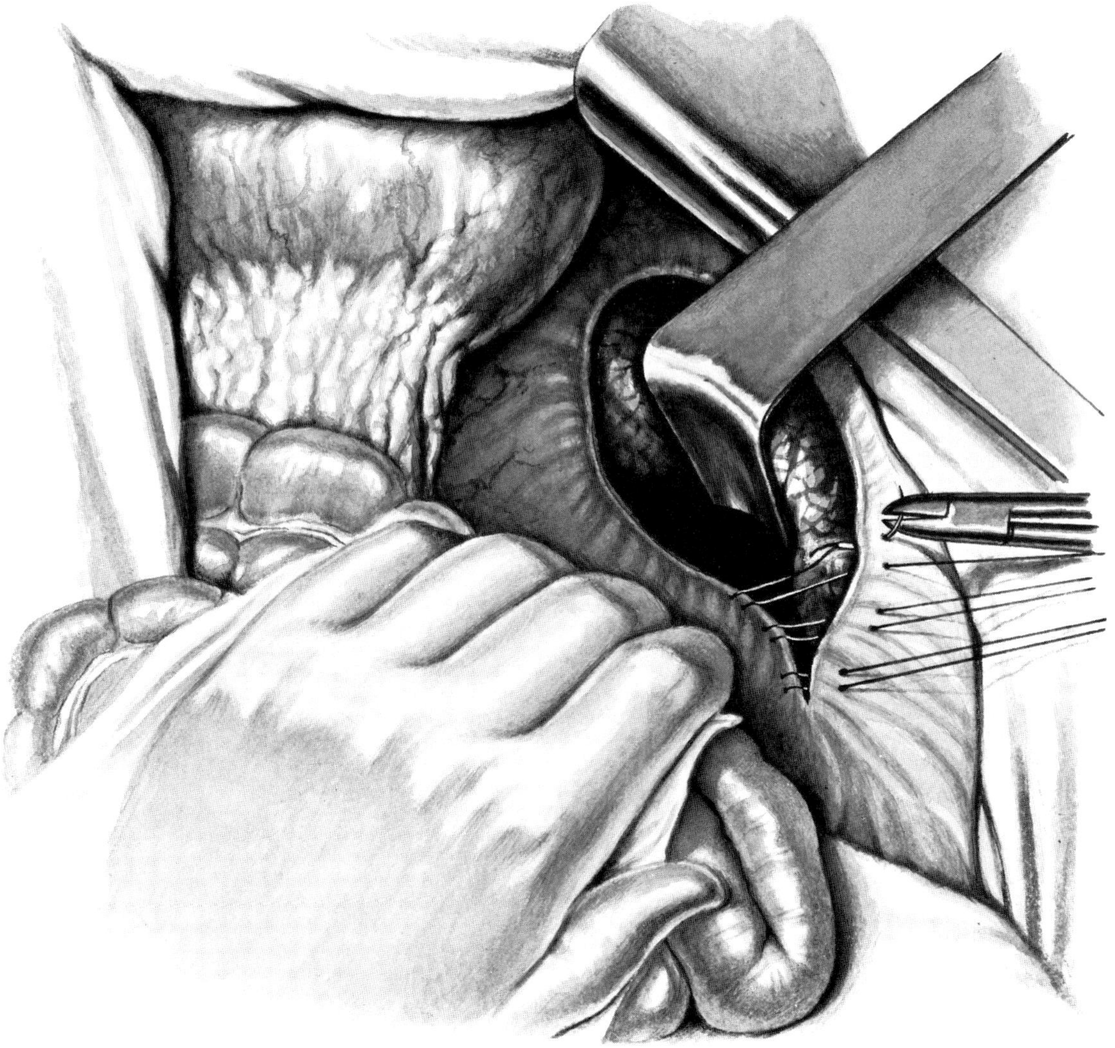

Fig. 758. Defect in diaphragm is closed with Halsted sutures.

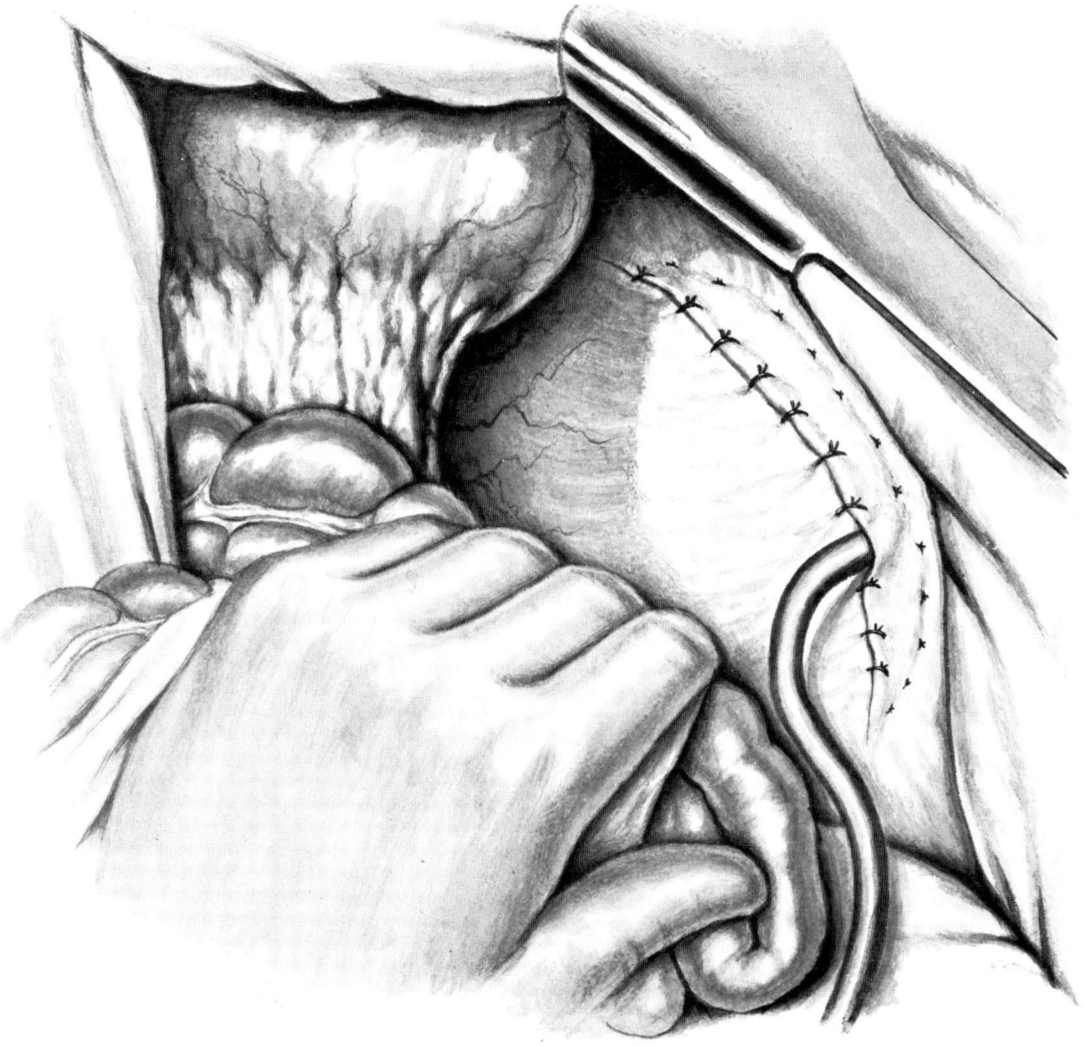

Fig. 759. Catheter is left between layers of diaphragm.

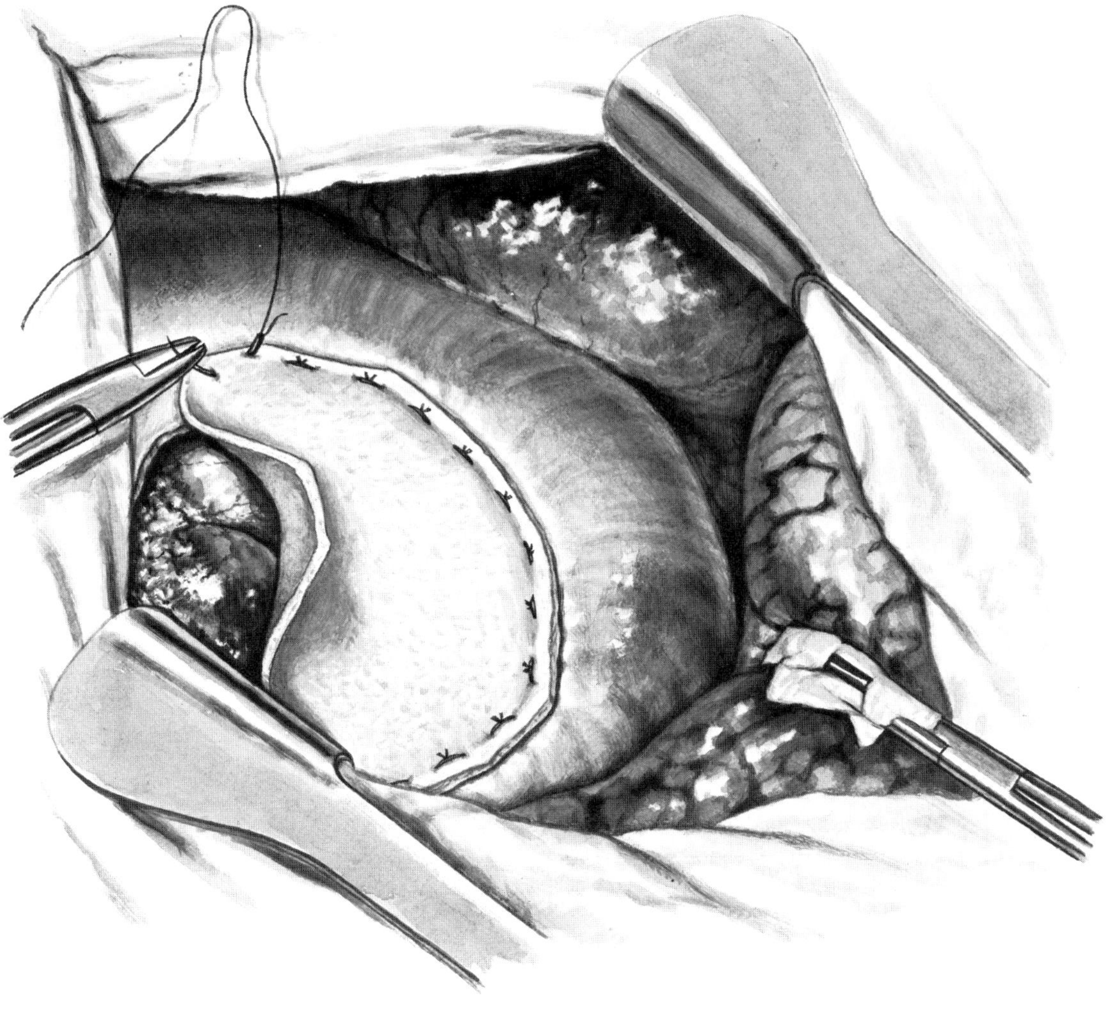

Fig. 760. Large defect in diaphragm is repaired with alloplastic material.

PLASTIC SURGERY IN PARASTERNAL (RETROSTERNAL AND RETROCOSTOSTERNAL) DIAPHRAGMATIC HERNIAS

In retrosternal and retrocostosternal hernias the transperitoneal approach is least traumatic and most convenient. Medial laparotomy is performed. The contents of the hernial sac are reduced into the abdominal cavity (Fig. 761). The hernial sac is grasped from inside with several forceps and inverted into the abdominal cavity. Then the sac is cut away at the level of the hernial aperture (Fig. 762). A large sac firmly fastened in the thoracic cavity need not be removed.

The hernial aperture is closed with interrupted Halsted sutures (Figs. 763 and 764). If there are no muscular tissues in the anterior margin of the aperture, the diaphragm is stitched to the periosteum of the posterior sternal surface or to the perichondrium of the adjacent ribs.

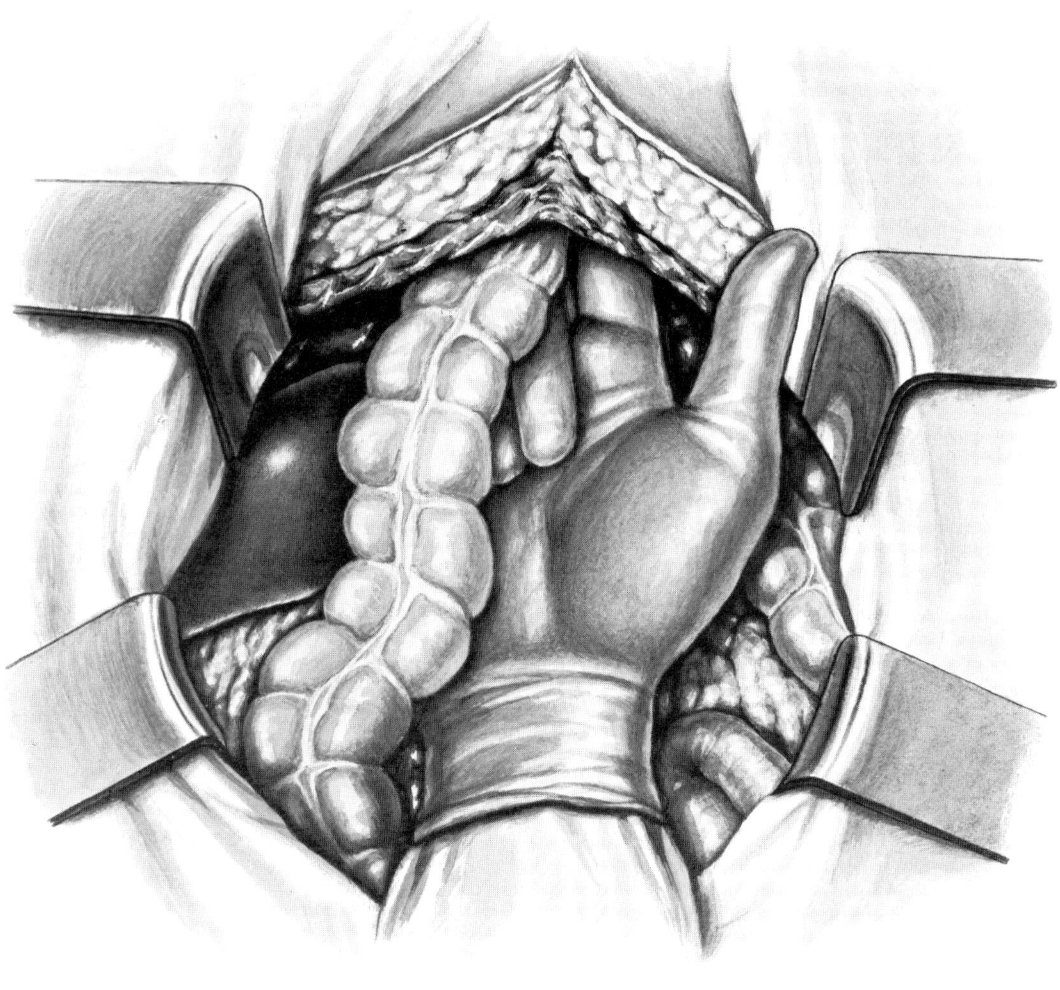

Fig. 761. Reduction of herniated structures into abdominal cavity.

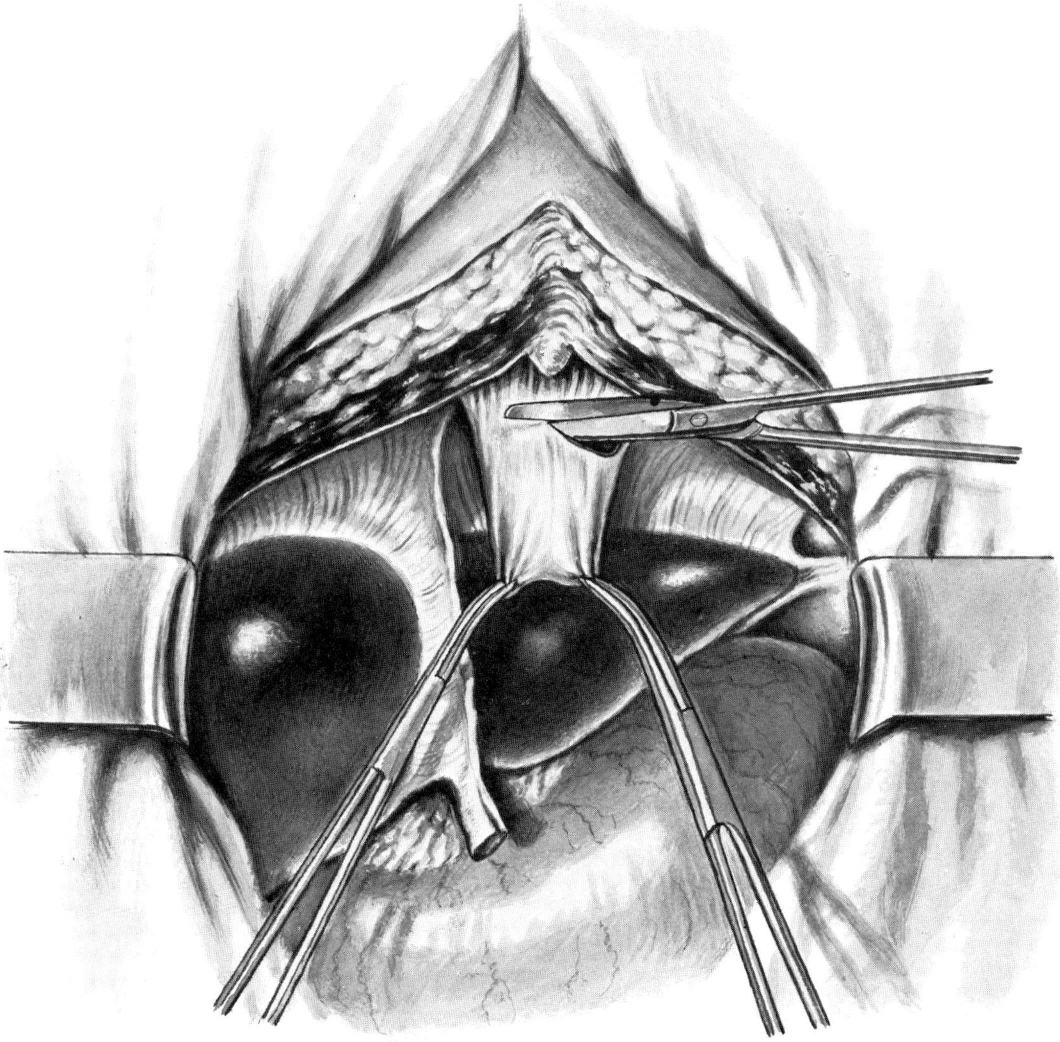

Fig. 762. Hernial sac, which has been turned inside out, is cut away.

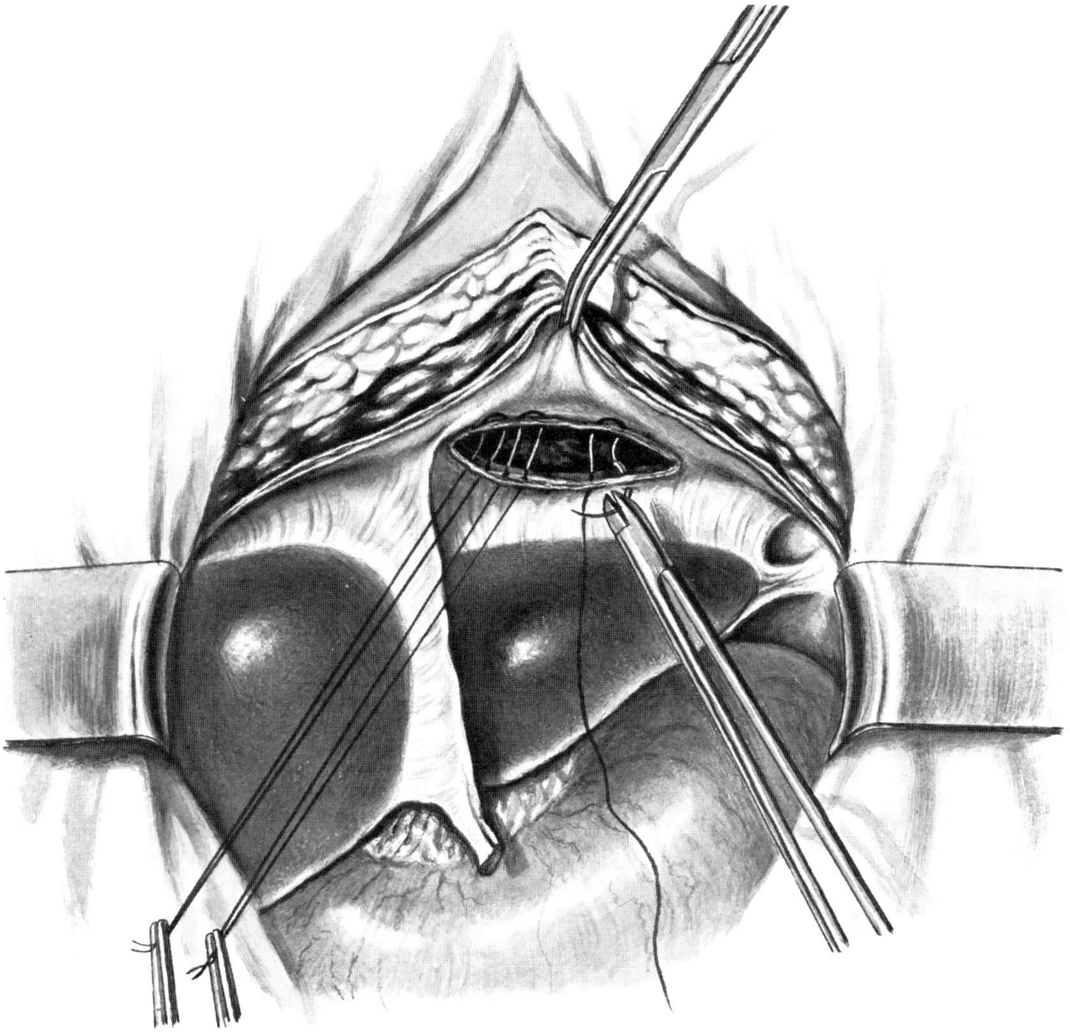

Fig. 763. Application of Halsted sutures to hernial aperture.

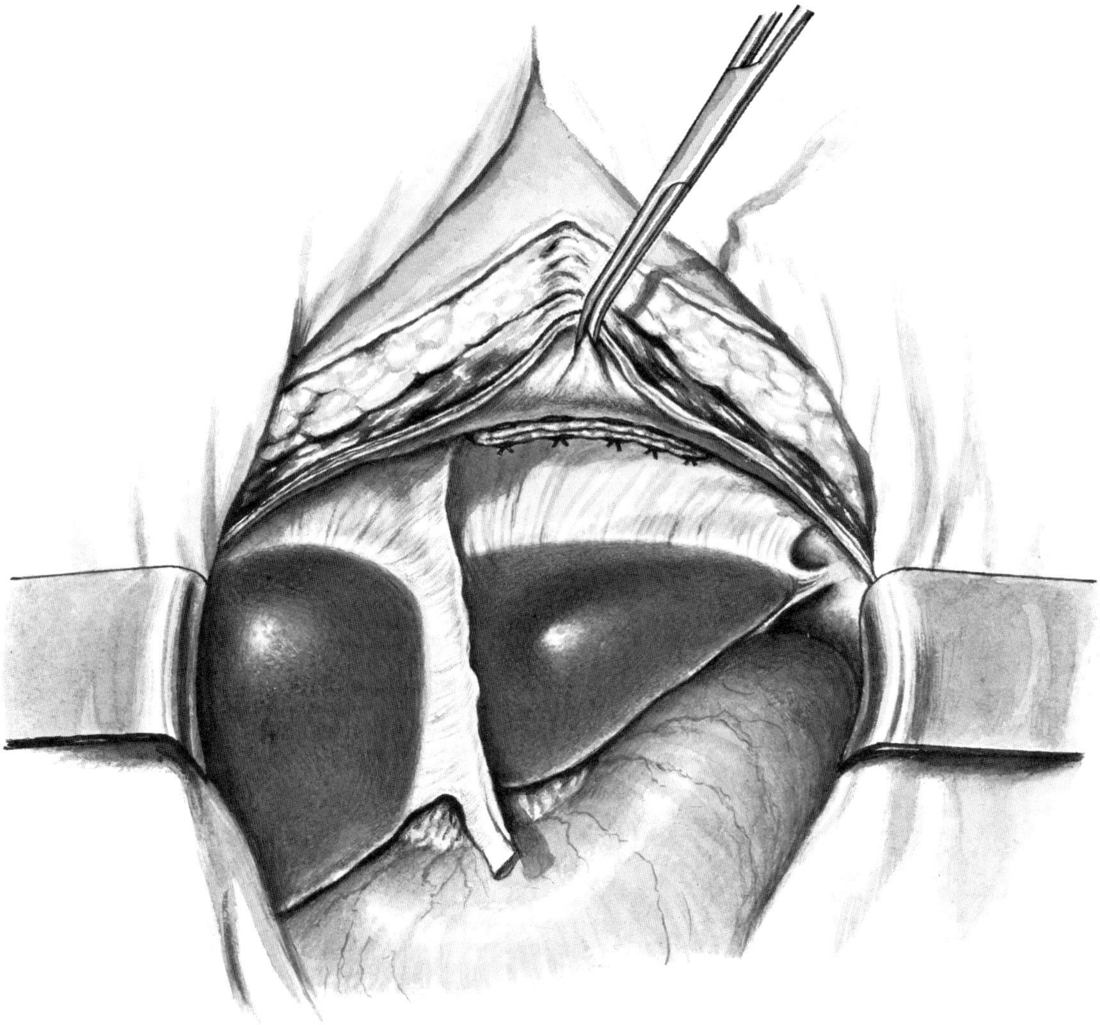

Fig. 764. Hernial aperture is closed with sutures.

PLASTIC SURGERY IN STRANGULATED DIAPHRAGMATIC HERNIAS

The operative approach and the method of surgical intervention are determined by the character and the location of the hernia. The transthoracic approach is commonly used (with the exception of operations for a parasternal hernia). The greater omentom, the stomach, and an intestinal loop may be strangulated in a diaphragmatic hernia (Fig. 765). A cut must be made in the hernial aperture to free the strangulated organs. In severe swelling of the strangulating ring the cut is made along Kocher's probe inserted into the ring to avoid injuring the adjacent organs (Fig. 766). If the probe cannot be inserted, the dome of the diaphragm is first cut, and the incision is then extended to the hernial aperture. The viable strangulated organs are reduced into the abdominal cavity. They are resected if they have suffered irreparable changes. The defect in the diaphragm is closed with interrupted sutures, preferably with duplication of the edges as it is commonly done in nonstrangulated diaphragmatic hernias.

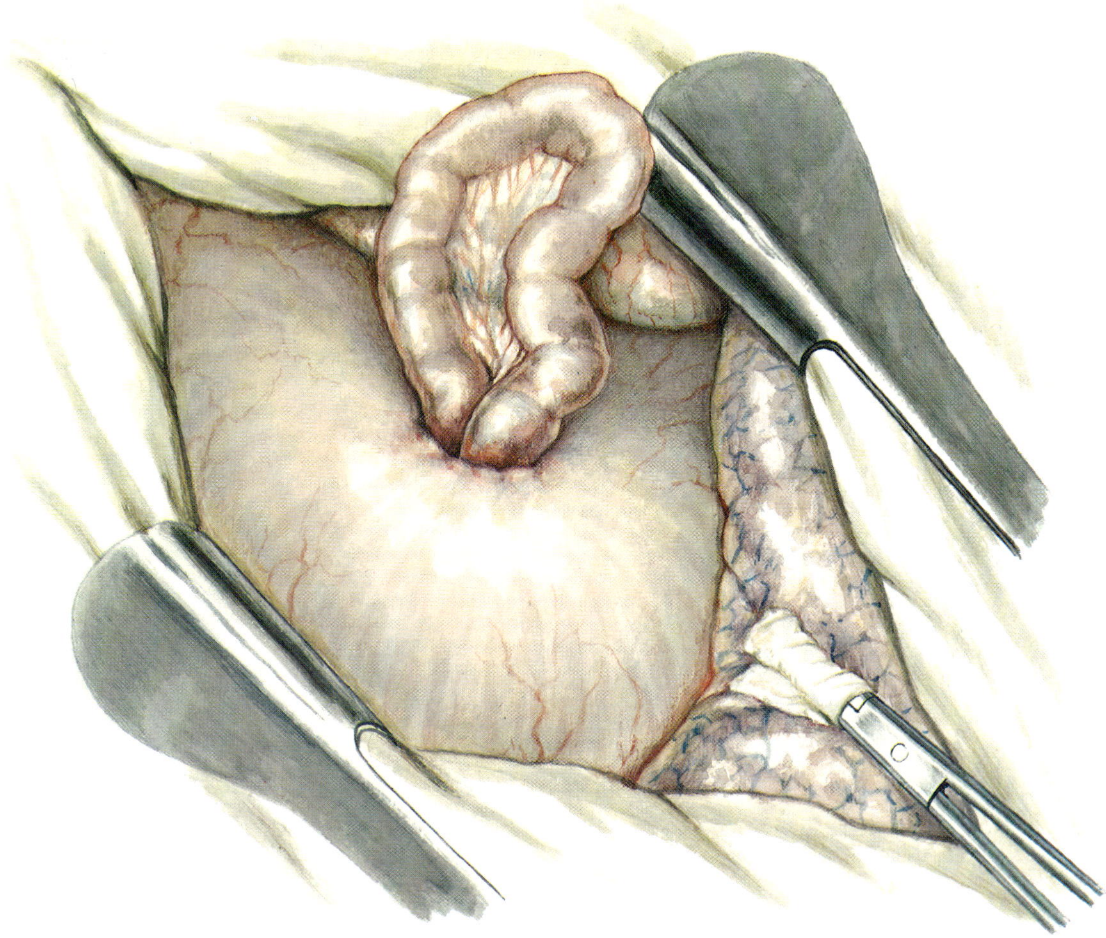

Fig. 765. Strangulated false diaphragmatic hernia on left side.

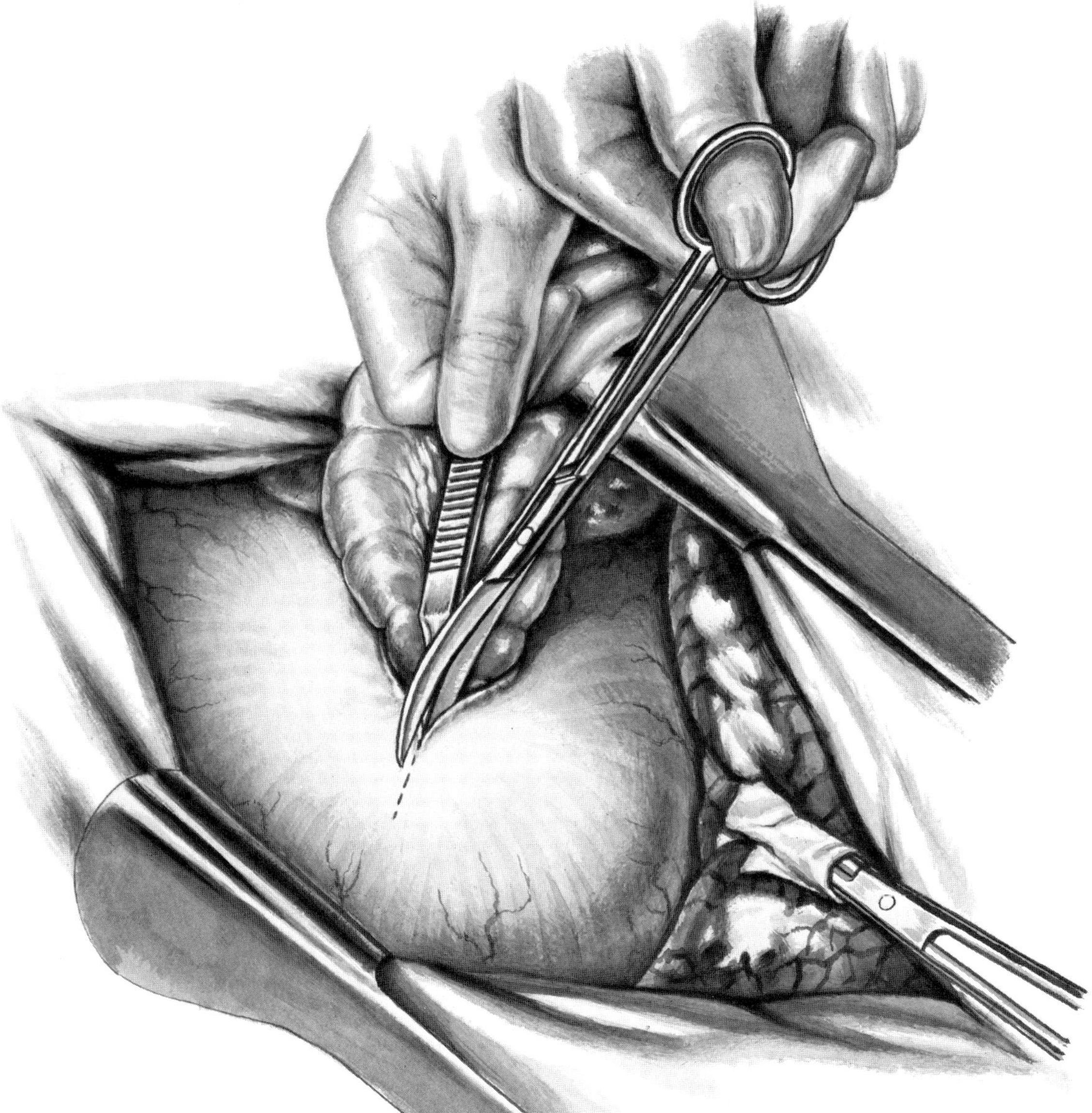

Fig. 766. Strangulating ring is cut.

PLASTIC SURGERY IN RELAXATION OF DIAPHRAGM

Subtotal or localized relaxation of the left diaphragmatic dome with retained muscles along its periphery may be managed by the method of phrenicoplication. Thoracotomy is conducted in the left eighth intercostal space. The lung is drawn aside, and the elevated thinned-out diaphragmatic dome is exposed. It is grasped by the hand so that a wide fold is formed. Pressing back the abdominal organs the surgeon gradually takes firm hold of the entire defective part of the diaphragm. The edges of the fold are held with two fenestrated clamps. The

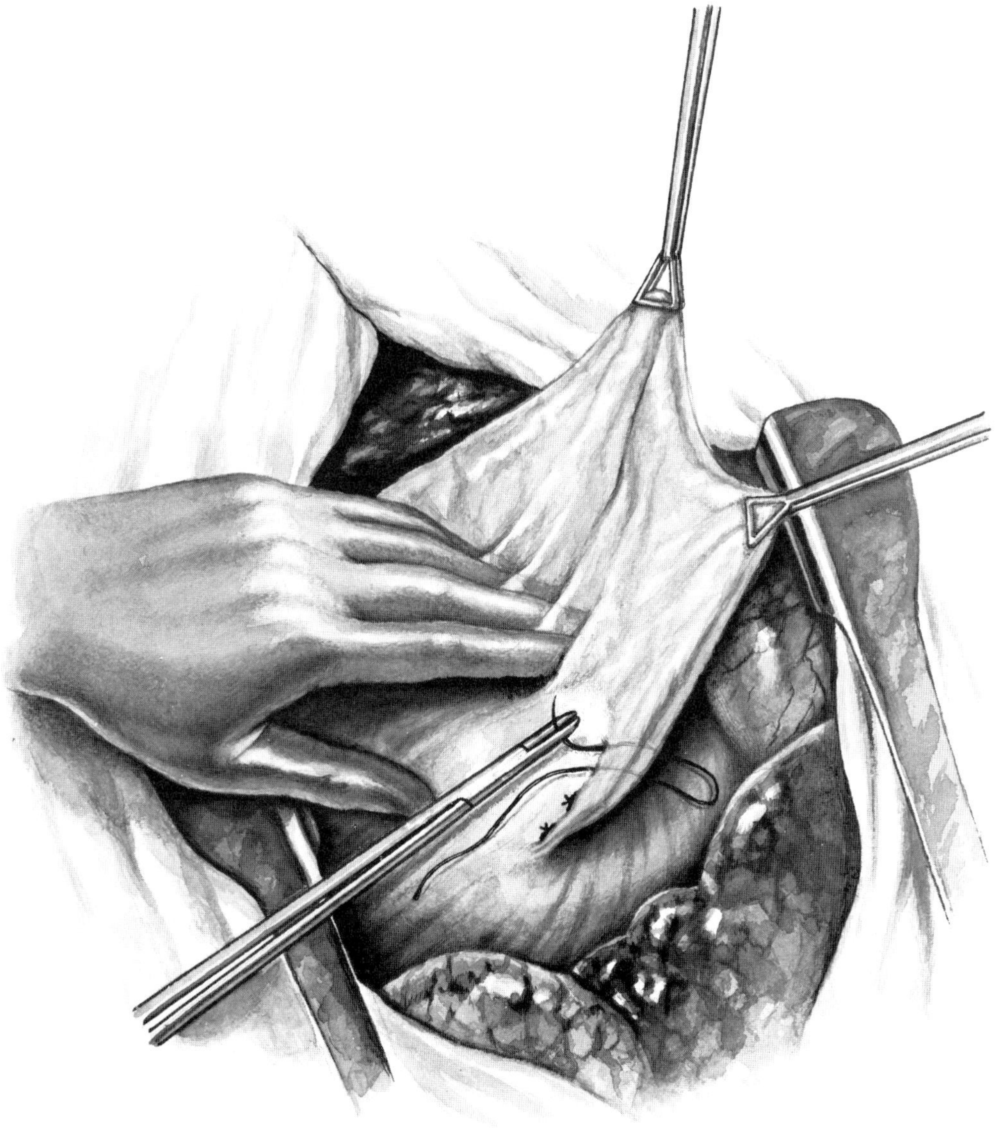

Fig. 767. Base of fold of relaxed diaphragm is stitched with Halsted sutures.

surgeon pushes back the base of the fold with his left hand and stitches it with Halsted sutures (Fig. 767) along its whole length. The duplicated portion of the diaphragm thus formed is folded over to cover the defective part of the diaphragm and sutured to the intact muscle fibers (Fig. 768).

During phrenicoplication special care should be taken to avoid passing the thread through the abdominal organs when the fold is stitched and sutured to the diaphragm. This becomes a real danger if the abdominal organs are fused with the diaphragm. In such cases the diaphragm is cut lengthwise to form two flaps, a lateral and a medial (Fig. 769). The edge of the lateral flap is stitched with interrupted sutures to the base of the medial flap (Fig. 770). The medial flap is then placed over the lateral one as a duplication and fastened to the diaphragm with interrupted sutures (Fig. 771).

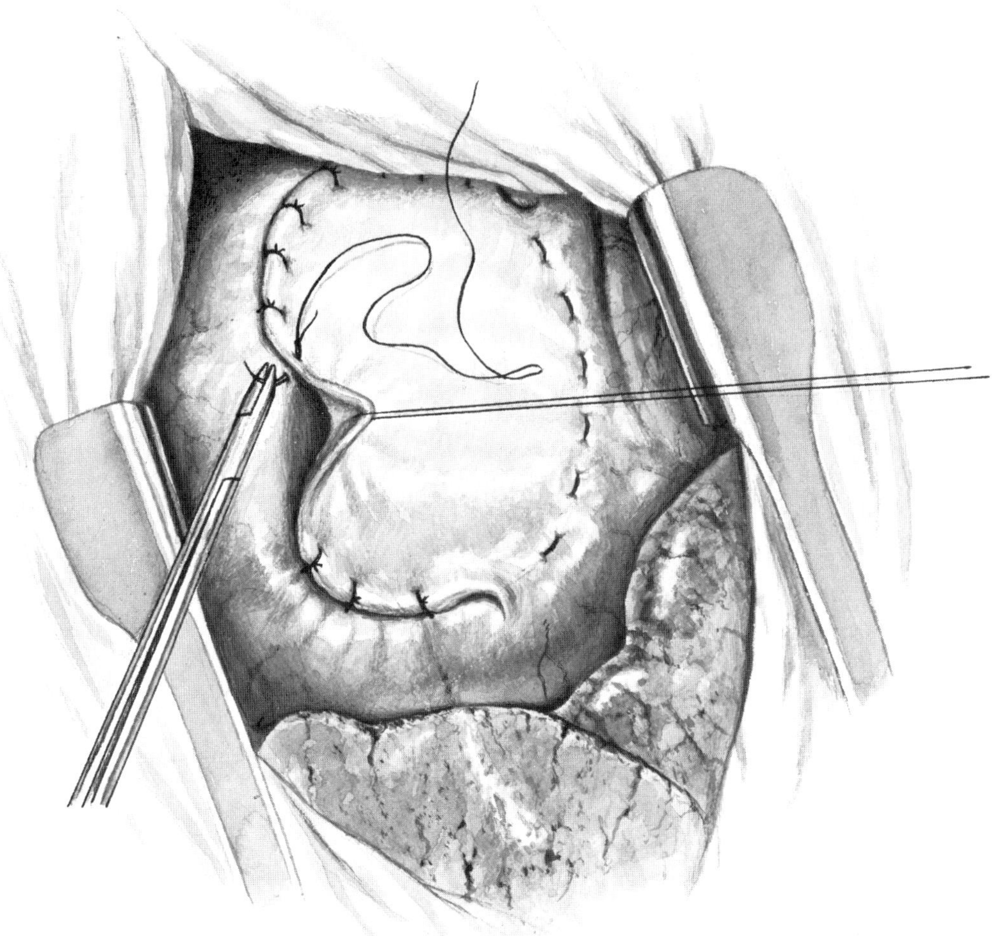

Fig. 768. Fold of relaxed diaphragm is stitched to intact muscles of diaphragm.

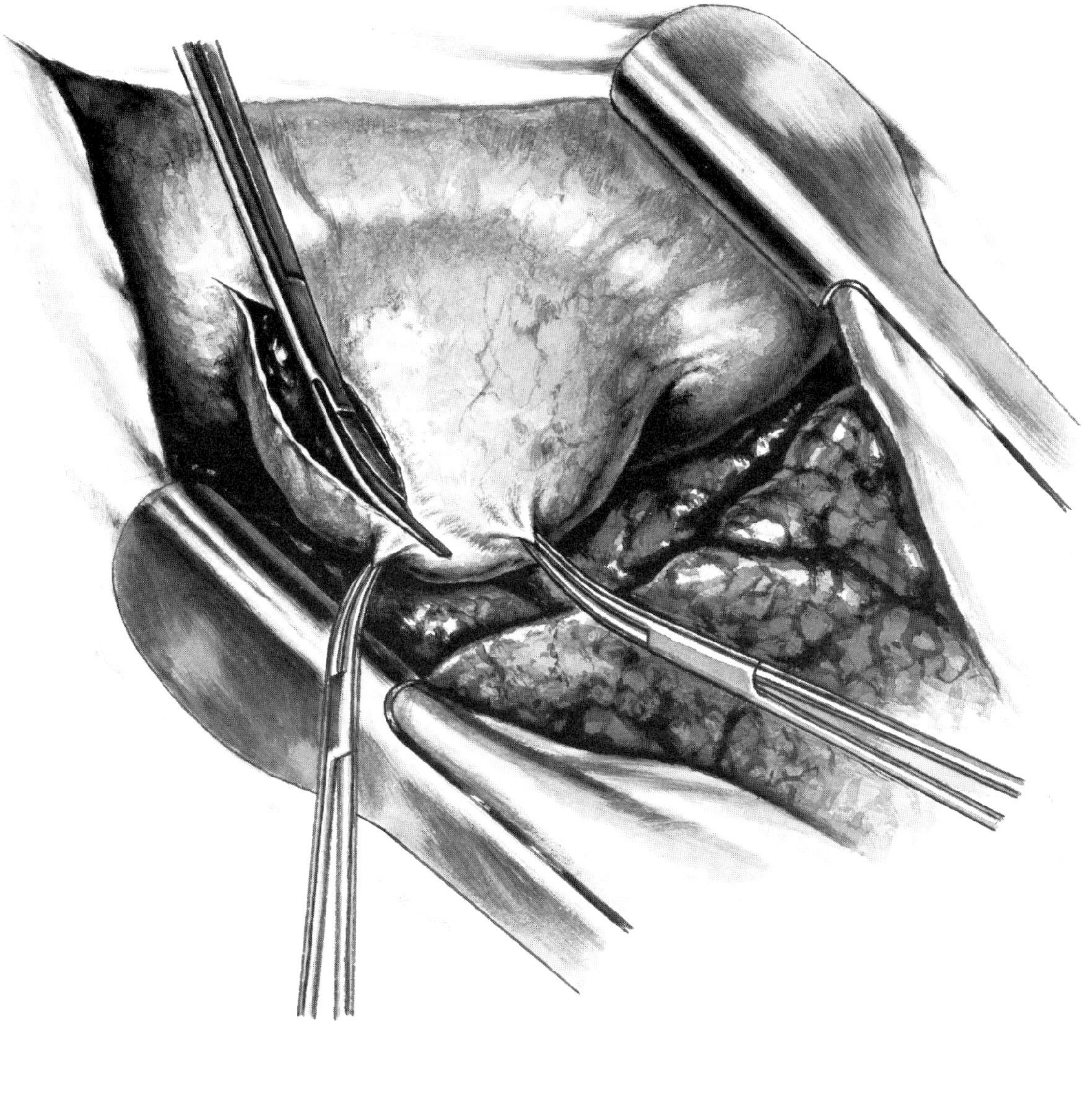

Fig. 769. Relaxed area of diaphragmatic dome is cut.

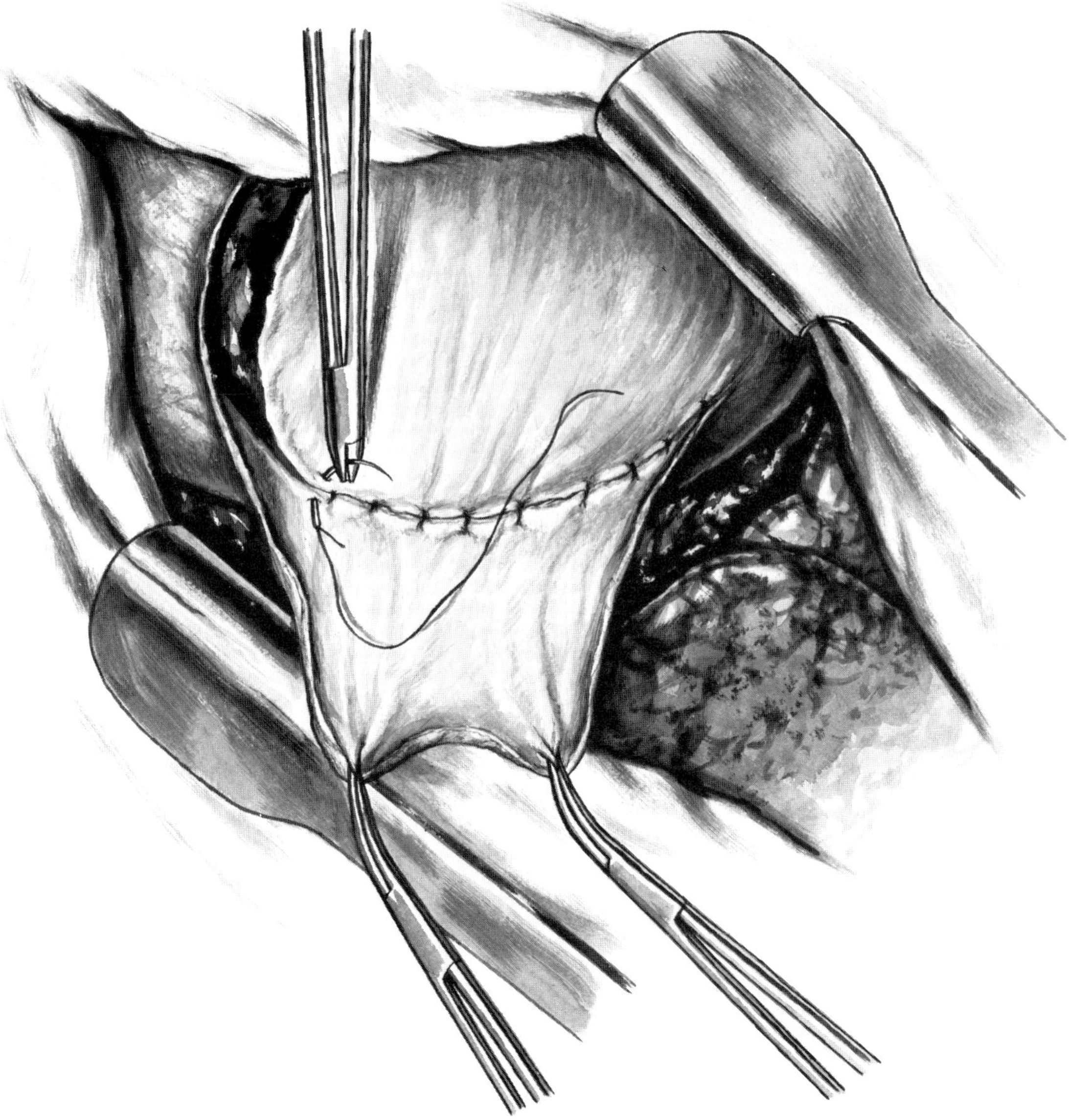

Fig. 770. Incision in diaphragmatic dome is sutured.

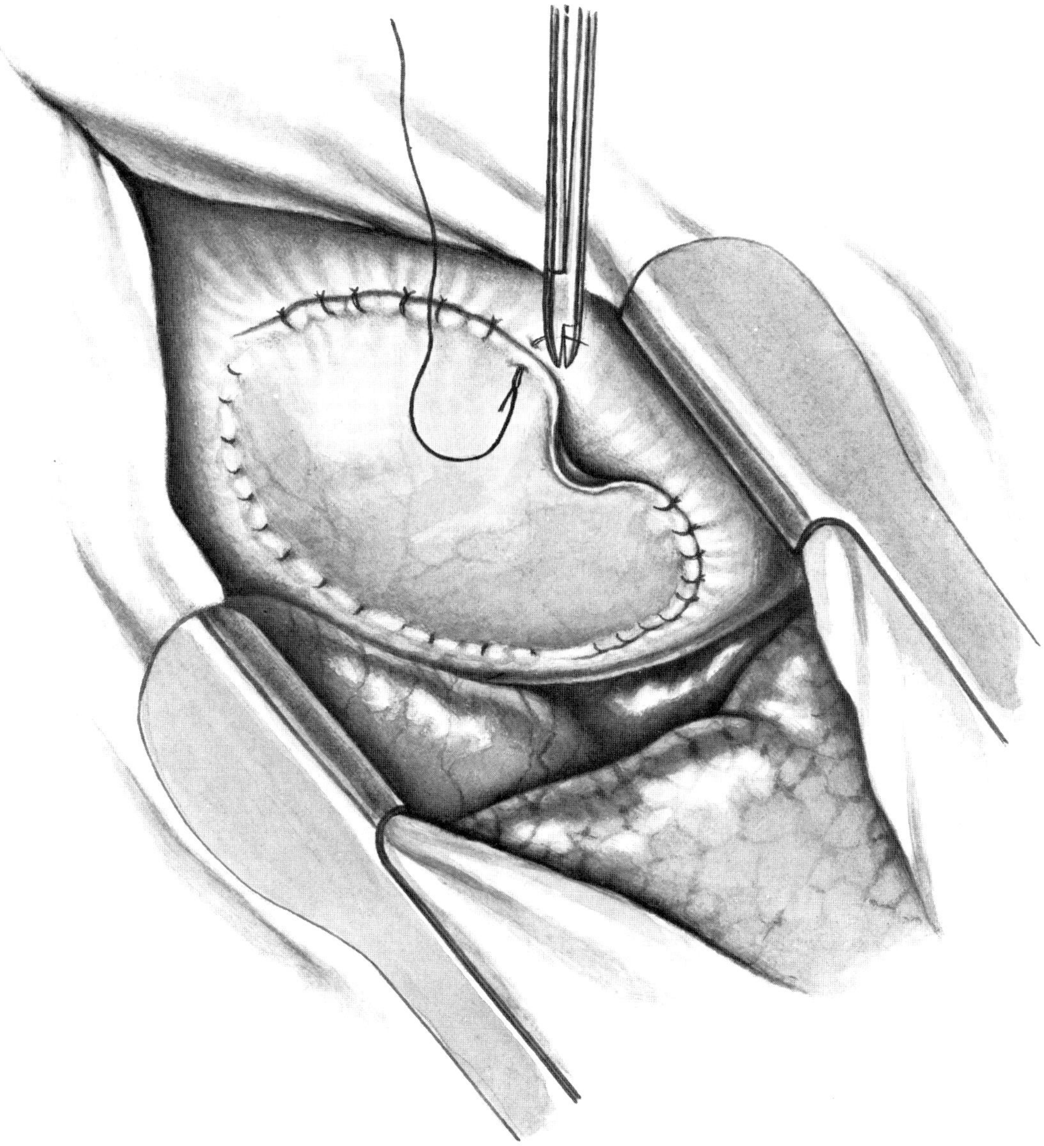

Fig. 771. Duplication of diaphragm.

ALLOPLASTIC REINFORCEMENT OF RELAXED DIAPHRAGMATIC DOME

When the whole dome of the diaphragm is relaxed, it is reinforced with alloplastic material. The dome is cut longitudinally (Fig. 772), and one of its flaps, together with a plate of polyvinyl-alcohol sponge 0.3 to 0.5 cm thick, is stitched with interrupted sutures to the base of the other flap and the intercostal tissues along the entire line of attachment of the diaphragm (Fig. 773). A free graft is sutured over it with the threads also passed through the alloplastic prosthesis (Fig. 774). As a result of the operation a ''triple-layer'' diaphragm is formed of polyvinyl-alcohol sponge and two layers of diaphragmatic tissue, isolating the alloplastic material from the pleural and abdominal cavities.

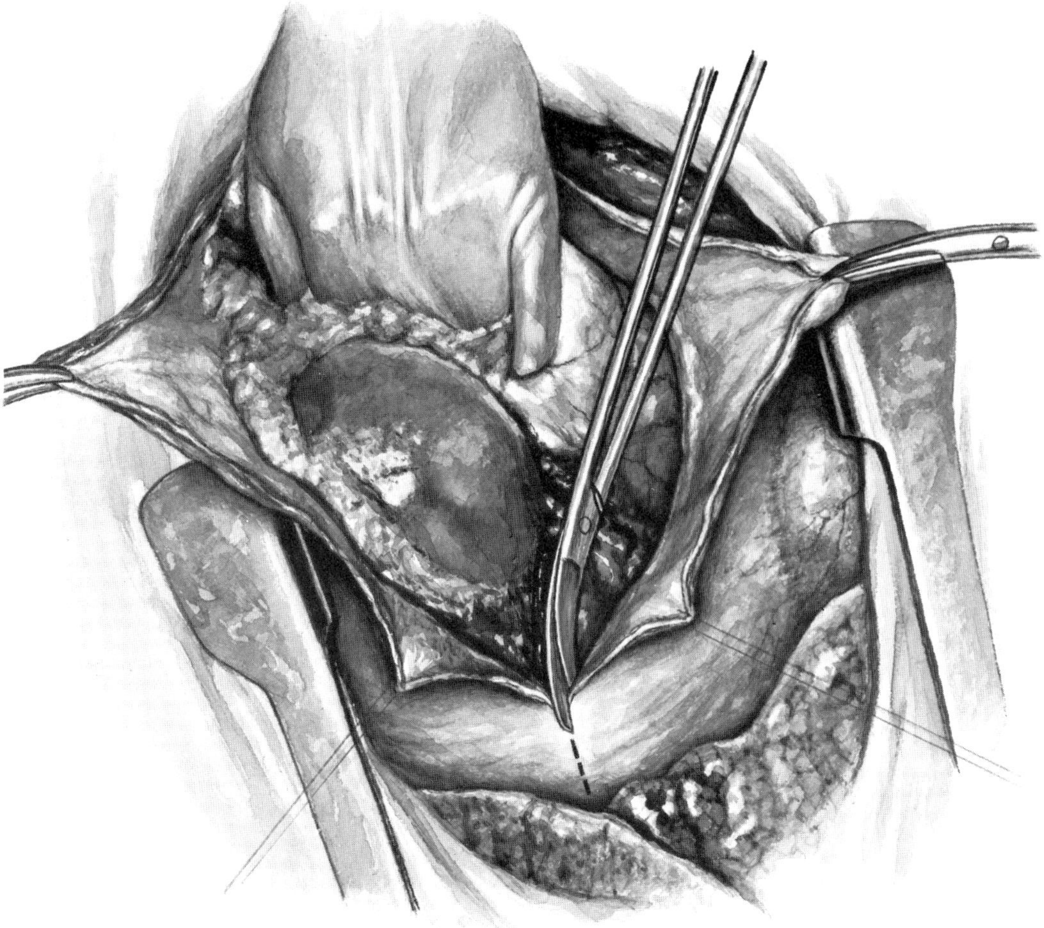

Fig. 772. Relaxed dome of diaphragm is cut.

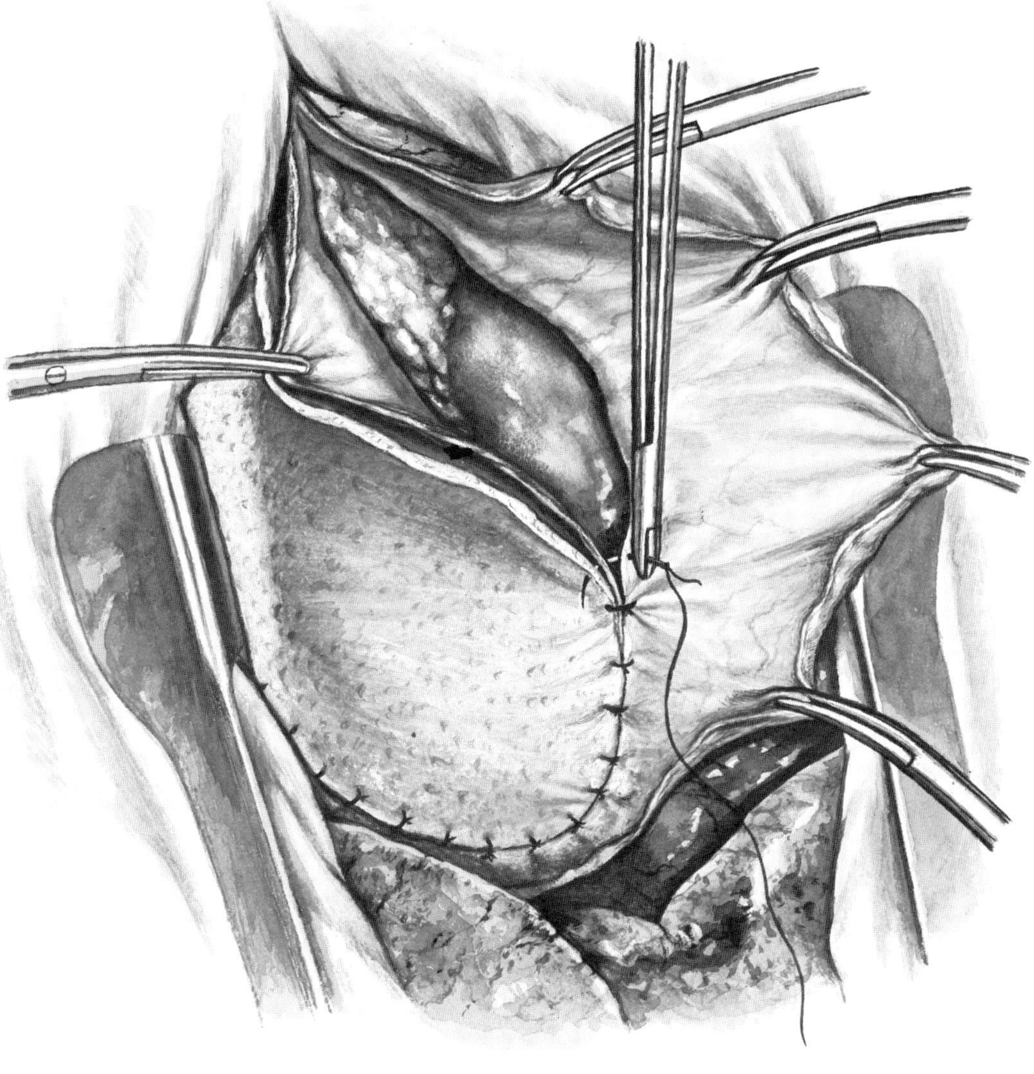

Fig. 773. One flap together with alloplastic prosthesis is stitched to base of other diaphragmatic flap.

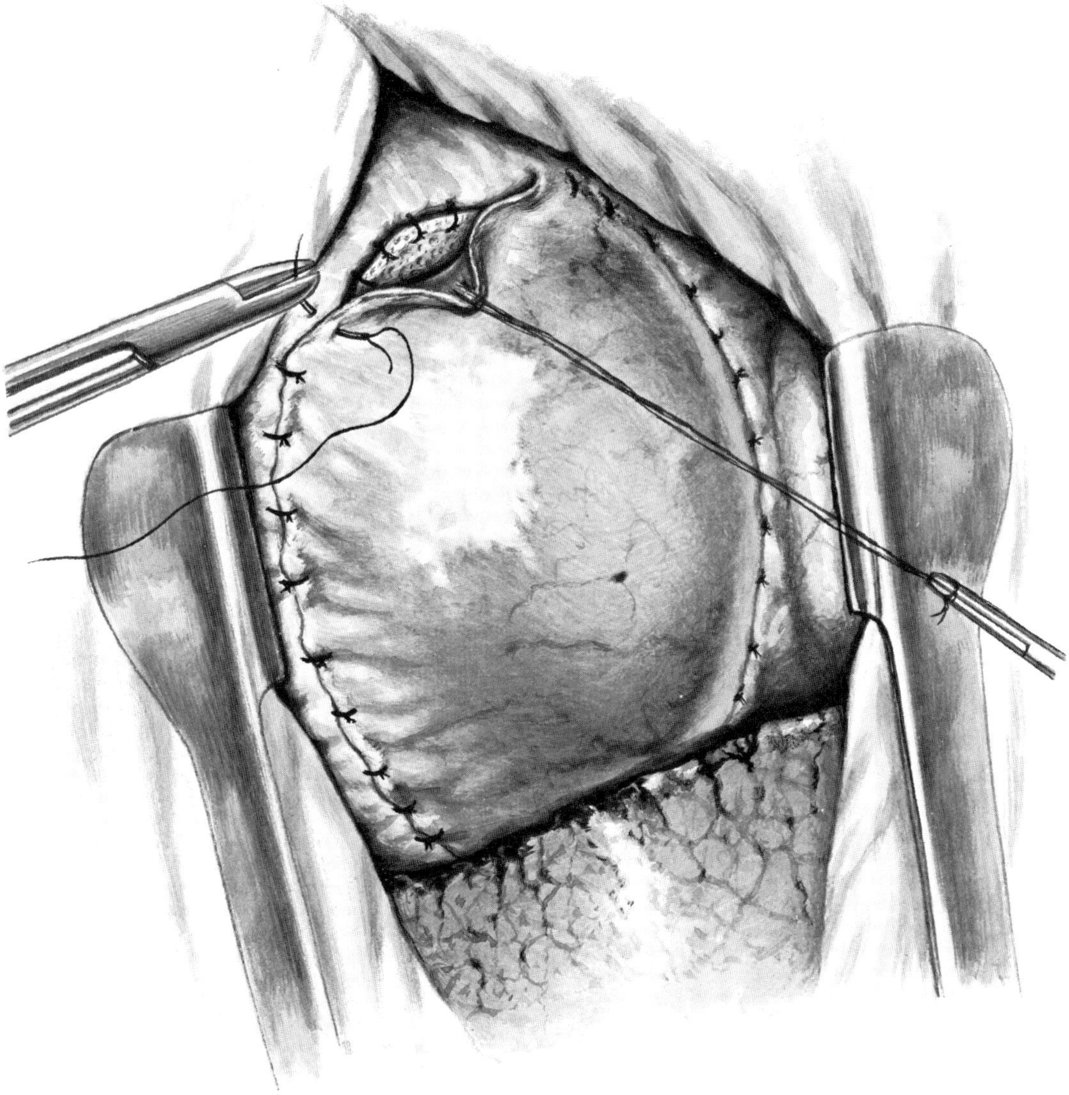

Fig. 774. Interrupted sutures are applied to diaphragmatic graft and prosthesis.

Operations in hiatal hernias

GENERAL PRINCIPLES

In paraesophageal hiatal hernia, which as a rule does not cause disturbances in the activity of the cardia, transperitoneal reduction of the stomach into the abdominal cavity is performed and the medial crura of the diaphragm are sutured to each other behind the esophagus (crurorhaphy). A similar operation is also conducted for a large sliding (cardiofundal) hernia with no considerable attendant disturbances in the function of the cardia.

Correction of cardiac insufficiency is the main purpose of operation for sliding hernia complicated by severe reflux esophagitis. Esophagofundorhaphy with no less than half the esophageal circumference wrapped in the gastric fundus is a sufficiently radical intervention when only the valvular function of the cardia is disturbed, while the esophagocardiac sphincter is only moderately relaxed (which may be determined by esophagomanometry). In severe paresis of the sphincter preference should be given to Nissen's fundoplication. It is expedient to supplement both these operations with pyloroplasty.

The tendency of the esophagus to longitudinal spastic contraction is one of the main causes of recurrent sliding hiatal hernia and recurrent gastroesophageal reflux following Nissen's fundoplication. In view of this, when performing transperitoneal fundoplication, it is expedient to refrain from correcting the hernia, but to carry out sagittal diaphragmotomy according to Savinykh; having partially shifted the fundoplication cup into the mediastinum (''mediastinalization of the cardia'') the surgeon fastens the stomach to the margins of the opening in the diaphragm. A sliding hernia with marked shortening of the esophagus is managed by Nissen's transpleural fundoplication, but the surgeon, in this case, is obliged to leave part of the stomach in the mediastinum. Transperitoneal valvular gastroplication, which is undertaken in the presence of contraindictions for a transpleural operation, is usually quite effective too. The same can be said of distal gastric resection with the creation of a Y-shaped anastomosis or replacement of the removed portion of the stomach by a loop of the small intestine.

In sliding hernia complicated by peptic esophageal stricture, Nissen's fundoplication or valvular gastroplication is indicated in the early stages since a fresh peptic stricture undergoes involution after the reflux is corrected. In later periods, with the cicatricial stricture already formed, the stenosed terminal part of the esophagus has to be resected. Purse-string valvular esophagogastrostomy prevents recurrent reflux.

Transperitoneal operations are carried out through median laparotomy or a left oblique subcostal approach. Transpleural operations are performed by means of left thoracotomy in the seventh intercostal space. In combination of hiatal hernia with a diverticulum of the right esophageal wall, both abnormalities may be corrected through a right transpleural approach.

TRANSABDOMINAL CRURORHAPHY WITH ESOPHAGOFUNDORHAPHY

Median laparotomy is performed. The right hepatic lobe is mobilized and moved aside to the right (Fig. 775). The fundus of the stomach is reduced into the abdominal cavity (Fig. 776). Loops are drawn under the esophagus, with which it is moved either to the left or to the right side. The hernial sac is cut away from the hiatus and is usually left in the mediastinum.

The medial crura of the diaphragm are sutured together behind the esophagus (Fig. 777). Esophagofundorhaphy is carried out for the prevention of gastroesophageal reflux (Fig. 778).

The esophagus is stitched to the margin of the opening in the diaphragm with a few sutures, with caution exercised so as not to injure the vagus nerves.

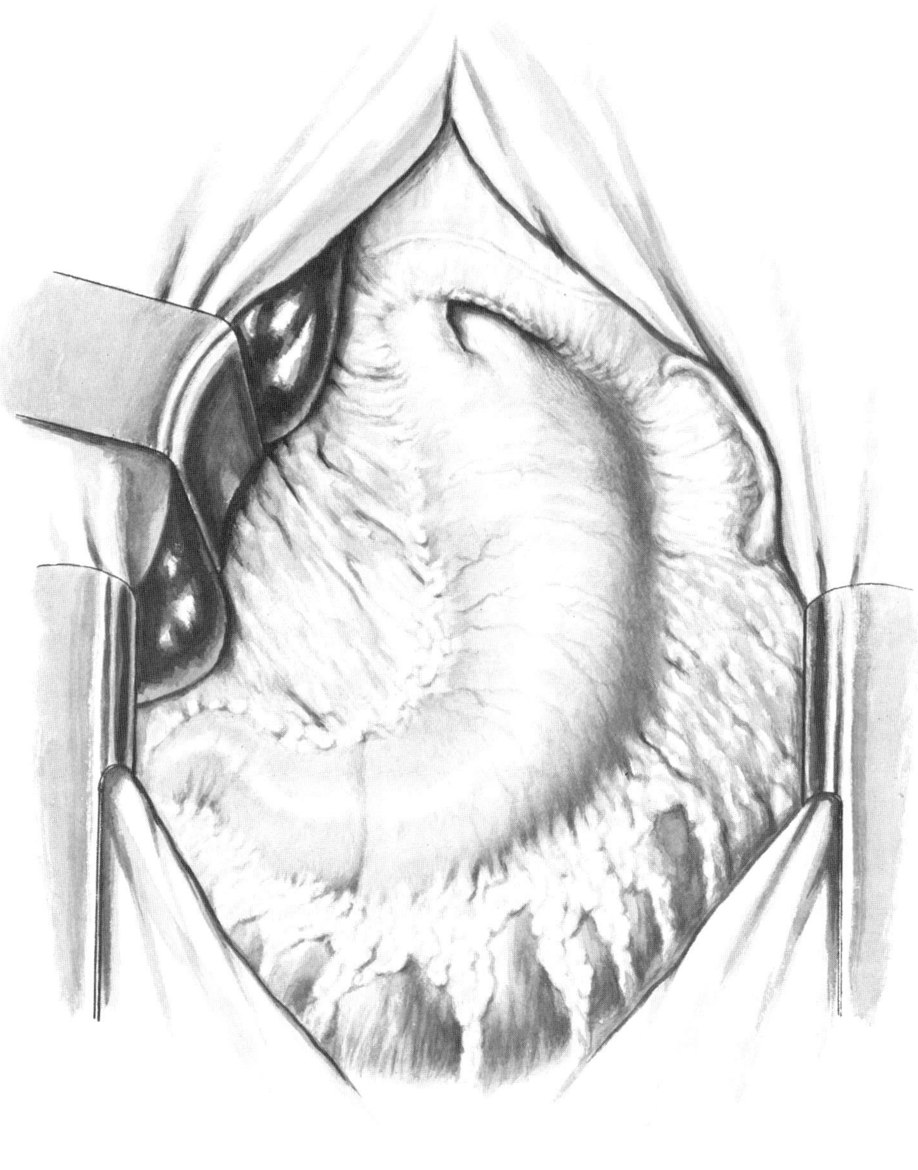

Fig. 775. Left lobe of liver is mobilized.

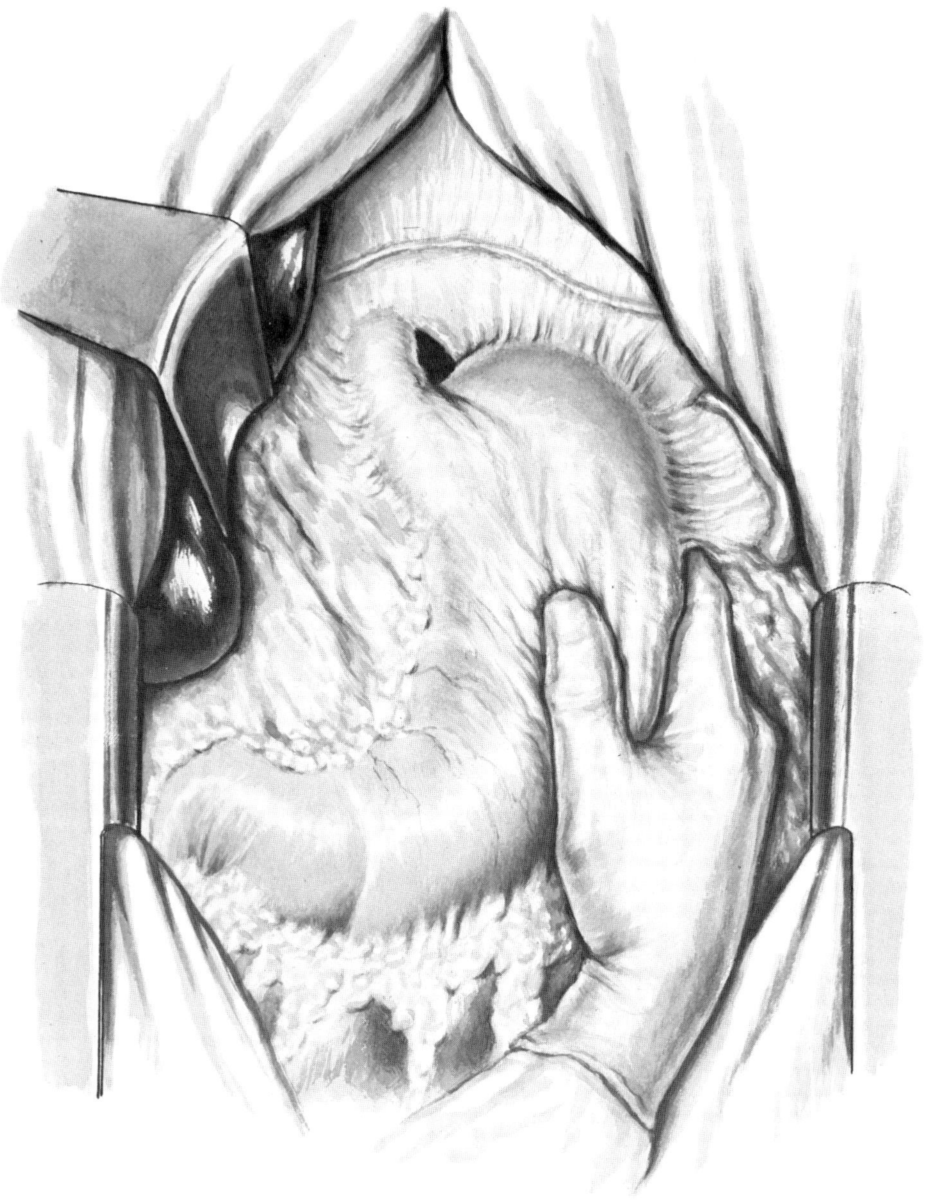

Fig. 776. Reduction of stomach into abdominal cavity.

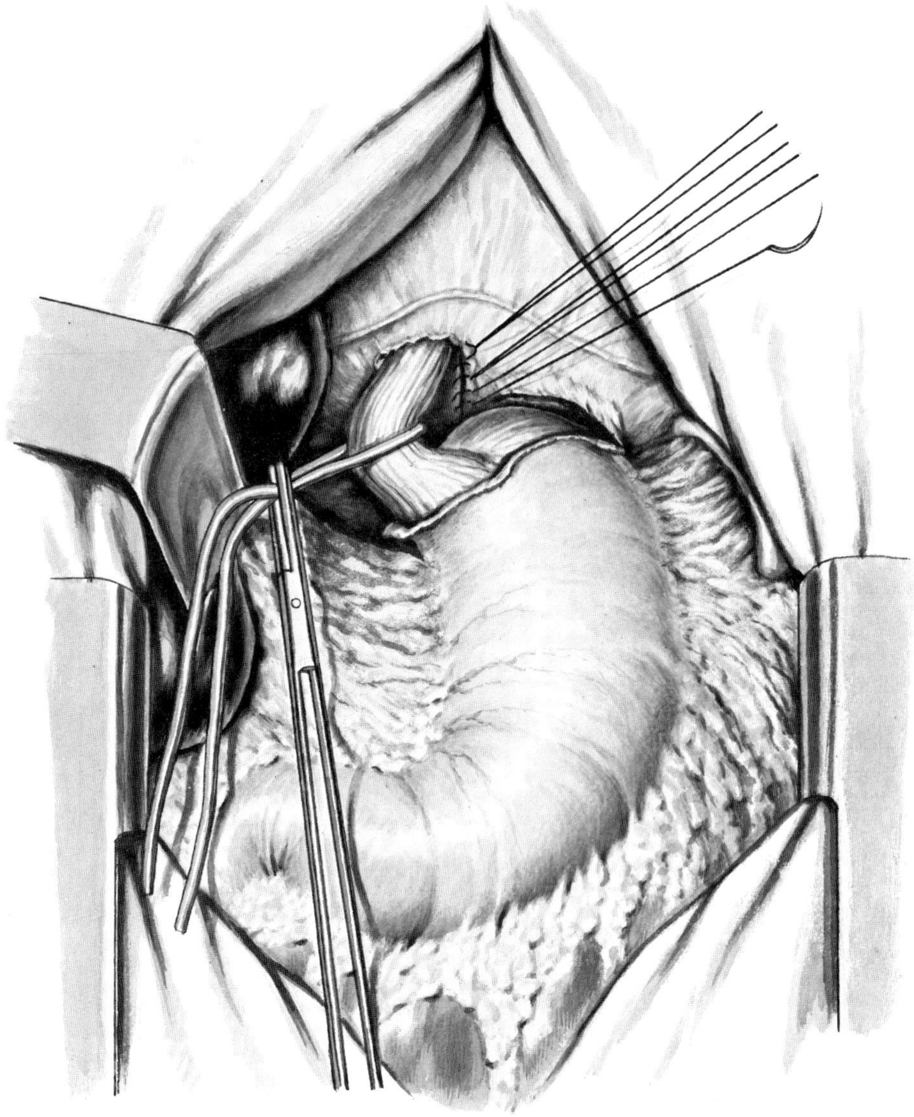

Fig. 777. Medial crura of diaphragm are stitched together.

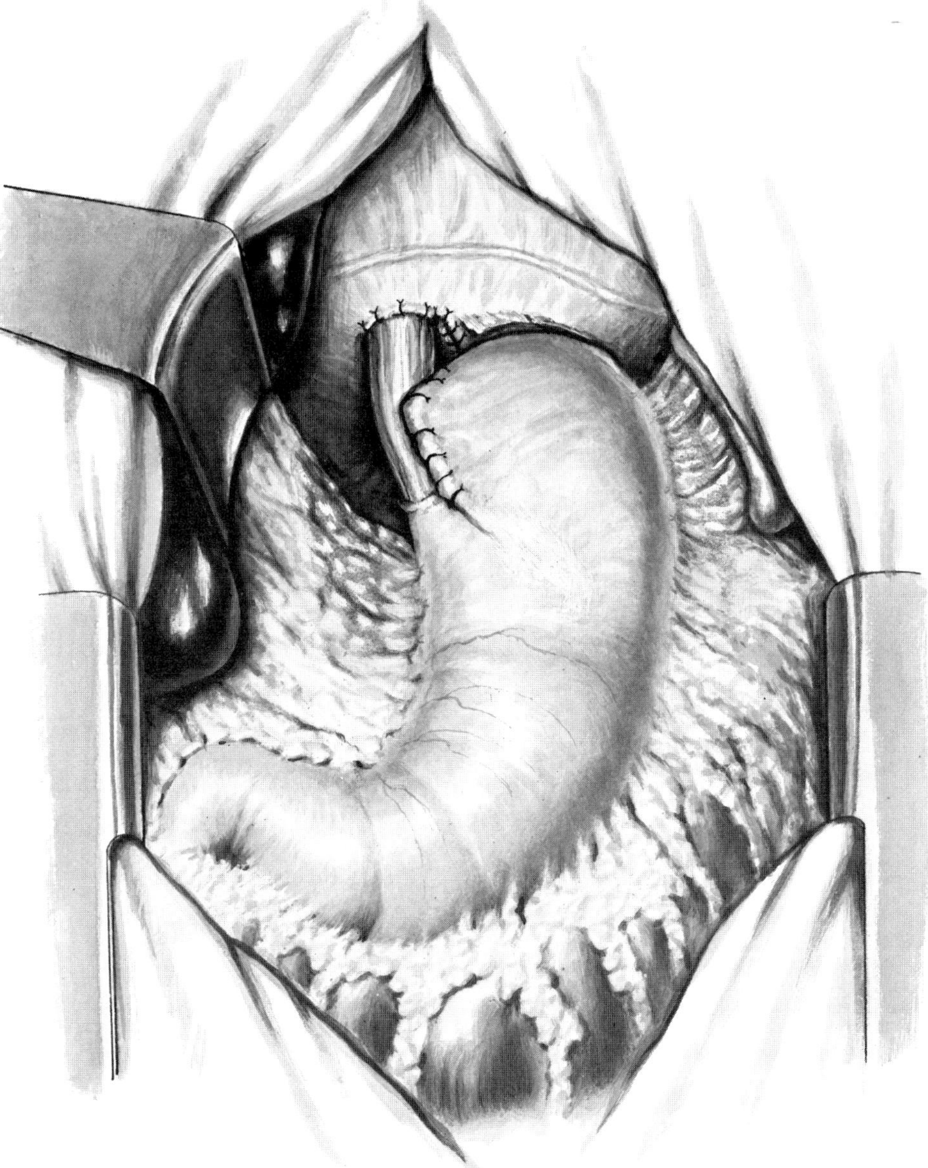

Fig. 778. Esophagofundorhaphy.

TRANSABDOMINAL FUNDOPLICATION WITH MEDIASTINALIZATION OF THE CARDIA

Median laparotomy is accomplished. The left hepatic lobe is mobilized and moved aside to the right (Fig. 779). When there is a hernia, the fingers are easily advanced through the widened hiatus into the posterior mediastinum (Fig. 780). The peritoneum is cut along the edge of the esophageal hiatus. The stretched esophagodiaphragmatic membrane is cut lengthwise, and a loop is drawn around the esophagus. A small sagittal diaphragmotomy is made for additional widening of the hiatus with transection of the phrenic vein between

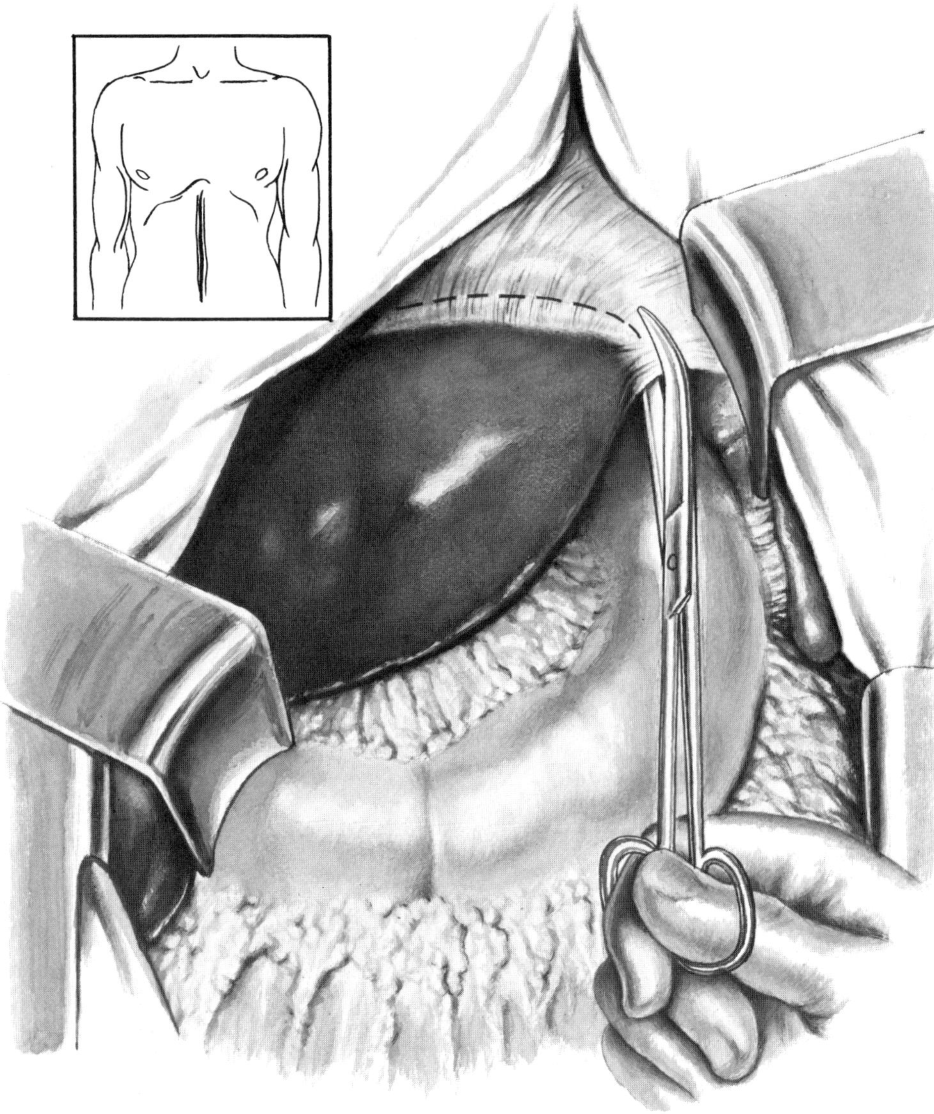

Fig. 779. Left lobe of liver is mobilized.

ligatures (Fig. 781). The upper part of the lesser omentum is incised, and the fundus of the stomach mobilized. The mobilized fundus is drawn behind the esophagus, and a cuff is formed with the threads passed through the coats of the stomach and the esophagus (Fig. 782). To prevent the gastric wall from unfolding later, it is desirable to apply a second row of sutures. Both rows may be stitched with a continuous thread on an atraumatic needle. The fundoplication cuff is moved into the mediastinum (''mediastinalization of the cardia''), and the stomach is stitched to the margins of the wide hiatus (Fig. 783). Pylorplasty completes the operation.

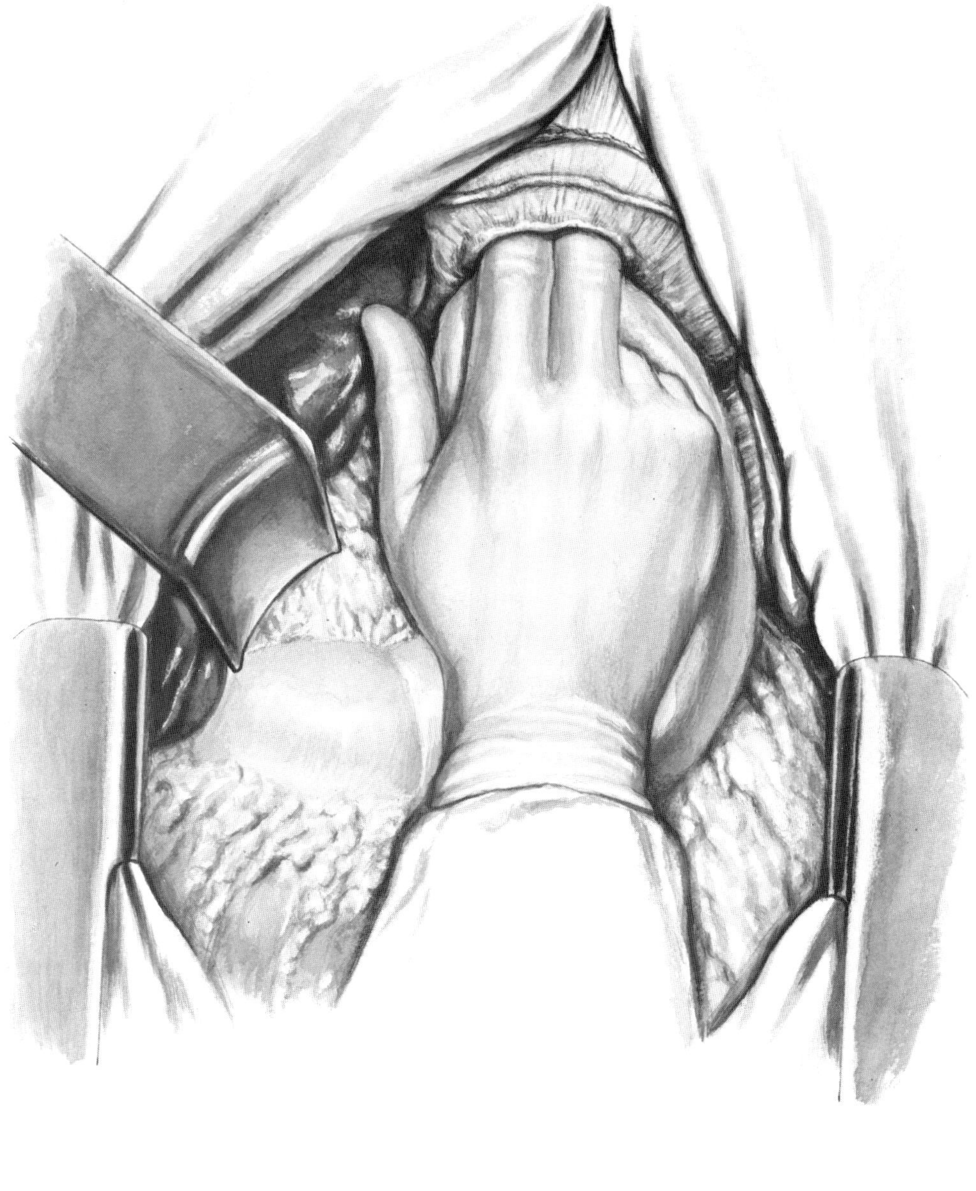

Fig. 780. Exploration of hiatus.

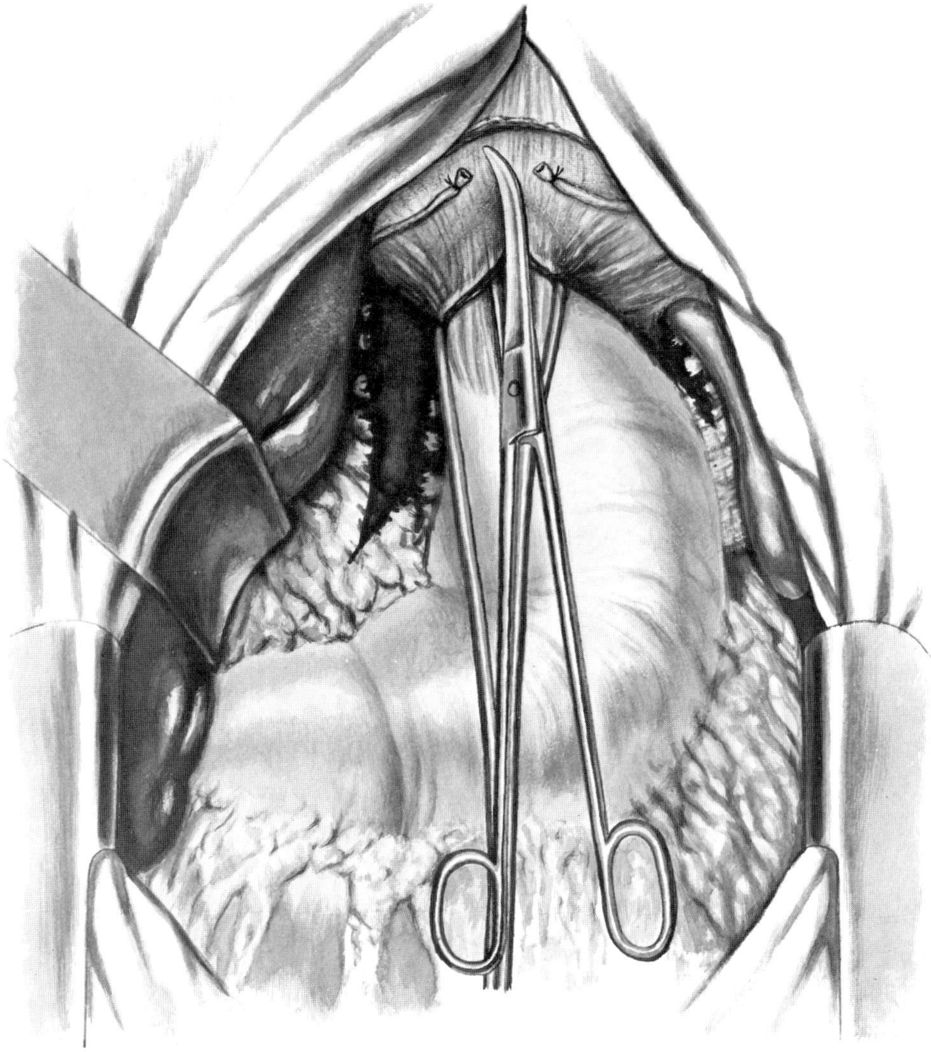

Fig. 781. Sagittal diaphragmotomy for widening hiatus. Phrenic vein is transected and esophagus held with loop.

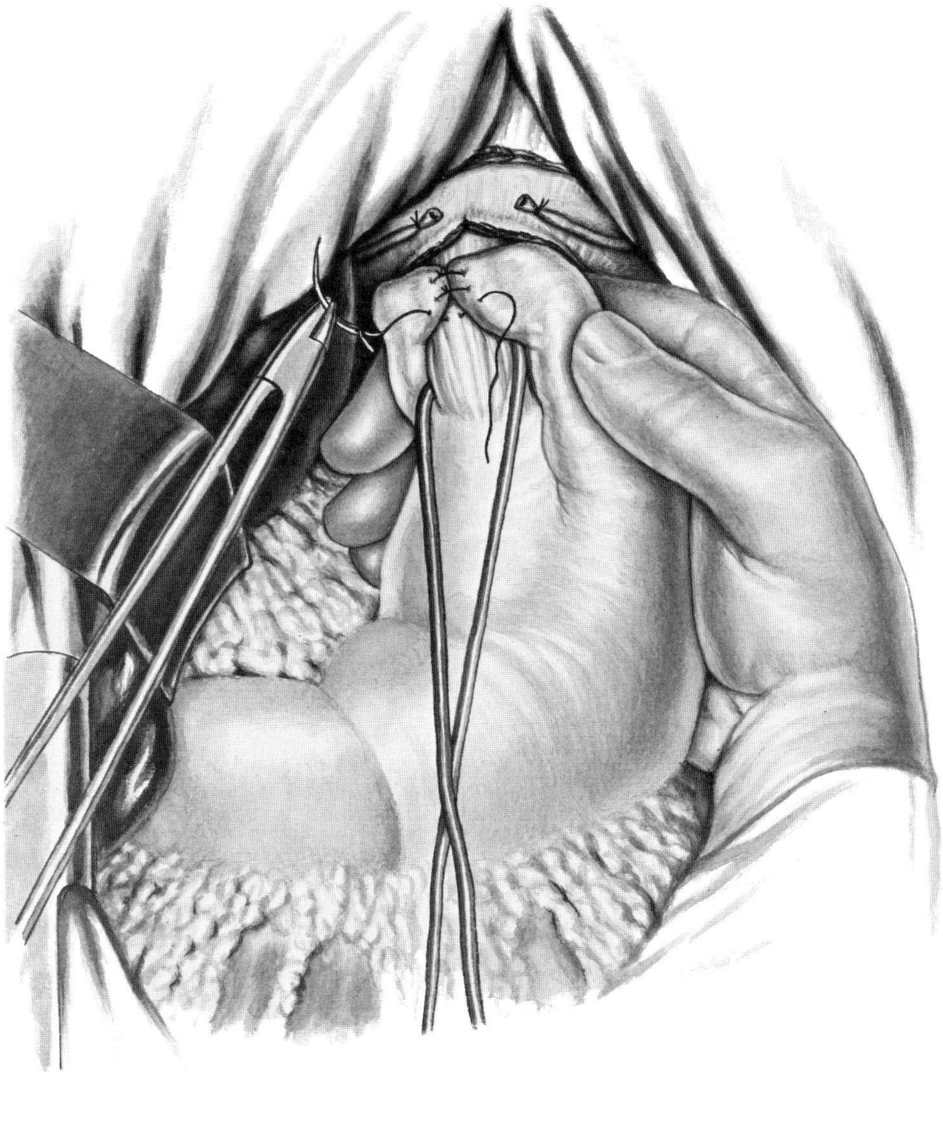

Fig. 782. Fundoplication after Nissen is performed.

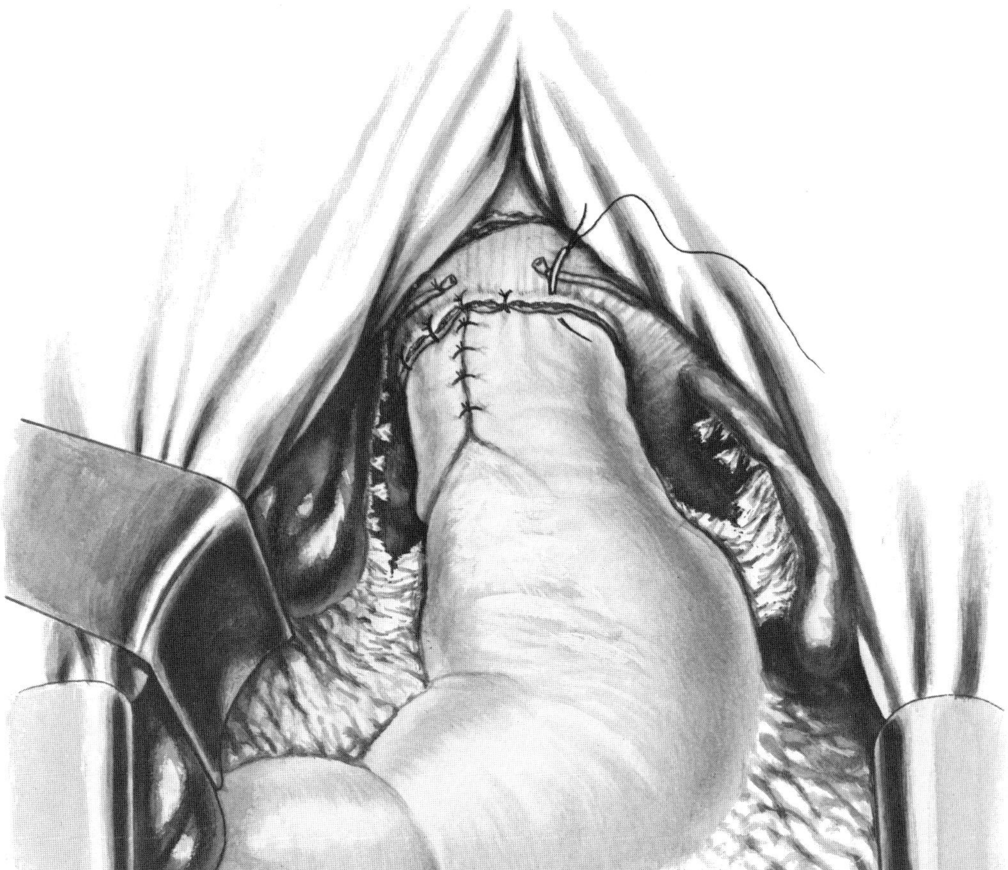

Fig. 783. Stomach is stitched to widened hiatus.

TRANSPLEURAL FUNDOPLICATION IN SLIDING HERNIA WITH SHORTENING OF ESOPHAGUS

Left thoracotomy is performed. A small incision is made in the diaphragmatic dome, through which a finger is inserted into the hernial sac (Fig. 784). The sac is detached with a circular incision from the edges of the hiatus, which is then stretched with hooks. The fundus of the stomach is moved into the posterior mediastinum, and fundoplication is accomplished (Fig. 785). The edges of the hiatus are stitched to the walls of the stomach (Fig. 786). The opening made earlier in the diaphragm is sutured.

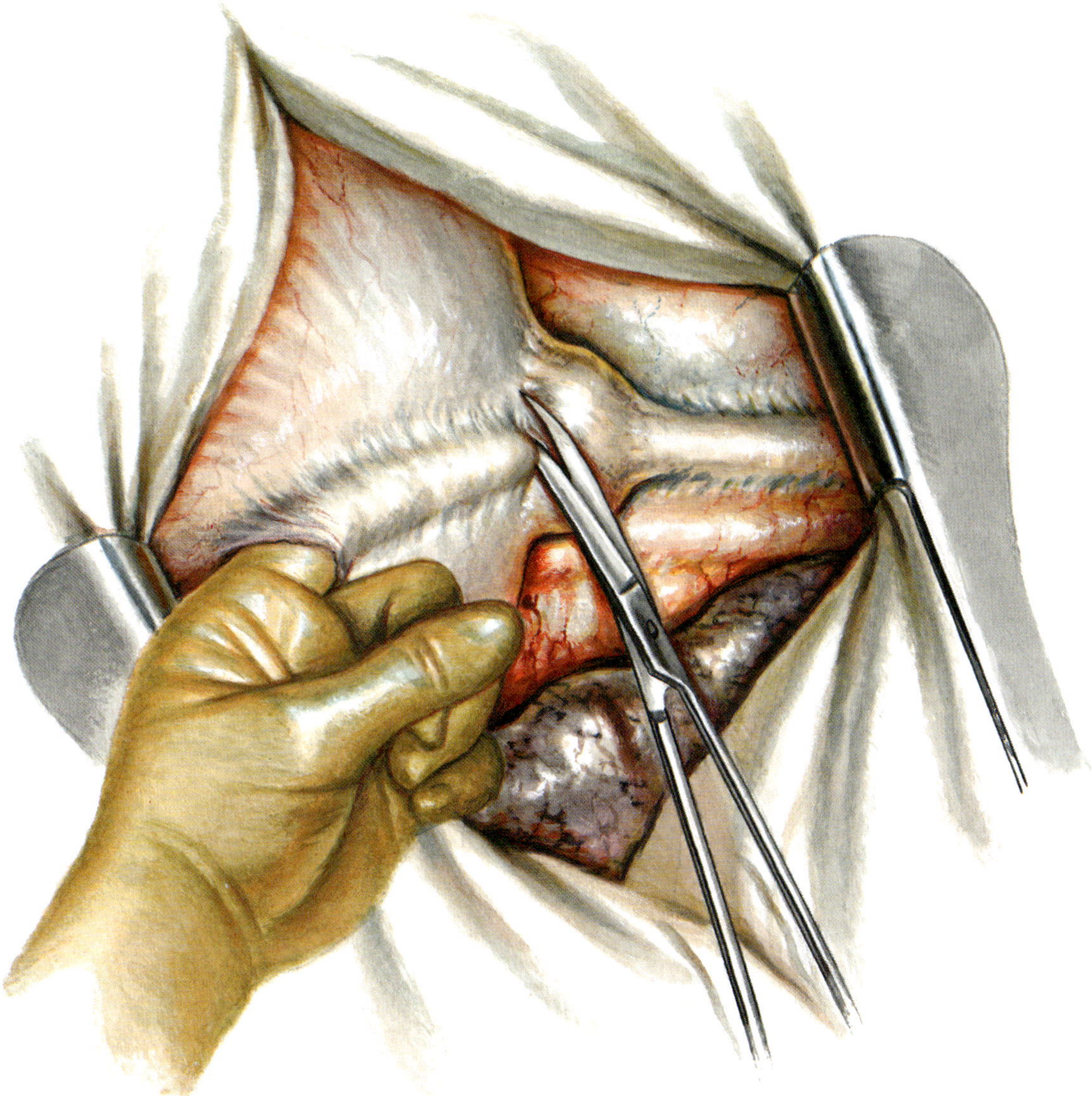

Fig. 784. Finger is inserted into hernial sac through additional incision in diaphragm.

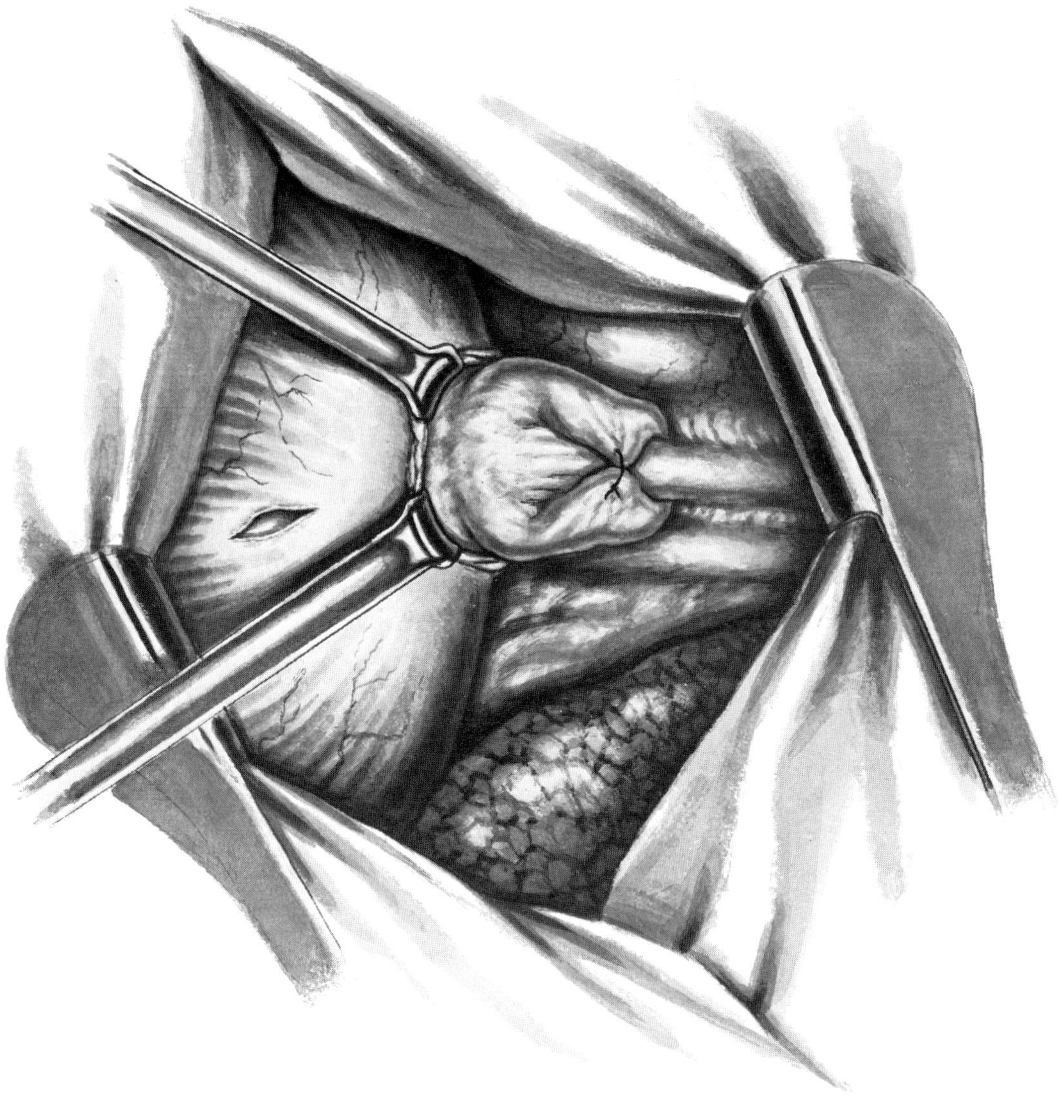

Fig. 785. Fundoplication after Nissen.

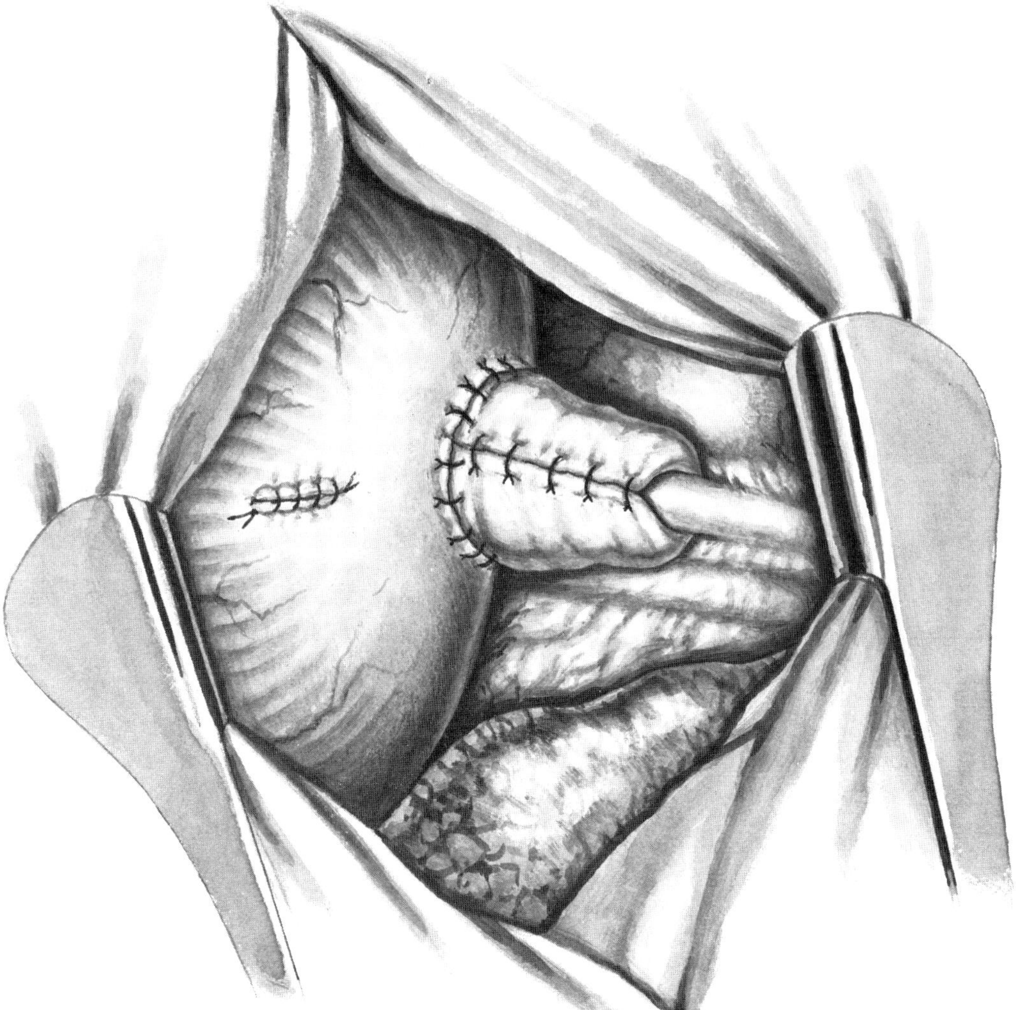

Fig. 786. Additional incision in diaphragm is sutured; stomach is stitched to edges of hiatus.

TRANSABDOMINAL VALVULAR GASTROPLICATION IN HERNIA WITH SHORTENING OF ESOPHAGUS

The operation is undertaken when a thoracic intervention is contraindicated. Laparotomy is performed, and the left hepatic lobe is mobilized and drawn aside to the right. The fact that the cardia of the stomach is located in the mediastinum due to a short esophagus is established (Fig. 787). The cranial part of the stomach is mobilized. Sagittal diaphragmotomy is carried out to make the hiatus still wider. The stomach is held with a

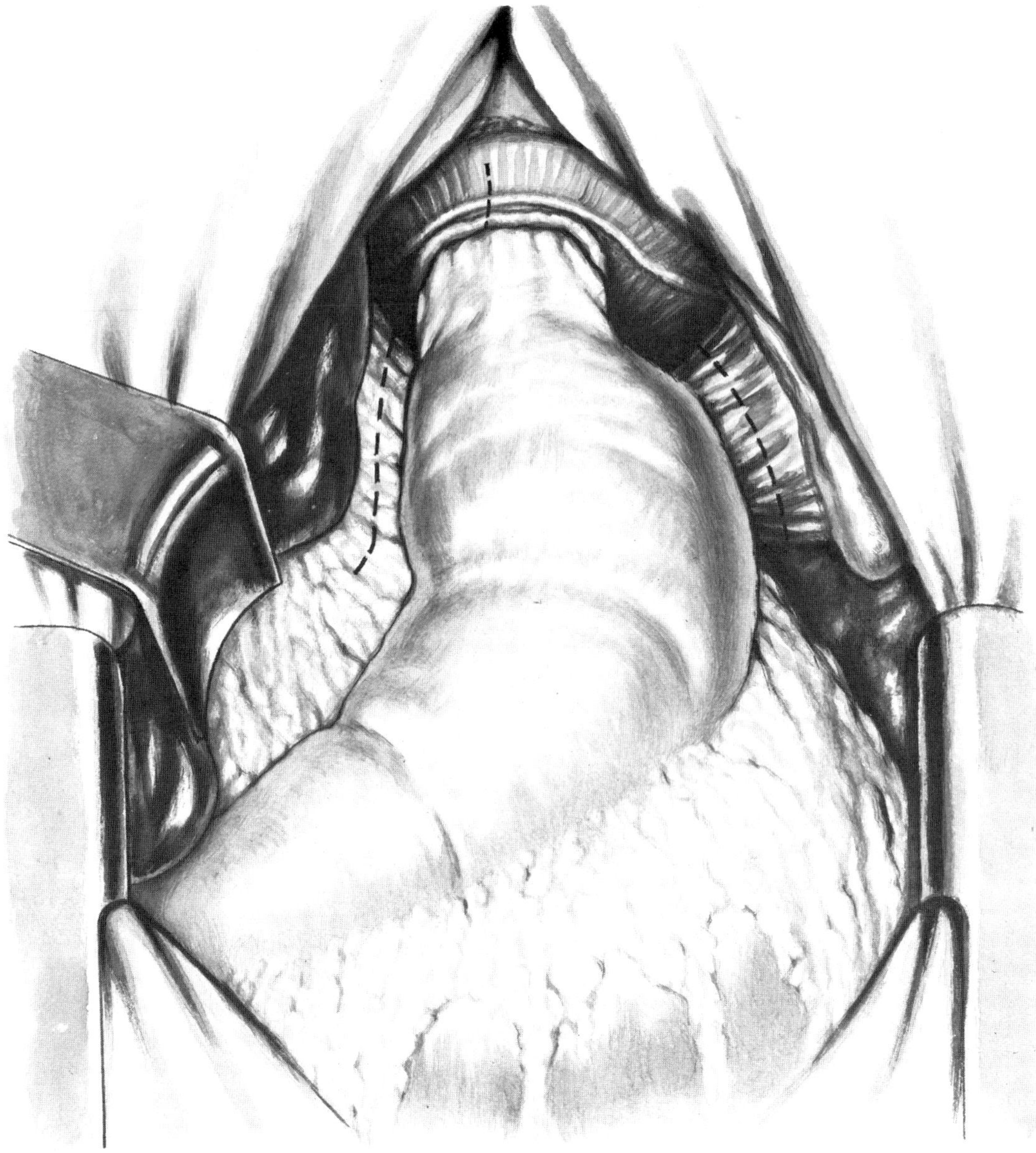

Fig. 787. Left hepatic lobe is moved aside to right. Dotted lines show where cardiac part of stomach and esophagus are mobilized.

loop just below the diaphragm (Fig. 788). The part of the stomach above the loop is shaped into a tube by applying several longitudinal rows to gather its walls (Fig. 789). The tube formed from the stomach and continuous with the esophagus is surrounded by the mobilized fundus of the stomach as in Nissen's fundoplication (Fig. 790). The edges of the hiatus are sutured to the gastric walls. As a result of this operation the cardiac opening is transposed 5 to 6 cm caudally. The valve is formed only out of the walls of the stomach (Fig. 791).

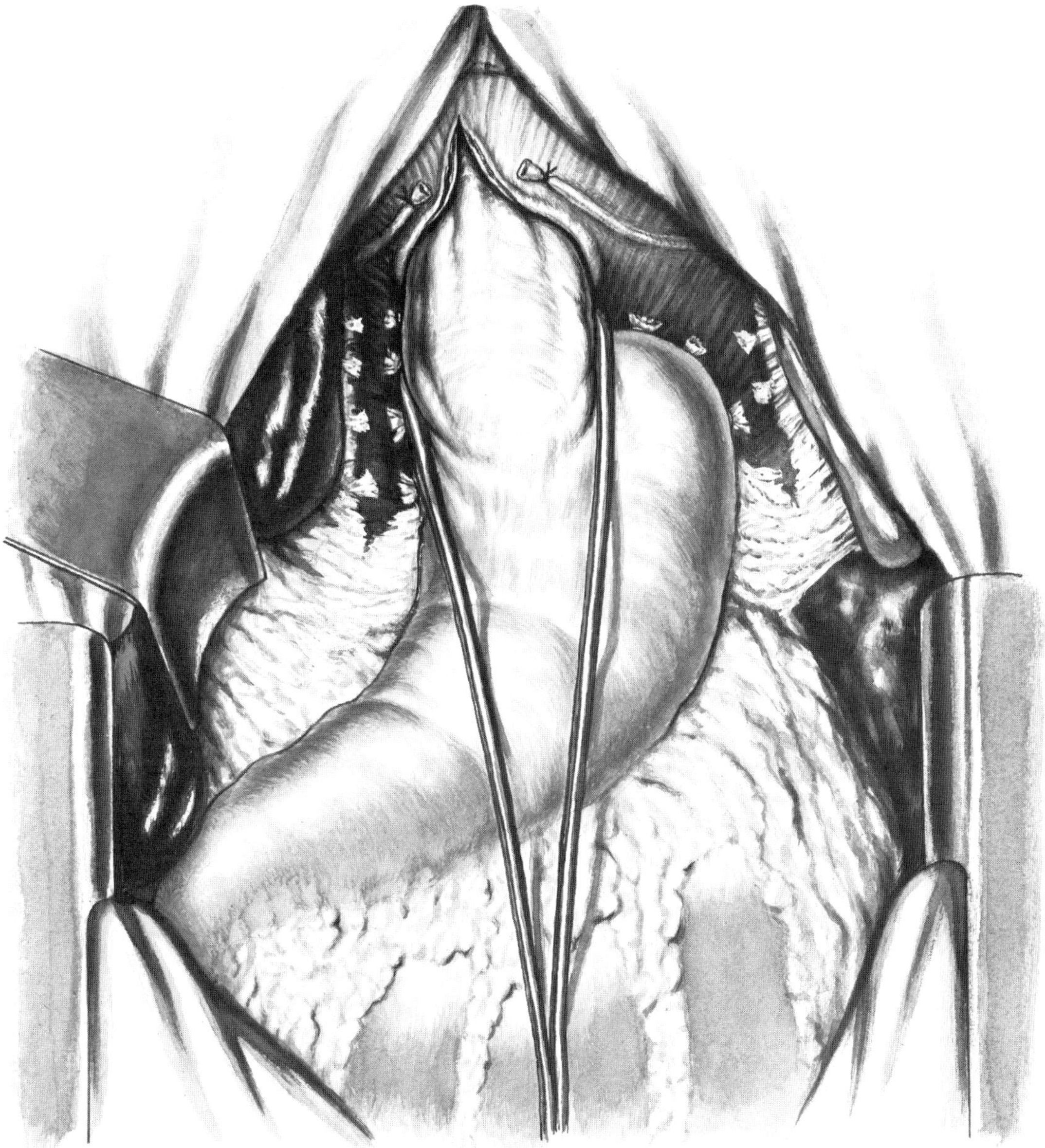

Fig. 788. Stomach is held by loop below diaphragm.

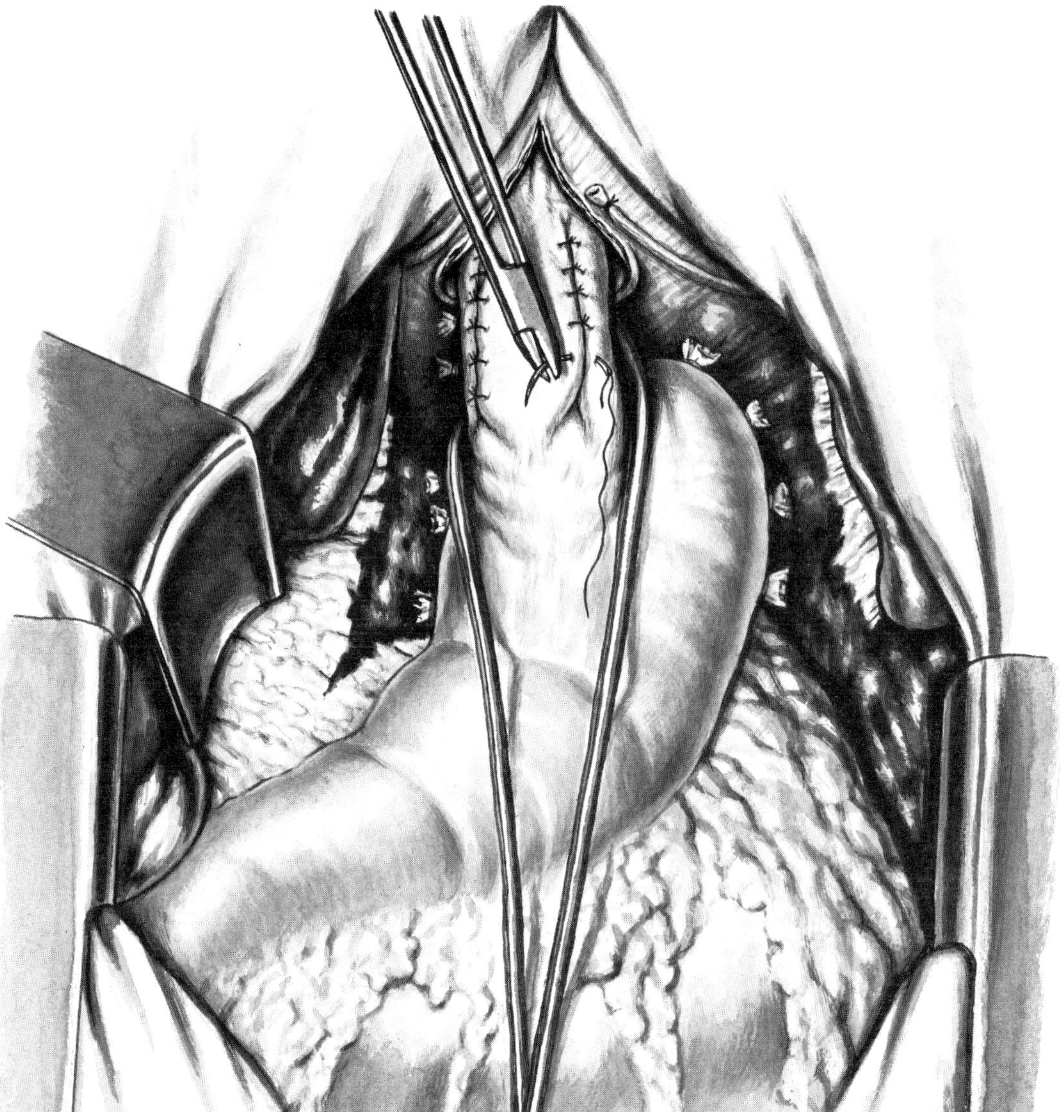

Fig. 789. Gathering sutures are applied to gastric wall.

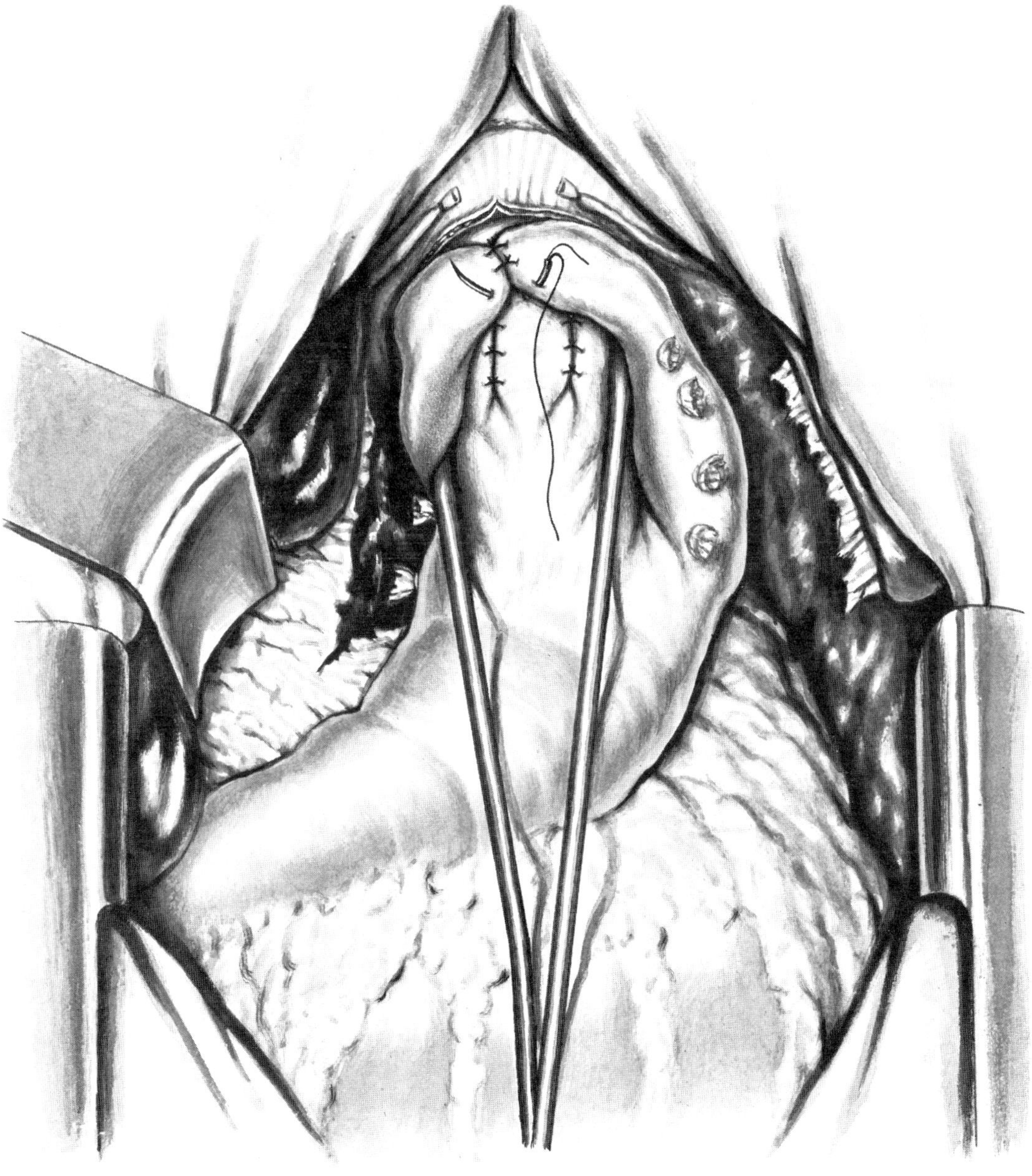

Fig. 790. Formation of gastroplication valve.

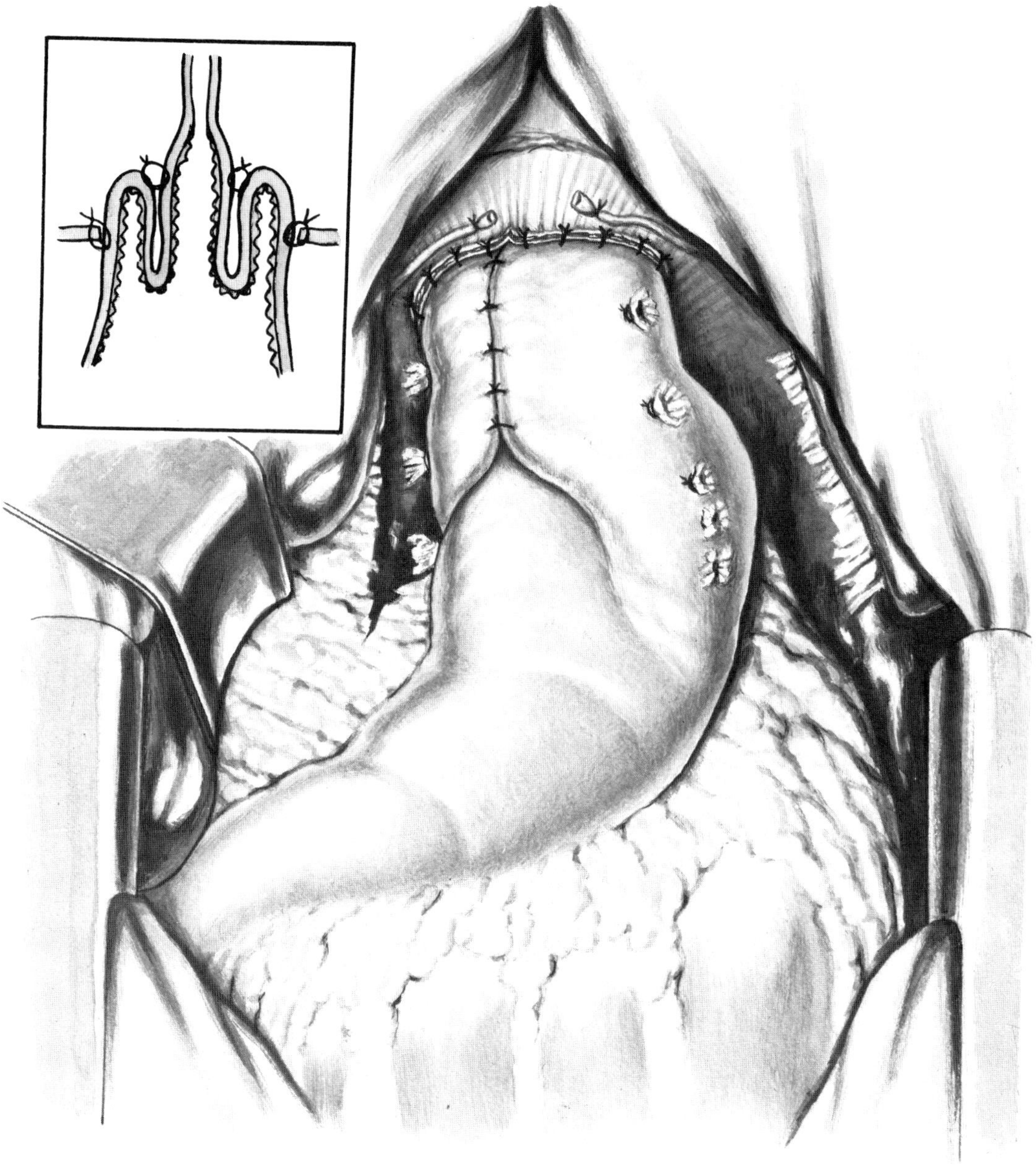

Fig. 791. Stomach is stitched to edges of hiatus.

TRANSPLEURAL ESOPHAGOFUNDORHAPHY THROUGH A RIGHT APPROACH

The operation is performed when a hernia is combined with a diverticulum of the right esophageal wall. Right thoracotomy is carried out in the seventh intercostal space. The right diaphragmatic dome is drawn caudally with a wide hook; the lung is moved cranially and medially. The mediastinal pleura is transected above the lower portion of the esophagus and the herniation (Fig. 792). The esophagus is held with a loop. The cardiac part of the stomach is brought out into the mediastinum through the widened esophageal hiatus (Fig. 793). The fundus of the stomach is stitched with two sutures (Fig. 794). With these sutures as guiding ligatures, esophagofundorhaphy is performed with no less than two thirds of the esophageal circumference wrapped in the fundus (Fig. 795). The edges of the esophageal hiatus are stitched to the stomach (Fig. 796). Fundoplication may be performed in a similar manner. The esophageal diverticulum is corrected at the same time as the hernia.

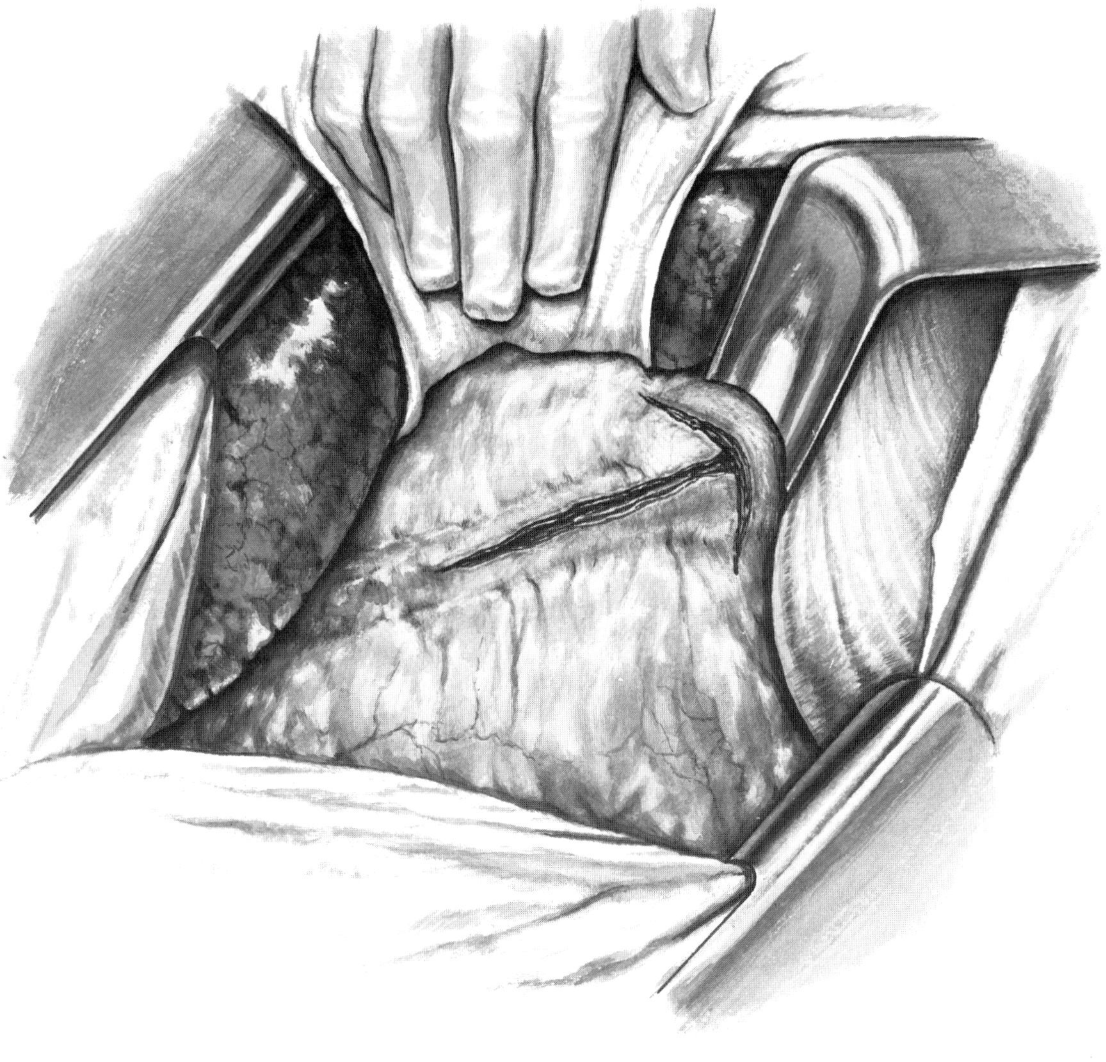

Fig. 792. Mediastinal pleura is cut above esophagus and along edge of hiatus.

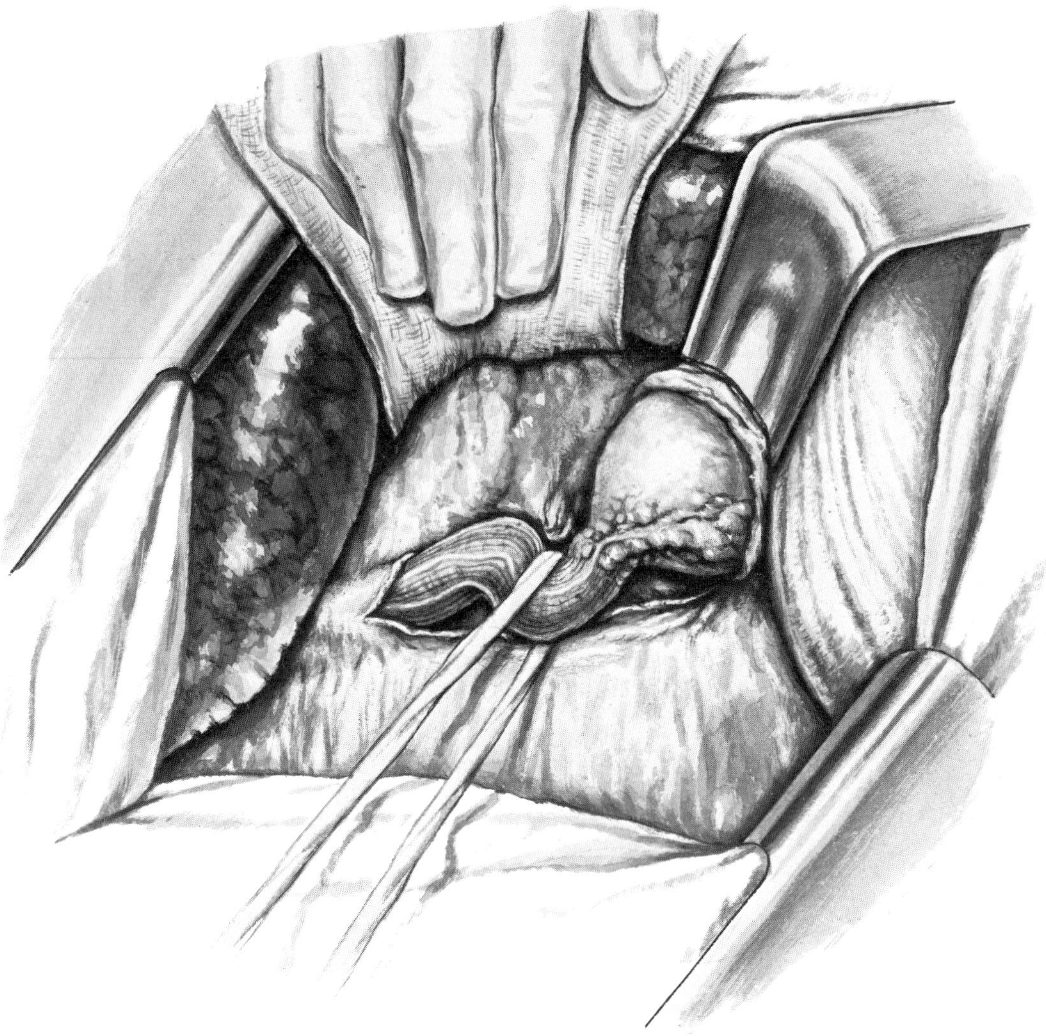

Fig. 793. Esophagus is held with loop.

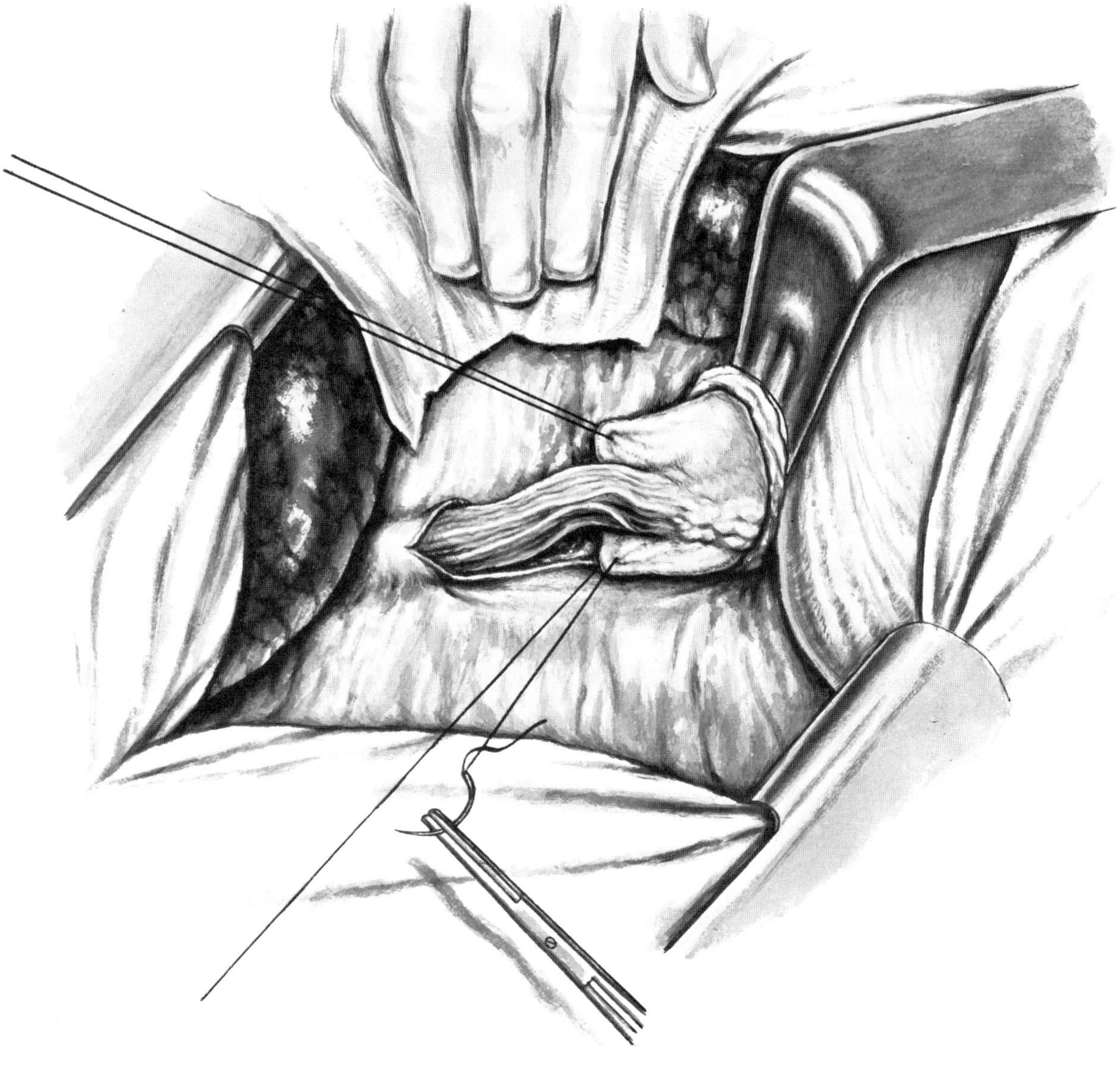

Fig. 794. Traction sutures are stitched through fundus of stomach.

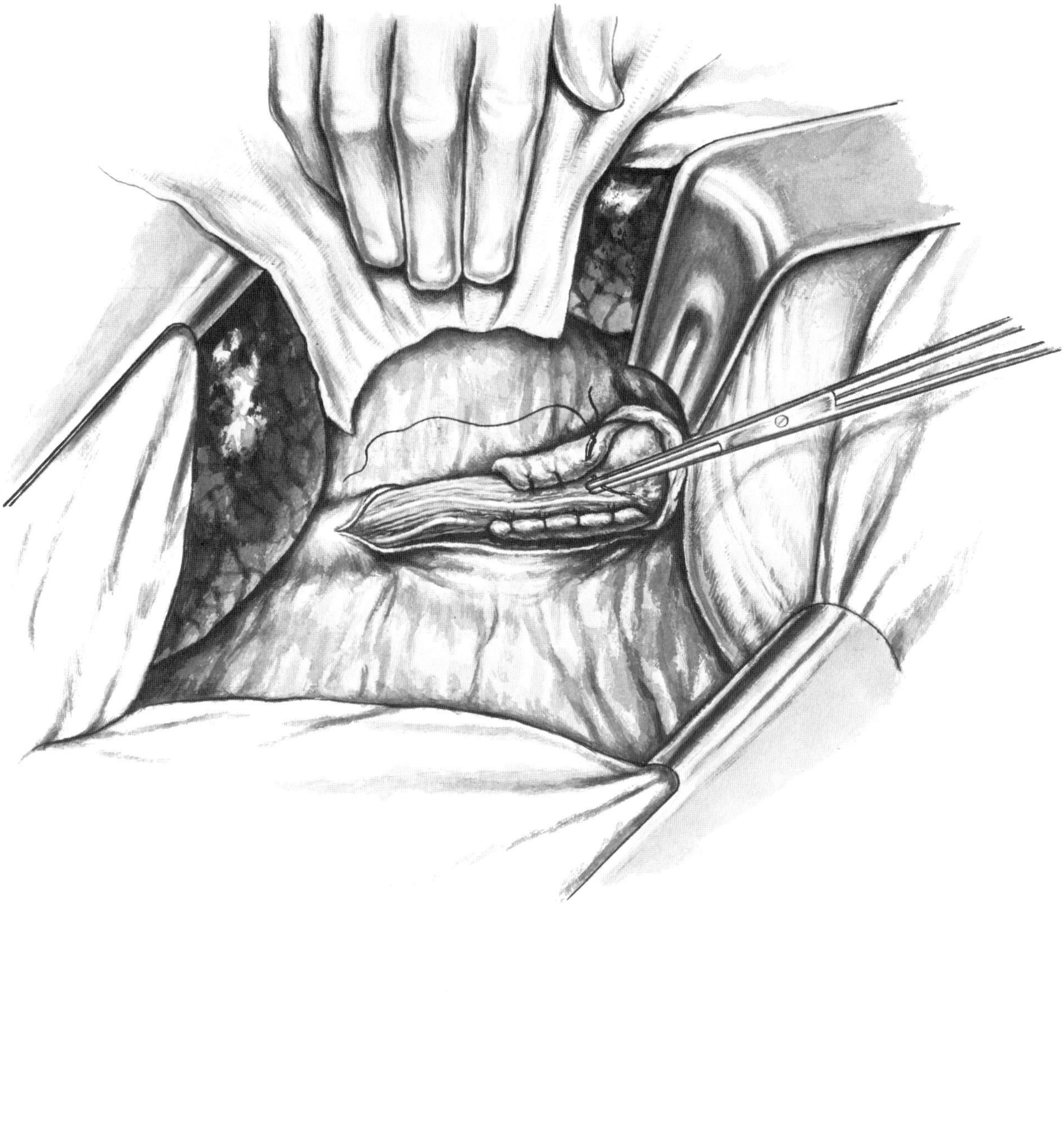

Fig. 795. Esophagofundorhaphy is carried out.

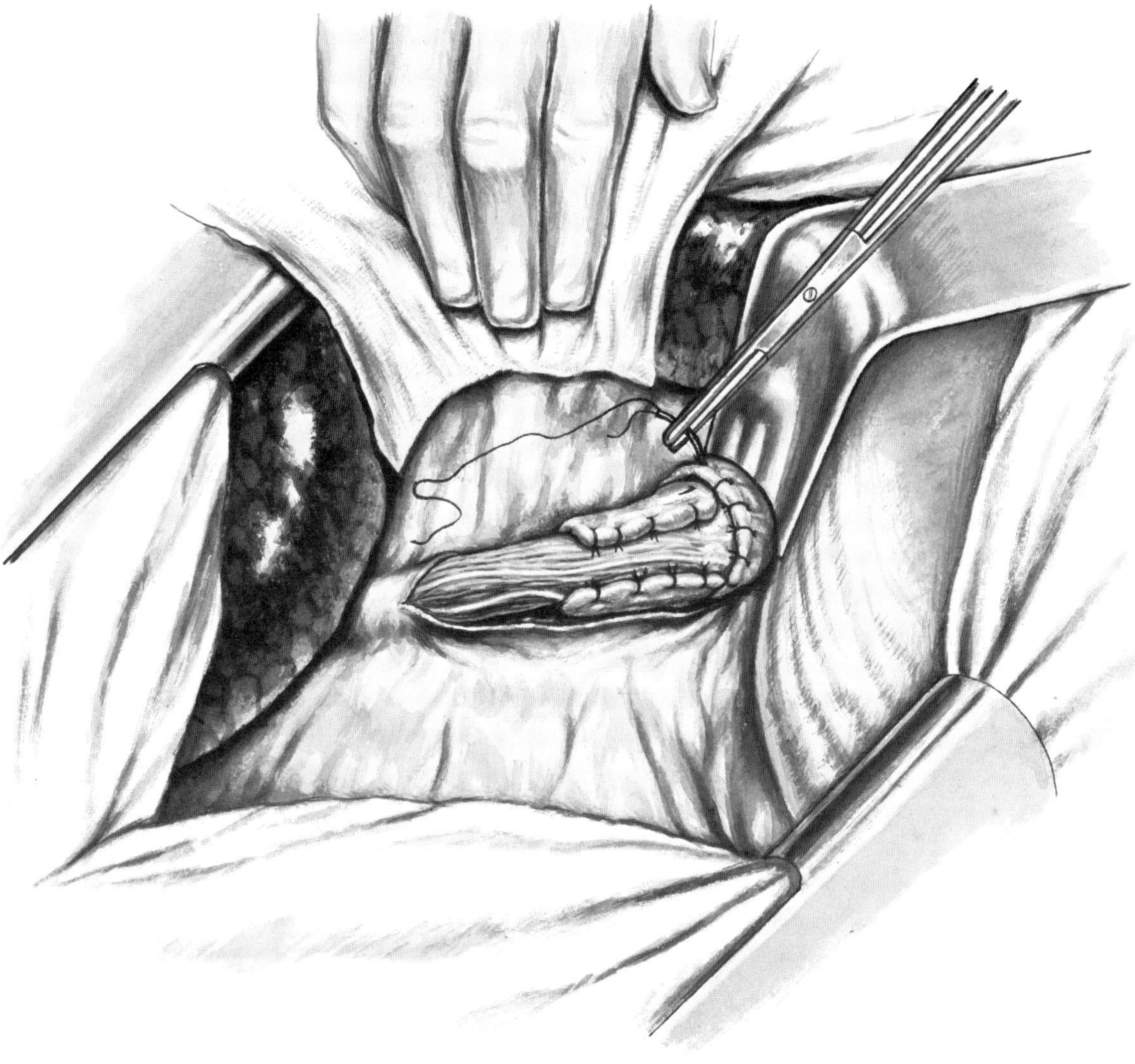

Fig. 796. Stomach is stitched to edges of hiatus.

PLASTIC SURGERY OF ESOPHAGEAL HIATUS WITH DIAPHRAGMATIC GRAFT AFTER PETROVSKY

Thoracotomy in the seventh intercostal space is performed. The lung is moved cranially. The mediastinal pleura is cut, and a pedicle diaphragmatic graft is tailored to repair the hiatus by Petrovsky's method (Fig. 797). Fundoplication is performed. The diaphragmatic graft is fitted around the esophagus (Fig. 798). The wound is sutured with a cuff formed around the esophagus with the graft (Fig. 799). The esophagus is stitched to the diaphragm with a few sutures.

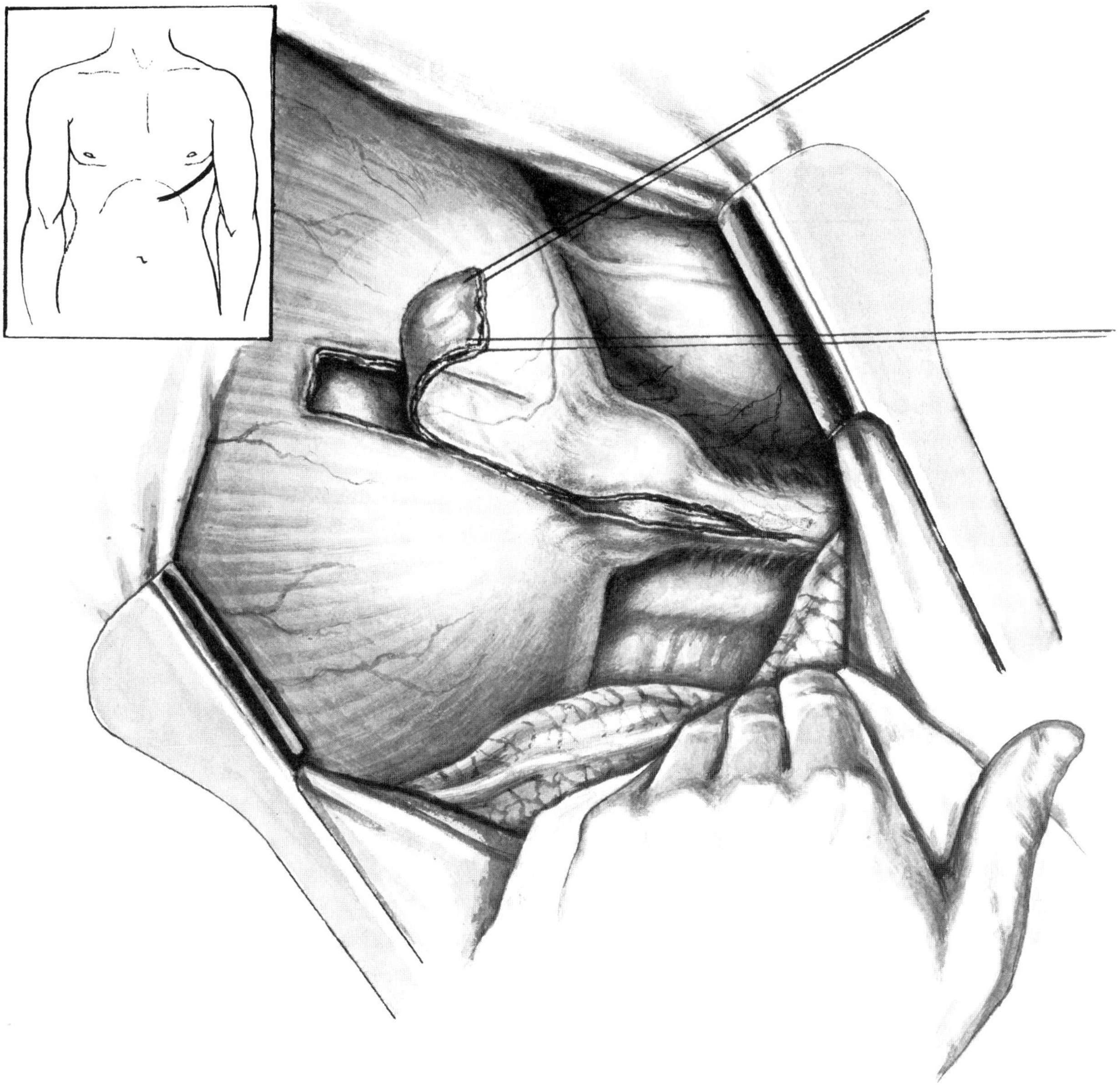

Fig. 797. Pedicle graft is tailored from diaphragm.

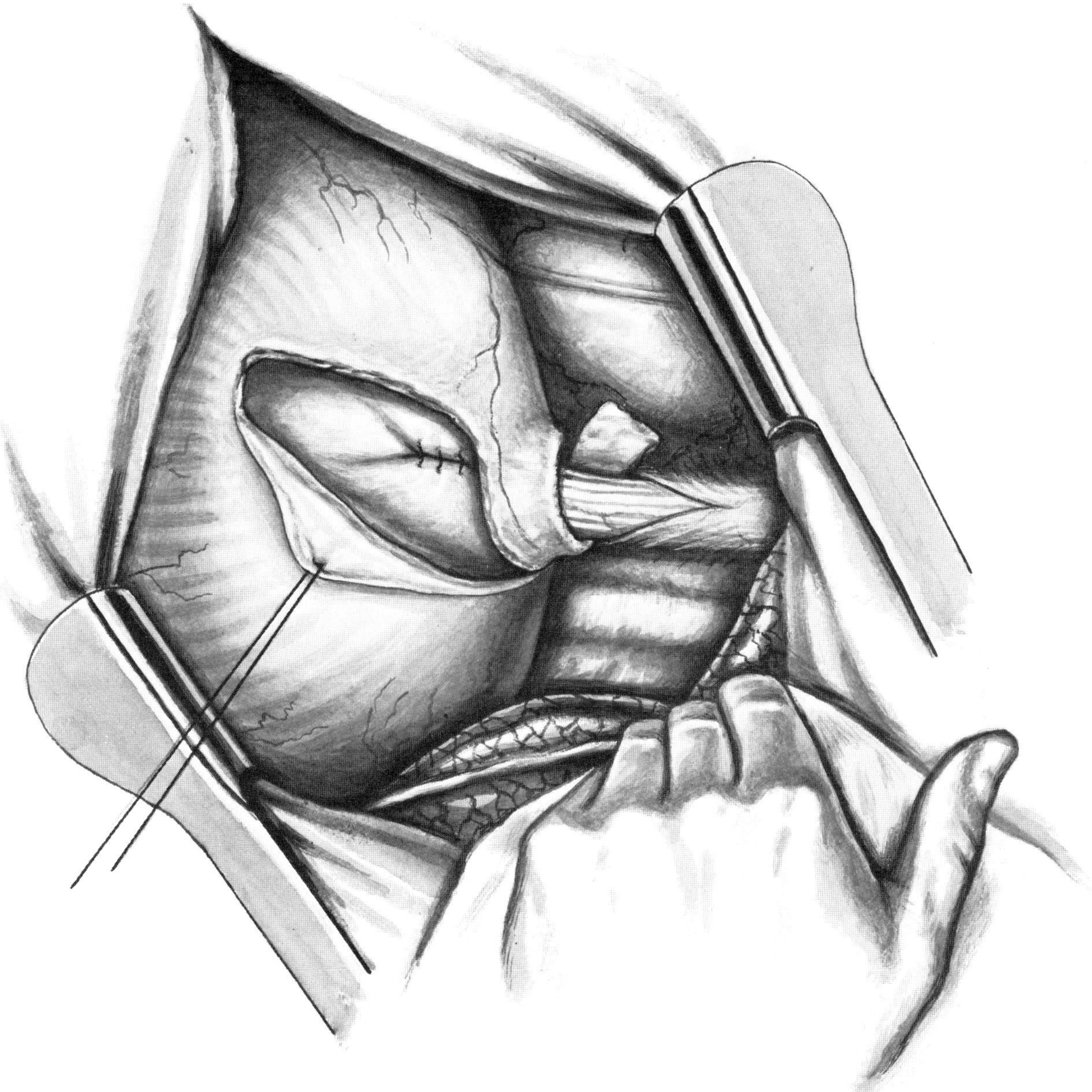

Fig. 798. After fundoplication is completed, esophagus is wrapped in diaphragmatic graft.

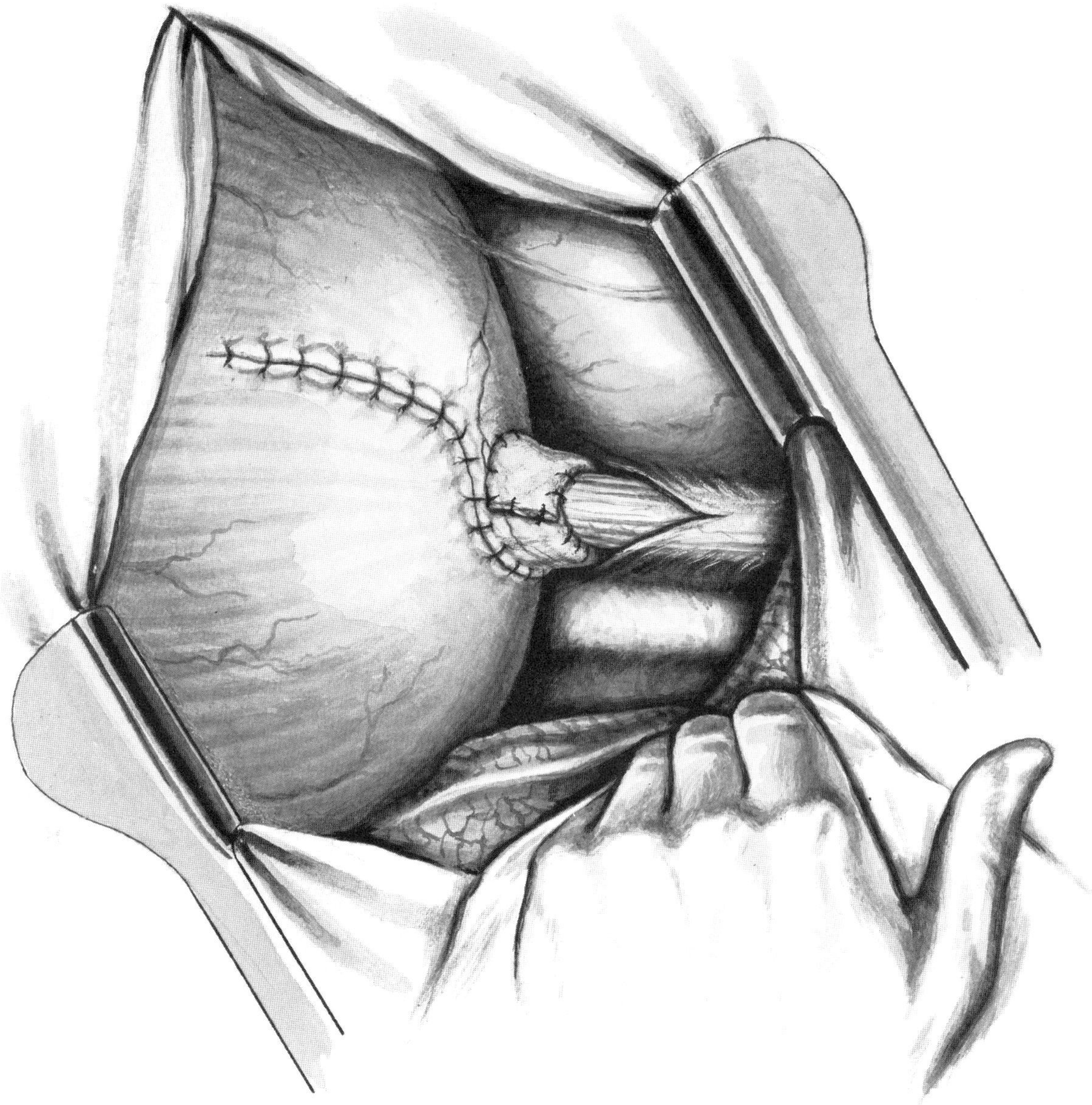

Fig. 799. Hiatal hernia has been corrected by plastic surgery with diaphragmatic graft.

PURSE-STRING VALVULAR ESOPHAGOGASTROSTOMY

The operation is indicated in hiatal hernia complicated by total peptic stricture of the esophagus.

Left thoracotomy is carried out. The esophagus is held with a loop (Fig. 800). The diaphragm is incised for some distance. Clamps are applied to the cardia and to the esophagus above the stricture, which nearly always occupies only the terminal part of the esophagus (Fig. 801). The esophagus is cut away from the stomach, and the opening in the latter is sutured (Fig. 802). Six or eight traction sutures are stitched through the free wall of the stomach demarcating a round area about 8 cm in diameter. Cuts are made with a scalpel through the serous and muscular coats down to the submucous coat between the traction sutures (Fig. 803). The seromus-

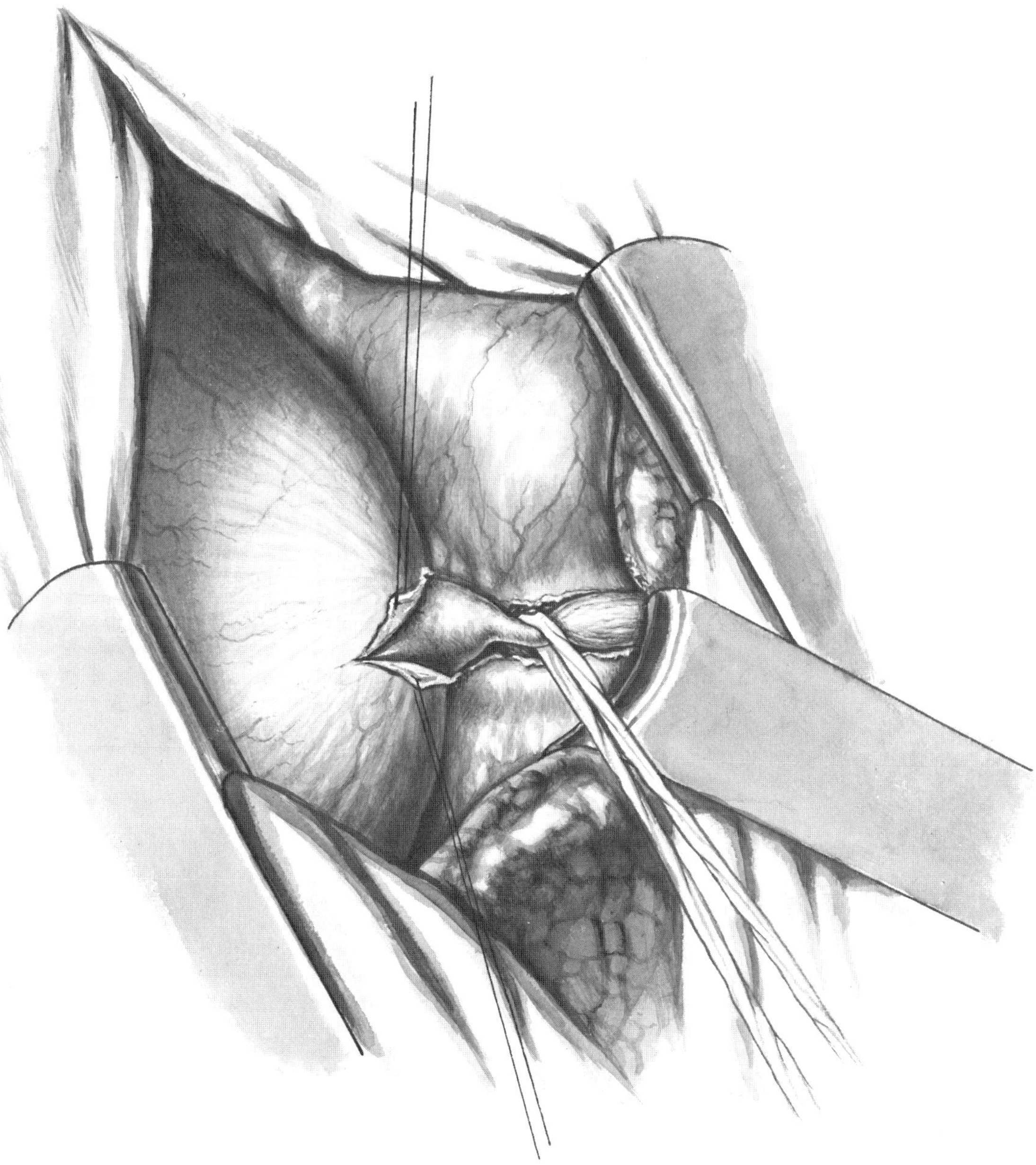

Fig. 800. Esophagus is held with loop cranial to stricture.

cular flap delineated by the incision is removed without injuring the mucous membrane and the submucous coat in which the vessels pass. A continuous blanket seromuscular suture is applied to the edge of the incision, and 1.5 to 2.0 cm from it a second seromuscular purse-string suture is placed with a synthetic thread (Fig. 804). The inner (first) suture is tightened to a width equal to the esophageal lumen; the manipulation is checked with the index finger (inset in Fig. 804).

A small perforating opening is made in the center of the gastric area with the bared submucous coat (Fig. 805), and the edges of this opening are stitched to the seromuscular coat in the region of the partly tightened (first) purse-string suture (Fig. 806). The constricted part

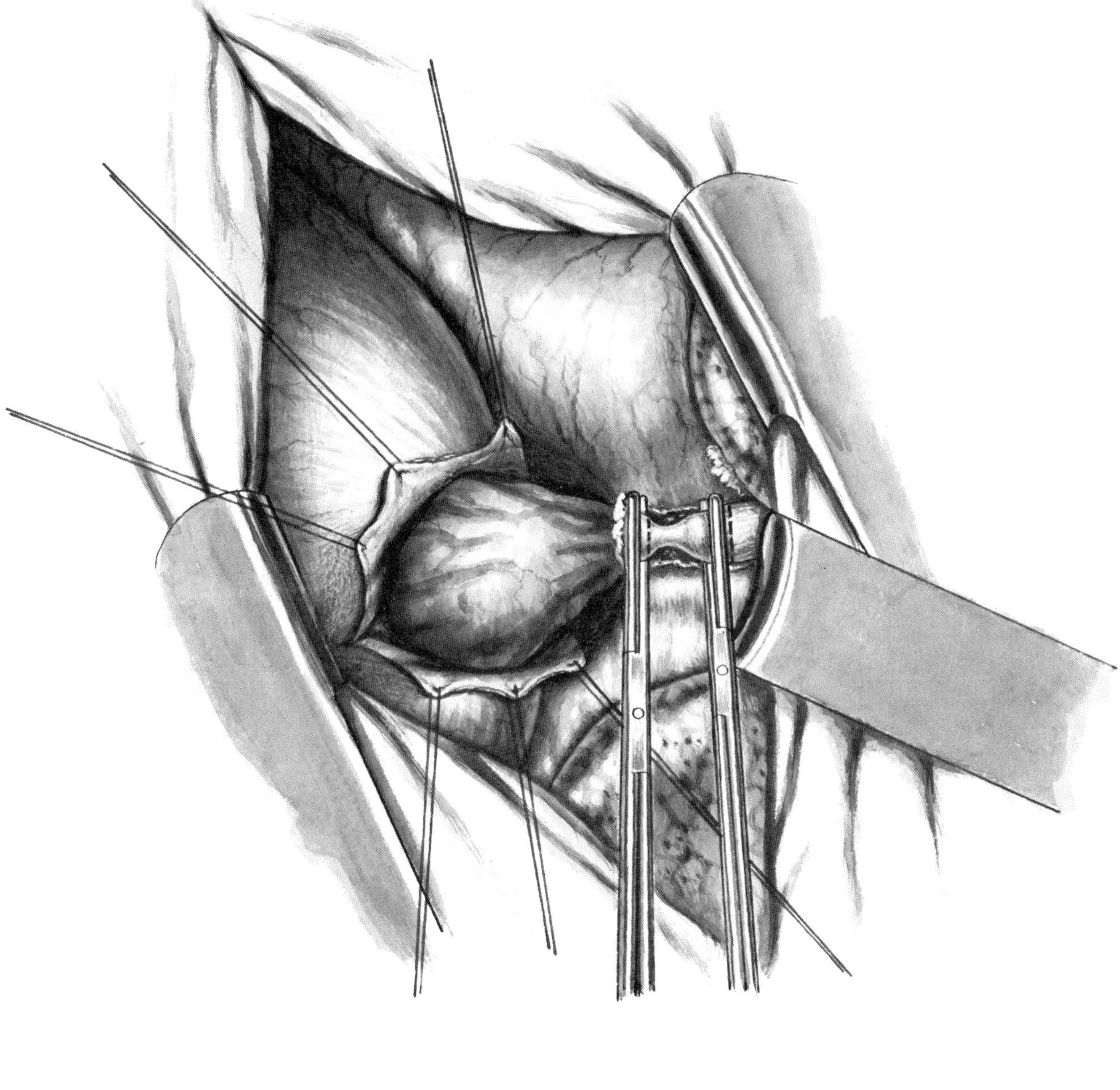

Fig. 801. Diaphragm is cut and held with traction sutures. Esophagus is clamped above and below stricture.

of the esophagus is resected, and the esophagus is stitched into the opening prepared in the stomach (Fig. 807). The outer (second) purse-string suture is tightened to a width permitting insertion of the esophagus, and the site of the anastomosis between the esophagus and the stomach is invaginated into it (Fig. 808). A valve is thus formed in the region of the anastomosis (inset in Fig. 809). The stomach is sutured to the edges of the opening in the diaphragm (Fig. 810). It is unnecessary to transect the muscular edge of the esophageal hiatus during this operation; the intervention may be performed (after the esophagus is cut away from the stomach) through an incision in the diaphragmatic dome. The esophageal hiatus in this case is completely sutured.

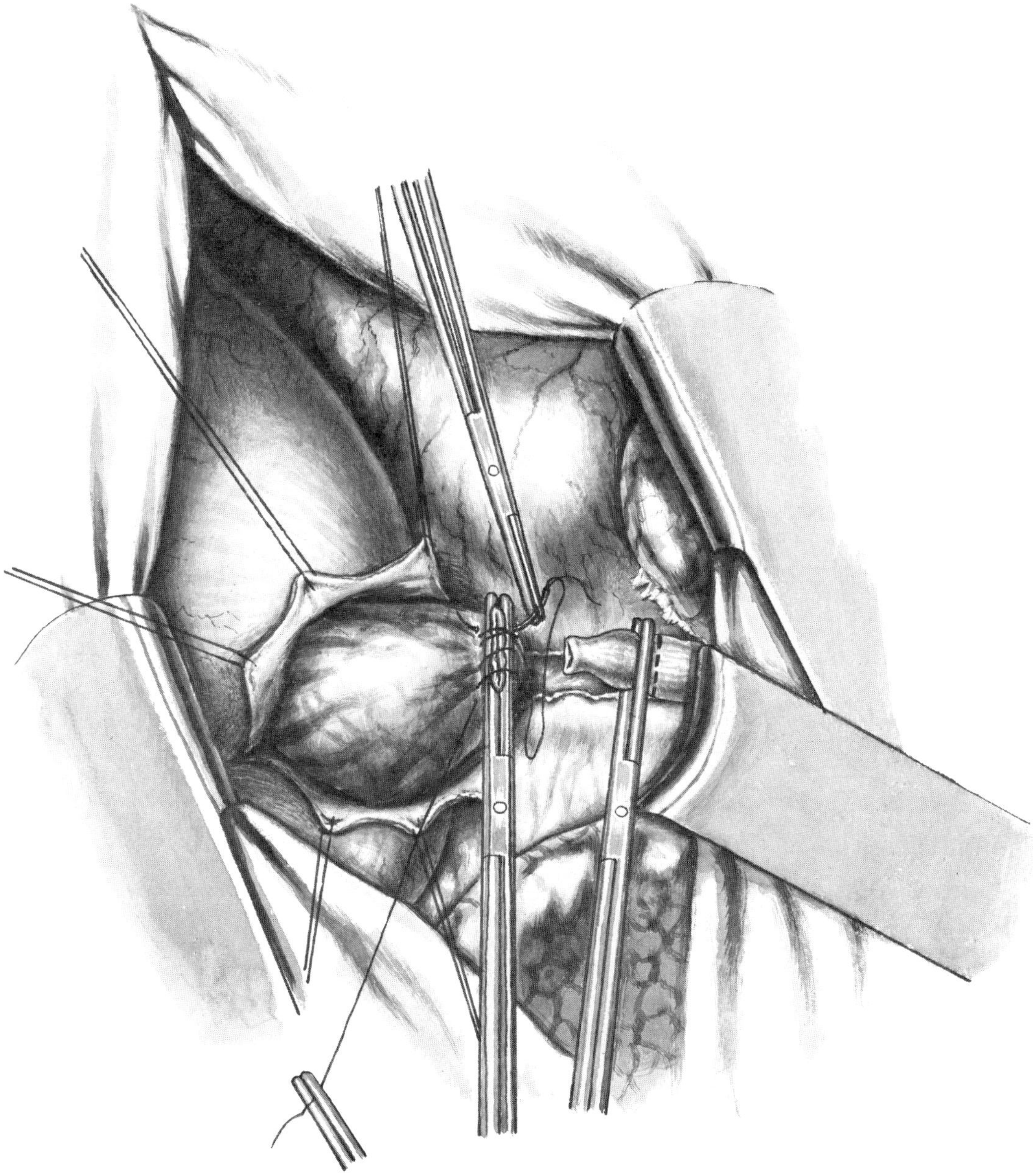

Fig. 802. Esophagus is transected. Opening in stomach is closed with continuous suture.

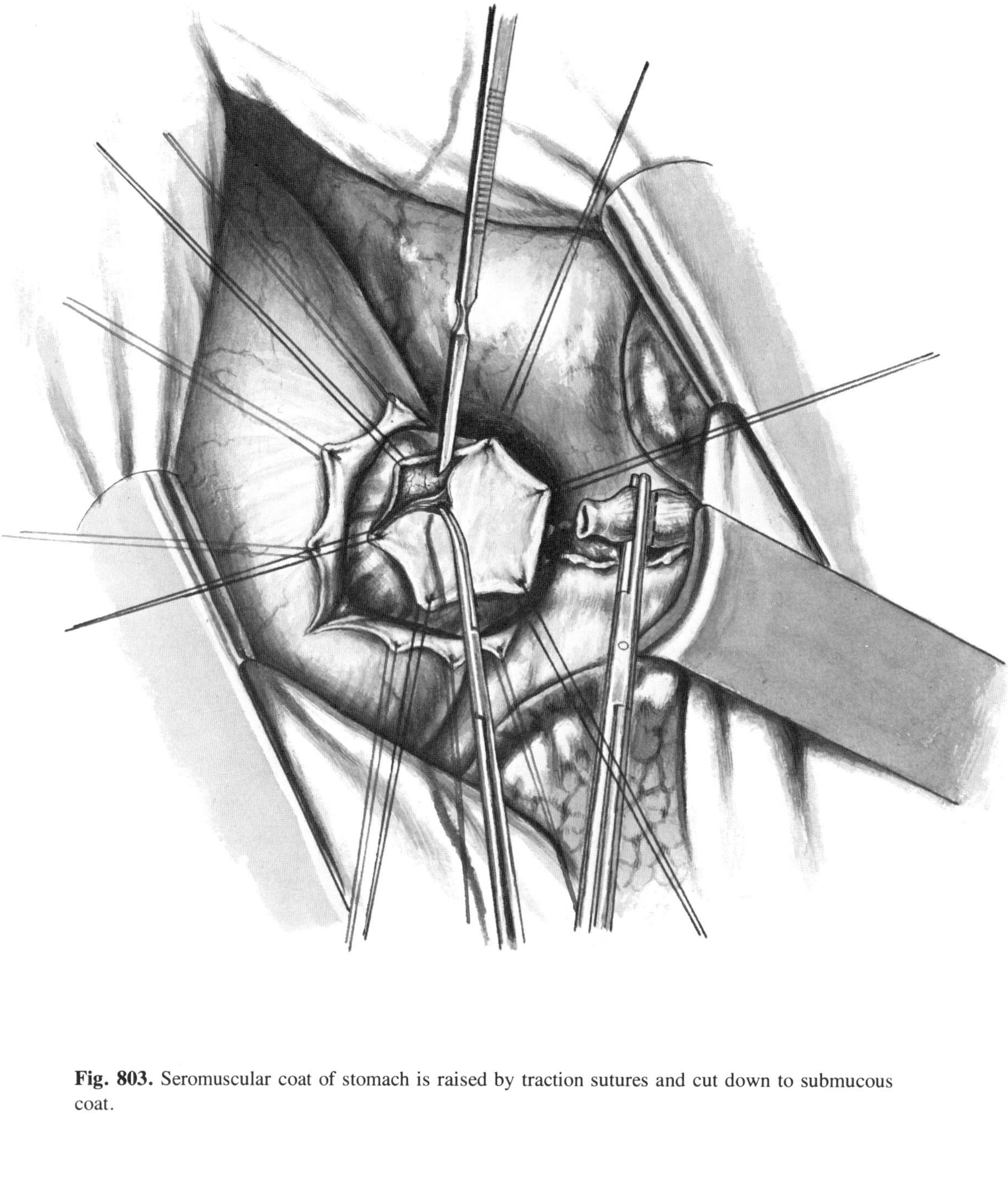

Fig. 803. Seromuscular coat of stomach is raised by traction sutures and cut down to submucous coat.

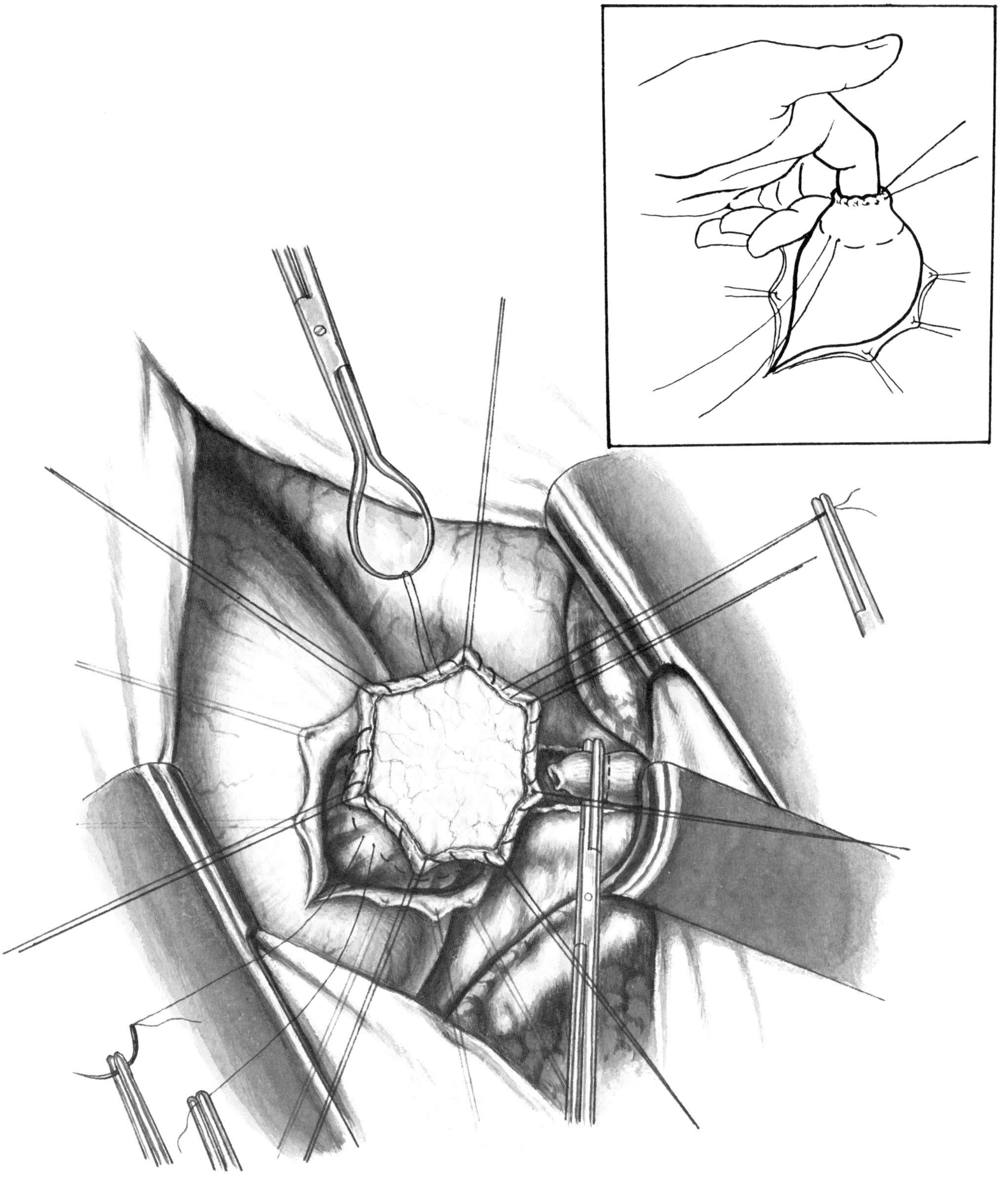

Fig. 804. First and second purse-string sutures have been applied. *Inset,* tightening of first purse-string suture.

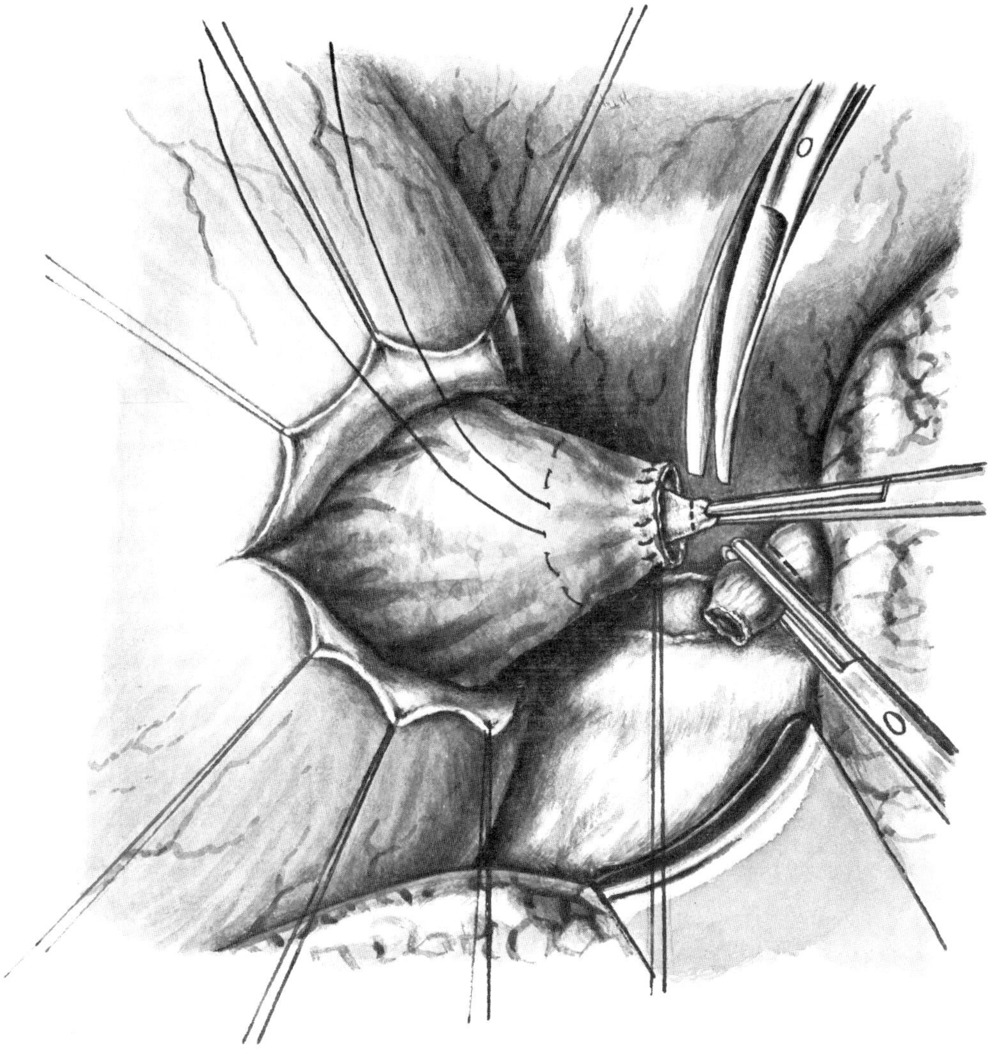

Fig. 805. Mucous coat of stomach is cut.

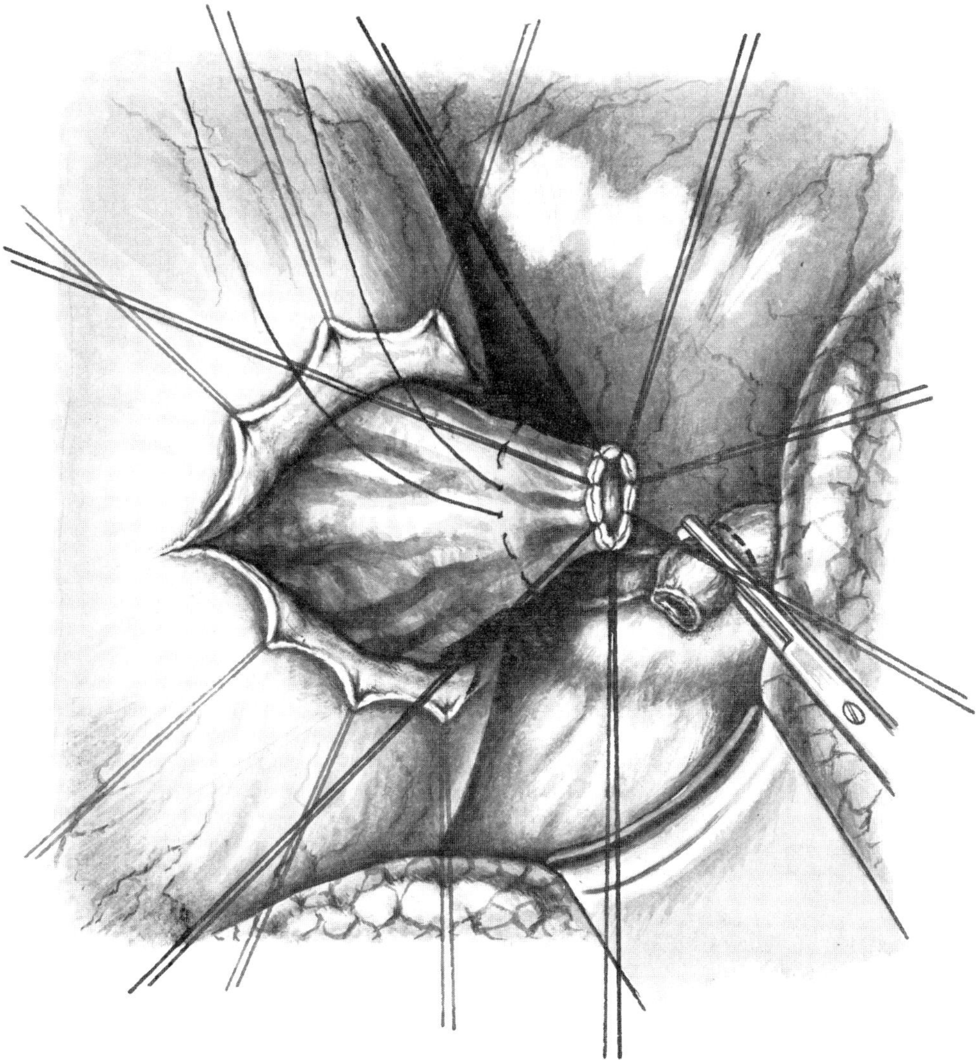

Fig. 806. Mucous coat is stitched to edges of incised serous and muscular coats, which were narrowed by means of purse-string suture.

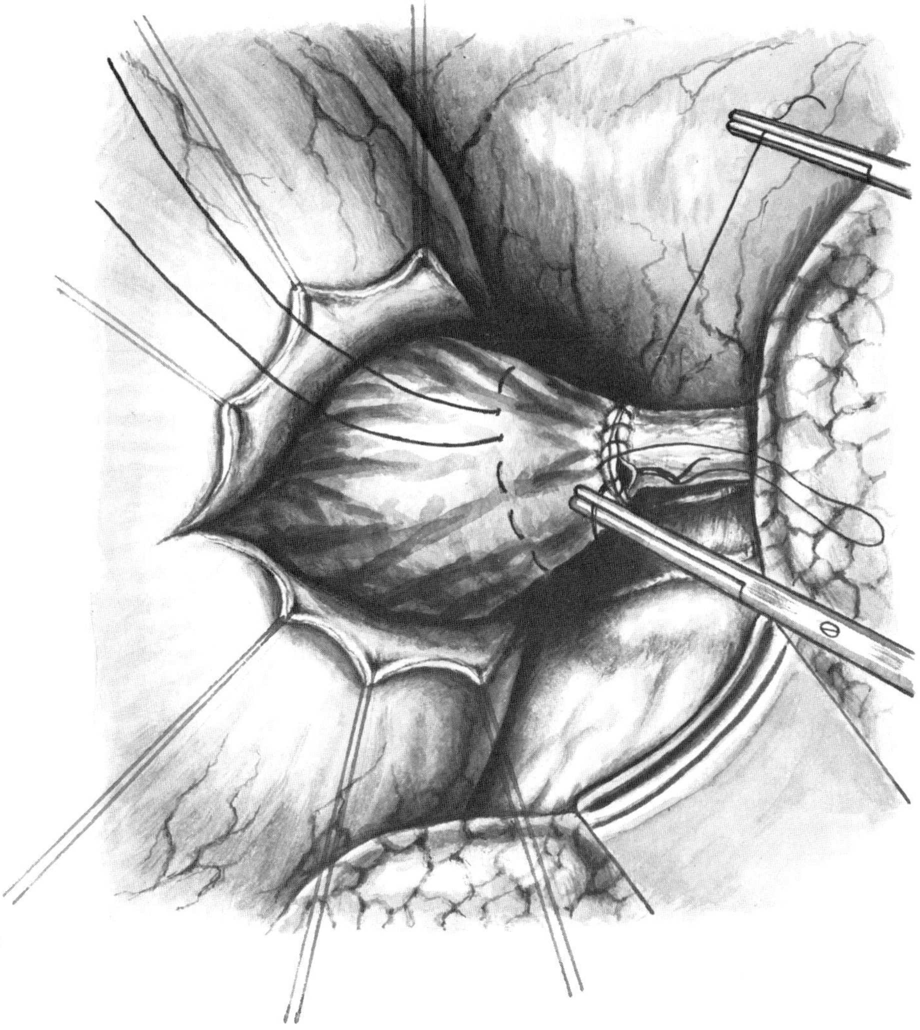

Fig. 807. First row of sutures of esophagogastricanastomosis are applied.

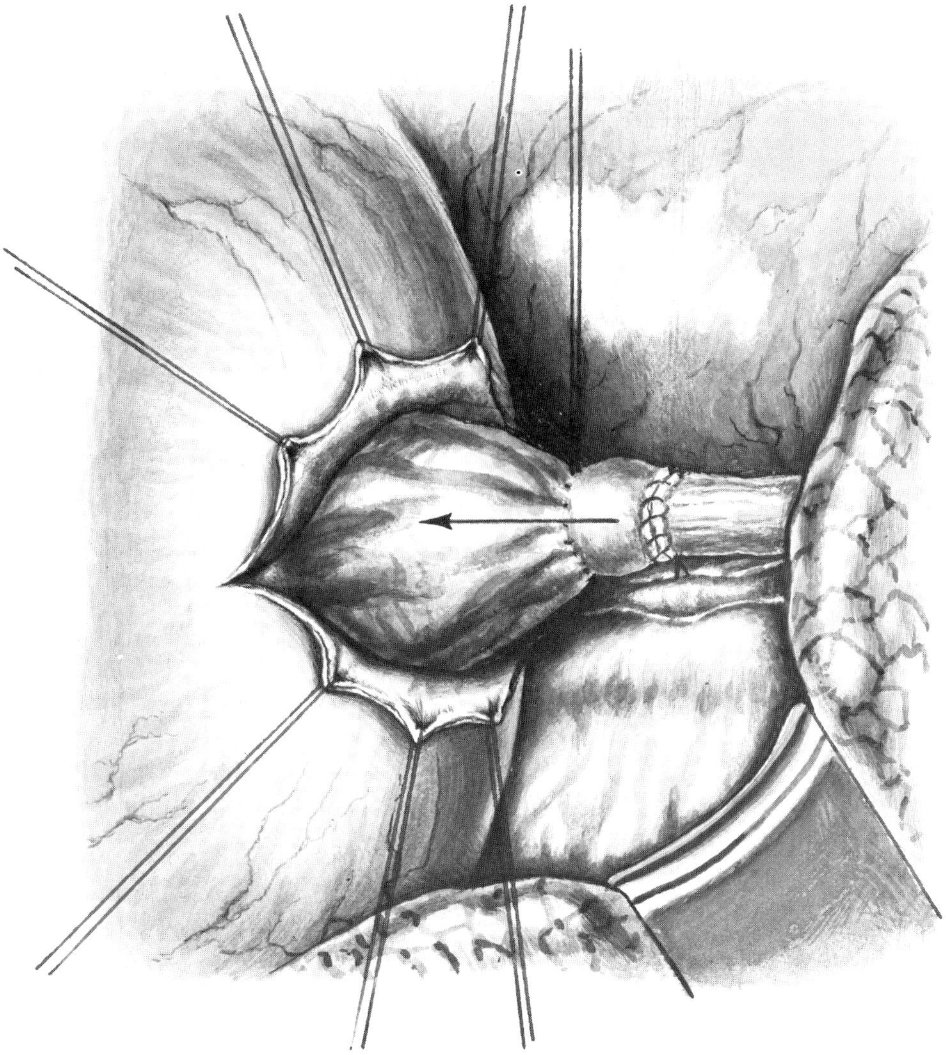

Fig. 808. Second purse-string suture is tightened to width of esophagus.

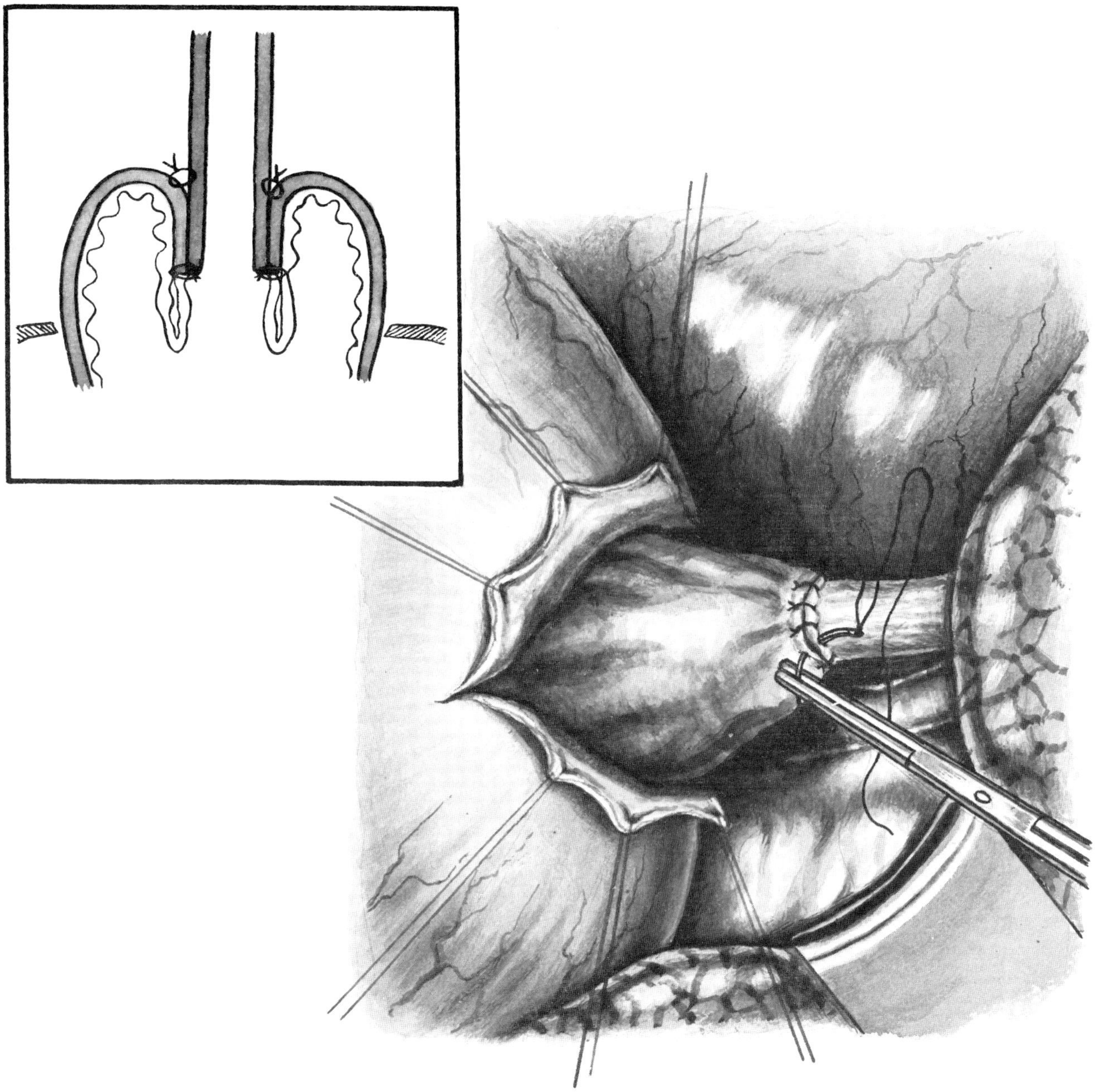

Fig. 809. Application of second row of sutures of purse-string valvular esophagogastricanastomosis.

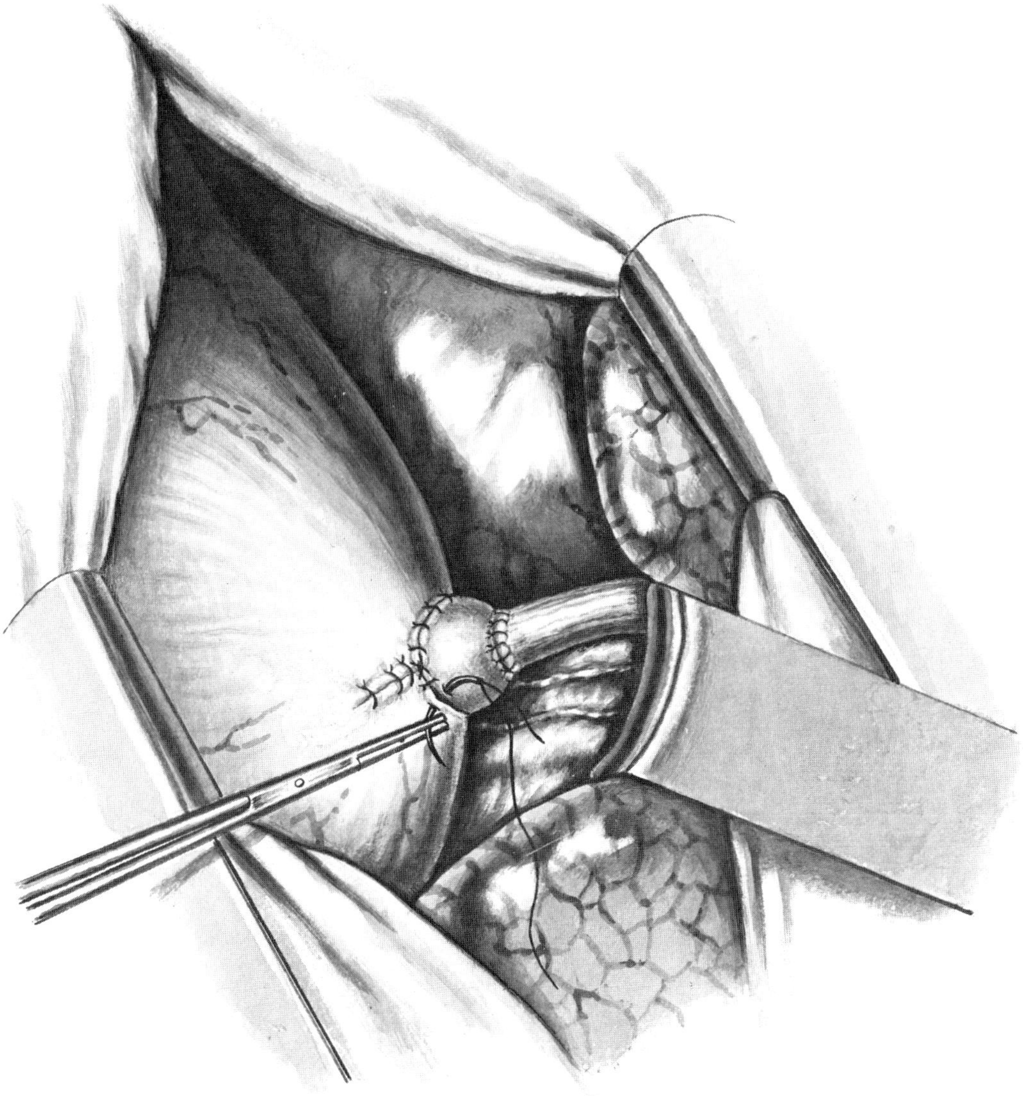

Fig. 810. Stomach is stitched to edges of esophageal hiatus.